Clinical Therapy
in Breastfeeding Patients

Clinical Therapy
in Breastfeeding Patients

Third Edition

Thomas W. Hale, RPh, PhD

Professor of Pediatrics

Associate Dean of Research

Texas Tech University School of Medicine

Amarillo, Texas 79106

Pamela D. Berens, MD, FACOG, IBCLC

Professor

Department of Obstetrics, Gynecology and Reproductive Sciences

University of Texas

Houston, Texas 77030

Clinical Therapy in Breastfeeding Patients
Third Edition

DISCLAIMER

The information contained in this publication is intended to supplement the knowledge of healthcare professionals regarding drug use during lactation. This information is advisory only and is not intended to replace sound clinical judgment or individualized patient care. The authors disclaim all warranties, whether expressed or implied, including any warranty as to the quality, accuracy, safety, or suitability of this information for any particular purpose.

Library of Congress Control Number: 2010921903

ISBN-13: 978-0-9823379-8-1

Printing and Binding: Malloy

Cover Printing: Malloy

Printed in the USA

Preface

The number of women who leave the hospital breastfeeding has risen to an all-time high. Virtually all of these women will at one time or another use a medication. Many will require treatment for severe and complicated syndromes. Thus one of the most common questions we get is, "What medications can we use in this patient with this syndrome?" In the ensuing decade, much more data have been published on the various medications, and we can now provide good evidence of safety for many medications.

The purpose of this work is to provide the clinician a guide not only into the best types of medications in breastfeeding mothers, but also a guide in the current therapy of various syndromes as well. The data on treatment and choice of medications for various syndromes have been thoroughly reviewed in the literature and should be accurate with present treatment protocols. It is by no means our intent to guide therapy with these suggestions, but only to provide safety data on the medications commonly found to be useful for various syndromes and conditions.

We fully understand that certain conditions require the use of very specific medications, and they may not be suitable for a breastfeeding mother. This is the domain of the clinician who is treating the patient. We simply hope to provide some suitable alternative medications available that have published data on their transmission into human milk. Why not choose a medication fully effective for the syndrome, and one that is safe for a breastfeeding infant?

In medicine we sometimes have a tendency to use the newest and most advertised medication. Unfortunately, these are the exact medications for which we have limited or no data on their use in breastsfeeding mothers. Science is a slow process. It takes a lot of time before we know the complications and levels of these same medications in human milk. We, therefore, respectfully suggest that if an older, better, studied medication will work and we know it is safe for breastfed infants, then it should be the clinician's first choice in this situation.

Because we have limited data on the many thousands of medications available, if it is not included in this text, then we probably do not have any breastfeeding data available, otherwise we would have included it. This does not mean that the drug cannot be used safely in breastfeeding mothers, only that we could not find any data to support its entry in this work.

Everyone now knows that breastfed infants are infinitely more healthy. Numerous research trials in the last decade confirm this. We urge that the reader always opt to assist the breastfeeding mother in choosing medications that are compatible with breastfeeding. Even brief interruptions of breastfeeding for unfounded reasons may predispose the mother to loosing her milk supply.

THE AUTHORS MAKE NO RECOMMENDATIONS AS TO THE SAFETY OF THESE MEDICATIONS DURING LACTATION, BUT ONLY REVIEWS WHAT IS CURRENTLY KNOWN IN THE SCIENTIFIC LITERATURE.

The references enclosed are primarily review articles that summarize the current standard of care for the various syndromes or conditions. For exact references concerning drug levels in milk, please consult *Medications and Mothers' Milk* where each medication is thoroughly referenced.

Thomas W. Hale and Pamela D. Berens

How to Use this Book

Principles of Therapy:

This section describes the basics of the syndrome or condition and a few principles of therapy.

Treatment

This section describes the current most accepted treatment for this disease or syndrome.

Medications:

This section describes those medications which can be used to treat the syndrome and those that have evidence-based information on their transfer into human milk. In essence, these are medications generally accepted as compatible with breastfeeding.

Generic and Trade Name.

Each of the medications listed begins with their respective generic name followed by common Trade names in the USA.

AAP:

This entry lists the recommendation provided by the American Academy of Pediatrics as published in their document, "The Transfer of Drugs and Other Chemicals into Human Milk" (*Pediatrics* 108:776-789, 2001). Drugs are listed in tables according to the following recommendations: Drugs that are contraindicated during breastfeeding; Drugs of abuse: Contraindicated during breastfeeding; Radioactive compounds that require temporary cessation of breastfeeding; Drugs whose effects on nursing infants is unknown but may be of concern; Drugs that have been associated with significant effects on some nursing infants and should be given to nursing mothers with caution; and Maternal medication usually compatible with breastfeeding. In this book the AAP recommendations have been paraphrased to reflect these recommendations. Not Reviewed simply implies that the drug has not yet been reviewed by this committee. The author recommends that each user review these recommendations for further detail.

Hale's Lactation Risk Category (LRC):

L1 SAFEST:

Drug which has been taken by a large number of breastfeeding mothers without any observed increase in adverse effects in the infant. Controlled studies in breastfeeding women fail to demonstrate a risk to the infant and the possibility of harm to the breastfeeding infant is remote; or the product is not orally bioavailable in an infant.

L2 SAFER:

Drug which has been studied in a limited number of breastfeeding women without an increase in adverse effects in the infant. And/or the evidence of a demonstrated risk which is likely to follow use of this medication in a breastfeeding woman is remote.

L3 MODERATELY SAFE:

There are no controlled studies in breastfeeding women; however, the risk of untoward effects to a breastfed infant is possible, or controlled studies show only minimal non-threatening adverse effects. Drugs should be given only if the potential benefit justifies the potential risk to the infant.

L4 POSSIBLY HAZARDOUS:

There is positive evidence of risk to a breastfed infant or to breastmilk production, but the benefits from use in breastfeeding mothers may be acceptable despite the risk to the infant (e.g., if the drug is needed in a life-threatening situation or for a serious disease for which safer drugs cannot be used or are ineffective).

L5 CONTRAINDICATED:

Studies in breastfeeding mothers have demonstrated that there is significant and documented risk to the infant based on human experience, or it is a medication that has a high risk of causing significant damage to an infant. The risk of using the drug in breastfeeding women clearly outweighs any possible benefit from breastfeeding. The drug is contraindicated in women who are breastfeeding an infant.

Relative Infant Dose:

The relative infant dose (RID) is calculated by dividing the infant's dose via milk in "mg/kg/day" by the maternal dose in "mg/kg/day". This weight-normalizing method indicates approximately how much of the "maternal dose" the infant is receiving. Many authors now use this preferred method because it gives a better indication of the relative dose transferred to the infant. In this edition, I now report RID ranges, which is the RID published by various authors. This gives the reader an estimate of all the relative infant doses published by the various authors.

Please understand, however, that many authors use different methods for calculating RID. Some are not weight-normalized. In these cases, their estimates may differ slightly from this book. While I often place the 'authors' estimates of relative infant dose, the RID range that I calculate is based on a 70 Kg mother and is weight-normalized in all instances. So RID may be slightly different according to who calculates it.

Many researchers now suggest that anything less than 10% of the maternal dose is probably safe. This is usually correct. However, some drugs (metronidazole, fluconazole) actually have much higher relative infant doses, but because they are quite non-toxic, they do not often bother an infant. To calculate this dose, I chose the data I felt was best, and this often included larger studies with AUC calculations of mean concentrations in milk. I also chose an average body weight of 70 kg for an adult. Thus the RIDs herein are calculated assuming a maternal average weight of 70 kg and a daily milk intake of 150 mL/kg/day in the infant. Please note, many authors fail to normalize their data for weight. Others provide a RID for 'each' feeding, not a daily average. Therefore, our values may vary slightly from others simply due to differences in the method of calculation.

Pregnancy Risk Category:

This is the A through X category provided by the manufacturer to the FDA pertaining to risk during gestation.

Comment:

This section provides a very brief review of the drug and its levels in milk. A more thorough review is provided in the textbook, *Medications and Mothers' Milk*, 2010.

Clinical Tips:

These tips are provided the clinician as the most current recommendations by the preponderence of evidence-based publications. This tips section provides the authors' recommendations for various drugs that are more suitable for treating these syndromes/conditions in breastfeeding mothers. Accordingly, the healthcare professional must make the final recommendations as to the suitability of these drugs and therapy in each individual patient.

Table of Contents

Acne

Principles of Therapy

Acne is one of the most prevalent skin diseases. It generally occurs in mid to late teens, but even adults are susceptible. The etiology of the syndrome is still elusive. Acne begins in the prepubertal periods with the onset of secretion of adrenal androgens that initiate increased sebum production. Early changes in acne occur in the pilosebaceous follicles of the face and trunk, with abnormal keratinization occurring in the follicular epithelium. Desquamation of the epithelial cells from follicle walls become impacted. Proliferation of anaerobic diphtheroids (Propionibacterium acnes) that require sebaceous lipids to grow is the next step in the inflammatory process that ensues. This bacteria subsequently releases chemo-attractive factors for neutrophils that initiate the inflammatory process. Treatment of acne largely depends on the severity of symptoms, but begins with therapies to suppress follicular hyperkeratosis that is the earliest event in the formation of the acne lesion. Treatments involve the use of topical agents, such as tretinoin and others, to suppress hyperkeratosis, possibly in conjunction with antimicrobial drugs to suppress bacterial growth and subsequent inflammation. Systemic estrogens may be used in females to assist in reducing sebaceous gland secretions. While reserved for severe nodulocystic acne, isotretinoin (Accutane) is remarkably effective, aside from the fact that it is horribly teratogenic (25 fold increase). Prevention of pregnancy while receiving isotretinoin and for one month following therapy is mandatory. Treatment of acne begins with the recognition that the disease involves not only the skin, but the whole patient, due largely to the many psychosocial aspects of this process. Acne treatment requires time. It is important to present the patient with a reasonable time table. Frequently six to eight weeks of therapy is needed to evaluate clinical response. Long term maintainance therapy is often recommended.

Treatment

- Topical treatments that remove the excess sebum from the affected skin to prevent bacterial overgrowth, and/or target the bacteria itself.

- Systemic treatments can be used with extreme caution; many of these treatments are teratogenic or use antibiotics that are contraindicated in pregnancy and lactation.

Medications

- ADAPALENE   (*Differin*)
  - AAP = Not reviewed
  - LRC = L3
  - RID =
  - Pregnancy = C
  - Comment: Adapalene is a retinoid-like compound (similar to Tretinoin) used topically for treatment of acne. No data are available on its transfer into human milk. However, adapalene is virtually

unabsorbed when applied topically to the skin. Plasma levels are almost undetectable (<0.25 ng/mL plasma), so milk levels would be infinitesimally low and probably undetectable. Some recent data suggest this retinoid is less irritating than tretinoin.

- AZELAIC ACID   (*Azelex, Finevin*)
  - ○ AAP = Not reviewed
  - ○ LRC = L3
  - ○ RID =
  - ○ Pregnancy = B
  - ○ Comment: Azelaic is a dicarboxylic acid derivative normally found in whole grains and animal products. Azelaic acid, when applied as a cream, produces a significant reduction of P. acnes and has an antikeratinizing effect as well. Small amounts of azelaic acid are normally present in human milk. Azelaic acid is only modestly absorbed via skin (<4%), and it is rapidly metabolized. Due to its poor absorption and rapid half-life (45 min), it is not likely to penetrate milk or produce untoward effects in a breastfed infant.

- BENZOYL PEROXIDE (*Benzac AC, Benzac W, Desquam-X, Foxtex, PanOxyl*)
  - ○ AAP = Not reviewed
  - ○ LRC = L3
  - ○ RID =
  - ○ Pregnancy = C
  - ○ Comment: While small amounts of benzoyl peroxide are absorbed through the skin, the peroxide is rapidly destroyed in the skin. The antibacterial effect is presumed due to the release of active or free-radical oxygent which oxidize proteins and destroy bacteria. Small amouts of benzoic acid are excreted in the skin. There is no risk to the use of benzoyl peroxide in a breastfeeding mother.

- CLINDAMYCIN, TOPICAL (*Cleocin T, Clinda-Derm*)
  - ○ AAP = Not reviewed (topical)
  - ○ LRC = L2
  - ○ RID = 1.6% (oral)
  - ○ Pregnancy = B
  - ○ Comment: Topically applied clindamycin is poorly absorbed. Cleocin T topical solution or lotion contains clindamycin phosphate equivalent to 10 mg/mL. Transcutaneous absorption is minimal (<1-4%) and reported plasma levels are low to nil. Some does appear in urine of treated patients. Due to low maternal plasma levels, virtually none should be expected in breastmilk.

- ERYTHROMYCIN (*E-Mycin, Ery-Tab, Eryc, Ilosone*)
  - ○ AAP = Maternal Medication Usually Compatible with Breastfeeding
  - ○ LRC = L2
  - ○ RID = 1.4-1.7%
  - ○ Pregnancy = B
  - ○ Comment: Erythromycin is an older, narrow-spectrum antibiotic. In one study of patients receiving 400 mg three times daily, milk levels varied from 0.4 to 1.6 mg/L. Doses as high as 2 gm per day

produced milk levels of 1.6 to 3.2 mg/L. One case of hypertrophic pyloric stenosis apparently linked to erythromycin administration has been reported. In a study of two to three patients who received a single 500 oral dose, milk levels at four hours ranged from 0.9 to 1.4 mg/L with a milk/plasma ratio of 0.92. Newer macrolide-like antibiotics (azithromycin) may preclude the use of erythromycin. A recent and large study now suggests a strong positive correlation between the use of erythromycin in breastfeeding mothers and hypertrophic pyloric stenosis in newborns.

- ERYTHROMYCIN+ BENZOYL PEROXIDE (*Benzamycin*)
  - AAP = Not reviewed
  - LRC = L2
  - RID = 1.6% (oral)
  - Pregnancy = B
  - Comment: See comments above.

- ERYTHROMYCIN TOPICAL (*Staticin, Del-Mycin, Eryderm, T-Stat, Akne-Mycin, Erygel*)
  - AAP = Not reviewed
  - LRC = L2
  - RID = 1.6% (oral)
  - Pregnancy = B
  - Comment: There are numerous topical formulations of erythromycin. Regardless, the absorption of topical erythromycin is considered minimal. With minimal transcutaneous absorption and a low RID of only 1.6%, the levels in breastmilk following topical use would be exceedingly low.

- METRONIDAZOLE TOPICAL GEL (*MetroGel Topical*)
  - AAP = Not reviewed
  - LRC = L3
  - RID =
  - Pregnancy = B
  - Comment: Metronidazole topical gel is primarily indicated for acne and is a gel formulation containing 0.75% metronidazole. Following topical application of 1 gm of metronidazole gel to the face (equivalent to 7.5 mg metronidazole base), the maximum serum concentration was only 66 nanograms/mL in only one of ten patients. (In three of the ten patients, levels were undetectible). This concentration is 100 times less than the serum concentration achieved following the oral ingestion of just one 250 mg tablet. Therefore, the topical application of metronidazole gel would produce only exceedingly low plasma levels in the mother and minimal to no levels in milk.

- TAZAROTENE (*Tazorac*)
  - AAP = Not reviewed
  - LRC = L3
  - RID =
  - Pregnancy = X
  - Comment: Tazarotene is a specialized retinoid for topical use and is used for the topical treatment of stable plaque psoriasis and acne. Following topical application, tazarotene is converted to an

active metabolite; transcutaneous absorption is minimal (<1%). Only 2-3% of the topically applied drug is absorbed transcutaneously. Tazarotene is metabolized to the active ingredient, tazarotenic acid. Following topical application, tazarotene is converted to an active metabolite; transcutaneous absorption is minimal (<1%). Little compound could be detected in the plasma. At steady state, plasma levels were only 0.09 ng/mL, although this value is largely a function of surface area treated. When applied to large surface areas, systemic absorption is increased. Data on transmission to breastmilk are not available. The manufacturer reports some is transferred to rodent milk, but it has not been tested in humans.

- TRETINOIN   (*Retin - A, Renova*)
  - ∘ AAP = Not reviewed
  - ∘ LRC = L3 if used topically
  - ∘ RID =
  - ∘ Pregnancy = C for topical
  - ∘ Comment: Tretinoin is a retinoid derivative similar to Vitamin A. It is primarily used topically for acne and wrinkling, and sometimes administered orally for leukemias and psoriasis. Blood concentrations measured 2-48 hours following application are essentially zero. Absorption of Retin-A via topical sources is reported to be minimal, and breastmilk would likely be minimal to none. However, if it is used orally, transfer into milk is likely and should be used with great caution in a breastfeeding mother.

- TRIAMCINOLONE ACETONIDE   (*Aristocort, Azmacort, Tri-Nasal*)
  - ∘ AAP = Not reviewed
  - ∘ LRC = L3
  - ∘ RID =
  - ∘ Pregnancy = C
  - ∘ Comment: Triamcinolone is a typical corticosteroid (see prednisone) that is available for topical, intranasal, injection, inhalation, and oral use. Although no data are available on triamcinolone secretion into human milk, it is likely that the milk levels would be exceedingly low and not clinically relevant when administered topically or via inhalation or intranasally. While the oral adult dose is 4-48 mg/day, the inhaled dose is 200 μg three times daily, and the intranasal dose is 220 μg/day. There is virtually no risk to the infant following use of the intranasal products in breastfeeding mothers. Applied topically, absorption depends on the site (1% from forearm, 4% from scalp, 7% from forehead, and 36% from scrotom). When applied to the face, it is unlikely to produce significant plasma levels and dose in milk should be minimal to nil.

Clinical Tips

The order of therapy of acne should begin with benzoyl peroxides, azelaic acid, and then retinoids (tretinoin, tazarotene and adapalene). Second line treatment would include topical (not oral in breastfeeding mothers) antibiotics, such as erythromycin or clindamycin (topically). Third-line of treatment is with isotretinoin (Accutane), although the teratologic risks are enormous with this product.

Retinoids are poorly absorbed through the skin and milk levels are likely low, if even detectable at all. Most patients can use retinoids if they begin therapy with low-strength cream formulations (0.025% tretinoin) and increase the strength later on. Other topical preparations, such as the peroxides (e.g., benzoyl peroxide), are absorbed to some degree and metabolized to oxygen free radicals and inactive benzoic acid byproducts almost instantly. While somewhat irritating, they are quite effective. The combination of benzoyl peroxide washes in the morning and a retinoid at bedtime is a good initial therapy. The peroxides are unlikely to harm a breastfeeding infant, as plasma enzymes, if absorbed, almost instantly degrade them.

Salicylic acid preparations are available, but are not considered as effective as the retinoids. A new combination of benzoyl peroxide and erythromycin is popular and would not be absorbed significantly. A perhaps preferred alternative to benzoyl peroxide is azelaic acid cream, which produces a significant reduction of *P. acnes* and an anti-keratinizing effect as well. Azelaic is only modestly absorbed via skin (< 4%), and it is rapidly metabolized. Azelaic acid is a normal dietary constituent in whole grains and animal products. Due to its poor penetration into plasma and rapid half-life (45 min.), it is probably safe for breastfeeding mothers. Antiandrogenic estrogens (certain birth control preparations) are effective therapy in reducing sebaceous gland production of lipids. Estrogens should be used only rarely, as they are known to suppress milk production. If estrogens are employed in breastfeeding mothers, they should only be used after mothers have established a good milk supply, and mothers should be advised to monitor their milk supply.

Topical antibiotic preparations include tetracycline, metronidazole, clindamycin, erythromycin, and meclocycline sulfosalicylate. The percutaneous absorption of all the above is almost nil. In many cases, plasma levels are undetectable. Therefore, topical application of the above antibiotics is probably safe for breastfeeding mothers. While clindamycin is commonly used, there is increasing resistance reported to erythromycin and metronidazole, although they are still useful. However, the 'chronic' oral use of these same antibiotics is problematic. Oral tetracycline, when ingested 'in milk' is poorly bioavailable (< 30-40%). While the absolute level of tetracycline in milk is low (< 2.58 mg/L) and bioavailability of this would be only 30-40%, taken over a long period of time, the amount of tetracycline reaching the infant could be significant. The newer tetracyclines are even more problematic. The bioavailability of the newer tetracyclines (minocycline, doxycycline) is much higher (80%), even in the presence of calcium salts, so that the chronic use of these two tetracyclines should be discouraged. Further, due to a chronic hypersensitivity syndrome now associated with minocycline, most dermatologists are using doxycycline instead for chronic acne. Chronic oral therapy with clindamycin is risky for both mother and infant due to higher risks of pseudomembranous colitis for the mother and infant. The use of isotretinoin (Accutane) in breastfeeding mothers is extremely risky. First, we have no data on its use in breastfeeding mothers, but due to its high lipid solubility, its transfer into milk is likely (see vitamin A). Second, the use of this incredibly teratogenic compound in a young breastfeeding mother who is at risk for pregnancy and who cannot readily use potent estrogen-containing birth control products is extraordinarily risky at best. Although controversial, some concern exists over the ability of isotretinoin to induce depression. We do not recommend the use of this product in breastfeeding mothers; the benefits of treatment do not justify the risks.

Finally, a number of reviews have found that treatment responses are highly individual and should be based entirely on the individual clinical response. Much of these data concludes that moderate severe acne should be initially treated with retinoids and topical antibiotics. Oral isotretinoin is indicated for severe nodular acne, although we do not recommend this therapy for breastfeeding mothers.

Suggested Reading

Cook-Bolden, F. E. (2008). Clinical presentation and diagnosis of acne: patient-centric considerations. *Cutis, 82*(2 Suppl 1), 4-8.

Del Rosso, J. Q., Leyden, J. J., Thiboutot, D., & Webster, G. F. (2008). Antibiotic use in acne vulgaris and rosacea: clinical considerations and resistance issues of significance to dermatologists. *Cutis, 82*(2 Suppl 2), 5-12.

Frangos, J. E., Alavian, C. N., & Kimball, A. B. (2008). Acne and oral contraceptives: update on women's health screening guidelines. *J Am Acad Dermatol, 58*(5), 781-786.

Ghali, F., Kang, S., Leyden, J., Shalita, A. R., & Thiboutot, D. M. (2009). Changing the face of acne therapy. *Cutis, 83*(2 Suppl), 4-15.

Gollnick, H., Cunliffe, W., Berson, D., Dreno, B., Finlay, A., Leyden, J. J., et al. (2003). Management of acne: a report from a Global Alliance to Improve Outcomes in Acne. *J Am Acad Dermatol, 49*(1 Suppl), S1-37.

Hale, E. K., & Pomeranz, M. K. (2002). Dermatologic agents during pregnancy and lactation: an update and clinical review. *Int J Dermatol, 41*(4), 197-203.

Strauss, J. S., Krowchuk, D. P., Leyden, J. J., Lucky, A. W., Shalita, A. R., Siegfried, E. C., et al. (2007). Guidelines of care for acne vulgaris management. *J Am Acad Dermatol, 56*(4), 651-663.

Thiboutot, D. M. (2008). Overview of acne and its treatment. *Cutis, 81*(1 Suppl), 3-7.

Tschen, E. (2008). Addressing patient variability: clinical challenges in the initiation of acne treatment. *Cutis, 82*(2 Suppl 1), 9-17.

Yan, A. C. (2006). Current concepts in acne management. *Adolesc Med Clin, 17*(3), 613-637.

Yan, A. C., & Treat, J. R. (2008). Beyond first-line treatment: management strategies for maintaining acne improvement and compliance. *Cutis, 82*(2 Suppl 1), 18-25.

Acute Sinusitis

Principles of Therapy

The clinical manifestations of acute sinusitis vary greatly, depending on the duration of infection (acute or chronic), and the age of the patient. Acute sinusitis is defined as inflammation of the sinuses with symptoms that have persisted for less than four weeks. Subacute sinusitis is defined as inflammation of the sinuses with symptoms lasting one to three months. Chronic sinusitis is associated with inflammatory symptoms lasting more than three months. Sinusitis generally develops because of impaired clearance of secretions resulting from obstruction of the sinus ostia by infection, inflammation, or anatomic abnormalities, or an increased viscosity of sinus secretions. Due to impaired drainage, an overgrowth of pathogenic bacteria results. Symptoms of infectious or acute sinusitis are difficult to distinguish from the symptoms of the common cold or allergic rhinitis. Because acute sinusitis often occurs soon after or in conjunction with allergic vasomotor rhinitis, it is generally believed that allergic rhinitis may in some cases predispose to acute infectious sinusitis. In adults, purulent postnasal discharge and facial pain over the affected sinus that worsens with movement are the typical symptoms. Fever occurs in fewer than 50% of cases. Jaw pain with chewing, nasal congestion and pressure, and a history of a recent upper respiratory tract infection are other manifestations. Most cases of acute sinusitis are of viral etiology and will resolve within seven to ten days. When symptoms persist outside of this time frame, the chances of a bacterial infection are increased. Symptoms of subacute or chronic infections are subtle and difficult to diagnose. Fever is usually absent. Fatigue, malaise, and irritability are most common. Chronic sinusitis may mimic asthma, allergic rhinitis, or chronic inflammatory bronchitis. Approximately 40% of chronic sinusitis patients have dental problems. Infectious etiologies: *Strep. Pneumonia* 40%, *H. influenzae* 30%, *M.Catarrhalis* 7%, anaerobes 8%, viruses 15%, and *Staph. Aureus* 4%.

Treatment

- Acute viral sinusitis will typically resolve in seven to ten days. Treatment during this time can be managed in most cases by supportive care.

- When symptoms are relatively mild and have been present for less than eight weeks, treatment is optional in patients who are otherwise healthy.

- Antibiotic treatment options include amoxicillin, doxycycline, amoxicillin-clavulanate, trimethoprim/sulfamethoxazole, quinolones and macrolides.

Medications

- AMOXICILLIN + CLAVULANATE   (*Augmentin*)
  - AAP = Not reviewed

- ○ LRC = L1
- ○ RID = 1%
- ○ Pregnancy = B
- ○ Comment: Addition of clavulanate extends spectrum of amoxicillin by inhibiting beta lactamase enzymes. Small amounts of amoxicillin (0.9 mg/L milk) are secreted in breastmilk. No harmful effects were reported in one report. In another study of 67 breastfeeding mothers, 27 mothers were treated with amoxicillin/ clavulanic acid and 40 mothers were treated with only amoxicillin. In the amoxicillin/ clavulanic acid group, 22.3% of the infants had mild adverse effects. Only 7.5% of the control group (amoxicillin-only) infants had adverse effects. However, the authors suggest that this difference in untoward effects is not clinically significant.

- AZITHROMYCIN (*Zithromax*)
  - ○ AAP = Not reviewed
  - ○ LRC = L2
  - ○ RID = 5.9%
  - ○ Pregnancy = B
  - ○ Comment: Azithromycin belongs to the erythromycin family. It has an extremely long half-life, particularly in tissues. Azithromycin is concentrated for long periods in phagocytes, which are known to be present in human milk. In one study of a patient who received 1 gm initially followed by 500 mg doses each at 24 hour intervals, the concentration of azithromycin in breastmilk varied from 0.64 mg/L (initially) to 2.8 mg/L on day three. The predicted dose of azithromycin received by the infant would be approximately 0.4 mg/kg/day. This would suggest that the level of azithromycin ingested by a breastfeeding infant is not clinically relevant. New pediatric formulations of azithromycin have been recently introduced. Pediatric dosing is 10 mg/kg STAT, followed by 5 mg/kg per day for up to five days.

- CEFPROZIL (*Cefzil*)
  - ○ AAP = Maternal Medication Usually Compatible with Breastfeeding
  - ○ LRC = L1
  - ○ RID = 3.7%
  - ○ Pregnancy = B
  - ○ Comment: Cefprozil is a typical second-generation, cephalosporin antibiotic. Following an oral dose of 1000 mg, the breastmilk concentrations were 0.7, 2.5, and 3.4 mg/L at two, four, and six hours postdose, respectively. The peak milk concentration occurred at six hours and was lower thereafter. Milk/plasma ratios varied from 0.05 at 2 hours to 5.67 at 12 hours. However, the milk concentration at 12 hours was small (1.3 μg/mL). Using the highest concentration found in breastmilk (3.5 mg/L), an infant consuming 800 mL of milk daily would ingest about 2.8 mg of cefprozil daily. Because the dose used in this study is approximately twice that normally used, it is reasonable to assume that an infant would ingest less than 1.7 mg per day, an amount clinically insignificant. Pediatric indications for infants 6 months and older are available.

- CEFPODOXIME PROXETIL (*Vantin*)
  - ○ AAP = Not reviewed
  - ○ LRC = L2

- ○ RID =
- ○ Pregnancy = B
- ○ Comment: Cefpodoxime is a cephalosporin antibiotic that is subsequently metabolized to an active metabolite. Only 50% is orally absorbed. In a study of three lactating women, levels of cefpodoxime in human milk were 0%, 2%, and 6% of maternal serum levels at four hours following a 200 mg oral dose. At six hours post-dosing, levels were 0%, 9%, and 16% of concomitant maternal serum levels. Pediatric indications down to six months of age are available.

- **CEFUROXIME** (*Ceftin, Zinacef, Kefurox*)

  - ○ AAP = Not reviewed
  - ○ LRC = L2
  - ○ RID = 0.6-2%
  - ○ Pregnancy = B
  - ○ Comment: Cefuroxime is a broad-spectrum second-generation cephalosporin antibiotic that is available orally and IV. The manufacturer states that it is secreted into human milk in small amounts, but the levels are not available.

    In a study of 38 mothers who received cefuroxime, 2.6% reported mild side effects that were not significantly different from controls (9%). Cefuroxime has a very bitter taste. The IV salt form, cefuroxime sodium, is very poorly absorbed orally. Only the axetil salt form is orally bioavailable.

- **CLARITHROMYCIN** (*Biaxin*)

  - ○ AAP = Not reviewed
  - ○ LRC = L1
  - ○ RID = 2.1%
  - ○ Pregnancy = C
  - ○ Comment: Antibiotic that belongs to erythromycin family. In a study of 12 mothers receiving 250 mg twice daily, the Cmax occurred at 2.2 hours. The estimated average dose of clarithromycin via milk was reported to be 150 μg/kg/day, or 2% of the maternal dose. Clarithromycin is probably compatible with breastfeeding. Observe for diarrhea and thrush in the infant.

- **CO-TRIMOXAZOLE** (*TMP-SMZ, Bactrim, Cotrim, Septra*)

  - ○ AAP = Maternal Medication Usually Compatible with Breastfeeding
  - ○ LRC = L3
  - ○ RID =
  - ○ Pregnancy = C
  - ○ Comment: Co-trimoxazole is the mixture of trimethoprim and sulfamethoxazole. See individual monographs for each of these products.

- **DOXYCYCLINE** (*Doxychel, Vibramycin, Periostat*)

  - ○ AAP = Not reviewed
  - ○ LRC = L3
  - ○ RID = 4.2-13.3%
  - ○ Pregnancy = D

◦ Comment: Doxycycline is a long half-life tetracycline antibiotic. In a study of 15 subjects, the average doxycycline level in milk was 0.77 mg/L following a 200 mg oral dose. One oral dose of 100 mg was administered 24 hours later, and the breastmilk levels were 0.380 mg/L. Following a dose of 100 mg daily in 10 mothers, doxycycline levels in milk on day two averaged 0.82 mg/L (range 0.37-1.24 mg/L) at three hours after the dose, and 0.46 mg/L (range 0.3-0.91 mg/L) 24 hours after the dose. The relative infant dose in an infant would be < 6% of the maternal weight-adjusted dosage. Following a single dose of 100 mg in three women or 200 mg in three women, peak milk levels occurred between two and four hours following the dose. The average "peak" milk levels were 0.96 mg/L (100 mg dose) or 1.8 mg/L (200 mg dose). After repeated dosing for five days, milk levels averaged 3.6 mg/L at doses of 100 mg twice daily. In a study of 13 women receiving 100-200 mg doses of doxycycline, peak levels in milk were 0.6 mg/L (n=3 @100 mg dose) and 1.1 mg/L (n=11 @ 200 mg dose).

Tetracyclines administered orally to infants are known to bind in teeth, producing discoloration and inhibiting bone growth, although there is the least severe staining of teeth with doxycycline and oxytetracycline. Although most tetracyclines secreted into milk are generally bound to calcium, thus inhibiting their absorption, doxycycline is the least bound (20%), and may be better absorbed in a breastfeeding infant than the older tetracyclines. While the absolute absorption of older tetracyclines may be dramatically reduced by calcium salts, the newer doxycycline and minocycline analogs bind less and their overall absorption, while slowed, may be significantly higher than earlier versions. Prolonged use (> three weeks) could potentially alter GI flora and induce dental staining, although doxycycline produces the least dental staining. Short term use (three to four weeks) is not contraindicated. No harmful effects have yet been reported in breastfeeding infants, but prolonged use is not advised. For prolonged administration, such as for exposure to anthrax, check the CDC web site, as they have published specific dosing guidelines.

- LEVOFLOXACIN (*Levaquin, Quixin*)

  ◦ AAP = Not reviewed

  ◦ LRC = L3

  ◦ RID = 10.5-17.2%

  ◦ Pregnancy = C

  ◦ Comment: Levofloxacin is a pure (S) enantiomer of the racemic fluoroquinolone Ofloxacin. Its kinetics, including milk levels, should be identical to Ofloxacin. In one case report of a mother receiving 500 mg/day, the 24 hour average milk level was reported to be approximately 5 µg/mL. A peak level of 8.2 µg/mL was reported, and occurred at five hours after the dose. The half-life of levofloxacin in milk was estimated to be seven hours, which would result in undetectable amounts in milk after 48 hours. The authors report the absolute infant dose would be 1.23 mg/kg/day, although this was calculated from the highest milk level of eight samples. While the peak levels were reported to be 8.2 µg/mL, the average milk level reported was 5 µg/mL. Using these data, the relative infant dose would range from 10.5% to 17%. However, the time-to-peak interval reported in this case was five hours, rather than 1-1.8 hours reported following both oral and IV doses in the prescribing information. Of the 10 reported levels in this study, only one was above 5 µg/mL. Thus the reported average level of 5 µg/mL is probably consistent with other data. This suggests a Milk/Plasma ratio of approximately 0.95, which is probably correct. Thus levofloxacin concentrations in milk peak around 1-1.8 hours and at levels close to plasma levels. Observe the infant for changes in gut flora, candida overgrowth, or diarrhea.

- OFLOXACIN   (*Floxin*)
  - AAP = Maternal Medication Usually Compatible with Breastfeeding
  - LRC = L2
  - RID = 3.1%
  - Pregnancy = C
  - Comment: Ofloxacin is a typical fluoroquinolone antimicrobial. Breastmilk concentrations are reported equal to maternal plasma levels. In one study in lactating women who received 400 mg oral doses twice daily, drug concentrations in breastmilk averaged 0.05-2.41 mg/L in milk (24 hours and two hours postdose, respectively). The drug was still detectable in milk 24 hours after a dose. The fluoroquinolones are becoming more popular in pediatrics due to recent studies and reviews showing their safe use. It is very unlikely that arthropathy would ensue following the dose received via milk. The only probable risk is a change in gut flora, diarrhea, and a remote risk of overgrowth of *C. difficile*. Ofloxacin levels in breastmilk are consistently lower (37%) than ciprofloxacin. If a fluoroquinolone is required, ofloxacin, levofloxacin, or norfloxacin are probably the better choices for breastfeeding mothers.

Clinical Tips

Acute infections of viral etiology may resolve spontaneously and may need only symptom relief. When a bacterial infection is suspected, goals of treatment are to eradicate the offending organism, clear sinuses, provide symptomatic relief, and prevent intracranial complications. Suitable analgesics would include acetaminophen, ibuprofen, or hydrocodone in cases of severe pain. The choice of antibiotic varies due to the age of patients. In adults, empiric therapy should be initially directed against H. influenza and Strep. pneumoniae. While a 10-14 day course of amoxicillin may be tried, current studies show most strains are resistant and response is no better than placebo. First choice is probably amoxicillin + clavulanic acid (500/125 mg TID or 875/125 mg BID PO x 10 days), or cefuroxime axetil (250 mg BID x 10 days), or TMP-SMX (160/800 mg q 12 hours). The CDC recommends amoxicillin, doxycycline, or trimethoprim/sulfamethoxazole as first-line choices. Alternative treatments include cefprozil or cefpodoxime. In penicillin-allergic patients, clarithromycin (500 mg po BID x 10 days) or azithromycin (250 mg daily for five days) may be used. All of the above chemotherapeutic agents have been studied in breastfeeding mothers and levels in milk are low. While the incidence of resistance is growing, the use of fluoroquinolone antibiotics is increasing as well. Although ciprofloxacin is useful, it may produce higher milk levels (40%) than other fluoroquinolones, and it should be used cautiously in breastfeeding mothers. Pseudomembranous colitis has been reported in one infant. In patients needing fluoroquinolones, ofloxacin (400 mg q 12 hours x 10 days) or levofloxacin (750 mg orally once daily for five days) would be preferred due to lower levels in milk, although studies do not show that fluoroquinolones are more effective than amoxicillin. The only consequence of using the fluoroquinolones is the possibility of overgrowth of C. difficile, which at these doses via milk is low.

Suggested Reading

Lim, M., Citardi, M. J., & Leong, J. L. (2008). Topical antimicrobials in the management of chronic rhinosinusitis: a systematic review. *Am J Rhinol, 22*(4), 381-389.

Longworth, D. L. (2008). Update in infectious disease treatment. *Cleve Clin J Med, 75*(8), 584-590.

Lund, V. J. (2008). Therapeutic targets in rhinosinusitis: infection or inflammation? *Medscape J Med, 10*(4), 105.

Pearlman, A. N., & Conley, D. B. (2008). Review of current guidelines related to the diagnosis and treatment of rhinosinusitis. *Curr Opin Otolaryngol Head Neck Surg, 16*(3), 226-230.

Schumann, S. A., & Hickner, J. (2008). Patients insist on antibiotics for sinusitis? Here is a good reason to say "no". *J Fam Pract, 57*(7), 464-468.

Allergic Rhinitis

Principles of Therapy

Allergic rhinitis is characterized by symptoms of nasal and ocular itching, repetitive sneezing, watery rhinorrhea, and nasal congestion. It is most often seasonal, occurring during spring or fall, depending on the source of the allergen. Perennial allergic rhinitis, which occurs independent of season, is most likely due to animal dander, house dust, and insect allergens, particularly the dust mite or cockroach. Treatment of the various types of allergic rhinitis should be initially directed toward avoidance of the irritant. While significantly effective, avoidance is not always possible. Pharmacotherapy thus becomes the mainstay of treatment in most patients. Drug therapy includes the use of antihistamines, topical and oral decongestants, mast-cell stabilizers, oral or topical corticosteroids, and lastly, immunotherapy. Because many of the older antihistamines are sedating (including the infant), the new non-sedating antihistamines are preferred for breastfeeding mothers. One major decongestant, phenylpropanolamine, was just removed from the US market, thus leaving only pseudoephedrine, which is a problem for breastmilk production. Intranasal corticosteroids may be used safely with breastfeeding mothers, as the maternal plasma levels are low, and milk levels would be virtually undetectable. Although immunotherapy has not been studied in breastfeeding mothers, the passage of minuscule levels of plant and animal proteins into milk is very unlikely.

Treatment

- Allergen avoidance

- Topical nasal steroids

- Topical nasal antihistamines

- Topical nasal decongestants

- Antihistamines

Medications

- AZELASTINE   (*Astelin, Optivar*)
    - AAP = Not reviewed
    - LRC = L3
    - RID =
    - Pregnancy = C
    - Comment: Azelastine (Astelin) is an antihistamine for oral, intranasal, and ophthalmic administration. It is effective in treating seasonal and perennial rhinitis and nonallergic vasomotor rhinitis.

Ophthalmically, it is effective for allergic conjunctivitis (itchy eyes). Oral bioavailability is 80%, and intranasal bioavailability is only 40%. No data are available on the transfer of azelastine into human milk. The doses used intranasally and ophthalmically are so low that it is extremely unlikely to produce clinically relevant levels in human milk. Oral administration could potentially lead to slightly higher levels, but azelastine is relatively devoid of serious side effects, and it is doubtful that any would occur in a breastfed infant. However, this is an extremely bitter product. It is possible that even miniscule amounts in milk could alter the taste, leading to rejection by the infant.

- BECLOMETHASONE   (*Vanceril, Beclovent, Beconase*)
    - AAP = Not reviewed
    - LRC = L2
    - RID =
    - Pregnancy = C
    - Comment: Beclomethasone is a potent steroid that is generally used via inhalation in asthma or via intranasal administration for allergic rhinitis. Due to its potency, only very small doses are generally used and, therefore, minimal plasma levels are attained. Intranasal absorption is generally minimal. Due to small doses administered, absorption into maternal plasma is extremely small. Therefore, it is unlikely that these doses would produce clinically relevant levels in breastmilk.

- BROMPHENIRAMINE   (*Dimetane, Brombay, Dimetapp, Bromfed*)
    - AAP = Not reviewed
    - LRC = L3
    - RID =
    - Pregnancy = C
    - Comment: Brompheniramine is a popular antihistamine sold as Dimetane or numerous other products, including pseudoephedrine. Although untoward effects appear limited, some reported side effects from Dimetapp preparations are known. Although only insignificant amounts of brompheniramine appear to be secreted into breastmilk, there are a number of reported cases of irritability, excessive crying, and sleep disturbances that have been reported in breastfeeding infants. In breastfeeding mothers, pseudoephedrine has been documented to reduce milk production, so caution is recommended (see pseudoephedrine). Non-sedating antihistamines are recommended instead of this product.

- CETIRIZINE   (*Zyrtec*)
    - AAP = Not reviewed
    - LRC = L2
    - RID =
    - Pregnancy = B
    - Comment: Cetirizine is a popular new antihistamine useful for seasonal allergic rhinitis. It is a metabolite of hydroxyzine and is one of the most potent of the antihistamines. It is rapidly and extensively absorbed orally and due to a rather long half-life is used only once daily. It penetrates the CNS poorly and, therefore, produces minimal sedation. Studies in dogs suggests that only 3% of the dose is transferred into milk. Cetirizine is a suitable antihistamine for use in breastfeeding mothers.

Levocitirizine, or Xyxal, is the active form of cetirizine. It has twice the binding affinity at the H1-receptor compared to cetirizine. No data on its transfer into human milk are available at this time.

- CHLORPHENIRAMINE (*Aller Chlor, Chlor-Tripolon, Chlor-Trimeton*)
    - ◦ AAP = Not reviewed
    - ◦ LRC = L3
    - ◦ RID =
    - ◦ Pregnancy = B
    - ◦ Comment: Chlorpheniramine is an old, but commonly used, antihistamine. Although no data are available on secretion into breastmilk, it has not been reported to produce side effects. Sedation is the only likely side effect. Non-sedating antihistamines are recommended instead of this product.

- CROMOLYN SODIUM (*Nasalcrom, Gastrocrom, Intal*)
    - ◦ AAP = Not reviewed
    - ◦ LRC = L1
    - ◦ RID =
    - ◦ Pregnancy = B
    - ◦ Comment: Cromolyn is an extremely safe drug that is used clinically as an antiasthmatic, an antiallergic, and to suppress mast cell degranulation and allergic symptoms. No data on penetration into human breastmilk are available, but it has an extremely low pKa, and minimal levels would be expected. Less than 0.001% of a dose is distributed into milk of the monkey. No harmful effects have been reported on breastfeeding infants. Less than 1% of this drug is absorbed from the maternal (and probably the infant's) GI tract, so it is unlikely to produce untoward effects in nursing infants. This product is frequently used in pediatric patients and poses no risk for an infant when used in a breastfeeding mother.

- FEXOFENADINE (*Allegra*)
    - ◦ AAP = Maternal Medication Usually Compatible with Breastfeeding
    - ◦ LRC = L2
    - ◦ RID = 0.5-0.7%
    - ◦ Pregnancy = C
    - ◦ Comment: Fexofenadine is a non-sedating histamine-1 receptor antagonist and is the active metabolite of terfenadine (Seldane). It is indicated for symptoms of allergic rhinitis and other allergies. Unlike Seldane, no cardiotoxicity has been reported with this product. In a study of four women receiving 60 mg/d terfenadine, no terfenadine was found in milk. The authors estimate that only 0.45% of the weight-adjusted maternal dose would be ingested by the infant.

- FLUTICASONE (*Flonase, Flovent, Cutivate, Veramyst*)
    - ◦ AAP = Not reviewed
    - ◦ LRC = L3
    - ◦ RID =
    - ◦ Pregnancy = C
    - ◦ Comment: Fluticasone is a typical steroid primarily used intranasally for allergic rhinitis and intrapulmonary for asthma. The intranasal form is called Flonase or Veramyst, the inhaled form is

Flovent. When instilled intranasally, the absolute bioavailability is less than 2%, so virtually none of the dose is absorbed systemically. Oral absorption following inhaled fluticasone is approximately 30%, although almost instant first-pass absorption virtually eliminates plasma levels of fluticasone. Peak plasma levels following inhalation of 880 µg is only 0.1 to 1.0 nanogram/mL. Adrenocortical suppression following oral or even systemic absorption at normal doses is extremely rare due to limited plasma levels. Plasma levels are not detectable when using suggested doses. With the above limited oral and systemic bioavailability and rapid first-pass uptake by the liver, it is not likely that milk levels will be clinically relevant, even with rather high doses.

- LEVOCABASTINE   (*Livostin*)
  - ◦ AAP = Not reviewed
  - ◦ LRC = L2
  - ◦ RID =
  - ◦ Pregnancy = C
  - ◦ Comment: Levocabastine is an antihistamine primarily used via nasal spray and eye drops. It is used for allergic rhinitis and ophthalmic allergies. After application to eye or nose, very low levels are attained in the systemic circulation (<1 ng/mL). In one nursing mother, it was calculated that the daily dose of levocabastine in the infant was about 0.5 µg, far too low to be clinically relevant.

- LORATADINE   (*Claritin*)
  - ◦ AAP = Maternal Medication Usually Compatible with Breastfeeding
  - ◦ LRC = L1
  - ◦ RID = 0.3%
  - ◦ Pregnancy = B
  - ◦ Comment: Loratadine is a long-acting antihistamine with minimal sedative properties. During 48 hours following administration, the amount of loratadine transferred via milk was 4.2 µg, which was 0.01% of the administered dose. Through 48 hours, only 6.0 µg of descarboethoxyloratadine (metabolite) (7.5 µg loratadine equivalents) were excreted into breastmilk, or 0.029% of the administered dose of loratadine or its active metabolite were transferred via milk to the infant. A kg infant would receive only 0.46% of the loratadine dose received by the mother on a mg/kg basis (2.9 µg/kg/day). It is very unlikely this dose would present a hazard to infants. Loratadine does not transfer into the CNS of adults, so it is unlikely to induce sedation, even in infants.

- MOMETASONE   (*Elocon, Nasonex*)
  - ◦ AAP = Not reviewed
  - ◦ LRC = L3
  - ◦ RID =
  - ◦ Pregnancy = C
  - ◦ Comment: Mometasone is a corticosteroid primarily intended for intranasal and topical use. It is considered a medium-potency steroid, similar to betamethasone and triamcinolone. Following topical application to the skin, less than 0.7% is systemically absorbed over an eight hour period. It is very unlikely that mometasone would be excreted into human milk in clinically relevant levels following topical or intranasal administration.

- OXYMETAZOLINE (*Afrin, Allerest, Anefrin At-Eze, Aturgyl, Af-Tipa, Alerjon*)
  - AAP = Not reviewed
  - LRC = L3
  - RID =
  - Pregnancy = Hazardous
  - Comment: Oxymetazoline is a potent alpha-adrenergic agonist. Absorption from nasal mucosa is significant. High doses could lead to maternal and infant toxicity. Caution is recommended.

- PHENYLEPHRINE (*Neo-Synephrine, AK-Dilate, Vicks Sinex Nasal, Neofrin*)
  - AAP = Not reviewed
  - LRC = L3
  - RID =
  - Pregnancy = C
  - Comment: Phenylephrine is a sympathomimetic most commonly used as a nasal decongestant due to its vasoconstrictive properties. It is also used for treatment of ocular uveitis, inflammation, and glaucoma as a mydriatic agent to dilate the pupil during examinations, and for cardiogenic shock. Phenylephrine is a potent adrenergic stimulant and systemic effects (tachycardia, hypertension, arrhythmias), although rare, have occurred following ocular administration in some sensitive individuals. Numerous pediatric formulations are in use, and it is generally considered safe in pediatric patients. Used ophthalmically in eye exams, the maternal dose of the medication would be very low, and it is not likely to pose a problem for a breastfeeding infant. Although no data are available on its secretion into human milk, it is probable that very small amounts will be transferred into milk, but due to its poor oral bioavailability (<38%), it is not likely that it would produce clinical effects in a breastfed infant unless the maternal doses were quite high.

- PHENYLPROPANOLAMINE (*Dexatrim, Acutrim*)
  - AAP = Not reviewed
  - LRC = L2
  - RID =
  - Pregnancy = C
  - Comment: Phenylpropanolamine is an adrenergic agonist frequently used in nasal decongestants and also diet pills. It produces significant constriction of nasal mucosa and is a common ingredient in cold preparations. No data are available on its secretion into human milk, but due to its low molecular weight and its rapid entry past the blood-brain-barrier, it should be expected. It has recently been withdrawn from the US market.

- PSEUDOEPHEDRINE (*Sudafed, Halofed, Novafed*)
  - AAP = Maternal Medication Usually Compatible with Breastfeeding
  - LRC = L3
  - RID = 4.7%
  - Pregnancy = C
  - Comment: Pseudoephedrine is an adrenergic compound primarily used as a nasal decongestant. It is secreted into breastmilk, but in low levels. In a study of three lactating mothers who received 60

mg of pseudoephedrine, the milk/plasma ratio was as high as 2.6-3.9. The average pseudoephedrine milk level over 24 hours was 264 µg/L. The calculated dose that would be absorbed by the infant was still very low (0.4 to 0.6% of the maternal dose).

In a study of eight lactating women who received a single 60 mg dose of pseudoephedrine, the 24 hour milk production was reduced by 24% from 784 mL/d in the placebo period to 623 mL/d in the pseudoephedrine period. While this study was done with a single 60 mg dose, if the normal dosing rate of 60 mg four times daily was used, the estimated infant dose of pseudoephedrine would have been 4.3% of the weight-adjusted maternal dose. While these results are preliminary, it is apparent that mothers in late-stage lactation may be more sensitive to pseudoephedrine and have greater loss in milk production. Therefore, breastfeeding mothers with poor or marginal milk production should be exceedingly cautious in using pseudoephedrine. While there are anecdotal reports of its use in mothers with engorgement, we do not know if it is effective or recommend its use for this purpose at this time.

- TRIPROLIDINE   (*Actidil, Actacin*)
  - ○ AAP = Maternal Medication Usually Compatible with Breastfeeding
  - ○ LRC = L1
  - ○ RID = 1.8%
  - ○ Pregnancy = C
  - ○ Comment: Triprolidine is an antihistamine. It is secreted into milk, but in very small levels, and is marketed with pseudoephedrine as Actifed. In a study of three patients who received 2.5 mg triprolidine, the average concentration in milk ranged from 1.2 to 4.4 µg/L over 24 hours. The relative infant dose is less than 1.8% of the weight-normalized maternal dose. This dose is far too low to be clinically relevant.

Clinical Tips

While antihistamines have been used in infants and breastfeeding mothers for many years, the clinician should attempt to use the newer non-sedating varieties as sedation in breastfed infants may increase the risk of SIDS. Numerous meta-analysis of these studies have suggested that intranasal steroids are far superior to antihistamines. Current data suggest loratadine, fexofenadine, and cetirizine are preferred antihistamines due to minimal sedation and their documented safe use in infants. Ocular antihistamines, such as Azelastine and Levocabastine, may be useful to control eye symptoms associated with allergy.

Astemizole has a long half-life, numerous drug-drug interactions, and has been reported to induce sedation in breastfed infants and should be avoided. Clemastine has been reported to induce drowsiness, irritability, refusal to feed, and neck stiffness and should be avoided. Chlorpheniramine and brompheniramine are probably safe to use, but should be avoided for long-term therapy due to sedation of the infant. While diphenhydramine (Benadryl) has been used for many years both in infants and breastfeeding mothers, its ability to induce sedation makes it less ideal for long-term therapy during breastfeeding. Its short-term use is safe in mother's of normal (non-apneic) infants. A newer non-sedating antihistamine azelastine (Astelin) may be useful when used intranasally, as it poorly absorbed (only 40%) and has minimal side effects. However, we do not have breastfeeding data as of yet on this product and recent studies suggest it is largely ineffective for rhinitis. Oral decongestants, including phenylephrine and phenylpropanolamine, have been used for many years in breastfeeding mothers, largely without reported side effects, although phenylpropranolamine was recently removed from the US market due to cardiovascular toxicity. Recent data from our laboratories suggests that pseudoephedrine may significantly suppress milk production in some mothers, particularly those long postpartum. While it may be useful for engorgement and for short-term use, long-term use may suppress milk production and lead to reduced weight gain in infants. While the other decongestants transfer into milk to some degree, they have not been reported to produce significant problems. Nevertheless, they should only be used on a short-term basis.

Topical, intranasal decongestant sprays, such as oxymetazoline and naphazoline, have not been studied in breastfeeding mothers, but their plasma levels, while not high at recommended doses, can lead to adrenergic side effects if overdosed. While the intranasal absorption is reported as significant, no oral data seems to be available, so the oral absorption in a breastfeeding infant may or may not be possible. Regardless, it is not overly likely that the amount of oxymetazoline or naphazoline absorbed via the nasal mucosa would cause overt side effects in a breastfed infant. But rebound congestion and a syndrome called rhinitis medicamentosa, in which a progressively shorter duration of action leads to continuous use, is well known and patients are generally advised to avoid chronic use of these medications. Cromolyn is virtually nontoxic and non-absorbed, but it is poorly efficacious. It is unlikely to produce untoward effects in a breastfed infant. At present, we do not have data on the topical use of nasal steroids in breastfeeding women. Of the group, fluticasone is not bioavailable and, therefore, would be an ideal choice. Further, it is cleared by the FDA for use in young infants. Although we do not have data on the other nasal steroids (triamcinolone, mometasone, budesonide, beclomethasone), most are unlikely to transfer to human milk in clinically relevant amounts if the mother uses normal therapeutic doses. Of the above remedies, maternal use of cromolyn and the topical nasal steroids are the least likely to produce long-term problems in breastfed infants. However, the nasal steroids are by far more effective.

The use of plant and animal allergens for immunotherapy to treat allergies have not really been studied in breastfeeding mothers. However, it is unlikely any of this antigenic material would ever enter milk, nor would it likely cause problems for a breastfeeding infant. Allergy shots containing antigenic material would not be contraindicated in breastfeeding mothers. Immunotherapy typically takes months of therapy to achieve success.

Suggested Reading

Antonicelli, L., Micucci, C., Voltolini, S., Feliziani, V., Senna, G. E., Di Blasi, P., et al. (2007). Allergic rhinitis and asthma comorbidity: ARIA classification of rhinitis does not correlate with the prevalence of asthma. *Clin Exp Allergy, 37*(6), 954-960.

Apter, A. J. (2008). Advances in the care of adults with asthma and allergy in 2007. *J Allergy Clin Immunol, 121*(4), 839-844.

Bousquet, J., Bodez, T., Gehano, P., Klossek, J. M., Liard, F., Neukirch, F., et al. (2009). Implementation of guidelines for allergic rhinitis in specialist practices. A randomized pragmatic controlled trial. *Int Arch Allergy Immunol, 150*(1), 75-82.

Brozek, J. L., Baena-Cagnani, C. E., Bonini, S., Canonica, G. W., Rasi, G., van Wijk, R. G., et al. (2008). Methodology for development of the Allergic Rhinitis and its Impact on Asthma guideline 2008 update. *Allergy, 63*(1), 38-46.

Demoly, P., Concas, V., Urbinelli, R., & Allaert, F. A. (2008). Spreading and impact of the World Health Organization's Allergic Rhinitis and its impact on asthma guidelines in everyday medical practice in France. Ernani survey. *Clin Exp Allergy, 38*(11), 1803-1807.

Douglass, J. A., & O'Hehir, R.E. (2006). 1. Diagnosis, treatment and prevention of allergic disease: the basics. *Med J Aust., 185*(4), 228-233.

Karafilidis, J. G., & Andrews, W. T. (2008). Allergic rhinitis practice parameter update: correction to information regarding OMNARIS (ciclesonide) nasal spray. *J Allergy Clin Immunol, 122*(6), 1236.

Anesthetic Agents

Principles of Therapy

Medications used in anesthesia comprise an unusual array of compounds, consisting of those with local effects, such as lidocaine or bupivacaine, those with widespread systemic effects, such as the benzodiazepines, opioid analgesics, and gaseous general anesthetics, such as nitrous oxide and others. Although the data concerning many of these products and their transfer into human milk is still rather limited, there are data on most of these medications. It is important to remember that virtually all medications transfer into human milk to some degree. The absolute amount of transfer of drugs into milk is determined largely by equilibrium forces between the maternal plasma and the milk compartment. Because many anesthetic medications have brief plasma half-lives and rapidly redistribute from the plasma compartment to other remote compartments (adipose, muscle), the overall degree of exposure of the breastfeeding infant via breastmilk to these agents is often quite minimal. Because of this rapid redistribution from the plasma to other compartments in breastfeeding mothers, most anesthetic drugs attain minimal levels in milk. The anesthetic agents that follow have been studied in breastfeeding mothers and their milk levels are for the most part quite low. As such, they are unlikely to induce clinical effects in a breastfeeding infant. Regional anesthetics (spinal or epidural anesthesia) may be a safe option depending on the clinical scenario and may minimize maternal plasma and milk drug levels. Regional anesthesia frequently uses both a local anesthetic and an analgesic.

Treatment

General recommendations for anesthesia in breastfeeding mothers are:

- **Premedication:** Therapeutic doses of temazepam, lorazepam, midazolam, opioids, and glycopyrrolate may be safely used. Preferred H_2 blockers include ranitidine or famotidine. Avoid premedication with meperidine (pethidine) due to long-lasting residual effects of its metabolite.

- **Induction:** Thiopental sodium, midazolam, and propofol have both been shown to be safe.

- **Muscle Relaxants:** We have little data on these agents, but thus far no untoward effects have been reported.

- **Anesthetic gases:** Anesthetic gases by design clear rapidly from the systemic circulation. Most are gone in minutes. Few would enter milk or even reside in milk after plasma levels have dropped. Anesthetic gases should not be a problem for a breastfed infant following a brief (<1 hour) period for clearance.

- **Antinauseants:** We do not yet have breastmilk levels on ondansetron or granisetron, although they are routinely used in pediatric oncology. It is unlikely their milk levels will be high enough to induce clinical effects in a breastfeeding infant. Metoclopramide (brief use) has been extensively studied and is largely without clinical effect in a breastfed infant.

- **Postoperative analgesia:** Preferred opiates vary with the procedure, but morphine, fentanyl, sufentanil, or others may be used safely. Meperidine has been implicated in neonatal sedation and behavioral delay and should be used cautiously. NSAIDs of choice include ketorolac, ibuprofen, or diclofenac. Kappa opioids, such as nalbuphine (Nubain), can be used safely in postpartum women, as milk levels are low. In infants with respiratory difficulties, opioids should be used cautiously. Use naloxone or naltrexone cautiously, as they may produce rapid withdrawal in an infant dependent on opiates following gestational exposure.

- **Local anesthetics:** Thus far without exception, the transfer of local anesthetics into human milk has been extremely low in those studied. Studies with lidocaine and bupivacaine show milk levels to be subclinical. While ropivacaine is gaining in popularity due to its reduced hypotensive, cardiotoxic, and CNS side effects in patients, we still do not have data on its transfer to human milk.

- **Breastfeeding:** Mothers should be able to breastfeed their infants safely after a brief interval following surgery. While dependent on the specific drug, most drugs are largely cleared from the plasma compartment by the time a mother is awake, alert, and not heavily sedated.

Medications

- ALFENTANIL   (*Alfenta*)
  - AAP = Not reviewed
  - LRC = L2
  - RID = 0.4%
  - Pregnancy = C
  - Comment: Alfentanil is secreted into breastmilk. Following a dose of 50 µg/kg IV (plus several additional 10 µg/kg doses), the mean levels of alfentanil in colostrum at four hours varied from 0.21 to 1.56 µg/L of colostrum, levels probably too small to produce overt toxicity in breastfeeding infants. Mean levels 28 hours post-alfentanil were 0.05 µg/L.

- BUPIVACAINE   (*Marcaine*)
  - AAP = Not reviewed
  - LRC = L2
  - RID = 0.9%
  - Pregnancy = C
  - Comment: Bupivacaine is the most commonly employed regional anesthetic used in delivery because its placental transfer to the fetus is the least of the local anesthetics. In one study of five patients, levels of bupivacaine in breastmilk were below the limits of detection (<0.02 mg/L) at 2-48 hours postpartum. These authors concluded that bupivacaine is a safe drug for perinatal use in mothers who plan to breastfeed. In another study of 27 patients who received an average of 183.3 mg lidocaine and 82.1 mg bupivacaine via an epidural catheter, lidocaine milk levels at 2, 6, and 12 hours post administration were 0.86, 0.46, and 0.22 mg/L, respectively. Levels of bupivacaine in milk at 2, 6, and 12 hours were 0.09, 0.06, 0.04 mg/L, respectively. Bupivacaine has been used in millions of breastfeeding mothers without documented complications.

- BUTORPHANOL   (*Stadol*)
  - AAP = Maternal Medication Usually Compatible with Breastfeeding
  - LRC = L2
  - RID = 0.5%
  - Pregnancy = C during first and second trimester
  - Comment: Butorphanol is a potent narcotic analgesic. It is available as IV, IM, and a nasal spray. Butorphanol passes into breastmilk in low to moderate concentrations. The amount an infant would receive from breastmilk is probably clinically insignificant (estimated 4 µg/L of milk in a mother receiving 2 mg IM four times a day). Levels produced in infants are considered very low to insignificant. Butorphanol undergoes first-pass extraction by the liver, thus only 17% of the oral dose reaches the plasma. Butorphanol has been frequently used in labor and delivery in women who subsequently nursed their infants, although it has been noted to produce a sinusoidal fetal heart rate pattern and dysphoric or psychotomimetic responses in infants. This is probably very rare.

- DIAZEPAM   (*Valium*)
  - AAP = Drugs whose effect on nursing infants is unknown but may be of concern
  - LRC = L3
  - RID = 7.1%
  - Pregnancy = D
  - Comment: Diazepam is a powerful CNS depressant and anticonvulsant. Published data on milk and plasma levels are highly variable and many are poor studies. In three mothers receiving 10 mg three times daily for up to six days, the maternal plasma levels of diazepam averaged 491 ng/mL (day 4) and 601 ng/mL (day six). Corresponding milk levels were 51 ng/mL (day fourw) and 78 ng/mL (day 6). In a study of nine mothers receiving diazepam postpartum, milk levels of diazepam varied from approximately 0.01 to 0.08 mg/L. Taken together, most studies suggest that the dose of diazepam and its metabolite, desmethyldiazepam, to a suckling infant will be on average 0.78-9.1% of the weight-adjusted maternal dose of diazepam. The acute use of diazepam, such as in surgical procedures, is not likely to lead to significant accumulation. Long-term, sustained therapy may prove troublesome. The benzodiazepine family, as a rule, is not ideal for breastfeeding mothers due to relatively long half-lives and the development of dependence. However, it is apparent that the shorter-acting benzodiazepines (lorazepam, alprazolam) are safest during lactation provided their use is short-term or intermittent, low dose, and after the first week of life.

- FENTANYL (*Sublimaze*)
  - AAP = Maternal Medication Usually Compatible with Breastfeeding
  - LRC = L2
  - RID = 3-5%
  - Pregnancy = C
  - Comment: The transfer of fentanyl into human milk has been documented, but is low. In a group of ten women receiving a total dose of 50 to 400 µg fentanyl IV during labor, the concentration of fentanyl in milk was exceedingly low, generally below the level of detection (<0.05 ng/mL). In a few samples, the levels were between 0.05 and 0.15 ng/mL. Using these data, an infant would ingest less than 3% of the weight-adjusted maternal dose per day. In another study of 13 women who received 2 µg/kg IV after delivery and cord clamping, fentanyl concentration in colostrum was extremely low.

Colostrum levels dropped rapidly and were undetectable after 10 hours. The authors conclude that with these small concentrations and fentanyl's low oral bioavailability, intravenous fentanyl analgesia may be used safely in breastfeeding women. It is apparent that fentanyl transfer to milk under most clinical conditions is poor and is probably clinically unimportant.

- GRANISETRON   (*Kytril*)
  - AAP = Not reviewed
  - LRC = L3
  - RID =
  - Pregnancy = B
  - Comment: Granisetron is an antinauseant and antiemetic agent commonly used with chemotherapy. Following a 1 mg IV dose, the peak plasma concentration was only 3.63 ng/mL. No data are available on its transfer into human milk, but its levels are likely to be low. Further, this family of products (see ondansetron) are not highly toxic and are commonly used in children (two years +). It is unlikely that this product will be overtly toxic to a breastfed infant. However, when used with chemotherapeutic agents, long waiting periods should be used for elimination of the chemotherapeutic agents anyway.

- GLYCOPYRROLATE   (*Robinul*)
  - AAP = Not reviewed
  - LRC = L3
  - RID =
  - Pregnancy = B
  - Comment: Glycopyrrolate is a quaternary ammonium anticholinergic used prior to surgery to dry secretions. After administration, its plasma half-life is exceedingly short (<5 min.) with most of the product being distributed out of the plasma compartment rapidly. No data are available on its transfer into human milk, but due to its short plasma half-life and its quaternary structure, it is very unlikely that significant quantities would penetrate milk. In addition, due to its poor oral bioavailability, it is unlikely that glycopyrrolate would pose a significant risk to a breastfeeding infant.

- HALOTHANE   (*Fluothane*)
  - AAP = Maternal Medication Usually Compatible with Breastfeeding
  - LRC = L2
  - RID =
  - Pregnancy = C
  - Comment: Halothane is an anesthetic gas similar to enflurane, methoxyflurane, and isoflurane. Approximately 60-80% is rapidly eliminated by exhalation the first 24 hours postoperative, and only 15% is actually metabolized by the liver. In one study after a three hour surgery, only 2 ppm was detected in milk. At another exposure in one week, only 0.83 and 1.9 ppm were found. The authors assessed the exposure to the infant as negligible.

- KETOROLAC   (*Toradol, Acular*)
  - AAP = Maternal Medication Usually Compatible with Breastfeeding
  - LRC = L2
  - RID = 0.2%

- Pregnancy = C in first and second trimesters
- Comment: Ketorolac is a popular, nonsteroidal analgesic. In a study of 10 lactating women who received 10 mg orally four times daily, milk levels of ketorolac were not detectable in four of the subjects. The maximum daily dose an infant could absorb (maternal dose = 40 mg/day) would range from 3.16 to 7.9 µg/day, assuming a milk volume of 400 mL or 1000 mL. An infant would, therefore, receive less than 0.2% of the daily maternal dose.

- **LIDOCAINE** (*Xylocaine*)
  - AAP = Maternal Medication Usually Compatible with Breastfeeding
  - LRC = L2
  - RID = 0.5-3.1%
  - Pregnancy = B
  - Comment: Lidocaine is an antiarrhythmic and a local anesthetic. In one study of a breastfeeding mother who received IV lidocaine for ventricular arrhythmias, the mother received approximately 965 mg over seven hours, including the bolus starting doses. At seven hours, breastmilk samples were drawn and the concentration of lidocaine was 0.8 mg/L or 40% of the maternal plasma level (2.0 mg/L). Assuming that the mothers' plasma was maintained at 5 µg/mL (therapeutic= 1.5-5 µg/mL), an infant consuming 1 L per day of milk would ingest approximately 2 mg/day. This amount is exceedingly low in view of the fact that the oral bioavailability of lidocaine is very poor (35%). Once absorbed by the liver, lidocaine is rapidly metabolized. These authors suggest that a mother could continue to breastfeed while on parenteral lidocaine.

    Recommended doses are as follows: Caudal blockade, <300 mg; Epidural blockade, <300 mg; Dental nerve block, <100 mg; Tumescent liposuction, 4200 mg. When administered as a local anesthetic for dental and other surgical procedures, only small quantities are used, generally less than 40 mg. However, following liposuction, the amount used via instillation in the tissues is quite high. Nevertheless, maternal plasma and milk levels do not seem to approach high concentrations and the oral bioavailability in the infant would be quite low (<35%).

- **LORAZEPAM** (*Ativan*)
  - AAP = Drugs whose effect on nursing infants is unknown but may be of concern
  - LRC = L3
  - RID = 2.9%
  - Pregnancy = D
  - Comment: In one prenatal study, it has been found to produce a high rate of depressed respiration, hypothermia, and feeding problems in newborns. Newborns were found to secrete lorazepam for up to 11 days postpartum. In another study, the infants were unaffected following the prenatal use of 2.5 mg IV prior to delivery. Plasma levels of lorazepam in infants were equivalent to those of the mothers. The rate of metabolism in mother and infant appears slow but equal following delivery. In this study, there were no untoward effects noted in any of the infants. The benzodiazepine family, as a rule, is not ideal for breastfeeding mothers, due to relatively long half-lives and the development of dependence. However, it is apparent that the shorter-acting benzodiazepines are safer during lactation provided their use is short-term or intermittent, low dose, and after the first week of life.

- MEPERIDINE   (*Demerol*)
  - ◦ AAP = Maternal Medication Usually Compatible with Breastfeeding
  - ◦ LRC = L2
  - ◦ RID = 1.4-13.9%
  - ◦ Pregnancy = C
  - ◦ Comment: Meperidine is a potent opiate analgesic. It is rapidly and completely metabolized by the adult and neonatal liver to an active form, normeperidine. Significant but small amounts of meperidine are secreted into breastmilk. In a study of nine nursing mothers two hours after a 50 mg IM injection, the average concentration of meperidine in milk was 82 μg/L and a milk/plasma ratio of 1.12. The highest concentration of meperidine in breastmilk at two hours after dose was 0.13 mg/L. Published half-lives for meperidine in neonates (13 hours) and normeperidine (63 hours) are long and with time could concentrate in the plasma of a neonate. Wittel's studies clearly indicate that infants from mothers treated with meperidine (PCA post-cesarean) were neurobehaviorally depressed after three days. Infants from similar groups treated with morphine were not affected. Meperidine should be avoided, if possible, in breastfeeding mothers.

- METOCLOPRAMIDE   (*Reglan*)
  - ◦ AAP = Drugs whose effect on nursing infants is unknown but may be of concern
  - ◦ LRC = L2
  - ◦ RID = 4.7-14.3%
  - ◦ Pregnancy = B
  - ◦ Comment: Metoclopramide has multiple functions, but is primarily used for increasing the lower esophageal sphincter tone in gastroesophageal reflux in patients with reduced gastric tone. In breastfeeding, it is sometimes used in lactating women to stimulate prolactin release from the pituitary and enhance breastmilk production. Since 1981, a number of publications have documented major increases in breastmilk production following the use of metoclopramide, domperidone, or sulpiride. With metoclopramide, the increase in serum prolactin and breastmilk production appears dose-related up to a dose of 15 mg three times daily. Many studies show 66 to 100% increases in milk production, depending on the degree of breastmilk supply in the mother prior to therapy and maybe her initial prolactin levels. Doses of 15 mg/day were found ineffective, whereas doses of 30-45 mg/day were most effective. In most studies, major increases in prolactin were observed, such as from 125 ng/mL to 172 ng/mL in one patient. Metoclopramide is commonly used in breastfeeding women and is not contraindicated, although maternal depression is a common complication.

- MIDAZOLAM   (*Versed*)
  - ◦ AAP = Drugs whose effect on nursing infants is unknown but may be of concern
  - ◦ LRC = L2
  - ◦ RID = 0.6%
  - ◦ Pregnancy = D
  - ◦ Comment: Midazolam is a very short acting benzodiazepine primarily used as an induction or preanesthetic medication. The onset of action of midazolam is extremely rapid, its potency is greater than diazepam, and its metabolic elimination is more rapid. With a plasma half-life of only 1.9 hours, it is preferred for rapid induction and maintenance of anesthesia. After oral administration of 15 mg for up to six days postnatally in 22 women, the mean milk/plasma ratio was 0.15 and the maximum

level of midazolam in breastmilk was 9 μg/L and occurred one to two hours after administration. Therefore, the amount of midazolam transferred to an infant via early milk is minimal, particularly if the baby is breastfed more than four hours after administration. Midazolam is so rapidly redistributed to other tissues from the plasma compartment, milk levels will be exceedingly low.

- MORPHINE   (*Duramorph, Infumorph*)
    ◦ AAP = Maternal Medication Usually Compatible with Breastfeeding
    ◦ LRC = L3
    ◦ RID = 9.1%
    ◦ Pregnancy = C
    ◦ Comment: Morphine is a potent narcotic analgesic and a number of studies on its use in breastfeeding mothers are available. When used in normal clinical doses, it does not apparently sedate breastfeeding infants. While the highest reported RID has been 10.7%, virtually none of this passes the liver to enter the plasma compartment of the infant. Hence, present studies suggest morphine is a preferred potent analgesic for breastfeeding mothers. In summary, morphine is a preferred opiate in breastfeeding mothers primarily due to its poor oral bioavailability. It is unfortunate that the clinical studies above do not necessarily suggest this. High doses over prolonged periods could lead to sedation and respiratory problems in newborn infants.

- NALBUPHINE   (*Nubain*)
    ◦ AAP = Not reviewed
    ◦ LRC = L2
    ◦ RID = 0.6%
    ◦ Pregnancy = B
    ◦ Comment: Nalbuphine is a potent narcotic analgesic similar in potency to morphine. Nalbuphine is both an antagonist and agonist of opiate receptors. In a group of 20 postpartum mothers who received a single 20 mg IM nalbuphine dose, the total amount of nalbuphine excreted into human milk during a 24 hour period averaged 2.3 μg and was equivalent to 0.012% of the maternal dosage. According to the authors, an oral intake of 2.3 μg nalbuphine per day by an infant would not produce any measurable plasma concentrations in the neonate. In another study of 18 mothers who received 0.2 mg/kg every four hours over two to three days, the average concentration in breastmilk was 42 μg/L, with a maximum of 61 μg/L. The reported infant dose was an average of 7 μg/kg/day, with a maximum of 9 μg/kg/day. The authors estimate the RID = 0.6% of the weight-adjusted maternal daily dose and suggest breastfeeding is permissible. In summary, levels in milk are quite low.

- NITROUS OXIDE
    ◦ AAP = Not reviewed
    ◦ LRC = L3
    ◦ RID =
    ◦ Pregnancy =
    ◦ Comment: Nitrous oxide is a weak anesthetic gas. It provides good analgesia and a weak anesthesia. It is rapidly eliminated from the body due to rapid exchange with nitrogen via the pulmonary alveoli (within minutes). A rapid recovery generally occurs in three to five minutes. Due to poor lipid solubility, uptake by adipose tissue is relatively poor, and only insignificant traces of nitrous oxide

circulate in blood after discontinuing inhalation of the gas. No data are available on the entry of nitrous oxide into human milk, but it is probably quite low. Ingestion of nitrous oxide orally via milk is unlikely.

- ONDANSETRON   (*Zofran*)
  - ◦ AAP = Not reviewed
  - ◦ LRC = L2
  - ◦ RID =
  - ◦ Pregnancy = B
  - ◦ Comment: Ondansetron is used clinically for reducing the nausea and vomiting associated with chemotherapy. It has occasionally been used during pregnancy without effect on the fetus. It is available for oral and IV administration. Ondansetron is secreted in animal milk, but no data on humans are available. Four studies of ondansetron use in pediatric patients four-18 years of age are available.

- PALONOSETRON HCL   (*Aloxi*)
  - ◦ AAP = Not reviewed
  - ◦ LRC = L3
  - ◦ RID =
  - ◦ Pregnancy = B
  - ◦ Comment: Palonosetron is a selective 5HT3 receptor antagonist that blocks serotonin binding and reduces the vomiting reflex. It is used to reduce chemotherapy induced nausea and vomiting. It works similarly to ondansetron. No data are available on its transfer into human milk. Fortunately, this family of drugs is largely devoid of major side effects.

- PROPOFOL   (*Diprivan*)
  - ◦ AAP = Not reviewed
  - ◦ LRC = L2
  - ◦ RID = 4.4%
  - ◦ Pregnancy = B
  - ◦ Comment: Propofol is an IV sedative hypnotic agent for induction and maintenance of anesthesia. It is particularly popular in various pediatric procedures. Although the terminal half-life is long, it is rapidly distributed out of the plasma compartment to other peripheral compartments (adipose), so that anesthesia is short (three to ten minutes). Propofol is incredibly lipid soluble. However, only very low concentrations of propofol have been found in breastmilk. In one study of four women who received propofol 2.5 mg/kg IV followed by a continuous infusion, the breastmilk levels at four hours ranged from 0.04 to 0.24 mg/L during the induction phase only. Following continued infusion of propofol in some patients at 5 mg/kg/h, milk samples at four hours ranged from 0.04 to 0.74 mg/L. The second breastmilk level, obtained 24 hours after delivery, contained only 6% of the four-hour sample. From these data, it is apparent that only minimal amounts of propofol are transferred to human milk. No data are available on the oral absorption of propofol. Propofol is rapidly cleared from the neonatal circulation.

- ROPIVACAINE   (*Naropin*)
  - ◦ AAP = Not reviewed

- ◦ LRC = L2
- ◦ RID =
- ◦ Pregnancy = B
- ◦ Comment: Ropivacaine is a newer local anesthetic commonly used as a regional anesthetic and for epidural infusions. It is believed to produce less hypotension when compared to bupivacaine. No data are available on its transfer into human milk, but the manufacturer suggests it is probably much lower than the infant receives in utero. This agent is commonly used in obstetrics and probably poses few if any problems to a breastfeeding infant.

- **THIOPENTAL SODIUM** (*Pentothal*)
  - ◦ AAP = Maternal Medication Usually Compatible with Breastfeeding
  - ◦ LRC = L3
  - ◦ RID = 2.6%
  - ◦ Pregnancy = C
  - ◦ Comment: Thiopental is an ultra short-acting, barbiturate sedative. Used in the induction phase of anesthesia, it rapidly redistributes from the brain to adipose and muscle tissue; hence, the plasma levels are small, and the sedative effects are virtually gone in 20 minutes. Thiopental sodium is secreted into milk in low levels. In a study of two groups of eight women who received from 5.0 to 5.4 mg/kg thiopental sodium, the maximum concentration in breastmilk was 0.9 mg/L in mature milk and in colostrum was 0.34 mg/L. The milk/plasma ratio was 0.3 for colostrum and 0.4 for mature milk. The maximum daily dose to an infant would be 0.135 mg/kg or approximately 2.5% of the adult dose.

- **TROPISETRON**
  - ◦ AAP = Not reviewed
  - ◦ LRC = L3
  - ◦ RID =
  - ◦ Pregnancy = B3 (Australian)
  - ◦ Comment: Tropisetron is a serotonergic (5-HT3) receptor antagonist with antiemetic activity similar to ondansetron and many others. No data are available on its transfer to human milk. See ondansetron as an alternative in the USA.

Clinical Tips

Because most anesthetic agents are used for only brief periods during surgery, the absolute dose transferred into breastmilk is usually quite low. In general, agents that do not attain high levels in the plasma compartment do not attain high levels in the milk compartment. In addition, medications that are rapidly redistributed from the plasma to peripheral compartments do not usually produce high concentrations in milk either. Many anesthetic agents are rapidly cleared from the maternal plasma within minutes because they are redistributed to deep tissue compartments. Therefore, both the duration of exposure to the drug and the dose of medication in breastmilk are very brief. For this reason, the absolute daily dose transferred into milk is almost always low. This is fortuitous for breastfeeding mothers, as most all the literature thus far clearly suggests that the absolute amount of an anesthetic agent transferred into human milk is below clinical relevance. Based on the present literature, the early return to breastfeeding is advisable and advantageous for both mother and infant.

All of the above anesthetic agents have been studied in breastfeeding mothers. Most of these medications are only used once during the procedure, thus the volume of distribution is not filled at all. Because of the rapid redistribution to peripheral compartments, plasma levels of many of these agents are low and fleeting. For this reason, most all of the current studies indicate that milk levels of these drugs used in anesthesia are very low and barely detectable. Thus far, with exception of morphine, meperidine, and diazepam, we do not have any data suggesting that these agents transfer into milk in clinically relevant amounts. Of the opiate family, codeine has recently been involved in an infant death, due to its use in a mother who was a rapid metabolizer; hence, the morphine levels in milk were excessively high. Meperidine (pethidine) is now also in disfavor. It is known to produce neonatal sedation via breastmilk, and it should be avoided in labor and postnatally in breastfeeding mothers. It has also been implicated in adversely impacting latch and successful breastfeeding when used in the immediate postpartum period.

The Kappa opioids (nalbuphine and butorphanol) have been reported to induce psychotomimetic effects in adults. This is a possibility in infants as well, particularly following exposure prenatally.

Many anesthesiologists now recommend that as soon as a mother feels awake and alert, she can breastfeed. It is important to remember that the transport of drugs into milk is difficult, and most drugs penetrate milk poorly. However, it is always important to consider the age and stability of the infant. In a premature or weakened infant, the clinician may opt to withhold breastfeeding for a few hours to reduce the risk of any remaining medications in milk. In a healthy fullterm or older infant, these medications are not likely to produce any major side effects.

The reader requiring more information is referred to the Academy of Breastfeeding Medicine protocol on anesthetic drugs.

Suggested Reading

Chestnut, D. H. (2006). Cesarean delivery on maternal request: implications for anesthesia providers. *Int J Obstet Anesth, 15*(4), 269-272.

Courtney, K. (2007). Maternal anesthesia: what are the effects on neonates? *Nurs Womens Health, 11*(5), 499-502.

Cyna, A. M., & Dodd, J. (2007). Clinical update: obstetric anaesthesia. *Lancet, 370*(9588), 640-642.

Halpern, S. (2009). SOGC Joint Policy Statement on Normal Childbirth. *J Obstet Gynaecol Can, 31*(7), 602; author reply 602-603.

Hassan, Z. U., & Fahy, B. G. (2005). Anesthetic choices in surgery. *Surg Clin North Am, 85*(6), 1075-1089, vii-viii.

Hawkins, J. L. (2007). American Society of Anesthesiologists' Practice Guidelines for Obstetric Anesthesia: update 2006. *Int J Obstet Anesth, 16*(2), 103-105.

Kent, C. D., & Domino, K. B. (2007). Awareness: practice, standards, and the law. *Best Pract Res Clin Anaesthesiol, 21*(3), 369-383.

Kuczkowski, K. M. (2005). Anesthetic management of labor pain: what does an obstetrician need to know? *Arch Gynecol Obstet, 271*(2), 97-103.

Kuczkowski, K. M. (2009). Practice guidelines and prevention of obstetric anesthesia-related maternal mortality. *Middle East J Anesthesiol, 20*(2), 325-326.

Lyons, G. (2008). Saving mothers' lives: confidential enquiry into maternal and child health 2003-5. *Int J Obstet Anesth, 17*(2), 103-105.

Siddik-Sayyid, S., & Zbeidy, R. (2008). Practice guidelines for obstetric anesthesia--a summary. *Middle East J Anesthesiol, 19*(6), 1291-1303.

Wee, M. Y., Brown, H., & Reynolds, F. (2005). The National Institute of Clinical Excellence (NICE) guidelines for caesarean sections: implications for the anaesthetist. *Int J Obstet Anesth, 14*(2), 147-158.

Angina Pectoris

Principles of Therapy

Angina pectoris is precordial chest pain, usually associated with exercise, and is rapidly relieved by rest or nitrates. It presents in two forms: Stable and Unstable. Stable angina inevitably results from myocardial ischemia, most commonly associated with coronary artery disease and narrowing. Unstable angina is characterized by increasingly severe angina attacks, sudden-onset angina at rest, and angina lasting more than 15 minutes. Angina is due to increased oxygen requirements in the cardiac muscles with insufficient oxygen supply. When the patient rests, the oxygen requirement falls and the supply is again sufficient. Angina may present as pain or pressure in the chest, arm, jaw, shoulder, or back. Angina is usually due to myocardial ischemia secondary to poor vascular supply in the myocardium. Regardless of etiology, myocardial ischemia occurs when there is an imbalance between oxygen supply via the coronary arteries and myocardial oxygen demand.

Treatment

- Daily aspirin (81-325 mg)

- Administer clopidogrel when aspirin is contraindicated

- Generally, the treatment for stable angina targets relief of symptoms. Nitrates are very useful. Long term use of nitrates is not recommended, as rapid tolerance occurs.

- Angiotension converting enzyme inhibitors (ACE)

- Angiotension receptor blockers (ARB)

- Cholesterol-lowering agents, particularly statins

- Beta blockers

- Smoking cessation

- Coronary stenting or revascularization

Medication

- ASPIRIN   (*Anacin, Aspergum, Empirin, Genprin, Arthritis Foundation Pain Reliever, Ecotrin*)
    - AAP = Drugs associated with significant side effects and should be given with caution
    - LRC = L3
    - RID = 2.5 - 10.8%

- ○ Pregnancy = C during first and second trimester
- ○ Comment: Small amounts are secreted into breastmilk. In one study, salicylic acid (active metabolite of Aspirin) penetrated poorly into milk (dose =454 mg ASA), with peak levels of only 1.12 to 1.60 μg/mL, whereas peak plasma levels were 33 to 43.4 μg/mL. In another study of a rheumatoid arthritis patient who received 4 gm/day aspirin, none was detectable in her milk (<5mg/100cc). Because aspirin is implicated in Reye syndrome, it is a poor choice of analgesic to use in breastfeeding mothers. However, in rheumatic fever patients, it is still one of the anti-inflammatory drugs of choice and a risk-vs-benefit assessment must be done in this case.

  While the direct use of aspirin in infants and children is definitely implicated in Reye syndrome, the use of the 82 mg/d dose in breastfeeding mothers is unlikely to increase the risk of this syndrome. Unfortunately, we do not at present know of any dose-response relationship between aspirin and Reye syndrome, other than in older children where even low plasma levels of aspirin were implicated in Reye syndrome during viral syndromes, such as flu or chickenpox. Therefore, the use of aspirin in breastfeeding mothers is questionable, but the risk is probably low.

- BENAZEPRIL HCL   (*Lotensin, Lotrel*)
  - ○ AAP = Not reviewed
  - ○ LRC = L2
  - ○ RID = 0.00005%
  - ○ Pregnancy = C during first trimester. X during third trimester.
  - ○ Comment: Benazepril belongs to the ACE inhibitor family. Oral absorption is rather poor (37%). The active component (benazeprilat) reaches a peak at approximately two hours after ingestion. In a patient receiving 20 mg daily for three days, milk levels averaged 0.15 ng/L. Thus the levels in milk are almost unmeasurable. The manufacturer suggests a newborn infant ingesting only breastmilk would receive less than 0.1% of the mg/kg maternal dose of benazepril and benazeprilat. My calculations suggest much less, or a maximum of 0.00005% of the weight-adjusted maternal dose.

- CAPTOPRIL   (*Capoten*)
  - ○ AAP = Maternal Medication Usually Compatible with Breastfeeding
  - ○ LRC = L2
  - ○ RID = 0.02%
  - ○ Pregnancy = C in first trimester. X during third trimester.
  - ○ Comment: Captopril is a typical angiotensin converting enzyme inhibitor (ACE) used to reduce hypertension. In one report of 12 women treated with 100 mg three times daily, maternal serum levels averaged 713 μg/L, while breastmilk levels averaged 4.7 μg/L at 3.8 hours after administration. Data from this study suggest that an infant would ingest approximately 0.002% of the free captopril consumed by its mother (300mg) on a daily basis. No adverse effects have been reported in this study.

- CLOPIDOGREL   (*Plavix*)
  - ○ AAP = Not reviewed
  - ○ LRC = L3
  - ○ RID =
  - ○ Pregnancy = B

- Comment: Clopidogrel selectively inhibits platelet adenosine diphosphate-induced platelet aggregation. It is used to prevent ischemic events in patients at risk (e.g., cardiovascular disease, strokes, myocardial infarct). Clopidogrel is generally only used in those patients who are aspirin-intolerant. Although the plasma half-life is rather brief (eight hours), it's metabolite covalently bonds to platelet receptors with a half-life of 11 days. Because it produces an irreversible inhibition of platelet aggregation, any present in milk could inhibit an infant's platelet function for a prolonged period. Because aspirin affects platelet aggregation similarly, and its milk levels are quite low, it would appear to be an ideal alternative. The choice between using clopidogrel and aspirin must be made on clinical grounds and following a risk vs. benefit assessment until we know more about the levels secreted into human milk.

- DALTEPARIN SODIUM   (*Fragmin, Low Molecular Weight Heparin*)
  - AAP = Not reviewed
  - LRC = L2
  - RID = 15%
  - Pregnancy = B
  - Comment: Dalteparin is a low molecular weight polysaccharide fragment of heparin used clinically as an anticoagulant. In a study of two patients who received 5000-10,000 IU of dalteparin, none was found in human milk. In another study of 15 post-cesarean patients early postpartum (mean = 5.7 days), blood and milk levels of dalteparin were determined three to four hours post-treatment. Following subcutaneous doses of 2500 IU, maternal plasma levels averaged 0.074 to 0.308 IU/mL. Breastmilk levels of dalteparin ranged from <0.005 to 0.037 IU/mL of milk. Using these data, an infant ingesting 150 mL/kg/day would ingest approximately 5.5 IU/kg/day. Unfortunately, this study was done during the colostral phase, when virtually anything can enter milk. Thus the high RID is probably only for the first few days postpartum and would drop significantly after one week. More importantly, however, due to the polysaccharide nature of this production, oral absorption is unlikely, even in an infant.

- DILTIAZEM HCL   (*Cardizem SR, Dilacor-XR, Cardizem CD, Cartia XT*)
  - AAP = Maternal Medication Usually Compatible with Breastfeeding
  - LRC = L3
  - RID = 0.9%
  - Pregnancy = C
  - Comment: Diltiazem is a typical calcium channel blocker antihypertensive. In a report of a single patient receiving 240 mg/d on day 14 postpartum, levels in milk were parallel those of serum. Peak level in milk (and plasma) was slightly higher than 200 µg/L and occurred at eight hours. While nifedipine is probably a preferred choice calcium channel blocker, because of our experience with it, the relative infant dose with diltiazem is quite small, and it is not likely to be problematic.

- ENALAPRIL MALEATE   (*Vasotec*)
  - AAP = Maternal Medication Usually Compatible with Breastfeeding
  - LRC = L2
  - RID = 0.2%
  - Pregnancy = C in first trimester. X in third trimester.

- ◦ Comment: Enalapril maleate is an ACE inhibitor used as an antihypertensive. In one study of five lactating mothers who received a single 20 mg dose, the mean maximum milk concentration of enalapril and enalaprilat was only 1.74 μg/L and 1.72 μg/L, respectively. The author suggests that an infant consuming 850 mL of milk daily would ingest less than 2 μg of enalaprilat daily. In a study by Rush of a patient receiving 10 mg/day, the total amount of enalapril and enalaprilat measured in milk during the 24 hour period was 81.9 ng and 36.1 ng, respectively, or 1.44 μg/L and 0.63 μg/L of milk, respectively.

- **ENOXAPARIN** (*Lovenox, Low Molecular Weight Heparin*)
  - ◦ AAP = Not reviewed
  - ◦ LRC = L3
  - ◦ RID =
  - ◦ Pregnancy = B
  - ◦ Comment: Enoxaparin is a low molecular weight fraction of heparin used clinically as an anticoagulant. In a study of 12 women receiving 20-40 mg of enoxaparin daily for up to five days postpartum for venous pathology (n= 4) or cesarean section (n= 8), no change in anti-Xa activity was noted in the breastfed infants. Because it is a peptide fragment of heparin, its molecular weight is large (2000-8000 daltons). The size alone would largely preclude its entry into human milk at levels clinically relevant. Due to minimal oral bioavailability, any present in milk would not be orally absorbed by the infant. A similar compound, dalteparin, has been studied and milk levels are extremely low as well. See dalteparin.

- **HEPARIN** (*Heparin*)
  - ◦ AAP = Not reviewed
  - ◦ LRC = L1
  - ◦ RID =
  - ◦ Pregnancy = C
  - ◦ Comment: Although rarely used in angina, it may be initially used in some cases. Heparin is a large molecular weight protein use as an anticoagulant. It is used SC, IM, and IV because it is not absorbed orally. Due to its high molecular weight (range = 12,000-15,000 daltons), it is unlikely any would transfer into breastmilk. Any that did enter the milk would be rapidly destroyed in the gastric contents of the infant.

- **LISINOPRIL** (*Prinivil, Zestril*)
  - ◦ AAP = Not reviewed
  - ◦ LRC = L3
  - ◦ RID =
  - ◦ Pregnancy = C in first trimester. X in third trimester.
  - ◦ Comment: Lisinopril is a typical long-acting ACE inhibitor used as an antihypertensive. No breastfeeding data are available on this product. See enalapril, benazepril, captopril as alternatives.

- **METOPROLOL** (*Toprol-XL, Lopressor*)
  - ◦ AAP = Maternal Medication Usually Compatible with Breastfeeding
  - ◦ LRC = L3

- ○ RID = 1.4%
- ○ Pregnancy = C
- ○ Comment: At low doses, metoprolol is a very cardioselective beta-1 blocker and is used for the treatment of hypertension, angina, and tachyarrhythmias. In a study of three women four to six months postpartum who received 100 mg twice daily for four days, the peak concentration of metoprolol ranged from 0.38 to 2.58 μmol/L, whereas the maternal plasma levels ranged from 0.1 to 0.97 μmol/L. Assuming ingestion of 75 mL of milk at each feeding and the maximum concentration of 2.58 μmol/L, an infant would ingest approximately 0.05 mg metoprolol at the first feeding and considerably less at subsequent feedings. In another study of nine women receiving 50-100 mg twice daily, the maternal plasma and milk concentrations ranged from 4-556 nmol/L and 19-1690 nmol/L, respectively. Using these data, the authors calculated an average milk concentration throughout the day as 280 μg/L of milk. This dose is 20-40 times less than a typical clinical dose. These levels are probably too low to be clinically relevant.

- MORPHINE   (*Duramorph, Infumorph*)
  - ○ AAP = Maternal Medication Usually Compatible with Breastfeeding
  - ○ LRC = L3
  - ○ RID = 9.1%
  - ○ Pregnancy = C
  - ○ Comment: Morphine is a potent narcotic analgesic, and we have a number of studies on its use in breastfeeding mothers. When used in normal clinical doses, it does not apparently sedate breastfeeding infants. While the highest reported RID has been 10.7%, almost none of this would bypass the infant's liver and enter the plasma compartment of the infant. Hence, present studies suggest morphine is a preferred choice for breastfeeding mothers. In summary, morphine is probably the preferred opiate in breastfeeding mothers primarily due to its poor oral bioavailability. It is unfortunate that the clinical studies above do not necessarily suggest this. However, high doses over prolonged periods could lead to sedation and respiratory problems in newborn infants.

- NIFEDIPINE   (*Adalat, Procardia*)
  - ○ AAP = Maternal Medication Usually Compatible with Breastfeeding
  - ○ LRC = L2
  - ○ RID = 2.3-3.4%
  - ○ Pregnancy = C
  - ○ Comment: Nifedipine belongs to the calcium channel blocker family of antihypertensives. Two studies indicate that nifedipine is transferred to breastmilk in varying but generally low levels. In one study in which the dose was varied from 10-30 mg three times daily, the highest concentration (53.35 μg/L) was measured at one hour after a 30 mg dose. Other levels reported were 16.35 μg/L 60 minutes after a 20 mg dose and 12.89 μg/L 30 minutes after a 10 mg dose. In this study, using the highest concentration found and a daily intake of 150 mL/kg of human milk, the amount of nifedipine intake would only be 8 μg/kg/day (<1.8% of the therapeutic pediatric dose). The authors conclude that the amount ingested via breastmilk poses little risk to an infant.

- NITROGLYCERIN, NITRATES, NITRITES   (*Nitrostat, Nitrolingual, Nitrogard, Amyl Nitrite, Nitrong, Nitro-Bid, Nitroglyn, Minitran, Nitro-Dur*)
  - ○ AAP = Not reviewed

- ○ LRC = L4
- ○ RID =
- ○ Pregnancy = C
- ○ Comment: Nitroglycerin is a rapid and short acting vasodilator used in angina and other cardiovascular problems, including congestive heart failure. Nitrates come in numerous formulations, some for acute use (sublingual), others are more sustained (Nitro-Dur). At present, we do not know the degree of transfer of nitrates and nitrites into human milk. Two studies suggest that while nitrates/nitrites are well absorbed orally in the mother (approx. 50%), little seems to be transported to human milk. In another study, following a mean total nitrate intake from diet and water of 46.6, 168.1, and 272 mg/day, milk levels only averaged 4.4, 5.1, and 5.2 mg/L, respectively. Thus higher maternal intake did not necessarily correlate with higher milk levels. The authors conclude that mothers who ingest nitrates of 100 mg/day or less do not produce milk with elevated nitrate levels. Mothers who consume nitrates should breastfeed with caution at higher doses and with prolonged exposure. Observe the infant for methemoglobinemia.

- PROPRANOLOL   (*Inderal*)
  - ○ AAP = Maternal Medication Usually Compatible with Breastfeeding
  - ○ LRC = L2
  - ○ RID = 0.3-0.5%
  - ○ Pregnancy = C
  - ○ Comment: Propranolol is a popular beta blocker used in treating hypertension, cardiac arrhythmia, migraine headache, and numerous other syndromes. In general, the maternal plasma levels are exceedingly low; hence, the milk levels are low as well. In a study of a patient receiving 20 mg twice daily, milk levels varied from 4 to 20 μg/L, with an estimated average dose to the infant of 3 μg/day. In another patient receiving 40 mg four times daily, the peak concentration occurred at 3 hours after dosing. Milk levels varied from zero to 9 μg/L. After a 30 day regimen of 240 mg/day propranolol, the predose and postdose concentration in breastmilk was 26 and 64 μg/L, respectively. No symptoms or signs of beta blockade were noted in this infant. The above amounts in milk would likely be clinically insignificant. Long term exposure has not been studied. Of the beta blocker family, propranolol is probably preferred in lactating women. Use with great caution, if at all, in mothers or infants with asthma.

- VERAPAMIL   (*Calan, Isoptin, Covera-HS*)
  - ○ AAP = Maternal Medication Usually Compatible with Breastfeeding
  - ○ LRC = L2
  - ○ RID = 0.2%
  - ○ Pregnancy = C
  - ○ Comment: Verapamil is a typical calcium channel blocker used as an antihypertensive. It is secreted into milk, but in very low levels, which is highly controversial. Anderson reports that in one patient receiving 80 mg three times daily, the average steady-state concentrations of verapamil and norverapamil in milk were 25.8 and 8.8 μg/L, respectively. No verapamil was detected in the infant's plasma. Inoue reports that in one patient receiving 80 mg four times daily, the milk level peaked at 300 μg/L at approximately 14 hours. These levels are considerably higher than the aforementioned. In another study of a mother receiving 240 mg daily, the concentrations in milk were never higher

than 40 µg/L. From these three studies, the relative infant dose would vary from 0.15%, 0.98%, and 0.18%, respectively. Regardless of the variability, the relative amount transferred to the infant is still quite small.

Clinical Tips

The primary goal of treating angina is to reduce the workload on the heart or reduce the etiology of restricted blood flow caused by an infarct narrowed lumen of the coronary vessels. Although eliminating anginal symptoms is a stated goal, simply abolishing angina may not be effective in prolonging patient survival. The major goal must, therefore, be to eliminate the reason for myocardial ischemia. In essence, pharmacotherapy generally consists of multiple avenues of attack and includes beta-blockers, nitrates, and calcium channel blockers. The beta-blockers have for years been important in reducing myocardial ischemia, as they generally reduce total peripheral resistance, thus reducing overall workload on the heart. The goal of beta-blocker therapy is to lower the resting heart rate to 50-60 beats/minute. Atenolol, propranolol, metoprolol, labetalol, and carvedilol all seem to be effective in reducing myocardial ischemia. Pindolol has been documented to be ineffective and should not be used in ischemic patients. Of these agents, most have been studied in breastfeeding patients. Atenolol and acebutolol should be avoided in breastfeeding mothers due to high milk levels.

Propranolol reduces anginal pain by reducing heart rate and probably blood pressure. Propranolol is transferred into milk in extremely low amounts and is an ideal beta-blocker for breastfeeding mothers. Metoprolol levels in breastmilk are also quite low, and it is more cardioselective. While some side effects in breastfed infants have been noted with atenolol, it is probably safe when used carefully, although metoprolol is preferred. Observe infants for sedation, apnea, and hypoglycemia if long-term, higher doses are used. Of the beta-blockers, avoid acebutolol and perhaps atenolol, although they can be used, but only cautiously. Of the calcium channel blockers, nifedipine is the least preferred (for angina), due to questioned efficacy, although it transfers into milk minimally. Numerous other calcium channel blockers are available, but most have not been studied in this syndrome. Diltiazem has been found effective, but its transfer into milk is significant and caution is recommended. At present, we have no data on the transfer of nitroglycerin into human milk, but nitrates present in water have been found to transfer into milk poorly and are not contraindicated. While some caution is recommended with nitrates, until we get more data, they are not likely to cause overt side effects in infants. Due to the extremely short half-life of nitroglycerin, a brief interval prior to breastfeeding (two to three hours) would probably eliminate any risk. Long-acting nitrates (isosorbide dinitrate) are subject to tolerance and may not justify the risk to the breastfeeding infant.

ACE inhibitors are a mainstay in the treatment of angina and heart attack. Benazepril, captopril, and enalapril are suitable and reported milk levels are quite low.

Antiplatelet agents, such as ticlopidine and clopidogrel, have been poorly studied and are only marginally more effective than aspirin. Long-term aspirin therapy in breastfeeding mothers is generally not ideal. Data from the last decade clearly suggest that therapeutic doses of aspirin (administered directly to children) may significantly increase the risk of Reye syndrome in children and less so in infants. Although milk levels of aspirin are extraordinarily low, it should be used cautiously in breastfeeding mothers for long periods. Low molecular weight heparins, such as enoxaparin, tinzaparin and dalteparin, are presently popular and have been found to significantly reduce MI, recurrent angina, and death in patients with unstable angina. New data also suggests that dalteparin levels in milk (5.5 IU/kg/day) are extraordinarily low and would not affect a nursing infant. This is not unexpected, as it is a large molecular weight protein and would not be bioavailable even if ingested by the infant.

Suggested Reading

Abrams, J. (2005). Clinical practice. Chronic stable angina. *N Engl J Med, 352*(24), 2524-2533.

Beaulieu, M. D., Dufresne, L., & LeBlanc, D. (1998). Treating hypertension. Are the right drugs given to the right patients? *Can Fam Physician, 44*, 294-298, 301-292.

Cannon, C. (2003). Improving acute coronary syndrome care: the ACC/AHA guidelines and critical pathways. *J Invasive Cardiol, 15* (Suppl B), 22B-27B; discussion 27B-29B.

Cannon, C. P. (2008). Updated Strategies and Therapies for Reducing Ischemic and Vascular Events (STRIVE) ST-segment elevation myocardial infarction critical pathway toolkit. *Crit Pathw Cardiol, 7*(4), 223-231.

Collinson, P. O., Rao, A. C., Canepa-Anson, R., & Joseph, S. (2003). Impact of European Society of Cardiology/American College of Cardiology guidelines on diagnostic classification of patients with suspected acute coronary syndromes. *Ann Clin Biochem, 40*(Pt 2), 156-160.

Crilly, M., Bundred, P., Hu, X., Leckey, L., & Johnstone, F. (2007). Gender differences in the clinical management of patients with angina pectoris: a cross-sectional survey in primary care. *BMC Health Serv Res, 7*, 142.

Hagberg, S. M., Woitalla, F., & Crawford, P. (2008). 2002 ACC/AHA guideline versus clinician judgment as diagnostic tests for chest pain. *J Am Board Fam Med, 21*(2), 101-107.

LaBresh, K. A., Ellrodt, A. G., Gliklich, R., Liljestrand, J., & Peto, R. (2004). Get with the guidelines for cardiovascular secondary prevention: pilot results. *Arch Intern Med, 164*(2), 203-209.

Schenck-Gustafsson, K. (2006). Are the symptoms of myocardial infarction different in men and women, if so, will there be any consequences? *Scand Cardiovasc J, 40*(6), 325-326.

Trevelyan, J., Needham, E. W., Smith, S. C., & Mattu, R. K. (2004). Impact of the recommendations for the redefinition of myocardial infarction on diagnosis and prognosis in an unselected United Kingdom cohort with suspected cardiac chest pain. *Am J Cardiol, 93*(7), 817-821.

Wenger, N. K., Shaw, L. J., & Vaccarino, V. (2008). Coronary heart disease in women: update 2008. *Clin Pharmacol Ther, 83*(1), 37-51.

Anticoagulation Therapy

Principles of Therapy

Long-term anticoagulation therapy is becoming increasingly common for a widening range of illnesses. Due to the efficacy of anticoagulant therapy in ischemic syndromes, as well as in syndromes with atrial fibrillation and arrhythmias, the number of patients undergoing chronic anticoagulant therapy has risen. The number of agents used to inhibit coagulation has increased, as well, with the introduction of newer low molecular weight heparins. While the choice of anticoagulant as a function of the syndrome is largely outside the realm of this text, the number of breastfeeding mothers exposed to these compounds is significant and warrants coverage. The mechanism of action of these compounds varies enormously. Warfarin is a typical competitive inhibitor of vitamin K-dependent carboxylation of factors II, VII, IX, and X, and thus depletes the procoagulant factors. Heparin inhibits coagulation by its action on antithrombin III, which is a natural inhibitor of factors XIIa, XIa, Xa, IXa, IIa (thrombin), and plasmin. The low molecular weight heparins (enoxaparin, dalteparin) work similarly, but with fewer side effects than heparin. Platelet-inhibitory drugs, both reversibly or irreversibly, inhibit platelet cyclo-oxygenase, thus inhibiting platelet aggregation or synthesis of platelet factors, such as thromboxane A2. Aspirin is a typical irreversible antiplatelet medication. Heparin-induced thrombocytopenia (HIT) and heparin-induced thrombosis (HITTS) are rare complications related to heparin therapy and require discontinuation of heparin and the choice of an alternative anti-coagulant, such as argatroban. Low molecular weight heparin medications are less likely to be associated with these complications, but do not completely eliminate the risk.

Medications

- ARGATROBAN   (*Argatroban*)
  - AAP = Not reviewed
  - LRC = L4
  - RID =
  - Pregnancy = B
  - Comment: Argatroban is a synthetic inhibitor of thrombin and is derived from L-arginine. It reversibly binds to the thrombin active site and exerts an anticoagulant effect by inhibiting thrombin-catalyzed reactions. It is primarily indicated as an anticoagulant for treatment of thrombosis in patients with heparin-induced thrombocytopenia. No data are available on its transfer to human milk, but it is reported present in rodent milk. It is not known if this product is orally bioavailable, but probably not. The presence of this product in milk could potentially induce GI hemorrhage in weak or susceptible infants, including newborns, premature infants, infants with NEC, and other infants. Extreme caution is recommended until we know levels present in milk and more about its GI stability, absorption.

- ASPIRIN   (*Anacin, Aspergum, Empirin, Genprin, Arthritis Foundation Pain Reliever, Ecotrin*)
  - ○ AAP = Drugs associated with significant side effects and should be given with caution
  - ○ LRC = L3
  - ○ RID = 2.5 - 10.8%
  - ○ Pregnancy = C during first and second trimester
  - ○ Comment: Small amounts are secreted into breastmilk. Few harmful effects have been reported. In one study, with a dose of 454 mg of Aspirin, salicylic acid (active metabolite of Aspirin) penetrated poorly into milk, with peak levels of only 1.12 to 1.60 μg/mL, whereas peak plasma levels were 33 to 43.4 μg/mL.

    In another study of a rheumatoid arthritis patient who received 4 gm/day aspirin, none was detectable in her milk (<5mg/100cc). It is possible that extremely high doses in the mother could potentially produce slight bleeding in the infant. Because aspirin is implicated in Reye syndrome, it is not a suitable choice as an analgesic in breastfeeding mothers. However, in rheumatic fever patients, it is still one of the anti-inflammatory drugs of choice, and a risk-vs-benefit assessment must be done in this case with breastfeeding mothers. While the direct use of aspirin in infants and children is definitely implicated in Reye syndrome, the use of the 82 mg/d dose in breastfeeding mothers is unlikely to increase the risk of this syndrome (although this is unstudied). Unfortunately, we do not at present know of any dose-response relationship between aspirin and Reye syndrome, other than in older children where even low plasma levels of aspirin were implicated in Reye syndrome during viral syndromes, such as flu or chickenpox. Therefore, the use of aspirin in breastfeeding mothers is questionable, but the risk is probably low. While ibuprofen or acetaminophen are better choices as analgesics, they do not replace the use of aspirin for it antiplatelet function. Never use these products if the infant has a viral syndrome.

- DALTEPARIN SODIUM   (*Fragmin, Low Molecular Weight Heparin*)
  - ○ AAP = Not reviewed
  - ○ LRC = L2
  - ○ RID = 15%
  - ○ Pregnancy = B
  - ○ Comment: Dalteparin is a low molecular weight polysaccharide fragment of heparin used clinically as an anticoagulant. In a study of two patients who received 5000-10,000 IU of dalteparin, none was found in human milk. In another study of 15 post-cesarean patients 'early postpartum' (mean= 5.7 days), blood and milk levels of dalteparin were determined three to four hours post-treatment. Following subcutaneous doses of 2500 IU, maternal plasma levels averaged 0.074 to 0.308 IU/mL. Breastmilk levels of dalteparin ranged from <0.005 to 0.037 IU/mL of milk. The milk/plasma ratio ranged from 0.025 to 0.224. Using these data, an infant ingesting 150 mL/kg/day would ingest approximately 5.5 IU/kg/day. Due to the polysaccharide nature of this production, oral absorption is unlikely. Further, because this study was done early postpartum, it is possible that the levels in 'mature' milk would be lower. The authors suggest that "it appears highly unlikely that puerperal thromboprophylaxis with LMWH has any clinically relevant effect on the nursing infant." Although the RID appears high, it would be largely unabsorbable.

- DIPYRIDAMOLE   (*Persantine*)
  - ○ AAP = Not reviewed
  - ○ LRC = L3

- RID =
- Pregnancy = B
- Comment: Dipyridamole is most commonly used in addition to coumarin anticoagulants to prevent thromboembolic complications of cardiac valve replacement. According to the manufacturer, only small amounts are believed to be secreted in human milk. No reported untoward effects have been reported.

- **ENOXAPARIN** (*Lovenox, Low Molecular Weight Heparin*)
  - AAP = Not reviewed
  - LRC = L3
  - RID =
  - Pregnancy = B
  - Comment: Enoxaparin is a low molecular weight fraction of heparin used clinically as an anticoagulant. In a study of 12 women receiving 20-40 mg of enoxaparin daily for up to five days postpartum for venous pathology (n= 4) or cesarean section (n= 8), no change in anti-Xa activity was noted in the breastfed infants. Because it is a peptide fragment of heparin, its molecular weight is large (2000-8000 daltons). The size alone would largely preclude its entry into human milk at levels clinically relevant. Due to minimal oral bioavailability, any present in milk would not be orally absorbed by the infant. A similar compound, dalteparin, has been studied and milk levels are extremely low as well. See dalteparin.

- **HEPARIN** (*Heparin*)
  - AAP = Not reviewed
  - LRC = L1
  - RID =
  - Pregnancy = C
  - Comment: Heparin is a large protein molecule.. It is used SC, IM, and IV because it is not absorbed orally in mother or infant. Due to its high molecular weight (range= 12,000-15,000 daltons), it is unlikely any would transfer into breastmilk. Any that did enter the milk would be rapidly destroyed in the gastric contents of the infant.

- **TINZAPARIN SODIUM** (*Innohep*)
  - AAP = Not reviewed
  - LRC = L3
  - RID =
  - Pregnancy = B
  - Comment: Tinzaparin is a depolymerized heparin (low molecular weight heparin) similar to several others, such as dalteparin, enoxaparin, nadroparin, or parnaparin. The average molecular weight range of tinzaparin is approximately one-half that of regular (unfractionated) heparin (5500-7500 vs 12,000 daltons). No data are available on the transfer of this anticoagulant into human milk, but it is likely low. In studies with dalteparin, none was found in milk in one study and only small amounts in another (see dalteparin). In studies with enoxaparin, no changes in anti-Xa activity were noted in breastfed infants. It is very unlikely any would be orally bioavailable.

    Other typical low molecular weight heparins: Dalteparin (Fragmin), enoxaparin (Lovenox), nadroparin (Fraxiparin), parnaparin (Fluxum)

- WARFARIN   (*Coumadin, Panwarfin*)
  - ○ AAP =   Maternal Medication Usually Compatible with Breastfeeding
  - ○ LRC = L2
  - ○ RID =
  - ○ Pregnancy = X
  - ○ Comment: Warfarin is a potent anticoagulant. Warfarin is highly protein bound in the maternal circulation and, therefore, very little is secreted into human milk. Very small and insignificant amounts are secreted into milk, but it depends to some degree on the dose administered. In one study of two patients who were anticoagulated with warfarin, no warfarin was detected in the infant's serum nor were changes in coagulation detectable. In another study of 13 mothers, less than 0.08 μmol per liter (25 ng/mL) was detected in milk, and no warfarin was detected in the infants' plasma.

    According to these authors, maternal warfarin apparently poses little risk to a nursing infant, and thus far has not produced bleeding anomalies in breastfed infants. Other anticoagulants, such as phenindione, should be avoided. Observe infant for bleeding, such as excessive bruising or reddish petechia (spots). While the risks in breastfeeding premature infants (which are more susceptible to intracranial bleeding) is still low, oral supplementation with vitamin K1 will preclude any chance of hemorrhage. Even modest doses of Vitamin K1 counteract high doses of warfarin.

Clinical Tips

Warfarin has been extensively used in breastfeeding mothers, and in no cases have changes in the breastfed infant's coagulation been found, nor were warfarin levels in the neonate clinically relevant. Warfarin is extensively bound to protein in the maternal plasma compartment (> 99%) and does not penetrate into milk to any degree. Several studies have documented its safe use. Its effect is also reversed by the administration of vitamin K, which is routinely given to newborn infants. Heparin is a large molecular weight protein (40,000 daltons) and is unable to penetrate milk. Further, it would not be orally bioavailable in an infant, even if it did penetrate milk. The low molecular weight heparins (enoxaparin, dalteparin) are still 2000-9000 daltons in size and are far too large to enter milk in clinically relevant concentrations. They are not orally bioavailable. A new study shows that only minimal amounts of dalteparin are secreted into human milk (5.5 IU/kg/day). However, anticoagulant therapy in breastfeeding mothers should always be approached cautiously with close observation of the infant for signs of abnormal bleeding.

The use of antiplatelet medications in breastfeeding mothers is less well understood. While it is true that aspirin and dipyridamole levels in milk have been documented to be very low to undetectable, it is wise to remember that their effect on platelet cyclo-oxygenase is irreversible and requires re-synthesis of the platelet prior to a return of function. For this reason, very small levels of these agents could theoretically alter platelet aggregation to some degree. Some caution with these latter two drugs is advised in breastfeeding situations. The association of aspirin to Reye syndrome in children is also a possible risk factor, but the dose of aspirin via milk is so low that it seems unreasonable to assume it would increase the risk of Reye syndrome. Secondly, the age of highest incidence of Reye syndrome is six (4-12) years, which is sometimes beyond the breastfeeding period. Another antiplatelet drug, ticlopidine, is even more risky, due to severe neutropenia and is only used in those patients who are aspirin intolerant. At this time, without data, ticlopidine would not be a suitable choice for a breastfeeding patient.

Suggested Reading

Bowles, L., & Cohen, H. (2003). Inherited thrombophilias and anticoagulation in pregnancy. *Best Pract Res Clin Obstet Gynaecol, 17*(3), 471-489.

Clark, P., & Bates, S. M. (2009). North American and British guidelines for anti-thrombotic therapy: are we reaching consensus? *Thromb Res, 123*(Suppl 2), S111-123.

Shackford, S. R., Rogers, F. B., Terrien, C. M., Bouchard, P., Ratliff, J., & Zubis, R. (2008). A 10-year analysis of venous thromboembolism on the surgical service: the effect of practice guidelines for prophylaxis. *Surgery, 144*(1), 3-11.

Singh, P., Lai, H. M., Lerner, R. G., Chugh, T., & Aronow, W. S. (2009). Guidelines and the use of inferior vena cava filters: a review of an institutional experience. *J Thromb Haemost, 7*(1), 65-71.

Stone, S. E., & Morris, T. A. (2005). Pulmonary embolism during and after pregnancy. *Crit Care Med, 33*(10 Suppl), S294-300.

Weitz, J. I. (2009). Prevention and treatment of venous thromboembolism during pregnancy. *Catheter Cardiovasc Interv, 74*(Suppl 1), S22-26.

Anxiety Disorders

Principles of Therapy

Anxiety disorders compose a complex group of rather unique conditions, including generalized anxiety disorder, obsessive compulsive disorder, social phobias, panic disorder, post-traumatic stress disorders, and others. Symptoms include apprehension, tension, panic and stress, extreme fear and discomfort, sweating, trembling, chest pain, etc. Anxiety may be associated with environmental stress or even devoid of cause. Panic disorder (with or without agoraphobia) is the most common anxiety disorder, occurring in 2-6% of the population. When anxiety becomes disproportionate to reality, it may become pathologic. Attempts should be made to eliminate other associated diseases, such as depression, hyperthyroidism, pheochromocytoma, alcohol use and abuse, or psychiatric disorders.

Treatment

- Cognitive therapy may be helpful

- Antidepressants

- Benzodiazepines

Medications

- ALPRAZOLAM   (*Xanax*)
    - AAP = Drugs whose effect on nursing infants is unknown but may be of concern
    - LRC = L3
    - RID = 8.5%
    - Pregnancy = D
    - Comment: Alprazolam is a prototypic benzodiazepine drug similar to Valium, but is now preferred in many instances because of its shorter half-life. In a study of eight women who received a single oral dose of 0.5 mg, the peak alprazolam level in milk was 3.7 µg/L, which occurred at 1.1 hours; the observed milk/serum ratio (using AUC method) was 0.36. The neonatal dose of alprazolam in breastmilk is low. The author estimates the average between 0.3 to 5 µg/kg per day. While the infants in this study did not breastfeed, these doses would probably be too low to induce a clinical effect. In a brief letter, Anderson reports that the manufacturer is aware of withdrawal symptoms in infants following exposure in utero and via breastmilk. In a mother who received 0.5 mg 2-3 times daily (PO) during pregnancy, a neonatal withdrawal syndrome was evident in the breastfed infant the first week postpartum. These data suggests that the amount of alprazolam in breastmilk is insufficient to prevent a withdrawal syndrome following prenatal exposure. In another case of infant exposure

solely via breastmilk, the mother took alprazolam (dosage unspecified) for nine months while breastfeeding and withdrew herself from the medication over a three week period. The mother reported withdrawal symptoms in the infant including irritability, crying, and sleep disturbances. The benzodiazepine family, as a rule, are not ideal for breastfeeding mothers due to relatively long half-lives and the development of dependence. However, it is apparent that the shorter-acting benzodiazepines are safest during lactation provided their use is short-term or intermittent, low dose, and after the first week of life. Brief use is probably compatible with breastfeeding.

- BUSPIRONE   (*BuSpar*)
    - ◦ AAP = Not reviewed
    - ◦ LRC = L3
    - ◦ RID =
    - ◦ Pregnancy = B
    - ◦ Comment: No data exists on excretion into human milk. It is secreted into animal milk, so the same would be expected in human milk. BuSpar is said to be mg for mg equivalent to diazepam (Valium) in its anxiolytic properties, but does not produce significant sedation or addiction as the benzodiazepine family. Its metabolite is partially active, but has a brief half-life (4.8 hours) as well. Compared to the benzodiazepine family, this product would be a better choice for treatment of anxiety in breastfeeding women, although clinically, it is not very popular due to poor efficacy. Without accurate breastmilk levels, it is not known if the product is safe for breastfeeding women or the levels the infant would ingest daily. The rather brief half-life of this product and its metabolite would not likely lead to buildup in the infant's plasma.

- CLOMIPRAMINE   (*Anafranil*)
    - ◦ AAP = Drugs whose effect on nursing infants is unknown but may be of concern
    - ◦ LRC = L2
    - ◦ RID = 2.8%
    - ◦ Pregnancy = C
    - ◦ Comment: Clomipramine is a tricyclic antidepressant frequently used for obsessive-compulsive disorder. In one patient taking 125 mg/day, on the fourth and sixth day postpartum, milk levels were 342.7 and 215.8 μg/L, respectively. Maternal plasma levels were 211 and 208.4 μg/L at day four and six, respectively. Milk/plasma ratio varies from 1.62 to 1.04 on day four to six, respectively. Neonatal plasma levels continued to drop from a high of 266.6 ng/mL at birth to 127.6 ng/mL at day four, to 94.8 ng/mL at day six, to 9.8 ng/mL at 35 days. In a study of four breastfeeding women who received doses of 75 to 125 mg/day, plasma levels of clomipramine in the breastfed infants were below the limit of detection, suggesting minimal transfer to the infant via milk. No untoward effects were noted in any of the infants.

- CLONAZEPAM   (*Klonopin*)
    - ◦ AAP = Not reviewed
    - ◦ LRC = L3
    - ◦ RID = 2.8%
    - ◦ Pregnancy = D
    - ◦ Comment: Clonazepam is a typical benzodiazepine sedative, anticonvulsant. In one case report, milk levels varied between 11 and 13 μg/L (the maternal dose was omitted). Milk/maternal serum ratio

was approximately 0.33. In this report, the infant's serum level of clonazepam dropped from 4.4 μg/L at birth to 1.0 μg/L at 14 days while continuing to breastfeed, suggesting increasing clearance with time. In this case, excessive periodic breathing, apnea, and cyanosis occurred in this infant (36 weeks gestation) at six hours until ten days postpartum. The infant was exposed in utero as well as postpartum via breastmilk. In another study of a mother treated with 2 mg clonazepam, twice daily peak milk concentrations of 10.7 μg/L were reported at four hours postdose, with a maximum infant dose of 2.5% (weight-adjusted maternal dose). The infant's serum level of clonazepam at days two to four was 4.7 μg/L. In a group of 11 mothers receiving 0.25 to 2 mg clonazepam daily, ten of 11 breastfed infants had no detectable (limit of detection: 5-14 μg/L) clonazepam or metabolites in their serum. One infant (1.9 weeks old) had a serum concentration of 22 μg/L. Maternal dose was 0.5 mg daily. These data suggest the low incidence of toxicity with this medication in breastfeeding infants.

- DULOXETINE   (*Cymbalta*)
  - ○ AAP = Not reviewed
  - ○ LRC = L3
  - ○ RID = 0.141%
  - ○ Pregnancy = C
  - ○ Comment: Duloxetine is a selective serotonin and norepinephrine reuptake inhibitor (SNRI) that is indicated for depression and for patients with neuropathic pain. The primary role of SNRIs is as an alternative in patients with major depressive disorder who have responded poorly to other agents (e.g., tricyclics or SSRIs).

    The transfer of duloxetine into breastmilk was studied in six women who were at least 12 weeks postpartum and taking 40 mg twice daily for 3.5 days. Paired blood and breastmilk samples were taken at zero, one two, three, six, nine, and 12 hours postdose. The milk/plasma ratio was reported to be about 0.267. The daily dose of duloxetine was estimated to be 7 μg/day (range=4-15 μg/day). According to the manufacturer, the weight-adjusted infant dose would be approximately 0.141% of the maternal dose. Further, even this is unlikely absorbed, as duloxetine is unstable under acid conditions of the infant's stomach.

- ESCITALOPRAM   (*Lexapro*)
  - ○ AAP = Not reviewed
  - ○ LRC = L2
  - ○ RID = 5.2-8%
  - ○ Pregnancy = C
  - ○ Comment: Escitalopram is a selective serotonin reuptake inhibitor (SSRI) used in the treatment of depression. It is the active S(+)-enantiomer of citalopram (Celexa). While this agent is very specific for the serotonin receptor site, it does apparently have a number of other side effects which may be related to activities at other receptors. Antagonism of muscarinic, histaminergic, and adrenergic receptors has been hypothesized to be associated with various anticholinergic, sedative, and cardiovascular side effects.

    In a case report of a 32-year-old mother taking escitalopram (5 mg/day) while breastfeeding her newborn, the reported milk level was 24.9 ng/mL at one week postpartum. The infant's daily dose was estimated to be 3.74 μg/kg. At 7.5 weeks of age, the mother was taking 10 mg/day and the milk concentration level was 76.1 ng/mL. The infant daily dose was 11.4 µg/kg. There were no adverse events reported in the infant.

In a recent study of eight breastfeeding women taking an average of 10 mg/day, the total relative infant dose of escitalopram and its metabolite was reported to be 5.3% of the mother's dose. The mean M/P ratio (AUC) was 2.2 for escitalopram and 2.2 for demethylescitalopram. Absolute infant doses were 7.6 µg/kg/day for escitalopram and 3.0 µg/kg/day for demethylescitalopram. The drug and its metabolite were undetectable in most of the infants tested. No adverse events in the infants were reported. Because the absolute infant dose of escitalopram is less than an equivalent antidepressant dose of racemic citalopram (Celexa), it's use is preferred over citalopram in treating depression in lactating women.

- FLUOXETINE   (*Prozac*)
    - ◦ AAP = Drugs whose effect on nursing infants is unknown but may be of concern
    - ◦ LRC = L2
    - ◦ RID   = 1.6-14.6%
    - ◦ Pregnancy = C
    - ◦ Comment: Fluoxetine is a very popular serotonin reuptake inhibitor (SSRI) currently used for depression and a host of other syndromes. Fluoxetine absorption is rapid and complete, and the parent compound is rapidly metabolized to norfluoxetine, which is an active, long half-life metabolite (360 hours). Both fluoxetine and norfluoxetine appear to permeate breastmilk to levels approximately 1/5 to 1/4 of maternal plasma. In one patient at steady-state (dose =20mg/day), plasma levels of fluoxetine were 100.5 µg/L and levels of norfluoxetine were 194.5 µg/L. Fluoxetine levels in milk were 28.8 µg/L and norfluoxetine levels were 41.6 µg/L. Milk/plasma ratios were 0.286 for fluoxetine, and 0.21 for norfluoxetine. There are many other studies; consult *Medications and Mothers' Milk* for more data.

        Current data on Sertraline and escitalopram suggest these medications have difficulty entering milk, and more importantly, the infant. Therefore, they are preferred agents over fluoxetine for therapy of depression in breastfeeding mothers. However, it is important to remember that the risks of not breastfeeding far outweigh the risk of using fluoxetine, and women who can only take fluoxetine should be advised to continue breastfeeding and observe the infant for side effects. Finally, fluoxetine therapy during breastfeeding is by no means contraindicated and has been used in many thousands of women.

- FLUVOXAMINE   (*Luvox*)
    - ◦ AAP = Drugs whose effect on nursing infants is unknown but may be of concern
    - ◦ LRC = L2
    - ◦ RID   = 0.3-1.4%
    - ◦ Pregnancy = C
    - ◦ Comment: Although structurally dissimilar to the other serotonin reuptake inhibitors, fluvoxamine provides increased synaptic serotonin levels in the brain. It has several hepatic metabolites which are not active. Its primary indications are for the treatment of obsessive-compulsive disorders (OCD), although it also functions as an antidepressant. There are a number of significant drug-drug interactions with this product. In a case report of one 23-year-old mother and following a dose of 100 mg twice daily for two weeks, the maternal plasma level of fluvoxamine base was 0.31 mg/L

and the milk concentration was 0.09 mg/L. The authors reported a theoretical infant dose of 0.0104 mg/kg/day of fluvoxamine, which is only 0.5% of the maternal dose. According to the authors, the infant suffered no unwanted effects as a result of this intake and this dose poses little risk to a nursing infant. Numerous other studies are published. In summary, the data from at least eight studies suggest that only minuscule amounts of fluvoxamine are transferred to infants, that plasma levels in infants are too low to be detected, and no adverse effects have been noted.

- IMIPRAMINE (*Tofranil, Janimine*)
  - ◦ AAP = Drugs whose effect on nursing infants is unknown but may be of concern
  - ◦ LRC = L2
  - ◦ RID = 0.1-4.4%
  - ◦ Pregnancy = D
  - ◦ Comment: Imipramine is a classic tricyclic antidepressant. Imipramine is metabolized to desipramine, the active metabolite. Milk levels approximate those of maternal serum. In a patient receiving 200 mg daily at bedtime, the milk levels at 1, 9, 10, and 23 hours were 29, 24, 12, and 18 µg/L, respectively. However, in this previous study, the mother was not in a therapeutic range. In a mother with full therapeutic levels, it is suggested that an infant would ingest approximately 0.2 mg/L of milk. This represents a dose of only 30 µg/kg/day, far less than the 1.5 mg/kg dose recommended for older children. The long half-life of this medication in infants could, under certain conditions, lead to high plasma levels, although they have not been reported. Although no untoward effects have been reported, the infant should be monitored closely. Therapeutic plasma levels in children 6-12 years are 200-225 ng/mL. Two good reviews of psychotropic drugs in breastfeeding patients are available.

- LORAZEPAM (*Ativan*)
  - ◦ AAP = Drugs whose effect on nursing infants is unknown but may be of concern
  - ◦ LRC = L3
  - ◦ RID = 2.9%
  - ◦ Pregnancy = D
  - ◦ Comment: Lorazepam is a typical benzodiazepine from the Valium family of drugs. It is frequently used prenatally and presurgically as a sedative agent. In one prenatal study, it has been found to produce a high rate of depressed respiration, hypothermia, and feeding problems in newborns. Newborns were found to secrete lorazepam for up to 11 days postpartum. In McBrides's study, the infants were unaffected following the prenatal use of 2.5 mg IV prior to delivery. Plasma levels of lorazepam in infants were equivalent to those of the mothers. The rate of metabolism in mother and infant appears slow, but equal, following delivery. In this study, there were no untoward effects noted in any of the infants. In one patient receiving 2.5 mg twice daily for five days postpartum, the breastmilk levels were 12 µg/L. In another patient four hours after an oral dose of 3.5 mg, milk levels averaged 8.5 µg/L. Summerfield reports an average concentration in milk of 9 µg/L and an average milk/plasma ratio of 0.22. It would appear from these studies that the amount of lorazepam secreted into milk would be clinically insignificant under most conditions.

    The benzodiazepine family, as a rule, is not ideal for breastfeeding mothers due to relatively long half-lives and the development of dependence. However, it is apparent that the shorter-acting benzodiazepines are safer during lactation provided their use is short-term or intermittent, low dose, and after the first week of life. Lorazepam is apparently compatible with breastfeeding.

- PAROXETINE   (*Paxil*)
  - AAP = Drugs whose effect on nursing infants is unknown but may be of concern
  - LRC = L2
  - RID = 1.2-2.8%
  - Pregnancy = D
  - Comment: Paroxetine is a typical serotonin reuptake inhibitor. Although it undergoes hepatic metabolism, the metabolites are not active. Paroxetine is exceedingly lipophilic and distributes throughout the body with only 1% remaining in plasma. In one case report of a mother receiving 20 mg/day paroxetine at steady state, the breastmilk level at peak (four hours) was 7.6 µg/L. While the maternal paroxetine dose was 333 µg/kg, the maximum daily dose to the infant was estimated at 1.14 µg/kg or 0.34% of the maternal dose. In two studies of six and four nursing mothers respectively, the mean dose of paroxetine received by the infants in the first study was 1.13% (range 0.5-1.7) of the weight adjusted maternal dose. The mean M/P (AUC) was 0.39 (range 0.32-0.51) while the predicted M/P was 0.22. Numerous other studies exist. Consult *Mediations and Mother's Milk* for a complete review.

    These studies generally conclude that paroxetine can be considered relatively 'safe' for breastfeeding infants as the absolute dose transferred is quite low. Plasma levels in the infant were generally undetectable. Recent data suggests that a neonatal withdrawal syndrome may occur in newborns exposed in utero to paroxetine; although, there is significant difficulty in differentiating between withdrawal and toxicity. Symptoms include jitteriness, vomiting, irritability, hypoglycemia, and necrotizing enterocolitis. Suicide ideation and withdrawal symptoms seem worse with this product, and it should not be used in adolescent patients due to the risk of suicide. Other studies have suggested that paroxetine may produce cardiovascular problems in infants. These claims have been refuted in a much larger study. Regardless, levels of paroxtine in milk are quite low and it is probably compatible with breastfeeding.

- PROPRANOLOL   (*Inderal*)
  - AAP = Maternal Medication Usually Compatible with Breastfeeding
  - LRC = L2
  - RID = 0.3-0.5%
  - Pregnancy = C
  - Comment: Propranolol is a popular beta blocker used in treating hypertension, cardiac arrhythmia, migraine headache, and numerous other syndromes. In general, the maternal plasma levels are exceedingly low; hence, the milk levels are low as well. Milk/plasma ratios are generally less than one. In one study of three patients, the average milk concentration was only 35.4 µg/L after multiple dosing intervals. The milk/plasma ratio varied from 0.33 to 1.65. Using these data, the authors suggest that an infant would receive only 70 µg/L of milk per day, which is <0.1% of the maternal dose. In another study of a patient receiving 20 mg twice daily, milk levels varied from 4 to 20 µg/L, with an estimated average dose to the infant of 3 µg/day. In another patient receiving 40 mg four times daily, the peak concentration occurred at 3 hours after dosing. Milk levels varied from zero to 9 µg/L.

    After a 30 day regimen of 240 mg/day propranolol, the predose and postdose concentration in breastmilk was 26 and 64 µg/L, respectively. No symptoms or signs of beta blockade were noted in this infant. The above amounts in milk would likely be clinically insignificant. Long term exposure has not been studied, but propanolol is probably compatible with breastfeeding. Of the beta blocker family, propanolol or metoprolol are probably preferred in lactating women. Use with great caution, if at all, in mothers or infants with asthma.

- SERTRALINE   (*Zoloft*)
  - AAP = Drugs whose effect on nursing infants is unknown but may be of concern
  - LRC = L2
  - RID = 0.4-2.2%
  - Pregnancy = C
  - Comment: Sertraline is a typical serotonin reuptake inhibitor similar to Prozac and Paxil, but unlike Prozac, the longer half-life metabolite of sertraline is only marginally active. In one study of a single patient taking 100 mg of sertraline daily for three weeks postpartum, the concentration of sertraline in milk was 24, 43, 40, and 19 μg/L of milk at one, five, nine, and 23 hours, respectively, following the dose. The maternal plasma levels of sertraline after 12 hours was 48 ng/mL. Sertraline plasma levels in the infant at three weeks were below the limit of detection (<0.5 ng/mL) at 12 hours postdose. Routine pediatric evaluation after three months revealed a neonate of normal weight who had achieved the appropriate developmental milestones. In another study of three breastfeeding patients who received 50-100 mg sertraline daily, the maternal plasma levels ranged from 18.4 to 95.8 ng/mL, whereas the plasma levels of sertraline and its metabolite, desmethylsertraline, in the three breastfed infants were below the limit of detection (<2 ng/mL). Milk levels were not measured. Desmethylsertraline is poorly active, less than 10% of the parent sertraline. These studies generally confirm that the transfer of sertraline and its metabolite to the infant is minimal, and that attaining clinically relevant plasma levels in infants is remote at maternal doses less than 150 mg/day. Thorough reviews of antidepressant use in breastfeeding mothers are available in *Medications and Mothers' Milk*.

- TRAZODONE   (*Desyrel*)
  - AAP = Drugs whose effect on nursing infants is unknown but may be of concern
  - LRC = L2
  - RID = 2.8%
  - Pregnancy = C
  - Comment: Trazodone is an antidepressant whose structure is dissimilar to the tricyclics and to the other antidepressants. In six mothers who received a single 50 mg dose, the milk/plasma ratio averaged 0.14. Peak milk concentrations occurred at two hours and were approximately 110 μg/L (taken from graph) and declined rapidly thereafter. On a weight basis, an adult would receive 0.77 mg/kg whereas a breastfeeding infant, using these data, would consume only 0.005 mg/kg. The authors estimate that about 0.6% of the maternal dose was ingested by the infant over 24 hours.

- VENLAFAXINE   (*Effexor*)
  - AAP = Not reviewed
  - LRC = L3
  - RID = 6.8-8.1%
  - Pregnancy = C
  - Comment: Venlafaxine is a new serotonin reuptake inhibitor antidepressant. It inhibits both serotonin reuptake and norepinephrine reuptake. It is somewhat similar in mechanism to other

antidepressants, such as Prozac, but has fewer anticholinergic side-effects. In an excellent study of three mothers (mean age = 34.5 years, 84.5 kg) receiving venlafaxine (225-300 mg/d), the mean milk/plasma ratios for venlafaxine (V) and O-desmethylvenlafaxine (ODV) were 2.5 and 2.7, respectively. The mean maximum concentrations of V and ODV in milk were 1.16 mg/L and 0.796 mg/L. The Cmax for milk was 2.25 hours. The mean infant exposure was 3.2% for V and 3.2% for ODV of the weight-adjusted maternal dose. Venlafaxine was detected in the plasma of one of seven infants, while ODV was detected in four of the seven infants. The infants were healthy and showed no acute adverse effects.

However, recent data (MedWatch, FDA) has suggested that infants exposed in utero to various SNRIs, such as venlafaxine, may have profound adverse effects immediately upon delivery. These include respiratory distress, cyanosis, apnea, seizures, temperature instability, etc. It is not known if these adverse events are due to a direct toxic effect of venlafaxine on the fetus or to a discontinuation (withdrawal) syndrome. Studies have shown that these adverse effects may be partially relieved with venlafaxine received through breastmilk.

Clinical Tips

Panic Disorder

Panic disorder is an anxiety attack involving spontaneous attacks of panic which occur in situations not usually expected to produce anxiety. It consists of extreme fear and may be accompanied by agoraphobia, dizzinessness, collapse, breathlessness, trembling, chest pain, or hot flashes. The postpartum period is believed to be a time of increased risk for panic disorder. The psychopharmacological treatment of panic disorders has changed dramatically in the past decade. Treatment goals should initially include protecting the patient from hazards and relieving acute symptoms. Cognitive behavioral therapy has been shown to be quite effective and is a preferred treatment today. Previously, benzodiazepines were typical first line therapy, while today the antidepressants, especially the serotonin reuptake inhibitors (SSRIs), have become first-line therapy in many patients.

The preferred SSRIs are fluoxetine, venlafaxine, and sertraline, as these have been found to be very effective. Some tricyclic antidepressants, particularly imipramine, have been found effective, but due to side effects, they are not popular. Clinicians are advised to initiate therapy with lower doses of SSRIs, perhaps as little as one-fourth the normal dose and gently increase over time. Following the use of antidepressants, patients sometimes report a 'jitteriness syndrome' consisting of restlessness, sweating, flushing, or even increased anxiety. To avoid this response, many clinicians begin therapy with one-quarter to one-half the usual therapeutic dose and gently increase as tolerated. However, it is important to remember that the doses of SSRIs required in anxiety disorders are much higher than those used with depressive disorders, and the clinician should continue to increase the dose of the SSRI until symptoms abate.

Low doses of benzodiazepines, such as alprazolam, can be used temporarily to counteract this symptom. Because the SSRIs can induce manic symptoms in some patients, a careful family history of bipolar disorder should be obtained.

The benzodiazepines are known to be effective treatment for phobic disorder, panic attacks, and anticipatory anxiety. Several large studies of alprazolam found it clinically effective in reducing panic attacks. Diazepam, while effective, requires much larger doses (20-60 mg), which may be sedating. These doses would not be ideal for a breastfeeding mother, as diazepam has a long half-life and measurable milk levels. While alprazolam is more potent and effective than diazepam, it also suffers from a shorter half-life, thus requiring more frequent dosing or the use of a sustained-release product. Effective doses of alprazolam vary enormously between patients, but should be initiated at 0.25 to 0.5 mg three times daily, and then increased as symptoms require. The undesirable effects of benzodiazepines include sedation, potentiation of alcohol dependence, and significant withdrawal effects. Withdrawal can be severe and should be carried out over many days to weeks. Withdrawal symptoms include profound insomnia, anxiety, panic, tremor, and depersonalization. The presence of insomnia (which primarily only occurs in withdrawal) is a major means of differentiating between withdrawal and the return of anxiety symptoms. Because of the withdrawal effects, many patients refuse to stop benzodiazepines. Interestingly, in one breastfeeding mother who did withdraw, her breastfed infant subsequently exhibited withdrawal symptoms.

As a family, the benzodiazepines tend to have rather long half-lives and could potentially (after prolonged administration) build up in the plasma compartment of the breastfed infant, although this has not been reported. This could lead to sedation and increased risk of apnea. Therefore, recommend the shorter half-life medications, such as alprazolam or lorazepam, if a benzodiazepine is required. Use cautiously in premature infants or those subject to apnea. Remember, short intervals of use (one to three weeks) are less risky than long term therapy (months), especially with the longer half-life products like diazepam. We have no data on buspirone in breastmilk, but its unique lack of sedation or addiction may be useful in breastfeeding situations. However, while it may be effective for anxiety disorders, it is ineffective for panic disorder and in general is not a popular drug.

Generalized Anxiety Disorder

The main features of anxiety disorder are chronic, behavioral, and physiological symptoms of anxiety and hyperarousal.

Excessive worry, more days than not, is a cardinal feature. Somatic complaints, such as tension, fatigue, and insomnia, often coexist with this condition. Because anxiety disorders often coexist with depression and panic disorders, in this situation, depression and panic should be initially treated as above.

The treatment of anxiety disorders in the past has mainly required the use of the benzodiazepines, but newer data suggests that the SSRI family are quite effective. Benzodiazepines should only be used initially until the SSRI takes effect in several weeks. SSRIs should be started at approximately one-fourth to one-half the normal dose, and then gradually increased over time. It is well known that higher doses of SSRIs are ultimately required in anxiety disorders than for depression. The choice of SSRI is controversial, but less activating choices are preferred and include: sertraline, fluoxetine, escitalopram, and perhaps duloxetine. Response is generally seen in six weeks.

Buspirone has been found as effective as the benzodiazepines in some studies, although slower. At present, we do not have data on breastmilk levels of buspirone; however, it produces less drowsiness, psychomotor impairment, alcohol potentiation, and far less addiction than the benzodiazepines in patients, and it is probably a good candidate for breastfeeding mothers, even without clear milk levels.

As always, patients should be monitored for worsening depression or suicidality, especially the first two to four weeks of therapy with the SSRIs. Beta blockers have occasionally been used to treat some of the somatic symptoms of anxiety. Propranolol successfully reduces symptoms, such as tremor tachycardia and sweating. Do not use in pregnant or asthmatic women, or those with sinus bradycardia.

Obsessive-Compulsive Disorders

Obsessive-compulsive disorder (OCD) is a neuropsychiatric condition characterized by persistant, recurrent, unwanted, intrusive ideas and visions that induce severe anxiety and distress. It occurs in approximately 2-3%

of the population. The patient tries to resist these impulses, but this leads to the anxiety component of this syndrome. OCD may also worsen postpartum.

Treatment of this disorder is not that different from other anxiety disorders and includes the use of structured psychotherapy and the select serotonin reuptake inhibitors.

Sertraline, fluoxetine, fluvoxamine, paroxetine, escitalopram, and venlafaxine have been found to be effective and should be considered first line therapy, although many patients still suffer from symptoms to some degree. Recently, escitalopram has been found effective and may have a more favorable side effect profile.

While clomipramine and the SSRIs are apparently equally efficacious, the side effect profile of clomipramine is somewhat troublesome for some patients and includes anticholinergic effects (blurred vision, constipation, and dry mouth), sedation, and toxicity in overdose that is also common with the tricyclic antidepressants. Prior studies suggest therapy of at least six weeks is required at doses up to 300 mg/d to alleviate symptoms.

Therapy with the SSRIs, particularly fluvoxamine and fluoxetine, have been found equally effective, although they too require up to four to six weeks of therapy; 10-12 weeks of therapy are required prior to assuming these medications are ineffective. Doses are less clear. Some studies have found that 20 mg/d of fluoxetine is just as effective as 40-60 mg/d. Doses should initially be lower and gradually increased over one to two week intervals.

Clinical efficacy of various medications should not be discounted until the patient has been treated with a minimum daily dose of the following: clomipramine 250 mg, fluoxetine 60 mg, fluvoxamine 300 mg, paroxetine 60 mg, and sertraline 200 mg. In breastfeeding patients with young infants, the above higher doses could prove problematic, particularly with fluoxetine and clomipramine. Caution is recommended at the higher doses in breastfeeding mothers early postpartum. The use of neuroleptics is controversial. Although some patients may respond positively, numerous case reports of worsening symptoms can be found, particularly with risperidone and clozapine.

Social Phobia

Social phobia is described as severe and persistent fear of social situations, particularly with strangers. Its prevalence is approximately 5-10% of the population. It is typified by severe avoidance behavior leading to major social disruption. While social phobia may share several features with panic disorder, it has several unique phenomenologic features. The five most common fears of patients with social phobias are: 1) public speaking, 2) eating in public, 3) using public lavatories, 4) writing in public, and 5) being the object of attention. Shyness and avoidance are typical features of this syndrome.

Treament consists of cognitive behavioral therapy combined with SSRIs and short-term benzodiazepines. However, it is well known that pharmacotherapy alone is seldom effective and psychotherapy is almost mandatory for social phobias.

Paroxetine and fluvoxamine have been found to be very effective for these symptoms, although other SSRIs may be used, such as fluoxetine, escitalopram, or sertraline. The monamine oxidase inhibitors are also effective, but should be avoided due to major side effects. Other medications that have been found to be effective include the benzodiazepines, alprazolam, and clonazepam. Gabapentin also appears to be effective in the disorder.

Suggested Reading

Alexander, J. L. (2007). Quest for timely detection and treatment of women with depression. *J Manag Care Pharm, 13*(9 Suppl A), S3-11.

Brandes, M., Soares, C. N., & Cohen, L. S. (2004). Postpartum onset obsessive-compulsive disorder: diagnosis and management. *Arch Womens Ment Health, 7*(2), 99-110.

Brockington, I. (2004). Postpartum psychiatric disorders. *Lancet, 363*(9405), 303-310.

Burman, M. E., McCabe, S., & Pepper, C. M. (2005). Treatment practices and barriers for depression and anxiety by primary care advanced practice nurses in Wyoming. *J Am Acad Nurse Pract, 17*(9), 370-380.

Gorman, J. M. (2006). Gender differences in depression and response to psychotropic medication. *Gend Med, 3*(2), 93-109.

Levitt, C., Shaw, E., Wong, S., Kaczorowski, J., Springate, R., Sellors, J., et al. (2004). Systematic review of the literature on postpartum care: methodology and literature search results. *Birth, 31*(3), 196-202.

Steiner, M., Pearlstein, T., Cohen, L. S., Endicott, J., Kornstein, S. G., Roberts, C., et al. (2006). Expert guidelines for the treatment of severe PMS, PMDD, and comorbidities: the role of SSRIs. *J Womens Health (Larchmt), 15*(1), 57-69.

Asthma

Principles of Therapy

Asthma is defined as a chronic inflammatory disorder of the airways in which many cells play a role, particularly mast cells, eosinophils, and T lymphocytes. Asthma is characterized by periods of wheezing, cough, dyspnea, or chest tightness. Episodes are usually triggered by exercise, cold temperatures, or triggers such as animal dander or cigarette smoke. Asthma may be persistent rather than episodic. It is caused by airway hypersensitivity obstructing airflow; patients typically breathe at higher lung volumes and have prolonged expiration.

Most asthmatics are atopic. Increasingly, in the last decade, asthma has become recognized as an inflammatory process of the bronchi requiring anti-inflammatory treatment early on in the process. Initially, treatment consists of removal of offending allergens, such as cigarette smoke, animal dander, dust mites, and more recently, cockroaches. Asthmatics should avoid non-selective beta blockers as these medications can precipitate symptoms. The use of NSAID's can also trigger symptoms in some asthmatics. Early therapeutic intervention is presently aimed at controlling the inflammatory process. Presently, inhaled synthetic corticosteroids should be considered for first line therapy. Adjuncts to therapy also include the selective beta-2 agonists (e.g., albuterol, salmeterol) which provide relief of acute bronchoconstriction. The older beta agonist, isoproterenol, should not be used in asthmatics today. The anticholinergic agent ipratropium is useful in reflex cholinergic bronchoconstriction, particularly from cold air-induced asthma, sulfur dioxide-induced asthma, and cough-variant asthma. The newer leukotriene inhibitors (e.g., zafirlukast, montelukast), when used prophylactically, are useful in some patients in reducing the inflammatory response, but studies are inconclusive as to their overall usefulness. Influenza vaccination should be offered to asthmatic patients as they are at a greater risk of complications from infection.

Treatment

- Minimize impact of asthma on patient's life.

- Treatment is based on the severity of the symptoms.

- Beta-2 agonists as needed.

- Inhaled steroids as needed.

- Leukotriene inhibitors as needed.

- High dose oral steroid for severe attacks.

- Smoking cessation.

- Avoidance of asthma triggers.

- Administration of seasonal influenza vaccine

Medications

- ALBUTEROL   (*Proventil, Ventolin*)
  - ○ AAP = Not reviewed
  - ○ LRC = L1
  - ○ RID =
  - ○ Pregnancy = C
  - ○ Comment: Albuterol is a very popular beta-2 adrenergic agonist that is typically used to dilate constricted bronchi in asthmatics. It is active orally, but is most commonly used via inhalation. When used orally, high plasma levels are attained and transfer to breastmilk is possible. When used via inhalation, less than 10% is absorbed into maternal plasma. Small amounts are probably secreted into milk, although no reports exist. It is commonly used via inhalation in treating pediatric asthma. This product is safe to use in breastfeeding mothers.

- BECLOMETHASONE   (*Vanceril, Beclovent, Beconase*)
  - ○ AAP = Not reviewed
  - ○ LRC = L2
  - ○ RID =
  - ○ Pregnancy = C
  - ○ Comment: Beclomethasone is a potent steroid that is generally used via inhalation in asthma or via intranasal administration for allergic rhinitis. Due to its potency, only very small doses are generally used and, therefore, plasma levels are probably low. Intranasal absorption is generally minimal. It is unlikely that these doses will produce clinically relevant levels in a breastfeeding infant. Fluticasone and budesonide are preferred.

- BUDESONIDE   (*Rhinocort, Pulmicort Respules, Symbicort*)
  - ○ AAP = Not reviewed
  - ○ LRC = L1
  - ○ RID = 0.3%
  - ○ Pregnancy = C
  - ○ Comment: Budesonide is a potent corticosteroid used intranasally for allergic rhinitis, via inhalation for asthma, and in capsule form for Crohn's disease. As such, bioavailability via the lung is estimated to be less than 34% of the inhaled dose. Once absorbed systemically, budesonide is a weak systemic. In one five year study of children aged two to seven years, no changes in linear growth, weight, and bone age were noted following inhalation. Adrenal suppression at these doses is extremely remote. Using normal doses, it is unlikely that clinically relevant concentrations of budesonide would ever reach the milk nor be systemically bioavailable to a breastfed infant.

    One study tested samples from eight women before and after their first morning dose of 200 or 400 µg inhaled budesonide (Pulmicort Turbuhaler). Average milk level of budesonide (Cav) was 0.105-0.219 nmol/L with doses of 200 and 400 µg twice daily, respectively. Maternal plasma levels of budesonide reported (Cav) were 0.246-0.437 nmol/L at the doses above. Milk/plasma ratios were 0.428 and 0.502 at the doses above. Plasma samples from infants 1-1.5 hours after feeding showed levels below the limit of quantification. Therefore, the estimated daily infant dose is 0.3% of the mother's daily dose or approximately 0.0068-0.0142 µg/kg/day.

The new oral formulation of budesonide (Entocort EC) is used for Crohn's disease and is placed in special granules that pass the stomach before releasing the drug in controlled-release manner in the duodenum. Plasma budesonide has a high clearance rate due to high uptake by the liver. Plasma levels are low and brief, and its ability to suppress normal cortisol levels is about half that of prednisone. Because of its high first-pass clearance, it is rather unlikely to produce high or even significant levels in milk, nor be orally bioavailable to a significant degree in breastfeeding infants.

- CROMOLYN SODIUM   (*Nasalcrom, Gastrocrom, Intal*)
  - AAP = Not reviewed
  - LRC = L1
  - RID =
  - Pregnancy = B
  - Comment: Cromolyn is an extremely safe drug that is used clinically as an antiasthmatic, an antiallergic, and to suppress mast cell degranulation and allergic symptoms. No data on penetration into human breastmilk are available, but it has an extremely low pKa, and minimal levels would be expected. Less than 0.001% of a dose is distributed into milk of the monkey. No harmful effects have been reported on breastfeeding infants. Less than 1% of this drug is absorbed from the maternal (and probably the infant's) GI tract, so it is unlikely to produce untoward effects in nursing infants. This product is frequently used in pediatric patients and poses no risk for an infant when used in a breastfeeding mother.

- FLUNISOLIDE   (*Nasalide, Aerobid*)
  - AAP = Not reviewed
  - LRC = L3
  - RID =
  - Pregnancy = C
  - Comment: Flunisolide is a potent corticosteroid used to reduce airway hyperreactivity in asthmatics. It is also available as Nasalide for intranasal use for allergic rhinitis. Generally, only small levels of flunisolide are absorbed systemically (about 40%), thereby reducing systemic effects and presumably breastmilk levels as well. After inhalation of 1 mg flunisolide, systemic availability was only 40% and plasma level was 0.4-1 nanogram/mL. Adrenal suppression in children has not been documented, even after therapy of two months with 1600 µg/day. Once absorbed, flunisolide is rapidly removed by first-pass uptake in the liver. Although no data on breastmilk levels are yet available, it is unlikely that the level secreted in milk is clinically relevant.

- FLUTICASONE   (*Flonase, Flovent, Cutivate, Veramyst*)
  - AAP = Not reviewed
  - LRC = L3
  - RID =
  - Pregnancy = C
  - Comment: Fluticasone is a steroid primarily used intranasally for allergic rhinitis and via inhalation for asthma. The intranasal form is called Flonase or Veramyst, the inhaled form is Flovent. When instilled intranasally, the absolute bioavailability is less than 2%, so virtually none of the dose is absorbed systemically. Oral absorption following inhaled fluticasone is approximately 30%,

although its rapid first-pass absorption by the liver virtually eliminates plasma levels of fluticasone. Adrenocortical suppression following oral or even systemic absorption at normal doses is extremely rare due to limited plasma levels. Plasma levels are not detectable when using suggested doses. With the above limited oral and systemic bioavailability, and rapid first-pass uptake by the liver, it is not likely that milk levels will be clinically relevant, even with rather high doses.

- FORMOTEROL FUMARATE   (*Foradil Aerolizer, Symbicort*)
  - AAP = Not reviewed
  - LRC = L3
  - RID =
  - Pregnancy = C
  - Comment: Formoterol is a long-acting selective beta-2 adrenoceptor agonist used for asthma and COPD. Following inhalation of a 120 μg dose, the maximum plasma concentration of 92 picograms/mL occurred within five minutes. No data are available on its transfer into human milk, but the extremely low plasma levels would suggest that milk levels would be incredibly low, if even measurable. Studies of oral absorption in adults suggests that while absorption is good, plasma levels are still below detectable levels and may require large oral doses prior to attaining measurable plasma levels. It is not likely the amount present in human milk would be clinically relevant to a breastfed infant.

    Formoterol is also available in Symbicort, along with budesonide, as a long term treatment for asthma patients. It is available in 160/4.5 mcg and 80/4.5 mcg doses. See also budesonide.

- LEVALBUTEROL   (*Xopenex*)
  - AAP = Not reviewed
  - LRC = L2
  - RID =
  - Pregnancy = C
  - Comment: Levalbuterol is the active (R)-enantiomer of the drug substance racemic albuterol. It is a popular and new bronchodilator used in asthmatics. No data are available on breastmilk levels, but they will probably be low to nil. After inhalation, plasma levels are incredibly low, averaging 1.1 nanogram/mL. It is very unlikely that enough would enter milk to produce clinical effects in an infant. This product is commonly used in infancy for asthma and other bronchoconstrictive illnesses.

- METHYLPREDNISOLONE   (*Solu-Medrol, Depo-Medrol, Medrol*)
  - AAP = Maternal Medication Usually Compatible with Breastfeeding
  - LRC = L2
  - RID =
  - Pregnancy = C
  - Comment: Methylprednisolone (MP) is the methyl derivative of prednisolone. Four milligrams of methylprednisolone is roughly equivalent to 5 mg of prednisone. In general, the amount of methylprednisolone and other steroids transferred into human milk is minimal, as long as the dose does not exceed 80 mg per day. However, relating side effects of steroids administered via breastmilk and their maternal doses is rather difficult and each situation should be evaluated individually.

Extended use of high doses could predispose the infant to steroid side effects, including decreased linear growth rate, but these require rather high doses. Low to moderate doses are believed to have minimal effect on breastfed infants. See prednisone.

- MONTELUKAST SODIUM   (*Singulair*)
    ◦ AAP = Not reveiwed
    ◦ LRC = L3
    ◦ RID =
    ◦ Pregnancy = B
    ◦ Comment: Montelukast is a leukotriene receptor inhibitor similar to Accolate and is used as an adjunct in the treatment of asthma. The manufacturer reports that montelukast is secreted into animal milk, but no data on human milk are available. This product is cleared for use in children aged six and above. This product does not enter the CNS, nor many other tissues. Although the milk levels in humans are unreported, they are probably quite low.

- NEDOCROMIL SODIUM   (*Tilade*)
    ◦ AAP = Not reviewed
    ◦ LRC = L2
    ◦ RID =
    ◦ Pregnancy = B
    ◦ Comment: Nedocromil is believed to stabilize mast cells and prevent release of bronchoconstrictors in the lung following exposure to allergens. The systemic effects are minimal due to reduced plasma levels. Systemic absorption averages less than 8-17% of the total dose, even after continued dosing, which is quite low. The poor oral bioavailability of this product and the reduced side effect profile of this family of drugs suggest that it is unlikely to produce untoward effects in a nursing infant.

- SALMETEROL XINAFOATE   (*Serevent*)
    ◦ AAP = Not reviewed
    ◦ LRC = L2
    ◦ RID =
    ◦ Pregnancy = C
    ◦ Comment: Salmeterol is a long acting beta-2 adrenergic stimulant used as a bronchodilator in asthmatics. Maternal plasma levels of salmeterol after inhaled administration are very low (85-200 pg/mL) or undetectable. Studies in animals have shown that plasma and breastmilk levels are very similar. Oral absorption of both salmeterol and the xinafoate moiety are good. The terminal half-life of salmeterol is 5.5 hours, xinafoate is 11 days. No reports of use in lactating women are available. It should be considered compatible with breastfeeding.

- TERBUTALINE   (*Bricanyl, Brethine*)
    ◦ AAP = Maternal Medication Usually Compatible with Breastfeeding
    ◦ LRC = L2
    ◦ RID = 0.2-0.3%
    ◦ Pregnancy = B

- ○ Comment: Terbutaline is a popular Beta$_2$ adrenergic used for bronchodilation in asthmatics. It is secreted into breastmilk, but in low quantities. Following doses of 7.5 to 15 mg/day of terbutaline, milk levels averaged 3.37 µg/L. Assuming a daily milk intake of 165 mL/kg, these levels would suggest a daily intake of less than 0.5 µg/kg/day, which corresponds to 0.2 to 0.7% of maternal dose. In another study of a patient receiving 5 mg three times daily, the mean milk concentrations ranged from 3.2 to 3.7 µg/L. The author calculated the daily dose to infant at 0.4-0.5 µg/kg body weight. Terbutaline was not detectable in the infant's serum. No untoward effects have been reported in breastfeeding infants.

- **TRIAMCINOLONE ACETONIDE** (*Nasacort, Azmacort, Tri-Nasal*)
  - ○ AAP = Not reviewed
  - ○ LRC = L3
  - ○ RID =
  - ○ Pregnancy = C
  - ○ Comment: Triamcinolone is a typical corticosteroid (see prednisone) that is available for topical, intranasal, injection, inhalation, and oral use. It is commonly used in asthmatics. When applied topically to the nose (Nasacort) or to the lungs (Azmacort), only minimal doses are used and plasma levels are exceedingly low to undetectable. Although no data are available on triamcinolone secretion into human milk, it is likely that milk levels would be exceedingly low. While the oral adult dose is 4-48 mg/day, the inhaled dose is 200 µg three times daily, and the intranasal dose is 220 µg/day. There is virtually no risk to the infant following use of the intranasal products in breastfeeding mothers.

- **ZAFIRLUKAST** (*Accolate*)
  - ○ AAP = Not reviewed
  - ○ LRC = L3
  - ○ RID = 0.7%
  - ○ Pregnancy = B
  - ○ Comment: Zafirlukast is excreted into milk in low concentrations. Following repeated 40 mg doses twice daily (please note: average adult dose is 20 mg twice daily), the average steady-state concentration in breastmilk was 50 µg/L compared to 255 ng/mL in maternal plasma. Zafirlukast is poorly absorbed when administered with food. It is likely the oral absorption via ingestion of breastmilk would be low. The manufacturer recommends against using in breastfeeding mothers.

Clinical Tips

The goals of asthma therapy are to prevent bronchoconstriction and expiratory wheezing while maintaining normal lung function, normal quality of life, and minimizing pharmacologic side effects. In general, asthma is classified by the severity and frequency of attacks, varying from mild episodic, to mild persistent, to moderate persistent, and finally, to severe persistent attacks. Treatment is dependent on the classification within which the patient fits. In the last decade, more emphasis has been placed on treating the etiology of bronchoconstriction, namely inflammation, particularly using inhaled steroids. In the patient with mild episodic asthma, bronchodilators, such as albuterol or levalbuterol, are initially indicated. As the severity of attacks increase, the use of inhaled corticosteroids (budesonide, fluticasone), along with long-acting beta agonists (salmeterol, formoterol), have become the mainstay of treatment. The use of higher and higher doses of inhaled corticosteroids, such as fluticasone and budesonide, has become standard therapy.

In breastfeeding mothers, the mast-cell stabilizers (e.g., cromolyn and nedocromil) are some of the safest drugs one can use in asthmatics, although they must be used four times daily, which limits their popularity. They are not orally bioavailable and would not penetrate milk at all. However, they are not very efficacious and are seldom used today.

The most commonly used medications, albuterol, levalbuterol, salmeterol and formoterol, are poorly absorbed from the pulmonary mucosa. Less than 21-30% of albuterol is absorbed into the plasma compartment following administration via inhalation. Even then, peak plasma levels are in the low nanogram range. While not known, it is likely milk levels would be so low as to be undetectable. Levalbuterol (Xopenex) is the active R-isomer of albuterol, and its milk kinetics would be similar to albuterol. Salmeterol has a high binding affinity for lung tissue and is retained for many hours prior to elimination. These products have been used extensively in breastfeeding mothers without reported side effect in their infants.

The inhaled corticosteroids, particularly fluticasone and budesonide, are administered in microgram quantities. Because of poor bioavailability, and instant first pass uptake by the liver, plasma steroid levels in most asthmatics following intrapulmonary use are extremely low.

Of those studied (budesonide) in breastfeeding mothers, maternal plasma levels are incredibly low, as are milk levels. Hence, it is unlikely the small amount penetrating milk would be clinically relevant to a breastfed infant, as the oral bioavailability of these products are very low (ranging 1-10%). Thus far, no untoward effects on breastfed infants have been reported when exposed via milk. Of this family, budesonide and possibly fluticasone would appear to have the best kinetics (< 1% oral bioavailability) for breastfeeding mothers and their infants. The short-term use of oral or IV corticosteroids is not necessarily contraindicated because steroids are known to enter milk poorly. Even high oral doses of prednisone (120 mg daily) do not produce clinically relevant levels in milk. Short-term therapy with high doses would not likely affect a breastfed infant.

Of the leukotriene inhibitors, only Zafirlukast has been studied in breastfeeding mothers. Following repeated 40 mg doses twice daily, the average steady-state concentration in breastmilk was only 50 µg/L compared to 255 ng/mL in maternal plasma. Zafirlukast is poorly absorbed when administered with food. It is likely the oral absorption via ingestion of breastmilk would be low. Other leukotriene inhibitors, such as montelukast (Singulair), have not been studied.

Suggested Reading

Boskabady, M. H., Rezaeitalab, F., Rahimi, N., & Dehnavi, D. (2008). Improvement in symptoms and pulmonary function of asthmatic patients due to their treatment according to the Global Strategy for Asthma Management (GINA). *BMC Pulm Med, 8,* 26.

Brozek, J. L., Baena-Cagnani, C. E., Bonini, S., Canonica, G. W., Rasi, G., van Wijk, R. G., et al. (2008). Methodology for development of the Allergic Rhinitis and its Impact on Asthma guideline 2008 update. *Allergy, 63*(1), 38-46.

Busse, W. W., & Lemanske, R. F., Jr. (2007). Expert Panel Report 3: Moving forward to improve asthma care. *J Allergy Clin Immunol, 120*(5), 1012-1014.

Corrarino, J. (2008). New guidelines for diagnosis and management of asthma. *MCN Am J Matern Child Nurs, 33*(2), 136.

Demoly, P., Concas, V., Urbinelli, R., & Allaert, F. A. (2008). Spreading and impact of the World Health Organization's Allergic Rhinitis and its impact on asthma guidelines in everyday medical practice in France. Ernani survey. *Clin Exp Allergy, 38*(11), 1803-1807.

Kelly, H. W. (2007). Rationale for the major changes in the pharmacotherapy section of the National Asthma Education and Prevention Program guidelines. *J Allergy Clin Immunol, 120*(5), 989-994; quiz 995-986.

Kwok, R., Dinh, M., Dinh, D., & Chu, M. (2009). Improving adherence to asthma clinical guidelines and discharge documentation from emergency departments: implementation of a dynamic and integrated electronic decision support system. *Emerg Med Australas, 21*(1), 31-37.

Levy, M. L. (2008). Guideline-defined asthma control: a challenge for primary care. *Eur Respir J, 31*(2), 229-231.

Schatz, M., & Dombrowski, M. P. (2009). Clinical practice. Asthma in pregnancy. *N Engl J Med, 360*(18), 1862-1869.

Stoloff, S. W. (2008). Help patients gain better asthma control. *J Fam Pract, 57*(9), 594-602.

Thomas, M., Kay, S., Pike, J., Williams, A., Rosenzweig, J. R., Hillyer, E. V., et al. (2009). The Asthma Control Test (ACT) as a predictor of GINA guideline-defined asthma control: analysis of a multinational cross-sectional survey. *Prim Care Respir J, 18*(1), 41-49.

Wechsler, M.-E. (2009). Managing asthma in primary care: putting new guideline recommendations into context. *Mayo Clin Proc, 84*(8), 707-717.

Atopic Dermatitis

Principles of Therapy

Atopic dermatitis is a chronic, severely pruritic skin disorder characterized by dry skin, eczematous patches, and thickening of the skin. Diagnostic criteria must generally include dry skin; pruritus; weepy, shiny, or lichenified patches; and a tendency toward chronic or relapsing dermatitis. Patients frequently have elevated antibody levels (IgE) and a family or personal history of other allergic diseases, such as allergic rhinitis or asthma. Exacerbating factors in atopic dermatitis include dry skin, sensitivity to irritants (e.g., wool, sweat, saliva, foods, chemicals), infection (*Staphylococcus Aureus*), and stress. The distribution of lesions is characteristic, with involvement of the face, neck, and trunk. Elbows and knees are typically involved as well. Adult lesions are usually dry, leathery, hyperpigmented, or hypopigmented (particularly in black patients). Treatment includes removal of stress or irritating factors, less frequent bathing (brief and with mild soaps) followed by application of emollients or lotions, humidification of the home environment (during dry winters), mild topical corticosteroids, antipruritics (e.g., hydroxyzine, diphenhydramine), and topical or oral antibacterial preparations.

Treatment

- Treatments aim to keep skin moist: reduce bathing, bathe in cool water, use emollients.

- Topical steroids.

- Topical or oral immunosuppressants.

- Antibiotics for infected wounds.

Medications

- AZATHIOPRINE (*Imuran*)
    - AAP = Not reviewed
    - LRC = L3
    - RID = 0.25%
    - Pregnancy = D
    - Comment: Azathioprine is a powerful immunosuppressive agent that is metabolized to 6-Mercaptopurine (6-MP). In two mothers receiving 75 mg azathioprine, the concentration of 6-Mercaptopurine in milk varied from 3.5-4.5 µg/L in one mother and 18 µg/L in the second mother. The authors conclude that these levels would be too low to produce clinical effects in a breastfed infant. Using these data for 6-MP, an infant would absorb only 0.1% of the weight-adjusted maternal dose, which is probably too low to produce adverse effects in a breastfeeding infant. In another study of two infants who were breastfed by mothers receiving 75-100 mg/d

azathioprine, milk levels of 6-MP were not measured. But both infants had normal blood counts, no increase in infections, and above-average growth rate.

Four mothers who were receiving 1.2-2.1mg/kg/day of azathioprine throughout pregnancy and continued postpartum were studied while breastfeeding. Neither 6-TGN nor 6-MMPN could be detected in the exposed infants. Four case reports were performed with mothers taking between 50 to 100 mg/day of azathioprine. No adverse events were reported in any of the infants, and milk concentrations in two mothers proved to be undetectable.

- DIPHENHYDRAMINE   (*Benadryl, Cheracol*)
  - AAP = Not reviewed
  - LRC = L2
  - RID = 0.7-1.4%
  - Pregnancy = B
  - Comment: Small but unreported levels are thought to be secreted into breastmilk, although at present we do not have data on levels in breastmilk. However, the use of this sedating antihistamine in breastfeeding mothers is not ideal. Non-sedating antihistamines are generally preferred. There are anecdotal reports that diphenhydramine suppresses milk production. There are no data to support this theory.

- FLUTICASONE TOPICAL (*Cutivate*)
  - AAP = Not reviewed
  - LRC = L3
  - RID =
  - Pregnancy = C
  - Comment: In a group of normal individuals, transcutaneous absorption was minimal, with plasma levels below the limit of detection (0.05 ng/mL). In general, the topical use of this preparation would not pose a risk to a breastfeeding infant, although no data are yet available.

- HYDROCORTISONE TOPICAL   (*Westcort*)
  - AAP = Not reviewed
  - LRC = L2
  - RID =
  - Pregnancy = C
  - Comment: Absorption topically is dependent on placement; percutaneous absorption is 1% from the forearm, 2% from rectum, 4% from the scalp, 7% from the forehead, and 36% from the scrotal area. The amount transferred into human milk has not been reported, but as with most steroids, is believed minimal. Topical application to the nipple is generally approved by most authorities if amounts applied and duration of use are minimized. Only small amounts should be applied, and then only after feeding; larger quantities should be removed prior to breastfeeding. 0.5 to 1% ointments, rather than creams, are generally preferred.

- HYDROXYZINE (*Atarax, Vistaril*)
  - AAP = Not reviewed
  - LRC = L1

- RID =
- Pregnancy = C
- Comment: Hydroxyzine is an antihistamine structurally similar to cyclizine and meclizine. It produces significant CNS depression, anticholinergic side effects (drying), and antiemetic side effects. Hydroxyzine is largely metabolized to cetirizine (Zyrtec). No data are available on secretion into breastmilk.

- **MOMETASONE** (*Elocon, Nasonex*)
  - AAP = Not reviewed
  - LRC = L3
  - RID =
  - Pregnancy = C
  - Comment: Mometasone is a corticosteroid primarily intended for intranasal and topical use. It is considered a medium-potency steroid, similar to betamethasone and triamcinolone. Following topical application to the skin, less than 0.7% is systemically absorbed over an 8 hour period. It is extremely unlikely mometasone would be excreted into human milk in clinically relevant levels following topical or intranasal administration.

- **MUPIROCIN OINTMENT** (*Bactroban*)
  - AAP = Not reviewed
  - LRC = L1
  - RID =
  - Pregnancy = B
  - Comment: Mupirocin is a topical antibiotic used for impetigo, Staph, and other species. Mupirocin is only minimally absorbed following topical application. In one study, less than 0.3% of a topical dose was absorbed after 24 hours. Most remained adsorbed to the corneum layer of the skin. The drug is absorbed orally, but it is so rapidly metabolized that systemic levels are not sustained. It is quite safe for use in breastfeeding mothers.

- **PIMECROLIMUS** (*Elidel*)
  - AAP = Not reviewed
  - LRC = L2
  - RID =
  - Pregnancy = C
  - Comment: Pimecrolimus is a topical agent used as a cytokine inhibitor for atopic dermatitis. Systemic absorption following topical application is minimal, with reported blood concentrations consistently below 0.5 ng/mL following twice-daily application of the 1% cream. Oral absorption is unreported, but probably low to moderate as plasma levels of 54 ng/mL have been reported following twice daily oral doses of 30 mg. Pimecrolimus is cleared for use in pediatric patients 2 years and older. No data are available on its transfer to human milk, but because the maternal plasma levels are so low, it is extremely remote that this agent would penetrate milk in clinically relevant amounts. However, its use on or around the nipples should be avoided, as the clinical dose absorbed orally in the infant could be significant.

- TACROLIMUS (*Prograf, Protopic*)
    - AAP = Not reviewed
    - LRC = L3
    - RID = 0.1-0.5%
    - Pregnancy = C
    - Comment: Tacrolimus is an immunosuppressant. In one report of 21 mothers who received tacrolimus while pregnant, milk concentrations in colostrum averaged 0.79 ng/mL and varied from 0.3 to 1.9 ng/mL. Using these data and an average daily milk intake of 150 mL/kg, the average dose to the infant per day via milk would be <0.1 µg/kg/day. Because the oral bioavailability is poor (<32%), an infant would likely ingest less than 100 ng/kg/day. In a 32-year-old woman who had taken tacrolimus 0.1 mg/kg/d throughout pregnancy, the mean milk concentration was calculated to be 0.429 ng/mL. From these measurements, the exclusively breast-fed infant would ingest, on average, 0.06 µg/kg/d, which corresponds to 0.06% of the mother's weight-normalized dose.

        In a more recent study, a 29-year-old woman with a three-month-old breastfed infant was receiving 2 mg tacrolimus twice daily, in addition to azathioprine 100 mg, prednisone 5 mg, diltiazem 180 mg, atenolol 100 mg, and furosemide 20 mg daily. The milk-to-blood ratio was 0.23, and the average tacrolimus concentration in milk was 1.8 µg/L. The authors estimated the daily intake in the infant to be 0.5% of the maternal weight-adjusted dose (RID) or 0.27 µg/kg/day. This is less than 0.2% of the recommended pediatric dose for renal or liver transplant. The concentration-time profile of tacrolimus in milk was essentially flat. The highest concentration of tacrolimus in milk was at four and 8.5 hours postdose.

- TRIAMCINOLONE ACETONIDE (*Nasacort, Azmacort, Tri-Nasal*)
    - AAP = Not reviewed
    - LRC = L3
    - RID =
    - Pregnancy = C
    - Comment: Although no data are available on triamcinolone secretion into human milk, it is likely that the milk levels would be exceedingly low and not clinically relevant when administered via inhalation or intranasally. While the oral adult dose is 4-48 mg/day, the inhaled dose is 200 µg three times daily, and the intranasal dose is 220 µg/day. There is virtually no risk to the infant following use of the intranasal products in breastfeeding mothers.

Clinical Tips

Therapy of atopic dermatitis begins with education of the patient and includes instruction on reducing bathing and use of lubricants on the skin. Long showers, harsh detergents, shower brushes, and bubble baths should be avoided, although daily bathing is still recommended, depending on the climate. Bathing hydrates the stratum corneum and removes bacteria, but the application of a lubricant must be applied within three minutes to seal the moisture in the skin. Moisturizers of choice include Eucerin, Moisturel, Curel, Complex 15 creams or lotions. Avoid Vaseline Intensive Care lotion. Pure Vaseline, Aquaphor, and Crisco are back in fashion, but may be a bit heavy in some instances.

Topical steroids, particularly ointments (avoid lotions, gels), are preferred short-term therapy. Low to medium potency steroids are preferred (e.g., hydrocortisone, triamcinolone, mometasone, fluticasone). High potency steroids should be avoided. Hydroxyzine is the antihistamine/antipruritic of choice, although it produces significant sedation. Although we have no data on hydroxyzine transfer to milk, it is a commonly used pediatric antihistamine. Diphenhydramine is an effective antihistamine/antipruritic as well, but if used consistently could potentially produce sedation and/or hallucinations in the breastfed infant. As antipruritics, the antihistamines work poorly, and only those associated with significant sedation seem effective. Hydroxyzine and cetirizine (Zyrtec) are most effective. Doxepin is an effective antipruritic, but one report of dangerous sedation and apnea in a breastfeeding infant suggests that it may not be suitable for breastfeeding mothers.

The most common complication of atopic dermatitis is super-infection with *Staphylococcus aureus*. Topical neomycin is an allergic trigger and should be avoided. Mupirocin ointment would be an ideal choice for staphylococcus or streptococcus infections. Topical erythromycin or fusidic acid applied twice daily is effective. For severe infections, anti-staphylococcal systemic medications are required and could include Amoxicillin + clavulanate (Augmentin), cephalexin, cloxacillin, clindamycin, and others depending on sensitivity. However, recent reviews now suggest that topical antibiotic therapy may not be beneficial.

In severe refractory cases, the immunosuppressant azathioprine or cyclosporine may be effective. In addition, since patients with atopic dermatitis have defects in cell-mediated immunity, the immunosuppressant macrolides (cyclosporine, pimecrolimus, and tacrolimus) may prove to be beneficial in the treatment of this syndrome. Topical tacrolimus has been frequently studied in the treatment of atopic dermatitis because it was found to have better skin penetration and higher potency than topically applied cyclosporine. Numerous studies evaluating the use of topical tacrolimus are available and provide evidence that topical tacrolimus is effective in the treatment of this syndrome with no evidence thus far of systemic adverse effects. The FDA has approved a topical form of tacrolimus (Protopic) for use in moderate to severe eczema in those for whom standard eczema therapies are deemed inadvisable because of potential risks. Absorption via skin is minimal. In a study of 46 adult patients after multiple doses, plasma levels ranged from undetectable to 20 ng/mL with 45 of the patients having peak blood concentrations less than 5 ng/mL. In another study, the peak blood levels averaged 1.6 ng/mL, which is significantly less than the therapeutic range in kidney transplantation (7-20 ng/mL). While the absolute transcutaneous bioavailability is unknown, it is apparently very low ($< 0.5\%$). Combined with the poor oral bioavailability of this product, it is not likely a breastfed infant will receive enough following topical use (maternal) to produce adverse effects.

Recent data have suggested that probiotics may be useful in the prevention, but not necessarily the treatment of atopic dermatitis, particularly in allergic children.

Suggested Reading

Anstey, A. (2008). Therapeutic advances and shift in disease paradigm for atopic dermatitis. *Br J Dermatol, 159*(6), 1215-1216.

Dhar, S. (1999). Diagnostic criteria for atopic dermatitis. *Pediatr Dermatol, 16*(5), 413-414.

Kunz, B., Oranje, A. P., Labreze, L., Stalder, J. F., Ring, J., & Taieb, A. (1997). Clinical validation and guidelines for the SCORAD index: consensus report of the European Task Force on Atopic Dermatitis. *Dermatology, 195*(1), 10-19.

Nicol, N. H., & Boguniewicz, M. (2008). Successful strategies in atopic dermatitis management. *Dermatol Nurs, Suppl*, 3-18.

Williams, H. C. (2005). Clinical practice. Atopic dermatitis. *N Engl J Med, 352*(22), 2314-2324.

Wollenberg, A., & Bieber, T. (2009). Proactive therapy of atopic dermatitis--an emerging concept. *Allergy, 64*(2), 276-278.

Basal Cell Carcinoma

Principles of Therapy

Basal cell carcinoma is the most common malignancy arising from the epidermis. While they are considered malignant, they are only so in the immediate or local areas of the skin. They most commonly arise due to excessive past exposure to sun and largely only on the face. They arise slowly, presumably from stem cells within the hair follicle. They are most often excised surgically, but more recently topical therapy with imiquimod has become popular. However, it is not as effective as surgical excision according to new studies.

Treatment

- Surgical excision of the entire lesion (95+% cure rate). Cryotherapy alone provides unacceptable cure rates.

- Cryotherapy following excision (95+% cure rate)

- Radiation therapy rarely (90% cure rate)

- Mohs micrographic surgery (99% cure rate)

- Imiquimod topical therapy

Medications

- IMIQUIMOD (*Aldara*)
    - AAP = Not reviewed
    - LRC = L2
    - RID =
    - Pregnancy = C
    - Comment: Imiquimod is an immune response modifier used in the treatment of actinic keratoses and basal cell carcinoma. Mean peak serum levels following topical application three times weekly, ranged from 0.1 to 35 ng/mL and is to some degree a function of surface area treated. Less than 0.9% of the topically applied dose is transcutaneously absorbed into the plasma. Mean urinary recovery was less than 0.15% of the applied dose. No data are available on its transfer into human milk, but milk levels are probably low.

Clinical Tips

Cure rates generally depend on the size and location of the lesion. Most minimally involved basal cell carinomas may be successfully excised and treated in more than 90% of cases. Excision followed by cryosurgery is often used and affects a 95% cure rate. Mohs' micrographic surgery produce high cure rates as well and is recommended by the National Comprehensive Cancer Network for most high-risk lesions. Recent data suggests that imiquimod is effective, but only for lesions less than 2 cm in diameter. Cure rates may be lower.

Suggested Reading

Garg, S., Carroll, R. P., Walker, R. G., Ramsay, H. M., & Harden, P. N. (2009). Skin cancer surveillance in renal transplant recipients: re-evaluation of U.K. practice and comparison with Australian experience. *Br J Dermatol, 160*(1), 177-179.

Gudi, V., Ormerod, A. D., Dawn, G., Green, C., MacKie, R. M., Douglas, W. S., et al. (2006). Management of basal cell carcinoma by surveyed dermatologists in Scotland. *Clin Exp Dermatol, 31*(5), 648-652.

Mc Loone, N. M., Tolland, J., Walsh, M., & Dolan, O. M. (2006). Follow-up of basal cell carcinomas: an audit of current practice. *J Eur Acad Dermatol Venereol, 20*(6), 698-701.

Olsen, C. M., Hughes, M. C., Pandeya, N., & Green, A. C. (2006). Anthropometric measures in relation to basal cell carcinoma: a longitudinal study. *BMC Cancer, 6*, 82.

Rubin, A. I., Chen, E. H., & Ratner, D. (2005). Basal-cell carcinoma. *N Engl J Med, 353*(21), 2262-2269.

Telfer, N. R., Colver, G. B., Morton, C. A., & British Association of Dermatologists. (2008). Guidelines for the management of basal cell carcinoma. *Br J Dermatol, 159*(1), 35-48.

Bipolar Disorder - Mania

Principles of Therapy

The essential feature of bipolar disorder is the presence of chronic depression and occasional episodes of mania. Mania is characterized by inflated self-esteem or grandiosity, elation with hyperactivity, flight of ideas, overenthusiasm, easy distractability, and insomnia. The management of manic episodes has largely remained unchanged, and includes the use of lithium, valporate, and several atypical antipsychotic agents. The combination of olanzapine and carbamazepine is no longer recommended.

Compared with unipolar depression, the depressive phase of bipolar disorder includes symptoms such as hypersomnia, hyperphagia and weight gain, and decreased energy. Approximately one-half of all bipolar patients also have psychotic symptoms. Psychotic symptomatology is reduced more in divalproex-treated than in lithium-treated patients. The management of bipolar depression includes lithium, lamotrigine and quetiapine, or olanzapine, plus select serotonin reuptake inhibitors (SSRIs).

The mainstay of treatment of mania has been lithium, although acute episodes may require neuroleptics, such as haloperidol (Haldol), respiridone, or quetiapine. Although lithium use in breastfeeding mothers is controversial, some recent studies suggest that with close observation, lithium levels in the neonate are usually subclinical. More recently, the use of valproic acid or lamotrigine have been found to be effective alternatives to those who refuse or cannot take lithium. Bipolar disorder is strongly associated with several other disorders: migraine, obsessive-compulsive disorder, panic disorder, and attention-deficit/hyperactivity disorder. Valproic acid, because of its efficacy in treating migraine, mania, panic, and OCD, has assumed a more important role in the therapy of this disorder, particularly with the presence of the above comorbid conditions and in mania associated with substance abuse. Manic patients with mixed depressive symptoms respond less to lithium than those with pure or elated mania. Patients with coincident substance abuse respond less to lithium and better to valproate treatment.

Treatment

- First line treatment: Lithium, divalproex, olanzapine, risperidone, quetiapine, aripiprazole, ziprasidone

- Second line treatment: Carbamazepine, ECT, lithium + divalproex.

Medications

- ARIPIPRAZOLE   (*Abilify, Abilitat*)
  - AAP = Not reviewed
  - LRC = L3
  - RID = 1%
  - Pregnancy = C

- Comment: Aripiprazole is a second-generation antipsychotic, now first-line treatment for schizophrenia. In a small study of a single patient receiving 10 mg/day initially and then 15 mg subsequently, levels of aripiprazole in milk were reported to be 13 and 14 μg/L on two consecutive days (15 and 16 after initiation of therapy). Maternal plasma levels at the same time were 71 and 71μg/L. Levels were drawn in the morning before aripiprazole administration. Thus it appears from this brief report that they were drawn approximately 24 hours postdose.

- **CARBAMAZEPINE** (*Tegretol, Epitol, Carbatrol*)
  - AAP = Maternal Medication Usually Compatible with Breastfeeding
  - LRC = L2
  - RID = 3.8-5.9%
  - Pregnancy = D
  - Comment: Carbamazepine (CBZ) is a unique anticonvulsant commonly used for grand mal, clonic-tonic, simple, and complex seizures. It is also used in manic depression and a number of other neurologic syndromes. It is one of the most commonly used anticonvulsants in pediatric patients. In a brief study by Kaneko, with maternal plasma levels averaging 4.3 μg/mL, milk levels were 1.9 mg/L. In a study of three patients who received from 5.8 to 7.3 mg/kg/day carbamazepine, milk levels were reported to vary from 1.3 to 1.8 mg/L, while the epoxide metabolite varied from 0.5 to 1.1 mg/L. No adverse effects were noted in any of the infants. In another study by Niebyl, breastmilk levels were 1.4 mg/L in the lipid fraction and 2.3 mg/L in the skim fraction in a mother receiving 1000 mg daily of carbamazepine. This author estimated the daily intake of 2 mg carbamazepine daily (0.5 mg/kg) in an infant ingesting 1 liter of milk per day.

    In a study of CBZ and its epoxide metabolite (ECBZ) in milk, 16 patients received an average dose of 13.8 mg/kg/d. The average maternal serum levels of CBZ and ECBZ were 7.1 and 2.6 μg/mL, respectively. The average milk levels of CBZ and ECBZ were 2.5 and 1.5 mg/L, respectively. The relative percent of CBZ and ECBZ in milk were 36.4% and 53% of the maternal serum levels. A total of 50 milk samples in 19 patients were analyzed. Of these, the lowest CBZ concentration in milk was 1.0 mg/L; the highest was 4.8 mg/L. The CBZ level was determined in 7 infants 4-7 days postpartum. All infants had CBZ levels below 1.5 μg/mL. In a study of seven women receiving 250-800 mg/d carbamazepine, the CBZ level ranged from 2.8-4.5 mg/L in milk to 3.2-15.0 mg/L in plasma. The levels of ECBZ ranged from 0.5-1.7 mg/L in milk to 0.8-4.8 mg/L in plasma. The amount of CBZ transferred to the infant is apparently quite low. Although the half-life of CBZ in infants appears shorter than in adults, infants should still be monitored for sedative effects.

- **HALOPERIDOL** (*Haldol*)
  - AAP = Drugs whose effect on nursing infants is unknown but may be of concern
  - LRC = L2
  - RID = 2.1-12%
  - Pregnancy = C
  - Comment: Haloperidol is a potent antipsychotic agent that is reported to increase prolactin levels in some patients. In one study of a woman treated for puerperal hypomania and receiving 5 mg twice daily, the concentration of haloperidol in milk was 0.0, 23.5, 18.0, and 3.25 μg/L on day 1, 6, 7, and 21, respectively. The corresponding maternal plasma levels were 0, 40, 26, and 4 μg/L at day one, six, seven, and 21, respectively. The milk/plasma ratios were 0.58, 0.69, and 0.81 on days 6, 7, and 21, respectively. After four weeks of therapy, the infant showed no symptoms of sedation and was

feeding well. In another study, after a mean daily dose of 29.2 mg, the concentration of haloperidol in breastmilk was 5 µg/L at 11 hours postdose. In a study of three women on chronic haloperidol therapy receiving 3, 4, and 6 mg daily, milk levels were reported to be 32, 17, and 4.7 ng/mL. The latter levels(4.7) were taken from a patient believed to be noncompliant. Bennett calculates the relative infant dose to be 0.2-2.1% to 9.6% of the weight-adjusted maternal daily dose.

- LITHIUM CARBONATE   (*Lithobid, Eskalith*)
  - AAP = Drugs associated with significant side effects and should be given with caution
  - LRC = L3 with close observation
  - RID   = 12-30.1%
  - Pregnancy = D
  - Comment: Lithium is a potent antimanic drug used in bipolar disorder. Its use in the first trimester of pregnancy may be associated with a number of birth anomalies, particularly cardiovascular. If used during pregnancy, the dose required is generally elevated due to the increased renal clearance during pregnancy. Soon after delivery, maternal lithium levels should be closely monitored as the mother's renal clearance drops to normal in the next several days. Several cases have been reported of lithium toxicity in newborns. In a study of a 36-year-old mother who received lithium during and after pregnancy, the infant's serum lithium level was similar to the mother's level at birth (maternal dose = 400 mg), but dropped to 0.03 mmol/L by the sixth day. While the mother's dose increased to 800 mg/day postpartum, the infant's serum level did not rise above 10% of the maternal serum levels. At 42 days postpartum, the maternal and infant serum levels were 1.1 and 0.1 mmol/L, respectively.

    Some toxic effects have been reported. In a mother receiving 600-1200 mg lithium daily during pregnancy, the concentration of lithium in breastmilk at three days was 0.6 mEq/L. The maternal and infant plasma levels were 1.5 mEq/L and 0.6 mEq/L, respectively at three days. In this case, the infant was floppy, unresponsive, and exhibited inverted T waves, which are indicative of lithium toxicity. In another study done seven days postpartum, the milk and infant plasma levels were 0.3 mEq/L each, while the mother's plasma lithium levels were 0.9 mEq/L. In a case report of a mother receiving 300 mg three times daily and breastfeeding her infant at two weeks postpartum, the mother and infant's lithium levels were 0.62 and 0.31 mmol/L, respectively. The infant's neurobehavioral development and thyroid function were reported normal.

    From these studies, it is apparent that lithium can permeate milk and is absorbed by the breastfed infant. If the infant continues to breastfeed, it is strongly suggested that the infant be closely monitored for serum lithium levels. Lithium does not reach steady state levels for approximately 10+ days. Clinicians may wish to wait at least this long prior to evaluating the infant's serum lithium level, or sooner if symptoms occur. In addition, lithium is known to reduce thyroxine production, and periodic thyroid evaluation should be considered. Because hydration status of the infant can alter lithium levels dramatically, the clinician should observe changes in hydration carefully. A number of studies of lithium suggest that lithium administration is not an absolute contraindication to breastfeeding if the physician monitors the infant closely for elevated plasma lithium. Current studies, as well as unpublished experience, suggest that the infant's plasma levels rise to about 30-40% of the maternal level, most often without untoward effects in the infant. Recent evidence suggests that certain anticonvulsants, such as carbamazepine, valproic acid, lamotrigine, and others, may be effective in treating some forms of mania. Because these medications are probably safer to use in breastfeeding mothers, the clinician may wish to explore the use of these medications in certain manic breastfeeding mothers.

- LAMOTRIGINE   (*Lamictal*)
  - ◦ AAP = Drugs whose effect on nursing infants is unknown but may be of concern
  - ◦ LRC = L3
  - ◦ RID = 9.2-18.3%
  - ◦ Pregnancy = C
  - ◦ Comment: Lamotrigine is a newer anticonvulsant primarily indicated for treatment of simple and complex partial seizures. In a study of a 24-year-old female receiving 300 mg/day lamotrigine during pregnancy, maternal serum levels and cord levels of lamotrigine at birth were 3.88 μg/mL in the mother and 3.26 μg/mL in the cord blood. By day 22, the maternal serum levels were 9.61 μg/mL, the milk concentration was 6.51 mg/L, and the infant's serum level was 2.25 μg/mL. Following a reduction in dose, the prior levels decreased significantly over the next weeks. The milk/plasma ratio at the highest maternal serum level was 0.562. The estimated dose to the infant would be approximately 2-5 mg per day, assuming a maternal dose of 200-300 mg per day. The infant developed normally in every way. In another study of a single mother receiving 200 mg/day lamotrigine, milk levels of lamotrigine immediately prior to the next dose (trough) at steady state were 3.48 mg/L (13.6 uM). The authors estimated the daily dose to the infant to be 0.5 mg/kg/day. The above authors suggest that infants, while developing normally, should probably be monitored periodically for plasma levels of lamotrigine. The manufacturer reports that in a group of five women (no dose listed), breastmilk concentrations of lamotrigine ranged from 0.07-5.03 mg/L. Breastmilk levels averaged 40-45% of maternal plasma levels. No untoward effects were noted in the infants.

    In a study by Ohman of nine breastfeeding women at three weeks postpartum, the median milk/plasma ratio was 0.61, and the breastfed infants maintained lamotrigine concentrations of approximately 30% of the mother's plasma levels. The authors estimated the dose to the infant at = 0.2-1 mg/kg/d. No adverse effects were noted in the infants. One further study of six breastfeeding women consuming from 175-800 (mean = 400) mg/day resulted in average infant doses of 0.45 mg/kg/day, and an average infant plasma concentration of 0.6 mg/L. No adverse effects in the infants were noted. In a study of four mothers with partial epilepsy on lamotrigine monotherapy, serum levels of lamotrigine in nursing newborns ranged from <1.0 to 2.0 μg/mL on day 10 of life. Three babies had lamotrigine levels >1.0 μg/mL. Lamotrigine levels in newborns were on average 30% (range 20-43%) of the maternal drug level. Unfortunately, no decline was noted in two children with repeat levels at two months. The authors suggested significant genetic variability in the infants' ability to metabolize this drug. Close monitoring of the infant plasma levels was recommended.

    The use of lamotrigine in breastfeeding mothers produces significant plasma levels in some breastfed infants, although they are apparently not high enough to produce side effects. It is probably advisable to monitor the infant's plasma levels closely to insure safety.

- OLANZAPINE   (*Zyprexa, Symbyax*)
  - ◦ AAP = Not reviewed
  - ◦ LRC = L2
  - ◦ RID = 1.2%
  - ◦ Pregnancy = C
  - ◦ Comment: Olanzapine is a typical antipsychotic agent structurally similar to clozapine and may be used for treating schizophrenia and mania. In a recent and excellent study of seven mother-infant

nursing pairs receiving a median dose of olanzapine of 7.5 mg/day (range = 5-20 mg/day), the median infant dose ingested via milk was approximately 1.02% of the maternal dose. The median milk/plasma AUC ratio was 0.38. Olanzapine was undetected in the plasma of six infants tested. All infants were healthy and experienced no observable side effects. The maximum relative infant dose was approximately 1.2%. In a case report of a mother taking 20 mg/day, the milk/plasma ratio was 0.35, giving a relative infant dose of about 4% at steady state. This milk was not fed to the infant, so infant plasma levels were not performed. A study of five mothers receiving olanzapine at a dose of 2.5-20 mg/day reported milk/plasma ratios of 0.2 to 0.84, with an average relative infant dose of 1.6%. The authors reported no untoward effects on the infants attributable to olanzapine.

- QUETIAPINE FUMARATE   (*Seroquel*)

  ○ AAP = Not reviewed

  ○ LRC = L2

  ○ RID = 0.07-0.1%

  ○ Pregnancy = C

  ○ Comment: Quetiapine (Seroquel) is indicated for the treatment of psychosis and manic disorders. It has some affinity for histamine receptors, which may account for its sedative properties. It has been shown to increase the incidence of seizures, prolactin levels, and to lower thyroid levels in adults. In a patient (92 kg) receiving 200 mg/day of quetiapine throughout pregnancy, samples were expressed just before dosing, and at one, two, four, and six hours postdose. The average milk concentration (AUC) of quetiapine over the six hours was 13 µg/L, with a maximum concentration of 62 µg/L at one hour. Levels of quetiapine rapidly fell to almost predose levels by two hours. The authors report that an exclusively breastfed infant would ingest only 0.09% of the weight-adjusted maternal dose. At maximum, the infant would ingest 0.43% of the weight-adjusted maternal dose. Although only one patient was studied, the data suggests levels in milk are minimal at this maternal dose.

  One study of six mothers taking a combination of quetiapine, paroxetine, clonazepam, trazodone, and/or venlafaxine showed that no medication was detectable in three of the mothers' milk. In two of the other cases, quetiapine levels were below 0.01 mg/kg/day infant dose, while the final mother expressed an infant dose of less than 0.10 mg/kg/day. The mothers' doses of quetiapine ranged from 25-400 mg. The authors reported that no correlation was noted between drug exposure and developmental outcomes. In another study of one mother receiving 400 mg quetiapine per day three months postpartum, expressed milk contained an average drug concentration of 41 µg/L, and a milk-to-plasma ratio of 0.29. The relative infant dose reported was 0.09% of the mother's dose. The infant's plasma concentration was 1.4 µg/L, or 6% of the mother's plasma concentration. No adverse effects were reported in the infant, but the authors suggest monitoring the infant's progress and quetiapine serum concentration.

- RISPERIDONE   (*Risperdal, Invega*)

  ○ AAP = Not reviewed

  ○ LRC = L3

  ○ RID = 2.8-9.1%

  ○ Pregnancy = C

  ○ Comment: Risperidone is a potent antipsychotic agent belonging to a new chemical class. In a study of one patient receiving 6 mg/day of risperidone at steady state, the peak plasma level of approximately 130 µg/L occurred four hours after an oral dose. Peak milk levels of risperidone and 9-hydroxyrisperidone were approximately 12 µg/L, and 40 µg/L, respectively. The estimated daily dose of risperidone and metabolite (risperidone equivalents) was 4.3% of the weight-adjusted maternal dose. The milk/plasma ratios calculated from areas under the curve over 24 hours were 0.42 and 0.24, respectively, for risperidone and 6-hydroxyrisperidone. In another study, the transfer of risperidone and 9-hydroxyrisperidone into milk was studied in two breastfeeding women and one woman with risperidone-induced galactorrhea. In case two (risperidone dose = 42.1 µg/kg/d), the average concentration of risperidone and 9-hydroxyrisperidone in milk (Cav) was 2.1 and 6 µg/L, respectively. The relative infant dose was 2.8% of the maternal dose. In case three (risperidone dose = 23.1µg/kg/d), the average concentration of risperidone and 9-hydroxyrisperidone in milk (Cav) was 0.39 and 7.06 µg/L, respectively. The milk/plasma ratio determined in two women was <0.5 for both risperidone compounds. The relative infant doses were 2.3%, 2.8%, and 4.7% (as risperidone equivalents) of the maternal weight-adjusted doses in these three cases. Risperidone and 9-hydroxyrisperidone were not detected in the plasma of the two breastfed infants studied, and no adverse effects were noted. Paliperidone (Invega), the active metabolite of risperidone, is available in extended release tablets. This formulation has a volume of distribution of 6.95 L/kg, 74% protein binding, and a bioavailability of 28%.

- VALPROIC ACID   (*Depakene, Depakote*)
  - ○ AAP = Maternal Medication Usually Compatible with Breastfeeding
  - ○ LRC = L2
  - ○ RID   = 1.4-1.7%
  - ○ Pregnancy = D
  - ○ Comment: Valproic acid is a popular anticonvulsant used in grand mal, petit mal, myoclonic, and temporal lobe seizures. In a study of 16 patients receiving 300-2400 mg/d, valproic acid concentrations ranged from 0.4 to 3.9 mg/L (mean = 1.9 mg/L). The milk/plasma ratio averaged 0.05. In a study of one patient receiving 250 mg twice daily, milk levels ranged from 0.18 to 0.47 mg/L. The milk/plasma ratio ranged from 0.01 to 0.02. Alexander reports milk levels of 5.1 mg/L following a larger dose of up to 1600 mg/d. In a study of six women receiving 9.5 to 31 mg/kg/d valproic acid, milk levels averaged 1.4 mg/L, while serum levels averaged 45.1 mg/L. The average milk/serum ratio was 0.027. Most authors agree that the amount of valproic acid transferring to the infant via milk is low. Breastfeeding would appear safe. However, the infant may need monitoring for liver and platelet changes.

Clinical Tips

Acute Mania

For acute manic episodes, first line choices include lithium, divalproex, olanzapine, risperidone, quetiapine, aripiprazole, and other atypical antipsychotics and combinations of the above. At least two meta-analyses confirm the effectiveness of combining antipsychotics, such as aripiprazole, olanzapine, and others, plus lithium + divalproex. Second line treatment includes: carbamazepine or lithium + divalproex. Third line treatment includes: haloperidol, chlorpromazine, lithium or divalproex + haloperidol. Studies with breastfeeding mothers show milk levels with both of these drugs are moderate to low, with minimal effect on the infant.

Lithium, divalproex sodium (or valproic acid), and carbamazepine have well-documented efficacy in acute mania, although the data suggests that carbamazepine, while better than placebo, may in many cases be less effective than lithium for chronic control of mania. Recent studies also clearly show that adding antipsyhotics to lithium and divalproex is much more effective than lithium + divalproex alone in the treatment of acute mania. Haloperidol is as effective as other atypical antipsychotics in treating acute mania, but has a much higher incidence of tremor and other movement disorders. Due to these complications, it is now considered a third line treatment for acute mania.

Divalproex (valproic acid) has surpassed the use of lithium in the treatment of bipolar disorder, primarily because of safety issues, and because of a better therapeutic index. Valproate may also be more effective for various subtypes of bipolar disorder. It is apparently quite effective in patients with mixed mania, concurrent drug abuse, rapid cycling, and secondary mania. Doses and clinical plasma levels are virtually identical to those used in seizure disorders, and laboratory monitoring for liver function and plasma levels is recommended. Alopecia and cognitive dulling may sometimes occur at higher doses of valproate. Increased appetite and weight gain are common side effects. Carbamazepine and valproate have been studied in breastfeeding mothers and are considered relatively safe for use in these mothers. However, the concomitant use of valproate and carbamazepine may increase the hepatotoxic metabolites of valproate. Lithium is more effective for elated mania and less effective for mixed manic features. However, dropout rate due to side effects (GI irritation, metallic taste, tremor, polyuria, and cognitive dulling) in lithium-treated patients is higher than those in valproate-treated groups. Lithium transfer into milk is considered moderately high. Levels attained in the infant's plasma are generally about 30-40% of the maternal levels.

In a study of ten patients, maternal serum, breastmilk, and infant serum daily trough concentrations of lithium averaged 0.76, 0.35, and 0.16 mEq/L, respectively, with each lithium level lower than the preceding level by approximately one-half. If mothers are accurately maintained at around 0.6 – 1.0 mEq/L, then several studies suggest the infant's levels will be around 0.16 to 0.3 mEq/L, or 10-50% of the maternal level.

Lithium is known to inhibit thyroid function, thus occasional thyroid studies in the infant are suggested. Due to numerous drug-lithium interactions, be cautious of medicating the infant, as drug interactions could occur. Any change in hydration status of the infant could induce severe toxicity and should be closely monitored. If lithium is used in women who breastfeed, the infant will be exposed and should have routine monitoring of the indices affected by the particular medication. The frequency of monitoring depends on the age of the infant. A reasonable approach is monthly for two to three months, after any increase in maternal daily dose, or if side effects are observed in the infant. The available data indicates that the use of valproic acid during lactation is probably preferable to both carbamazepine and lithium. While the onset of activity of lithium is delayed (three to four weeks), valproate acts within days and the atypical antipsychotics within hours.

Recent data have found oxycarbazepine moderately ineffective, and it is no longer recommended for treatment of mania.

Bipolar Depression

Experimental data concerning the treatment of bipolar depression is somewhat poor. First line therapy of bipolar depression consists of the following: lithium, lamotrigine, quetiapine or quetiapine XR, lithium or divalproex + SSRI, or olanzapine + SSRI. The SSRIs are not considered first or even second line therapy in bipolar depression because they are known to trigger acute manic episodes, particularly if used alone (no antipsychotics). For more information on the SSRIs, see Postpartum Depression below.

Two recent large trials have suggested that lamotrigine is modestly effective in the treatment of bipolar depression, although it is weak. Untoward effects in patients include risk of Stevens-Johnson syndrome and toxic epidermal necrolysis. Risks to the breastfed infant appear low, even though levels in milk are moderately high.

There are now four large randomized controlled trials that show quetiapine is quite effective in treatment of bipolar depression.

The tricyclic antidepressants have fallen into disfavor due to the likelihood of sedation, weight gain, anticholinergic effects, and acute toxicity. Current studies also clearly suggest that prolonged use of antidepressants may significantly increase the risk of severe manic or hypomanic episodes and destabilize the course of illness. Hence, the use of antidepressants is presently only rarely advised.

Aripiprazole monotherapy has been recently found to be ineffective for bipolar depression, but studies are ongoing and this may change. It is cleared for treatment of monopolar depression.

Maintenance Treatment

Bipolar disorder is, in most instances, recurrent and chronic, with almost no tendency to mature out of the disorder. However, the long-term studies of lithium as maintenance therapy have been disappointing. In fact, some studies have found the outcome was no better on chronic lithium therapy than no therapy. While partially due to inadequate plasma levels, patient compliance with lithium is poor due to problems such as weight gain, hypothyroidism, polydipsia, acne, and polyuria. Recent studies have suggested that divalproex is just as effective, if not better than lithium and is generally better tolerated than lithium. With chronic use, divalproex has its problems as well, including transient hair loss (selenium and zinc may help), weight gain and increased appetite, and cognitive dulling (dose related).

First line therapy includes: lithium, lamotrigine monotherapy, divalproex, olanzapine, quetiapine, lithium or divalproex + quetiapine.

Second line therapy includes: carbamazepine, lithum + divalproex, lithium + carbamazpine, lithium or divalproex + olanzapine. Medications not recommended include antidepressants, gabapentin, topiramate, flupenthixol.

Complications: Data from numerous studies suggest that prolonged therapy with any of the atypical antipsychotics (quetiapine, risperidone, olanzapine, and other atypical antipsychotics) can cause a clinically significant increase in insulin resistance that may lead to clinical type II diabetes.

There have been four recent studies suggesting that Tamoxifen produced significant improvement in manic symptoms.

Recent data also suggest that cognitive therapy may be as effective as chronic lithium therapy. Adjunctive cognitive therapy produced less severe depression scores, longer times between replapses, and fewer disruptive attitudes.

Suggested Reading

ACOG Committee on Practice Bulletins-Obstetrics. (2008). ACOG Practice Bulletin: Clinical management guidelines for obstetrician-gynecologists number 92, April 2008 (replaces practice bulletin number 87, November 2007). Use of psychiatric medications during pregnancy and lactation. *Obstet Gynecol, 111*(4), 1001-1020.

Bauer, M. S., McBride, L., Williford, W. O., Glick, H., Kinosian, B., Altshuler, L., et al. (2006). Collaborative care for bipolar disorder: part I. Intervention and implementation in a randomized effectiveness trial. *Psychiatr Serv, 57*(7), 927-936.

Bauer, M. S., McBride, L., Williford, W. O., Glick, H., Kinosian, B., Altshuler, L., et al. (2006). Collaborative care for bipolar disorder: Part II. Impact on clinical outcome, function, and costs. *Psychiatr Serv, 57*(7), 937-945.

Beckford-Ball, J. (2006). An overview of the new NICE guidelines on bipolar disorder. *Nurs Times, 102*(34), 23-24.

Burt, V. K., & Rasgon, N. (2004). Special considerations in treating bipolar disorder in women. *Bipolar Disord, 6*(1), 2-13.

Cohen, L. S. (2007). Treatment of bipolar disorder during pregnancy. *J Clin Psychiatry, 68 Suppl 9*, 4-9.

Farrelly, N., Dibben, C., & Hunt, N. (2006). Current management of bipolar affective disorder: is it reflective of the BAP guidelines? *J Psychopharmacol, 20*(1), 128-131.

Gentile, S. (2006). Prophylactic treatment of bipolar disorder in pregnancy and breastfeeding: focus on emerging mood stabilizers. *Bipolar Disord, 8*(3), 207-220.

Payne, J. L. (2007). Antidepressant use in the postpartum period: practical considerations. *Am J Psychiatry, 164*(9), 1329-1332.

Perlis, R. H. (2007). Use of treatment guidelines in clinical decision making in bipolar disorder: a pilot survey of clinicians. *Curr Med Res Opin, 23*(3), 467-475.

Sharma, V. (2008). Treatment of postpartum psychosis: challenges and opportunities. *Curr Drug Saf, 3*(1), 76-81.

Stowe, Z. N. (2007). The use of mood stabilizers during breastfeeding. *J Clin Psychiatry., 68*(Suppl 9), 22-28.

Streeruwitz, A., Barnes, T. R., Fehler, J., Ohlsen, R., & Curtis, V. A. (2007). Pharmacological management of acute mania: does current prescribing practice reflect treatment guidelines? *J Psychopharmacol, 21*(2), 206-209.

Yatham, L. N., Kennedy, S. H., Schaffer, A., Parikh, S. V., Beaulieu, S., O'Donovan, C., et al. (2009). Canadian Network for Mood and Anxiety Treatments (CANMAT) and International Society for Bipolar Disorders (ISBD) collaborative update of CANMAT guidelines for the management of patients with bipolar disorder: update 2009. *Bipolar Disord, 11*(3), 225-255.

Breast Cancer

Principles of Therapy

Breast cancer is the most frequently diagnosed cancer in women and second most frequent cause of cancer death. Approximately 3-5% of breast cancer is associated with the BRCA1 or BRCA2 gene mutation. Thus the major portion of breast cancer is not necessarily gene-related and is inexplicable. Approximately 80% of invasive carcinomas of the breast are ductal adenocarcinomas, the rest are infiltrated lobal carcinomas. The lifetime risk for breast cancer in a woman is one in seven, but this includes elderly patients who are at higher risk. Thus the risk for a younger woman is much lower. Breast cancers during pregnancy and in the initial year after delivery are categorized as Pregnancy Associated Breast Cancer (PABC). The mean age of women with PABC is 32.

The diagnosis and treatment of breast cancer is an enormous field and is beyond the scope of this book. However, many of the chemotherapeutic options are listed below.

Treatment

- Breast conserving therapy (BCT), partial mastectomy, or full mastectomy. Axillary lymph node dissection or sentinel node biopsy (for clinically node negative women) as indicated.

- X-Radiation therapy.

- Chemotherapy.

- Hormone therapy (tamoxifen) for lobular carcinoma in situ.

- Breast-conserving therapy and radiation therapy for ductal carcinoma in situ.

- Early invasive disease requires surgery, radiation therapy, mastectomy in some cases.

- Monoclonal antibodies as adjuvant therapy.

Medications

- CYCLOPHOSPHAMIDE   (*Neosar, Cytoxan*)
    - AAP = Cytotoxic drug that may interfere with cellular metabolism of the nursing infant
    - LRC = L5
    - RID =
    - Pregnancy = D

- Comment: Cyclophosphamide is a powerful and toxic antineoplastic drug. A number of reports in the literature indicate that cyclophosphamide can transfer into human milk as evidenced by the production of leukopenia and bone marrow suppression in at least three breastfed infants. In one case of a mother who received 800 mg/week of cyclophosphamide, her infant was significantly neutropenic following six weeks of exposure via breastmilk. Major leukopenia was also reported in a second breastfed infant following only a brief exposure. The elimination kinetics are highly variable and depend on renal and liver function. Withhold breastfeeding for at least 72 hours following the use of this product.

- DOXORUBICIN   (*Adriamycin*)
  - AAP = Cytotoxic drug that may interfere with cellular metabolism of the nursing infant
  - LRC = L5
  - RID =
  - Pregnancy = D
  - Comment: Doxorubicin and its metabolite are secreted in significant amounts in breastmilk. Following a dose of 70 mg/meter sq., peak milk levels of doxorubicin and metabolite occurred at 24 hours and were 128 and 111 µg/L, respectively. The highest milk/plasma ratio was 4.43 at 24 hours. A classic anthracycline, doxorubicin is one of a number in this family. Doxorubicin, when administered, reaches a rapid C_{max} and disappears from the plasma compartment with a 3-exponential decay characterized by three differing half-lives, three to five minutes, one to two hours, and 24-36 hours. A fourth curve has been identified with a half-life of 110 hours, which accounts for approximately 30% of the total AUC. Because this product is detectable in plasma (and milk) for long periods, a waiting period of approximately seven to ten days is recommended.

- FLUOROURACIL   (*5FU, Adrucil, Efudex, Fluoroplex, Carac*)
  - AAP = Not reviewed
  - LRC = L5
  - RID =
  - Pregnancy = D during first and second trimesters
  - Comment: Fluorouracil is a potent antineoplastic agent generally used topically for various skin cancers and IV for various carcinomas. No data are available on its transfer into breastmilk. 5FU is an extremely toxic and dangerous compound and is probably contraindicated in breastfeeding women following IV therapy. It is rapidly cleared by the liver. 5FU is commonly used topically as a cream for actinic or solar keratosis. The topical absorption of 5FU is minimal, reported to be less than 10%. Although it is unlikely that significant quantities of 5FU would be transferred to a breastfed infant following topical application to small areas, caution is urged. If large body areas were exposed to this therapy, significant absorption could occur. Following IV therapy, a waiting period of at least 24 hours is recommended.

- GOSERELIN ACETATE IMPLANT   (*Zoladex*)
  - AAP = Not reviewed
  - LRC = L3
  - RID =
  - Pregnancy = X

- ° Comment: Goserelin is a synthetic decapeptide analogue of luteinizing hormone releasing factor, and it acts as a potent inhibitor of pituitary gonadotropin secretion. Following initial administration in males, goserelin causes an initial increase in serum luteinizing hormone (LH) and follicle stimulating hormone (FSH) levels. Chronic administration of goserelin leads to sustained suppression of pituitary gonadotropins and serum levels of testosterone in males. In females, a down-regulation of the pituitary gland following chronic exposure leads to suppression of gonadotropin secretion, a decrease in serum estradiol to levels consistent with the menopausal state. Serum LH and FSH are suppressed to follicular phase levels within four weeks. No data are available on its transfer into human milk, but due to its structure and molecular weight, it is very unlikely to enter milk or to be orally bioavailable in the infant.

- **LETROZOLE** (*Femara*)
  - ° AAP = Not reviewed
  - ° LRC = L4
  - ° RID =
  - ° Pregnancy = D
  - ° Comment: Letrozole is an aromatase inhibitor of estrogen synthesis and is used to treat estrogen-receptor positive breast cancer and other syndromes. No data are available on its transfer to human milk, but I would suspect the levels are low. However, it has a very long half-life, which is concerning in a breastfed infant and could lead to higher plasma levels over time. Therefore, the transfer of small amounts of this agent to an infant could seriously impair bone growth or sexual development of an infant, and for this reason, it is probably somewhat hazardous to use in a breastfeeding mother. Discontinue breastfeeding for at least 10 days.

- **METHOTREXATE** (*Folex, Rheumatrex*)
  - ° AAP = Cytotoxic drug that may interfere with cellular metabolism of the nursing infant
  - ° LRC = L3 for acute use
  - ° RID = 0.1%
  - ° Pregnancy = X
  - ° Comment: Methotrexate is a potent and potentially dangerous folic acid antimetabolite used in arthritic and other immunologic syndromes. It is also used as an abortifacient in tubal pregnancies. Methotrexate is secreted into breastmilk in small levels. Following a dose of 22.5 mg to one patient two hours postdose, the methotrexate concentration in breastmilk was 2.6 µg/L of milk, with a milk/plasma ratio of 0.08. The cumulative excretion of methotrexate in the first 12 hours after oral administration was only 0.32 µg in milk. These authors conclude that methotrexate therapy in breastfeeding mothers would not pose a contraindication to breastfeeding. However, methotrexate is believed to be retained in human tissues (particularly neonatal GI cells and ovarian cells) for long periods (months). Elimination of methotrexate is by a two-compartment model with a terminal elimination half-life of 8-15 hours. Patients with poor renal function have prolonged methotrexate half-lives. It is apparent that the concentration of methotrexate in human milk is minimal, although due to the toxicity of this agent, it is probably wise to pump and discard the mother's milk for a minimum of four days. This may require extending if the dose used is quite high.

- **MITOXANTRONE** (*Novantrone*)
  - ° AAP = Not reviewed

- ◦ LRC = L5
- ◦ RID =
- ◦ Pregnancy = D
- ◦ Comment: Mitoxantrone is an antineoplastic agent used in the treatment of relapsing multiple sclerosis. It is a DNA-reactive agent that intercalates into DNA via hydrogen bonding, causing crosslinks. In a study of a patient who received three treatments of mitoxantrone (6 mg/m^2) on days one to five, mitoxantrone levels in milk measured 120 ng/mL just after treatment (on the third day of treatment), and dropped to a stable level of 18 ng/mL for the next 28 days. This agent has an enormous volume of distribution and is sequestered in at least seven organs, including the liver and bone marrow. In another study, 15% of the dose remained 35 days after exposure. Assuming a mother were breastfeeding, these levels would provide about 18 μg/L of milk consumed after the first few days following exposure to the drug. In addition, it would be sequestered for long periods in the infant as well. As this is a DNA-reactive agent, and it has a huge volume of distribution leading to prolonged tissue, plasma, and milk levels, mothers should be strongly advised to not breastfeed following its use.

- TAMOXIFEN   (*Nolvadex*)
  - ◦ AAP = Not reviewed
  - ◦ LRC = L5
  - ◦ RID =
  - ◦ Pregnancy = D
  - ◦ Comment: Tamoxifen is a nonsteroidal antiestrogen. It attaches to the estrogen receptor and produces only minimal stimulation, thus it prevents estrogen from stimulating the receptor.

    Tamoxifen is metabolized by the liver and has an elimination half-life of greater than seven days (range 3-21 days). It is well absorbed orally, and the highest tissue concentrations are in the liver (60 fold). It is 99% protein-bound and normally reduces plasma prolactin levels significantly (66% after three months). At present, there are no data on its transfer into breastmilk; however, it has been shown to inhibit lactation early postpartum in several studies. In one study, doses of 10-30 mg twice daily early postpartum completely inhibited postpartum engorgement and lactation. In a second study, tamoxifen doses of 10 mg four times daily significantly reduced serum prolactin and inhibited milk production as well.

    This product has a very long half-life, and the active metabolite is concentrated in the plasma (two fold). This drug has all the characteristics that would suggest a concentrating mechanism in breastfed infants over time. Its prominent effect on reducing prolactin levels will inhibit early lactation and may ultimately inhibit established lactation. In this instance, the significant risks to the infant from exposure to tamoxifen probably outweigh the benefits of breastfeeding. Mothers receiving tamoxifen should not breastfeed until we know more about the levels transferred into milk and the plasma/tissue levels found in breastfed infants.

- TRASTUZUMAB   (*Herceptin*)
  - ◦ AAP = Not reviewed
  - ◦ LRC = L4
  - ◦ RID =
  - ◦ Pregnancy = B

○ Comment: Trastuzumab is recombinant DNA-derived humanized monoclonal antibody that selectively binds to receptors common on certain breast cancers. It is indicated in the treatment of patients with metastatic breast cancer whose tumors overexpress the HER2 protein. It is an IgG1 kappa that contains human framework regions that bind to the HER2 receptors on cancer cells. While IgG transfers minimally into human milk, we do not have data on the transfer of this recombinant product into human milk. Studies on cynomolgus monkeys at doses 25 times the weekly human dose demonstrated that trastuzumab is secreted in milk (levels were not reported). However, it was not associated with any adverse effects on the growth or development of these infant monkeys. It is not likely that this agent at doses used in humans would cause appreciable problems in a breastfeeding infant. However, it is not clear that mothers with breast cancer should breastfeed, as we do not yet understand how lactation would affect the mother's response to anticancer agents.

Clinical Tips

The treatment of breast cancer obviously depends on numerous factors far beyond the scope of this book. With noninvasive disease, such as lobular carcinoma in situ (LCIS), excision of the tumor following by tamoxifen therapy has been shown to decrease the risk of developing breast cancer. Other treatment options include close observation. The risk of subsequent invasive cancer in women with LCIS is approximately 1% per year. A more aggressive option would be bilateral prophylactic total mastectomy without axillary node dissection.

With ductal carcinoma in situ (DCIS), treatment options include breast-conserving surgery, followed by extensive radiation therapy and tamoxifen, and/or total mastectomy. DCIS is more likely to progress to invasive malignancy than LCIS. The role of tamoxifen in management of DCIS is less clear than in LCIS.

With early invasive breast cancer, procedures ranging from minimum breast-conserving surgery to total mastectomy are sometimes recommended. Additionally, axillary node dissection or possibly sentinel node dissection in those women without clinically apparent nodal disease is typically performed. Radiation therapy is usually employed with breast conserving therapy and may also be used after mastectomy. Adjuvant hormonal therapy, such as tamoxifen, in those women with estrogen or progesterone receptor positive breast tumors may also be recommended

Using the additional treatment options beyond surgery in breastfeeding patients with a diagnosis of cancer is risky and must be done carefully. Most, but not all, chemotherapeutic agents are rapidly cleared from the maternal circulation, and after a brief waiting period, breastfeeding mothers might be able to resume breastfeeding. This is solely determined by the clearance rate of the drug from the mother's circulation. Discussions regarding potential risks to the breastfed infant verses benefit to the mother with breast cancer must be individualized. The reader is advised to closely review the data on these individual agents in *Medications and Mothers' Milk* and discuss these data with the oncologist prior to considering resuming breastfeeding.

Frankly, we do not really know what effect, if any, breastfeeding has on the response of malignant tissues to chemotherapeutic agents. We more or less know how malignant tissues respond in non-breastfeeding mothers at various ages. However, does breastfeeding reduce or perhaps even increase the sensitivity of malignant tissues to the various treatments regimens? We simply do not know the answer to this question.

Suggested Reading

Cardoso, F., Bedard, P. L., Winer, E. P., Pagani, O., Senkus-Konefka, E., Fallowfield, L. J., et al. (2009). International guidelines for management of metastatic breast cancer: combination vs sequential single-agent chemotherapy. *J Natl Cancer Inst, 101*(17), 1174-1181.

Mayor, S. (2009). NICE updates guidance on early and advanced breast cancer. *BMJ, 338*, b815.

Murray, N., Brunt, M., Macbeth, F., & Winstanley, J. (2009). Advanced breast cancer: diagnosis and treatment. National Institute for Health and Clinical Excellence Guideline 2009 - a solid basis for good clinical practice. *Clin Oncol (R Coll Radiol), 21*(5), 368-370.

Ozanne, E. M., Loberg, A., Hughes, S., Lawrence, C., Drohan, B., Semine, A., et al. (2009). Identification and management of women at high risk for hereditary breast/ovarian cancer syndrome. *Breast J, 15*(2), 155-162.

Shah, S. S., Ketterling, R. P., Goetz, M. P., Ingle, J. N., Reynolds, C. A., Perez, E. A., et al. (2010). Impact of American Society of Clinical Oncology/College of American Pathologists guideline recommendations on HER2 interpretation in breast cancer. *Hum Pathol, 41*(1), 103-106.

Smith, I., & Chua, S. (2006). Medical treatment of early breast cancer. I: adjuvant treatment. *BMJ, 332*(7532), 34-37.

Smith, I., & Chua, S. (2006). Medical treatment of early breast cancer. III: chemotherapy. *BMJ, 332*(7534), 161-162.

Smith, R. A., Cokkinides, V., & Brawley, O. W. (2009). Cancer screening in the United States, 2009: a review of current American Cancer Society guidelines and issues in cancer screening. *CA Cancer J Clin, 59*(1), 27-41.

Souchon, R., Wenz, F., Sedlmayer, F., Budach, W., Dunst, J., Feyer, P., et al. (2009). DEGRO practice guidelines for palliative radiotherapy of metastatic breast cancer: bone metastases and metastatic spinal cord compression (MSCC). *Strahlenther Onkol, 185*(7), 417-424.

Tice, J. A., & Kerlikowske, K. (2009). Screening and prevention of breast cancer in primary care. *Prim Care, 36*(3), 533-558.

Veronesi, U., Zurrida, S., Viale, G., Galimberti, V., Arnone, P., & Nole, F. (2009). Rethinking TNM: a breast cancer classification to guide to treatment and facilitate research. *Breast J, 15*(3), 291-295.

Candida Albicans

Principles of Therapy

Candidiasis is the most common mucosal and invasive fungal infection in humans, and *Candida albicans* is the most common species. Fungal infections, particularly candida, have increased in incidence due to the extensive use of antibiotics. Other Candida species include *C. glabrata, C. tropicalis, C. parapisilosis,* and *C. krusei. C. albicans* is a normal flora and can be cultured from the mouth, feces, and vagina in most normal humans. The major risk factors for invasive candidiasis include diabetes, indwelling catheters, recent surgery, use of broad spectrum antibiotics, corticosteroid therapy, neutropenia and impaired cell-mediated immunity (HIV infection). Cutaneous candidiasis is most commonly associated with areas of increased moisture, such as intertriginous and inguinal areas, the vulva, and in breastfeeding mothers, possibly the nipple and areola.

Mucosal candidiasis can develop in the oropharynx, esophagus, gastrointestinal tract, vaginal mucosa, and urinary tract. Diagnosis of vulvovaginal Candidiasis (VVC) is made either by signs and symptoms or on the basis of inspection of vaginal discharge, using 10% KOH prepared slides under the microscope evaluating for budding hyphae.

The therapy of candidiasis largely depends on the location and severity of the infection. Topical candidiasis therapy includes reduction of moisture and the use of topical antifungals, such as nystatin, miconazole, butoconazole, tioconazole, terconazole, or clotrimazole. Multiple intravaginal versions of these agents are available over the counter for treatment of VVC. Recommended systemic therapy includes the use of fluconazole. Itraconazole or ketoconazole are less desirable alternatives. Hepatotoxicity related to ketoconazole is rare, but more common than with fluconazole. Drug–drug interactions are an important consideration to remember with the use of systemic medications. Some studies suggest that nystatin resistance has increased, and almost 45% of candida strains are resistant to Nystatin in certain populations. A study of oral candida in an otherwise healthy population found 88% of patients to be culture positive for *C. albicans,* with testing revealing that all strains were susceptible to fluconazole.

Numerous studies attest to the fact that upward of 37% or more of seven day old infants are colonized with Candida, and 82% of infants have culturable *Candida albicans* at four weeks postpartum. Even newborns delivered vaginally have Candida present in their oral cavity at seven days. One study on the occurrence of Candida in asymptomatic dyads found Candida in the oral cavity of 34.5% of predominately breastfed infants and in 34.5% of lactating mothers' breasts. In this study, 17 dyads had simultaneous occurrence of Candida, and 81.8% of these revealed the same species.

Fluconazole is cleared for use in infants six months and older. Epidemiologic information on candidemia from 1998 to 2001 done in Iowa found only 3% of Candida species to be resistant to fluconazole.

Vulvovaginal Candidiasis (VVC) is quite common with 75% of women experiencing at least one infection. Symptoms may include vaginal discharge, vulvar itching and irritation, and dysparunia.

Recurrent infections are defined as four or more episodes per year. Other indications of complicated candida infections include severe infections, non-candidal infections or those occurring in women with other risk factors such as pregnancy, poorly controlled diabetes, or immune suppression.

Treatment

- Most systemic antifungals are contraindicated in pregnancy and are generally used only in life-threatening infections. For invasive candidiasis, IV amphotericin B is recommended.

- Uncomplicated candida vulvovaginal vaginitis: topical therapy (duration dependent on agent) or oral treatment with fluconazole 150 mg single dose.

- Recurrent or complicated candida vulvovaginal vaginitis (> 4 episodes per year): topical therapy for 7-10 days or oral fluconazole 150 mg every third day for two doses.

- For minor issues, topical nystatin or azole treatments are suggested.

- Vaginitis: Topical intravaginal imidazole cream, lotion, or suppositories.

- Mucocutaneous: Nystatin powder or imidazole cream or lotion.

Medications

- BUTOCONAZOLE   (Femstat, Gynazole, Gynofort, Mycelex)
    - AAP = Not reviewed
    - LRC = L3
    - RID =
    - Pregnancy = C
    - Comment: Butoconazole is used for the treatment of vaginal candidiasis. It is not apparently any more effective than other azole antifungals. Only 5.5% is absorbed vaginally. Levels in milk, although not known, will probably be low. Myconazole is probably preferred in breastfeeding mothers.

- CLOTRIMAZOLE   (*Gyne-Lotrimin, Mycelex, Lotrimin, FemCare, Trivagizole*)
    - AAP = Not reviewed
    - LRC = L1
    - RID =
    - Pregnancy = B for topical/vaginal preparations
    - Comment: Clotrimazole is a broad-spectrum antifungal agent. It is generally used for candidiasis and various tinea species (athletes foot, ring worm). Clotrimazole is available in oral lozenges, topical creams, intravaginal tablets and creams. No data are available on penetration into breastmilk. However, after intravaginal administration, only 3-10% of the drug is absorbed (peak serum level= 0.01 to 0.03 µg/mL) and even less by oral lozenge. Hence, following vaginal administration, it seems unlikely that levels absorbed by a breastfeeding infant would be high enough to produce untoward effects. Safety of clotrimazole lozenges in children younger than three years of age has not been established. The risk of contact dermatitis with this agent may be higher.

- FLUCONAZOLE   (*Diflucan*)
    - AAP = Maternal Medication Usually Compatible with Breastfeeding
    - LRC = L2

- RID   =   16.4-21.5%
- Pregnancy = C
- Comment: Fluconazole is a synthetic triazole antifungal agent and is frequently used for vaginal, oropharyngeal, and esophageal candidiasis. Many of the triazole antifungals (itraconazole, terconazole) have similar mechanisms of action and are considered fungistatic in action. In vivo studies have found fluconazole to have fungistatic activity against a variety of fungal strains, including *C. albicans, C. tropicalis, T. glabrata*, and *C. neoformans.*

  The pharmacokinetics are similar following both oral and IV administration. The drug is almost completely absorbed orally (>90%). Peak plasma levels occur in one to two hours after oral administration. Unlike ketoconazole and itraconazole, fluconazole absorption is unaffected by gastric pH and does not require an acid pH to be absorbed. Steady state plasma levels are only attained after five to ten days of therapy, but can be achieved on day two with a loading dose (twice the daily dose) on the first day. Average plasma levels are 4.12 to 8.1 µg/mL. Fluconazole is widely and evenly distributed in most tissues and fluids and is distributed in total body water. Concentrations in skin and urine may be 10 fold higher than plasma levels. CSF concentrations are 50-94% of the plasma levels. Plasma protein binding is minimal at about 11%. Fluconazole is primarily excreted renally.

  Oral fluconazole is currently cleared for pediatric candidiasis for infants six months and older and has an FDA Safety Profile for neonates one day and older. Clinical cure rate for oropharyngeal candidiasis in pediatric patients is reported at 86% with fluconazole (2-3 mg/kg/day) compared to 46% of nystatin treated patients. Fluconazole is transferred into human milk with a milk/plasma ratio of approximately 0.85. Following a single 150 mg dose, milk levels at two, five, 24, and 48 hours were reported to be 2.93, 2.66, 1.76, and 0.98 µg/mL, respectively. Plasma levels at two, five, 24, and 48 hours were 6.4, 2.79, 2.52, and 1.19 µg/mL, respectively.

  From these data and assuming an average milk level of 2.3 mg/L, an infant consuming 150 mL/kg/d of milk would receive an average of 0.34 mg/kg/d of fluconazole or 16% of the weight-adjusted maternal dose, and less than 5.8% of the pediatric dose (6 mg/kg/d).

  In another study of one patient receiving 200 mg daily (1.5 times the above dose) for 18 days, the peak milk concentration was 4.1 mg/L at two hours following the dose. However, the mean concentration of fluconazole in milk was not reported.

  Pediatric Dosing: The recommended pediatric dosing for oral candidiasis is 6 mg/kg STAT followed by 3 mg/kg/day. For systemic candidiasis, 6-12 mg/kg/day is generally recommended. These current recommendations are for infants six months and older. The manufacturer states that a number of infants one day old and older have been safely treated. One study of premature infants suggests that the dose in very low birth weight infants should be 6 mg/kg every two to three days.

- GENTIAN VIOLET   (*Crystal Violet, Methylrosaniline chloride, Gentian Violet*)
  - AAP   =   Not reviewed
  - LRC   =   L3
  - RID   =
  - Pregnancy = C
  - Comment: Gentian violet is an older product that, when used topically and orally, is an exceptionally effective antifungal and antimicrobial. It is a strong purple dye that is difficult to remove. Gentian violet has been found to be equivalent to ketoconazole and far superior to nystatin in treating oral (not esophageal) candidiasis in patients with advanced AIDS. It is also useful in treating purulent

infections of the ear infected with methicillin-resistant Staphlococcus Aureus. Gentian violet (GV) solutions generally come as 1-2% Gentian violet dissolved in a 10% solution of alcohol. For use with infants, the solution should be diluted with distilled water to 0.25 to 0.5% Gentian violet. This reduces the irritant properties of GV and reduces the alcohol content as well. While the alcohol is irritating to the nipple, it is not detrimental to the infant. Higher concentrations of GV are known to be very irritating, leading to oral ulceration and necrotic skin reactions in children. If used, a small swab should be soaked in the solution, and then swabbed in the infant's gingivae. Apply it directly to the affected areas in the mouth no more than once or twice daily for no more than three to seven days. Direct application to the nipple has been reported.

- KETOCONAZOLE   (*Nizoral Shampoo, Nizoral*)
  - ○ AAP = Maternal Medication Usually Compatible with Breastfeeding
  - ○ LRC = L2
  - ○ RID = 0.3%
  - ○ Pregnancy = C
  - ○ Comment: Ketoconazole is an antifungal similar in structure to miconazole and clotrimazole. It is used orally, topically, and via shampoo. Ketoconazole is not detected in plasma after chronic shampooing. In a study of one patient (82 kg) receiving 200 mg daily for 10 days, milk samples were taken at 1.75, 3.25, 6.0, 8.0, and 24 hours after the tenth dose. The average concentration of ketoconazole over the 24 hours was 68 µg/L, while the Cmax at 3.25 hours was 0.22 mg/L. The absorption of ketoconazole is highly variable and could be reduced in infants due to the alkaline condition induced by milk ingestion. Ketoconazole requires acidic conditions to be absorbed, and its absorption and distribution in children is not known. Regardless, ketoconazole is probably safe in breastfeeding infants.

- MICONAZOLE   (*Monistat IV, Monistat 3, 7*)
  - ○ AAP = Not reviewed
  - ○ LRC = L2
  - ○ RID =
  - ○ Pregnancy = C
  - ○ Comment: Miconazole is an effective antifungal that is commonly used IV, topically, and intravaginally. After intravaginal application, approximately 1% of the dose is absorbed systemically. After topical application, there is little or no absorption (0.1%). It is unlikely that the limited absorption of miconazole from vaginal application would produce significant milk levels. Milk concentrations following oral and IV miconazole have not been reported. Oral absorption of miconazole is poor, only 25-30%. Miconazole is commonly used in pediatric patients less than one year of age.

- NYSTATIN   (*Mycostatin, Nilstat*)
  - ○ AAP = Not reviewed
  - ○ LRC = L1
  - ○ RID =
  - ○ Pregnancy = B
  - ○ Comment: Nystatin is an antifungal primarily used for candidiasis topically and orally. The oral absorption of nystatin is extremely poor, and plasma levels are undetectable after oral administration.

The likelihood of secretion into milk is remote due to poor maternal absorption. It is frequently administered directly to neonates in neonatal units for candidiasis. In addition, absorption into infant circulation is equally unlikely. Dose: neonates=100,000 units; younger children = 200,000 units, older children = 400,000-600,000 units, administered four times daily. Current studies suggest that resistance to nystatin is growing.

- TERCONAZOLE   (*Terazol 3, Terazol 7*)
  - ○ AAP = Not reviewed
  - ○ LRC = L3
  - ○ RID =
  - ○ Pregnancy = C
  - ○ Comment: Terconazole is an antifungal primarily used for vaginal candidiasis. It is similar to fluconazole and itraconazole. When administered intravaginally, only a limited amount (5-16%) is absorbed systemically (mean peak plasma level = 6 ng/mL). It is well absorbed orally. Even at high doses, the drug is not mutagenic, nor fetotoxic. At high doses, terconazole is known to enter breastmilk in rodents, although no data are available on human milk. The milk levels are probably too small to be clinically relevant.

- TIOCONAZOLE (*Monistat*)
  - ○ AAP = Not Reviewed
  - ○ LRC = L3
  - ○ RID =
  - ○ Pregnancy = C
  - ○ Comment: Only 2.9% systemically absorbed topically and less vaginally. Levels in plasma were low to undetectable. Levels in milk are unreported, but will probably be low to undetectable. However, this product has not been shown clinically to be superior to older azoles. Suggest miconazole as alternative, but tioconaozle is probably compatible with breastfeeding.

Clinical Tips

New data from our laboratories suggest that ductal (breast) candidiasis is unlikely. Candida may possibly exist on the nipple itself, although we do not have conclusive data. Oral manifestations of candida in infants may affect suckling and may induce nipple trauma, although this is unproven. Almost 80% of breastfeeding infants are colonized orally with *Candida albicans*, although this is seldom infectious.

Oral candidiasis is best treated with topical nystatin initially, but may require oral fluconazole in some instances of resistance. Vulvovaginal Candidiasis (VVC) in the breastfeeding patient can be treated with topical miconazole, butoconazole, tioconazole, or clotrimazole creams or one 150 mg tablet (PO) of fluconazole. Recurrent VVC is often treated by 150 mg oral fluconazole every 72 hours for three doses.

Suggested Reading

Gómez-López, A., Zaragoza, O., Rodríguez-Tudela, J. L., & Cuenca-Estrella, M. (2008). Pharmacotherapy of yeast infections. *Expert Opin Pharmacother, 9*(16), 2801-2816.

Hale, T. W., Bateman, T. L., Finkelman, M. A., & Berens, P. D. (2009). The absence of Candida albicans in milk samples of women with clinical symptoms of ductal candidiasis. *Breastfeed Med, 4*(2), 57-61.

Hassan, I., Powell, G., Sidhu, M., Hart, W. M., & Denning, D. W. (2009). Excess mortality, length of stay and cost attributable to candidaemia. *J Infect, 59*(5), 360-365.

Koh, A. Y., Kohler, J. R., Coggshall, K. T., Van Rooijen, N., & Pier, G. B. (2008). Mucosal damage and neutropenia are required for Candida albicans dissemination. *PLoS Pathog, 4*(2), e35.

Leon, C., Ruiz-Santana, S., Saavedra, P., Galvan, B., Blanco, A., Castro, C., et al. (2009). Usefulness of the "Candida score" for discriminating between Candida colonization and invasive candidiasis in non-neutropenic critically ill patients: a prospective multicenter study. *Crit Care Med, 37*(5), 1624-1633.

Pacini, D., Cerana, M., Beltrame, A., Di Biagio, A., & De Maria, A. (2007). Persistence of Candida albicans candidemia in non-neutropenic surgical patients: management of a representative patient in the absence of second-line treatment guidelines. *J Chemother, 19*(3), 335-338.

Zhang, H., Chen, H., Niu, J., Wang, Y., & Xie, L. (2009). Role of adaptive immunity in the pathogenesis of Candida albicans keratitis. *Invest Ophthalmol Vis Sci, 50*(6), 2653-2659.

Cardiac Arrhythmias

Principles of Therapy

Arrhythmias are primarily rapid or abnormal changes in rhythm of the heart. Symptoms include a pounding heart (palpitations), fatigue, dyspnea, syncope, angina, and heart failure. There are numerous types of arrhythmias and conditions that lead to such arrhythmias, which are largely beyond the scope of this text. Arrhythmias occur in numerous conditions, including premature ventricular complexes, ventricular tachycardia, atrial tachycardia, ventricular flutter, etc. Regardless, many of the same medications are used for these numerous conditions and will be discussed below. The medications used vary from the beta-blockers, calcium channel blockers, ACE and ARB inhibitors to a number of special antiarrhythmic agents. For the purposes of this section, all of the medications used for arrhythmias are included, but the list is shortened due to limited research in breastfeeding patients. Because arrhythmias present in a host of different patterns/conditions, certain medications are only used for certain arrhythmias, and the reader is cautioned that many of the included medications are not interchangeable.

Treatment

* Beta blockers, such as metoprolol, propranolol, atenolol, etc.

* Calcium channel blockers, such as diltiazem or verapamil

* Warfarin

* Antiarrhythmic drugs, such as flecainide, propafenone, sotalol, amiodarone

Medications

* ADENOSINE (*Adenocard*)
    ◦ AAP = Not reviewed
    ◦ LRC = L3
    ◦ RID =
    ◦ Pregnancy = C
    ◦ Comment: Adenosine has a brief half-life of only 10 seconds. It would not likely penetrate milk, nor last very long in the milk compartment. With a brief wait of a few minutes, it is probably compatible with breastfeeding.

* AMIODARONE (*Cordarone*)
    ◦ AAP = Drugs whose effect on nursing infants is unknown but may be of concern

- ◦ LRC = L5
- ◦ RID = 43.1%
- ◦ Pregnancy = D
- ◦ Comment: Amiodarone is a potent and sometimes dangerous antiarrhythmic drug and requires close supervision by clinicians. Although poorly absorbed by the mother (<50%), maximum serum levels are attained after three to seven hours. This drug has a very large volume of distribution, resulting in accumulation in adipose, liver, spleen, and lungs, and has a high rate of fetal toxicity (10-17%). It should not be given to pregnant mothers unless critically required.

    Significant amounts are secreted into breastmilk at levels higher than the plasma level. Breastmilk samples obtained at birth and at two and three weeks post-partum in two patients, contained levels of amiodarone and desethylamiodarone varying from 1.7 to 3.0 mg/L (mean= 2.3 mg/L) and 0.8 to 1.8 mg/L (mean= 1.1 mg/L), respectively. Despite the concentrations of amiodarone in milk, the amounts were apparently not high enough to produce plasma levels of both drugs higher than about 0.1 μg/mL, which are minimal compared to the maternal plasma levels of 1.2 μg/mL or higher.

    McKenna reported amiodarone milk levels in a mother treated with 400 mg daily. In this study, at six weeks postpartum, breastmilk levels of amiodarone and desethylamiodarone varied during the day from 2.8-16.4 mg/L and 1.1-6.5 mg/L, respectively. Reported infant plasma levels of amiodarone and desethylamiodarone were 0.4 and 0.25 mg/L, respectively. The dose ingested by the infant was approximately 1.5 μg/kg/day. The authors suggest that the amount of amiodarone ingested was moderate and could expose the developing infant to a significant dose of the drug and should be avoided. Because amiodarone inhibits extrathyroidal deiodinases, conversion of T4 to T3 is reduced. One reported case of hypothyroidism has been reported in an infant following therapy in the mother. Because of the long half-life and high concentrations in various organs, amiodarone could continuously build up to higher levels in the infant, although it was not reported in the above studies. This product should be used only under the most extraordinary conditions, and the infant should be closely monitored for cardiovascular and thyroid function. Thus breastfeeding should be avoided if this product is used chronically. Brief, three to seven days use is probably not contraindicated if a 24-48 hour interruption is used before reinstating breastfeeding.

    One case reported a mother who took 200 mg amiodarone three times daily to treat fetal ascites and tachycardia. Upon delivery, the mother stopped taking amiodarone. Breastmilk was tested to determine the levels of amiodarone, which were found to be 0.6 mg/L, 2.1 mg/L, and undetectable on days 5, 11, and 25, respectively. The baby was monitored closely during this period. The authors suggest that in some instances, with close monitoring, breastfeeding can occur during amiodarone therapy.

- ASPIRIN   (*Anacin, Aspergum, Empirin, Genprin, Arthritis Foundation Pain Reliever, Ecotrin*)
  - ◦ AAP = Drugs associated with significant side effects and should be given with caution
  - ◦ LRC = L3
  - ◦ RID = 2.5 - 10.8%
  - ◦ Pregnancy = C during first and second trimester
  - ◦ Comment: Extremely small amounts are secreted into breastmilk. Few harmful effects have been reported. In one study, salicylic acid (active metabolite of Aspirin) penetrated poorly into milk (dose =454 mg ASA), with peak levels of only 1.12 to 1.60 μg/mL, whereas peak plasma levels were 33 to 43.4 μg/mL.

In another study of a rheumatoid arthritis patient who received 4 gm/day aspirin, none was detectable in her milk (<5mg/100cc). Extremely high doses in the mother could potentially produce slight bleeding in the infant. Because aspirin is implicated in Reye syndrome, it is a poor choice of analgesic to use in breastfeeding mothers. However, in rheumatic fever patients, it is still one of the anti-inflammatory drugs of choice and a risk-vs-benefit assessment must be done in this case.

In a study of a patient consuming aspirin chronically, salicylate concentrations in milk peaked at three hours at a concentration of 10 mg/L following a maternal dose of 975 mg. Maternal plasma levels peaked at 2.25 hours at 108 mg/L.

While the direct use of aspirin in infants and children is definitely implicated in Reye syndrome, the use of the 82 mg/d dose in breastfeeding mothers is unlikely to increase the risk of this syndrome. Unfortunately we do not at present know of any dose-response relationship between aspirin and Reye syndrome other than in older children, where even low plasma levels of aspirin were implicated in Reye syndrome during viral syndromes, such as flu or chickenpox. Therefore, the use of aspirin in breastfeeding mothers is questionable, but the risk is probably low. Never use these products if the infant has a viral syndrome.

- ATENOLOL   (*Tenoretic, Tenormin*)
  - ○ AAP = Drugs associated with significant side effects and should be given with caution
  - ○ LRC = L3
  - ○ RID = 6.6%
  - ○ Pregnancy = D
  - ○ Comment: Atenolol is a potent cardio-selective beta-blocker. Data conflict on the secretion of atenolol into breastmilk. One author reports an incident of significant bradycardia, cyanosis, low body temperature, and low blood pressure in the breastfeeding infant of a mother consuming 100 mg atenolol daily, while a number of others have failed to detect plasma levels in the neonate or untoward side effects.

    In another study, women taking 50-100 mg/day were found to have M/P ratios of 1.5-6.8. However, even with high M/P ratios, the calculated intake per day (at peak levels) for a breastfeeding infant would only be 0.13 mg. In a study by White, breastmilk levels in one patient were 0.7, 1.2, and 1.8 mg/L of milk at doses of 25, 50, and 100 mg daily, respectively. In another study, the estimated daily intake for an infant receiving 500 mL milk per day would be 0.3 mg. In these five patients who received 100 mg daily, the mean milk concentration of atenolol was 630 μg/L. In a study by Kulas, the amount of atenolol transferred into milk varied from 0.66 mg/L with a maternal dose of 25 mg, 1.2 mg/L with a maternal dose of 50 mg, and 1.7 mg/L with a maternal dose of 100 mg per day. Although atenolol is approved by the AAP, some caution is recommended due to the milk/plasma ratios and the reported problem with one infant.

- CLOPIDOGREL   (*Plavix*)
  - ○ AAP = Not reviewed
  - ○ LRC = L3
  - ○ RID =
  - ○ Pregnancy = B
  - ○ Comment: Clopidogrel selectively inhibits platelet adenosine diphosphate-induced platelet aggregation. Aspirin is sometimes preferred as it is less expensive, quite tolerable, and very effective.

Clopidogrel is only used in those patients who are aspirin-intolerant. It is not known if it transfers into human milk. However, its plasma half-life is rather brief (eight hours), although it's metabolite covalently bonds to platelet receptors with a half-life of 11 days. Because it produces an irreversible inhibition of platelet aggregation, any present in milk could inhibit an infant's platelet function for a prolonged period. Because aspirin affects platelet aggregation similarly, and its milk levels are quite low, it would appear to be an ideal alternative. However, aspirin also inhibits platelet aggregation for long periods and may increase the risk of Reye syndrome in infants. The choice between using clopidogrel and aspirin must be made on clinical grounds and following a risk vs. benefit assessment until we know more about the levels secreted into human milk.

- DIGOXIN   (*Lanoxin, Lanoxicaps*)
  - ○ AAP = Maternal Medication Usually Compatible with Breastfeeding
  - ○ LRC = L2
  - ○ RID = 2.7-2.8%
  - ○ Pregnancy = C
  - ○ Comment: Digoxin is a cardiac stimulant used primarily to strengthen the contractile process. In one mother receiving 0.25 mg digoxin daily, the amount found in breastmilk ranged from 0.96 to 0.61 µg/L at four and six hours postdose, respectively. Mean peak breastmilk levels varied from 0.78 µg/L in one patient to 0.41 µg/L in another. Plasma levels in the infants were undetectable. In another study of five women receiving digoxin therapy, the average breastmilk concentration was 0.64 µg/L. From these studies, it is apparent that a breastfeeding infant would receive less than 1 µg/day of digoxin, too low to be clinically relevant. The small amounts secreted into breastmilk have not produced problems in nursing infants.

- DISOPYRAMIDE   (*Norpace, Napamide*)
  - ○ AAP = Maternal Medication Usually Compatible with Breastfeeding
  - ○ LRC = L2
  - ○ RID = 3.4%
  - ○ Pregnancy = C
  - ○ Comment: Disopyramide is used for treating cardiac arrhythmias similar to quinidine and procainamide. Small levels are secreted into milk. Following a maternal dose of 450 mg every eight hours for two weeks, the milk/plasma ratio was approximately 1.06 for disopyramide and 6.24 for its active metabolite. Although no disopyramide was measurable in the infant's plasma, the milk levels were 2.6-4.4 mg/L (disopyramide), and 9.6-12.3 mg/L (metabolite). Such levels are probably too small to affect an infant. No side effects were reported.

    In another study, in a woman receiving 100 mg five times daily, the maternal serum level was 10.3 µmol/L and the breastmilk level was 4.0 µmol/L, giving a milk/serum ratio of 0.4. From these levels, an infant ingesting 1 L of milk would receive only 1.5 mg per day. Lowest milk levels are at six to eight hours postdose.

- ESMOLOL   (*Brevibloc*)
  - ○ AAP = Not reviewed
  - ○ LRC = L3

- RID =
- Pregnancy = C
- Comment: Esmolol is an ultra short-acting beta blocker agent with low lipid solubility. It is of the same family as propranolol. It is primarily used for treatment of supraventricular tachycardia. It is only used IV and has an extremely short half-life. It is almost completely hydrolyzed in 30 minutes. No data on breastmilk levels are available.

- **FLECAINIDE ACETATE** (*Tambocor*)
  - AAP = Maternal Medication Usually Compatible with Breastfeeding
  - LRC = L3
  - RID = 4.9-5.2%
  - Pregnancy = C
  - Comment: Flecainide is a potent antiarrhythmic used to suppress dangerous ventricular arrhythmias. In a group of 11 breastfeeding mothers receiving 100 mg oral flecainide (mean= 3.2 mg/kg/day) every 12 hours for 5.5 days beginning one day postpartum, apparent steady-state levels of flecainide in both milk and plasma were achieved in most cases by day four of the study. Highest daily average concentration of flecainide in milk ranged from 270 to 1529 μg/L (mean= 953 μg/L) for the 11 subjects. Based on the pharmacokinetics of flecainide in infants, the expected average steady-state plasma concentration of flecainide in a newborn infant consuming all of the milk production of its mother (approximately 700 mL/day at the highest flecainide level of 1529 μg/L), the average daily intake by the infant would be 1.07 mg. In a normal 4 kg infant, the average plasma concentration in a breastfed infant would not be expected to exceed about 62 ng/mL. The average plasma level in infants treated with therapeutic doses is 360 ng/mL.

    In another study of one patient receiving 100 mg every 12 hours, milk levels of flecainide averaged 0.99 mg/L on day four and five postpartum.

- **LIDOCAINE** (*Xylocaine*)
  - AAP = Maternal Medication Usually Compatible with Breastfeeding
  - LRC = L2
  - RID = 0.5-3.1%
  - Pregnancy = B
  - Comment: Lidocaine is an antiarrhythmic and a local anesthetic. In one study of a breastfeeding mother who received IV lidocaine for ventricular arrhythmias, the mother received approximately 965 mg over seven hours, including the bolus starting doses. At seven hours, the concentration of lidocaine in breastmilk was 0.8 mg/L or 40% of the maternal plasma level (2.0 mg/L). These authors suggest that a mother could continue to breastfeed while on parenteral lidocaine. In a study of 27 parturients who received an average of 82.1 mg bupivacaine and 183.3 mg lidocaine via an epidural catheter, lidocaine milk levels at two, six, and 12 hours post administration were 0.86, 0.46, and 0.22 mg/L, respectively. Levels of bupivacaine in milk at two, six, and 12 hours were 0.09, 0.06, 0.04 mg/L, respectively. Based on these data, the average milk concentration of these agents over 12 hours was 0.5 and 0.07 mg/L.

    In a study of seven nursing mothers who received 3.6-7.2 mL of 2% lidocaine without adrenaline, the concentration of lidocaine in milk three and six hours after injection averaged 97.5 μg/L and

52.7 µg/L, respectively. These authors suggest that mothers who receive local injections of lidocaine can safely breastfeed.

- METOPROLOL (*Toprol-XL, Lopressor*)
    - ◦ AAP = Maternal Medication Usually Compatible with Breastfeeding
    - ◦ LRC = L3
    - ◦ RID = 1.4%
    - ◦ Pregnancy = C
    - ◦ Comment: At low doses, metoprolol is a very cardioselective Beta$_1$ blocker used for hypertension, angina, and tachyarrhythmias. In a study of three women four to six months postpartum who received 100 mg twice daily for four days, the peak concentration of metoprolol ranged from 0.38 to 2.58 µmol/L, whereas the maternal plasma levels ranged from 0.1 to 0.97 µmol/L. Assuming ingestion of 75 mL of milk at each feeding, and the maximum concentration of 2.58 µmol/L, an infant would ingest approximately 0.05 mg metoprolol at the first feeding and considerably less at subsequent feedings.

        In another study of nine women receiving 50-100 mg twice daily, the maternal plasma and milk concentrations ranged from 4-556 nmol/L and 19-1690 nmol/L, respectively. Using these data, the authors calculated an average milk concentration throughout the day as 280 µg/L of milk. This dose is 20-40 times less than a typical clinical dose.

- MEXILETINE HCL (*Mexitil*)
    - ◦ AAP = Maternal Medication Usually Compatible with Breastfeeding
    - ◦ LRC = L2
    - ◦ RID = 1.4-1.6%
    - ◦ Pregnancy = C
    - ◦ Comment: Mexiletine is an antiarrhythmic agent with activity similar to lidocaine. In a study on one patient who was receiving 600 mg/day in divided doses, the milk level at steady state was 0.8 mg/L. Mexiletine was not detected in the infant nor were untoward effects noted. In another study on day two to five postpartum and in a patient receiving 200 mg three times daily, the mean peak concentration of mexiletine in breastmilk was 959 µg/L, and the maternal serum was 724 µg/L. It is unlikely this exposure would lead to untoward side effects in a breastfeeding infant.

- PHENYTOIN (*Dilantin*)
    - ◦ AAP = Maternal Medication Usually Compatible with Breastfeeding
    - ◦ LRC = L2
    - ◦ RID = 0.6-7.7%
    - ◦ Pregnancy = D
    - ◦ Comment: Phenytoin is an old and efficient anticonvulsant. It is secreted in small amounts into breastmilk. The effect on the infant is generally considered minimal if the levels in the maternal circulation are kept in the low-normal range (10 µg/mL). Phenytoin levels peak in milk at 3.5 hours. In one study of six women receiving 200-400 mg/day, plasma concentrations varied from 12.8 to 78.5 µmol/L, while their milk levels ranged from 1.61 to 2.95 mg/L. In only two of these infants were plasma concentrations of phenytoin detectible (0.46 and 0.72 µmol/L). No untoward effects were noted in any of these infants. In a mother receiving 250 mg twice daily, milk levels were 0.26

and the milk/plasma ratio was 0.45. The maternal plasma level of phenytoin was 0.58. In another study of two patients receiving 300-600 mg/d, the average milk level was 1.9 mg/L. The maximum observed milk level was 2.6 mg/L.

- ◦ The neonatal half-life of phenytoin is highly variable for the first week of life. Monitoring the infants' plasma may be useful, although it is not definitely required. All of the current studies indicate rather low levels of phenytoin in breastmilk and minimal plasma levels in breastfeeding infants.

- **PROCAINAMIDE** (*Pronestyl, Procan*)
  - ◦ AAP = Maternal Medication Usually Compatible with Breastfeeding
  - ◦ LRC = L3
  - ◦ RID = 5.4%
  - ◦ Pregnancy = C
  - ◦ Comment: Procainamide is an antiarrhythmic agent. Procainamide and its active metabolite are secreted into breastmilk in moderate concentrations. In one patient receiving 500 mg four times daily, the breastmilk levels of procainamide at zero, three, six, nine, and 12 hours were 5.3, 3.9, 10.2, 4.8, and 2.6 mg/L, respectively. The milk levels averaged 5.4 mg/L for parent drug and 3.5 mg/L for metabolite. Although levels in milk are still too small to provide significant blood levels in an infant, use with caution.

- **PROPAFENONE** (*Rythmol*)
  - ◦ AAP = Not reviewed
  - ◦ LRC = L2
  - ◦ RID = 0.1%
  - ◦ Pregnancy = C
  - ◦ Comment: Propafenone is a class 1C antiarrhythmic agent with structural similarities to propranolol. In a mother receiving 300 mg three times daily and at three days postpartum, maternal serum levels of propafenone and 5-OH-propafenone (active metabolite) were 219 μg/L and 86 μg/L, respectively. The breastmilk level of propafenone and 5-OH-propafenone was 32 μg/L and 47 μg/L, respectively. The authors estimate that the daily intake of drug and active metabolite in their infant (3.3 kg) would have been 16 μg and 24 μg per day, respectively.

- **PROPRANOLOL** (*Inderal*)
  - ◦ AAP = Maternal Medication Usually Compatible with Breastfeeding
  - ◦ LRC = L2
  - ◦ RID = 0.3-0.5%
  - ◦ Pregnancy = C
  - ◦ Comment: Propranolol is a popular beta blocker used in treating hypertension, cardiac arrhythmia, migraine headache, and numerous other syndromes. In general, the maternal plasma levels are exceedingly low, hence the milk levels are low as well. In one study of three patients, the average milk concentration was only 35.4 μg/L after multiple dosing intervals. Using these data, the authors suggest that an infant would receive only 70 μg/L of milk per day, which is <0.1% of the maternal dose.

    In another study of a patient receiving 20 mg twice daily, milk levels varied from 4 to 20 μg/L, with an estimated average dose to infant of 3 μg/day. In another patient receiving 40 mg four times daily, the peak concentration occurred at three hours after dosing. Milk levels varied from zero to 9 μg/L. After a 30 day regimen of 240 mg/day propranolol, the predose and postdose concentration in breastmilk was 26 and 64 μg/L, respectively. No symptoms or signs of beta blockade were noted in this infant. The above amounts in milk would likely be clinically insignificant.

- QUINIDINE   (*Quinaglute, Quinidex*)
  - ○ AAP = Maternal Medication Usually Compatible with Breastfeeding
  - ○ LRC = L2
  - ○ RID = 14.4%
  - ○ Pregnancy = C
  - ○ Comment: Quinidine is used to treat cardiac arrhythmias. Three hours following a dose of 600 mg, the level of quinidine in the maternal serum was 9.0 mg/L and the concentration in her breastmilk was 6.4 mg/L. Subsequently, a level of 8.2 mg/L was noted in breastmilk. Quinidine is selectively stored in the liver. Long-term use could expose an infant to liver toxicity.

- SOTALOL   (*Betapace*)
  - ○ AAP = Maternal Medication Usually Compatible with Breastfeeding
  - ○ LRC = L3
  - ○ RID = 25.5%
  - ○ Pregnancy = B
  - ○ Comment: Sotalol is a typical beta blocker antihypertensive with low lipid solubility. It is secreted into milk in high levels. Sotalol concentrations in milk ranged from 4.8 to 20.2 mg/L (mean = 10.5 mg/L) in five mothers. The mean maternal dose was 433 mg/day. Although these milk levels appear high, no evidence of toxicity was noted in 12 infants. Another study of a 22-year-old mother taking 120 to 240 mg daily reported an infant dose of 20-23% of the weight adjusted maternal dose in milk. This would relate to an infant dose of 0.41 to 0.58 mg/kg. However, there were no untoward effects noted in the infant. It is suggested that if a mother decides to breastfeed while taking sotalol, the baby should receive close monitoring for side effects.

- VERAPAMIL   (*Calan, Isoptin, Covera-HS*)
  - ○ AAP = Maternal Medication Usually Compatible with Breastfeeding
  - ○ LRC = L2
  - ○ RID = 0.2%
  - ○ Pregnancy = C
  - ○ Comment: Verapamil is a typical calcium channel blocker used as an antihypertensive. It is secreted into milk, but in very low levels, which are conflicting. Anderson reports that in one patient receiving 80 mg three times daily, the average steady-state concentrations of verapamil and norverapamil in milk were 25.8 and 8.8 μg/L, respectively. The respective maternal plasma level was 42.9 μg/L. No verapamil was detected in the infant's plasma. Inoue reports that in one patient receiving 80 mg four times daily, the milk level peaked at 300 μg/L at approximately 14 hours. These levels are considerably higher than the aforementioned. In another study of a mother receiving 240 mg daily, the concentrations in milk were never higher than 40 μg/L. See bepridil, diltiazem, nifedipine as alternates. From these three studies, the relative infant dose would vary from 0.15%, 0.98%, and 0.18%, respectively. Regardless of the variability, the relative amount transferred to the infant is still quite small.

- WARFARIN   (*Coumadin, Panwarfin*)
  - ◦ AAP = Maternal Medication Usually Compatible with Breastfeeding
  - ◦ LRC = L2
  - ◦ RID =
  - ◦ Pregnancy = X
  - ◦ Comment: Warfarin is a potent anticoagulant. Warfarin is highly protein bound in the maternal circulation and, therefore, very little is secreted into human milk. Very small and insignificant amounts are secreted into milk, but it depends to some degree on the dose administered. In one study of two patients who were anticoagulated with warfarin, no warfarin was detected in the infant's serum, nor were changes in coagulation detectable. In another study of 13 mothers, less than 0.08 μmol per liter (25 ng/mL) was detected in milk, and no warfarin was detected in the infants' plasma.

Clinical Tips

The choice of medication for treating arrhythmias is largely dependent on the type of arrhythmia. Of the numerous newer antiarrhythmic drugs, few have been studied in breastfeeding mothers. Of the beta-blockers, metoprolol and perhaps propranolol are preferred. While atenolol has been commonly used and is approved by the AAP, one case of neonatal bradycardia has been reported. No reports on esmolol have been found, but it is structurally similarly to propranolol, and its short half-life suggests that its milk levels may be low. Lidocaine has been studied in several breastfeeding mothers, some at high doses (965 mg over seven hours). The maximum dose via milk is generally less than 120 μg/kg/day. In four studies thus far, all the authors suggest it is safe to breastfeed following lidocaine therapy.

Studies on flecainide and propafenone indicate low milk levels, and the authors suggest that no untoward effects were noted. Reported milk levels of verapamil vary, but none has yet been detected in the infant's plasma compartment. Due to high milk levels and untoward effects, do not use amiodarone in breastfeeding mothers for long periods.. The acute use over a few days is not necessarily contraindicated. If the mother has discontinued amiodarone, it is safe to reinstitute breastfeeding. Omega-3 fatty acids have recently been found in some studies to have a direct effect on a variety of myocardial channels, particularly potassium and calcium channels. Some, but not all, studies in men with PVCs have found a decreased risk of PVCs by 70%. Other studies similarly show a potential benefit to the use of fish oils in patients with arrhythmias.

As for anticoagulants, warfarin transfers into milk poorly and is compatible with breastfeeding. Heparin is simply too large to transfer into milk, and it would not be orally bioavailable in an infant anyway. Thus heparin is of no risk to a breastfeeding infant. Low molecular weight heparins are likewise compatible with breastfeeding. Please refer to the section on anticoagulants for further information.

Aspirin, while it produces low levels in milk, is somewhat risky. It is known to be associated with Reye syndrome when administered directly to children, although we do not know if the miniscule doses present in milk would elevate this risk. It is probably unlikely. Virtually all reported cases were in adolescent children using therapeutic doses of aspirin, not infants.

Clopidogrel has not yet been studied in breastfeeding mothers. Unfortunately, it binds irreversibly to platelet receptors, and any present in milk might alter the breastfeeding infant's platelet function slightly. It is only a theoretical risk at this time as we do not know plasma levels in the infant.

Suggested Reading

Ashikaga, H., & Marine, J. E. (2009). Prevention of atrial fibrillation: another good reason to recommend statins to women? *Heart, 95*(9), 693-694.

Brunetti, J. (2008). A brief overview of some of the changes of the American Heart Association's Guidelines for Cardiopulmonary Resuscitation and Emergency Cardiovascular Care. *Crit Care Nurs Clin North Am, 20*(3), 245-250.

Dhillon, S. K., Rachko, M., Hanon, S., Schweitzer, P., & Bergmann, S. R. (2009). Telemetry monitoring guidelines for efficient and safe delivery of cardiac rhythm monitoring to noncritical hospital inpatients. *Crit Pathw Cardiol, 8*(3), 125-126.

Guadagnoli, E., Normand, S. L., DiSalvo, T. G., Palmer, R. H., & McNeil, B. J. (2004). Effects of treatment recommendations and specialist intervention on care provided by primary care physicians to patients with myocardial infarction or heart failure. *Am J Med, 117*(6), 371-379.

Loo, B., Parnell, C., Brook, G., Southall, E., & Mahy, I. (2009). Atrial fibrillation in a primary care population: how close to NICE guidelines are we? *Clin Med, 9*(3), 219-223.

Lopes, R. D., Piccini, J. P., Hylek, E. M., Granger, C. B., & Alexander, J. H. (2008). Antithrombotic therapy in atrial fibrillation: guidelines translated for the clinician. *J Thromb Thrombolysis, 26*(3), 167-174.

Nieuwlaat, R., Eurlings, L. W., Cleland, J. G., Cobbe, S. M., Vardas, P. E., Capucci, A., et al. (2009). Atrial fibrillation and heart failure in cardiology practice: reciprocal impact and combined management from the perspective of atrial fibrillation: results of the Euro Heart Survey on atrial fibrillation. *J Am Coll Cardiol, 53*(18), 1690-1698.

Qasqas, S. A., McPherson, C., Frishman, W. H., & Elkayam, U. (2004). Cardiovascular pharmacotherapeutic considerations during pregnancy and lactation. *Cardiol Rev, 12*(4), 201-221.

Sarasin, F. P., Maschiangelo, M. L., Schaller, M. D., Heliot, C., Mischler, S., & Gaspoz, J. M. (1999). Successful implementation of guidelines for encouraging the use of beta blockers in patients after acute myocardial infarction. *Am J Med, 106*(5), 499-505.

Tiongson, J., Robin, J., Chana, A., Shin, D. D., & Gheorghiade, M. (2006). Are the American College of Cardiology/Emergency Cardiac Care (ACC/ECC) guidelines useful in triaging patients to telemetry units? *Acute Card Care, 8*(3), 155-160.

Cervical Dysplasia and Cancer

Principles of Therapy

The cervix is the distal end of the uterus that lies below the internal os. The junction between the columnar epithelium (endocervix) and the squamous epithelium (ectocervix) referred to as the squamocolumnar junction is often predisposed to dysplasia and malignancy. These changes are predominately induced by human papilloma viral infections. Other factors, such as smoking, diethylstilbesterol exposure at a young age, high numbers of sexual partners, early onset of sexual activity, and alterations in immune function, may play a role. Depending on size of tumor and grade, the rate of five year survivorship for adenocarcinoma is presently 70%, for squamous cell carcinoma is 61%, and for small cell carcinoma is 36%.

The pap smear is used to screen for both pre-invasive and invasive disease. Iniation of cervical cytology screening is recommended at age 21. An abnormal pap smear is a frequent finding, with an estimated overall abnormal pap smear rate of approximately 3.8% in US women. Pre-invasive squamous disease is graded from atypical squamous cells of undetermined significance (ASCUS), to low grade squamous intraepithelial lesions(HPV change or cervical intraepithelial neoplasia CIN 1), to high-grade squamous intraepithelial lesions (encompassing CIN 2 to 3). Testing for high risk human papilloma virus may be useful in triaging ASCUS pap smear results. Atypical glandular cells (AGC) suggests either an endocervical or endometrial etiology of pathology.

Colposcopy with directed biopsy is useful in evaluating a pap smear interpreted as AGC, ASCUS with high risk HPV +, dysplasia or suggestive of malignancy. Colposcopy with biopsy and endocervical curettage is an office procedure which typically requires no medication. Low-grade squamous intraepithelial lesions (CIN 1) can be followed with close observation and will frequently resolve without further therapy. Loop electrosurgical excision (LEEP) can be performed for more extensive disease or that which cannot be adequately evaluated and followed colposcopically. LEEP can be performed in an office setting with a paracervical block with lidocaine and the use of NSAID's or in a day surgical setting. LEEP has the advantage of obtaining a surgical specimen for pathologic evaluation. Laser vaporization and cryotherapy, while both useful treatment, do not provide a surgical specimen. Cryotherapy additionally has the disadvantage of possible recession of the squamocolumnar junction into the endocervical canal after therapy which may make future colposcopy more difficult. Women requiring treatment for cervical dysplasia require more diligent cervical surveillance for the initial two years after therapy.

Minimally invasive cervical cancers involve lesions with invasion less than 3mm. Management in this situation will depend on desire for future fertility. Early invasive diseases may be treated with cervical conization, radical hysterectomy, pelvic / paraaortic lymph node dissection, adjuvant radiation, and chemotherapy, depending on the particular disease stage.

Vaccinations against certain viral types of HPV are available and can be considered for administration, preferably prior to the onset of sexual activity and potential viral exposure. HPV vaccination is recommended for females age 9 -26. Advisory Committee on Immunization Practices (ACIP) recommend routine vaccination of 11-12 year-old females, with catch up vaccination for those 13-26. It is currently recommended that women who have undergone vaccination still obtain cervical screening.

Treatment

- Urgent colposcopy and biopsy

- Close observation of low-grade squamous intraepithelial lesions

- Loop electrosurgical excision

- Laser vaporization of transformation zone

- Cryosurgery

- Topical fluoruracil

- Hysterectomy (simple and radical) for invasive disease

- Radiation and/or chemotherapy

Medications

- CISPLATIN (*Cisplatin, Abiplatin, Bioplatino, Cis-Gry, C-Platin, Placis, Platamine*)
  - AAP = Not reviewed
  - LRC = L5
  - RID = 3.6%
  - Pregnancy =
  - Comment: Cisplatin is a platinum-containing anticancer agent. Platinum agents have high affinity for plasma proteins. Approximately 90% of cisplatin is covalently bound to plasma proteins within four hours. Following administration of radioactive cisplatin, cisplatin levels were eliminated in a biphasic manner. $T\frac{1}{2}$(alpha) was 25 to 49 minutes. $T\frac{1}{2}$(beta) was 58 to 73 hours. Other estimates of the terminal elimination half-life of total plasma cisplatin range between five to ten days. The volume of distribution is high, about 0.5 L/kg. Platinum penetrates into tissues and is irreversibly bound to tissue proteins. Platinum can be found in these tissues for years afterward.

    Plasma and breastmilk samples were collected from a 24-year-old woman treated for three prior days with cisplatin (30mg/meter). On the third day, 30 minutes prior to chemotherapy, platinum levels in milk were 0.9 mg/L and plasma levels were 0.8 mg/L. In another study, no cisplatin was found in breastmilk following a dose of 100 mg/meter². Other studies suggest that milk levels are ten fold lower than serum levels in an older lactating woman. These studies generally support the recommendation that mothers should not breastfeed while undergoing cisplatin therapy or should withhold breastfeeding for many days (>20-30). Two options are suggested: One, the breastmilk should be tested for platinum levels and not used as long as they are measurable. Two, without measuring platinum levels, breastfeeding should be permanently interrupted for this infant.

- GEMCITABINE (*Gemzar*)
  - AAP = Not reviewed

- LRC = L4
- RID =
- Pregnancy = D
- Comment: Gemcitabine is a nucleoside analogue used for the treatment of metastatic breast cancer, non-small cell lung cancer, and pancreatic cancer. Gemcitabine elimination follows a two phase elimination curve. The terminal elimination half-life is reported to be 49 minutes in females, but can range as high as 638 minutes following long infusions. The volume of distribution following short infusions (< 70 min.) was 50 L/m², indicating that gemcitabine, after short infusions, is not extensively distributed into tissues. For long infusions, the volume of distribution rose to 370 L/m², reflecting slow equilibration of gemcitabine within the tissue compartment. Gemcitabine is metabolized to an active metabolite, gemcitabine triphosphate, which can be extracted from peripheral blood mononuclear cells. The half-life of the terminal phase for gemcitabine triphosphate from mononuclear cells ranges from 1.7 to 19.4 hours. Within one week, 92% to 98% of the dose was recovered, almost entirely in the urine. No data are available on its transfer to milk, but gemcitabine levels in milk are probably quite low due to its low pKa(3.6). Women should be advised to withhold breastfeeding for seven days.

- **IFOSFAMIDE** (*Holoxan, Ifex, Ifolem, Holoxane*)

  - AAP = Not reviewed
  - LRC = L4
  - RID =
  - Pregnancy = D
  - Comment: Ifosfamide (IF) is structurally similar to Cyclophosphamide and is used in breast cancer. This family requires activation (metabolism) by the liver to produce the active cytotoxic agents. The oral bioavailability of IF is near 100% and reaches a peak at one to two hours. IF is eliminated with a mono exponential curve. The elimination half-life (T½ beta) ranges from 3.8 to 8.6 hours. Active metabolites stay in the plasma compartment with brief half-lives of four to six hours or less. Transport of IF and its metabolites into the CNS is exceedingly low (approximately 1/6th of the plasma compartment). This would suggest milk levels will probably be low when they are ultimately determined. The kinetics of this agent are highly variable depending on renal function, creatinine clearance, liver function, etc. Waiting periods before returning to breastfeeding should be adjusted for this factor. Withhold breastfeeding for at least 72 hours.

- PACLITAXEL (*Taxol*)

  - AAP = Not reviewed
  - LRC = L5
  - RID = 13.9-22.9%
  - Pregnancy = D
  - Comment: Paclitaxel is a diterpene plant product with antineoplastic activity that is derived from the bark of the western yew tree. It is an antimicrotubule agent that promotes assembly of dimeric tubulin, which is stable to depolymerization. It is a large molecular weight, highly lipophilic agent with only minimal kinetic data available. It is not known if paclitaxel enters milk, but due to the extraordinary toxicity and lipophilicity of this compound, it would be inadvisable to breastfeed while under therapy with this drug.

Clinical Tips

Worldwide, cervical cancer is the second most common malignancy in women. While most of the advances in this field have been in screening and early detection, many newer options have helped in the treatment of this syndrome. Its etiology is most commonly associated with HPV infections, but other, perhaps genetic, causes may be involved with progression of disease. Many women infected with the HPV virus will achieve an effective immune response against the infection and never develop disease. Because cervical cancer spreads by direct extension to other tissues and via lymphatics, early detection is important.

Detection during pregnancy can be problematic. If severe, or stage IB, IIA, or IVA, a radical hysterectomy is recommended. If stage IA, then delay of treatment in pregnant patients does not seem to alter the outcome, and mothers can continue with their pregnancy. However, stage IA still may require postpartum radical total abdominal hysterectomy.

Chemotherapy, such as cisplatin, for invasive cervical cancer show survival benefit. However, in breastfeeding mothers, cisplatin is retained in the body for long periods and could transfer into human milk. Thus, most women should avoid breastfeeding following the use of this metallic compound.

The use of nucleotide analogs, such as gemcitabine, may only require a brief interruption of breastfeeding, as it is rapidly cleared. Over 98% is gone in seven days.

The prolonged use of paclitaxel while breastfeeding is probably unsafe due to its incredible toxicity and the probability that it will enter milk due to its pharmacolkinetic properties.

Suggested Reading

ACOG Committee on Practice Bulletins-Gynecology. (2009). ACOG Practice Bulletin no. 109: Cervical cytology screening. Obstet Genecol, 114(6), 1409-1420.

ASCCP. (2002). 2001 consensus guidelines for the management of women with cervical cytological abnormalities. *JAMA, 287*, 2120-2129.

ASCCP. (2003). 2001 consensus guidelines for the management of women with cervical intraepithelial neoplasia. *Am J Obstet Gynecol, 189*, 295-304.

Burghardt, E., Winter, R., Tamussino, K., Pickel, H., Lahousen, M., Haas, J., et al. (1994). Diagnosis and surgical treatment of cervical cancer. *Crit Rev Oncol Hematol, 17*(3), 181-231.

Creasman, W. T., Kohler, M., & Korte, J. E. (2009). How valid are current cervical cancer prognostic factors that are used to recommend adjunctive radiation therapy after radical surgery? *Am J Obstet Gynecol, 201*(3), 260 e261-263.

Grochow, L. B., & Ames, M. M. (1998). *A clinician's guide to chemotherapy pharmacokinetics and pharmacodynamics. 1st ed.* Baltimore, MD: Williams & Wilkins.

Hill, D. A. (2009). New guidelines: fewer PAP tests for women older than 30 years and less aggressive treatment for adolescents. *Am Fam Physician, 80*(2), 131.

Hughes, C. (2009). Cervical cancer: prevention, diagnosis, treatment and nursing care. *Nurs Stand, 23*(27), 48-56; quiz 58.

Jordan, J., Arbyn, M., Martin-Hirsch, P., Schenck, U., Baldauf, J. J., Da Silva, D., et al. (2008). European guidelines for quality assurance in cervical cancer screening: recommendations for clinical management of abnormal cervical cytology, part 1. *Cytopathology, 19*(6), 342-354.

Long, H. Jr., Laack, N. N., & Gostout, B. S. (2007). Prevention, diagnosis, and treatment of cervical cancer. *Mayo Clin Proc, 82*(12), 1566-1574.

McDonald, S. D., Faught, W., & Gruslin, A. (2002). Cervical cancer during pregnancy. *J Obstet Gynaecol Can, 24*(6), 491-498.

Petignat, P., & Roy, M. (2007). Diagnosis and management of cervical cancer. *BMJ, 335*(7623), 765-768.

Ronco, G., & Giorgi Rossi, P. (2008). New paradigms in cervical cancer prevention: opportunities and risks. *BMC Womens Health, 8*, 23.

Saslow, D., Runowicz, C. D., Solomon, D., & et al. (2002). American Cancer Society guideline for the early detection of cervical neoplasia and cancer. *CA Cancer J Clin, 52*, 342-362.

Smith, R. A., Cokkinides, V., & Brawley, O. W. (2009). Cancer screening in the United States, 2009: a review of current American Cancer Society guidelines and issues in cancer screening. *CA Cancer J Clin, 59*(1), 27-41.

Teitelman, A. M., Stringer, M., Averbuch, T., & Witkoski, A. (2009). Human papilloma virus, current vaccines, and cervical cancer prevention. *J Obstet Gynecol Neonatal Nurs, 38*(1), 69-80.

Warren, J. B., Gullett, H., & King, V. J. (2009). Cervical cancer screening and updated Pap guidelines. *Prim Care, 36*(1), 131-149, ix.

Wells, S. F. (2008). Cervical cancer: an overview with suggested practice and policy goals. *Medsurg Nurs, 17*(1), 43-50; quiz 51.

Chlamydia

Principles of Therapy

Infection with *Chlamydia trachomatis* is the second most prevalent sexually transmitted disease in women and the most common bacterial genitourinary tract infection occurring in adolescents and women in their 20's in the USA. *Chlamydia trachomatis* accounts for at least 50% of reported cases of non-gonococcal urethritis. Most women are asymptomatic, although vaginal discharge, dysuria, urinary frequency, pelvic pain, and dyspareunia may occur. Studies have shown that it is particularly infectious to infants, there is a 50% risk of transmission of this infection to an infant from a mother with a cervical infection, and it is associated with conjuncitivitis and pneumonia in the infant. Cervicitis, with the characteristic yellow, mucopurulent secretion, is often present. In women, gram stains of mucopurulent discharge often show many leukocytes, but no gonococci. Complications of *Chlamydia trachomatis* are numerous and include bartholinitis, perihepatitis, chlamydial salpingitis, Reiter's syndrome, chlamydial ophthalmia neonatorum, chronic pelvic pain, ectopic pregnancy, infertility, pregnancy complications, etc.

Treatment

- Azithromycin (1 gram orally once) or doxycycline 100 mg twice daily for seven days.

- For pregnant patients, azithromycin 1 gram orally or amoxicillin 500 mg three times daily for seven days.

- Erythromycin, ofloxacin, or levofloxacin are second-line treatments.

- Doxycycline and azithromycin are equally effective, but doxycycline is much cheaper. Both are ideal for breastfeeding mothers.

- When someone is diagnosed with gonorrhea, empiric Chlamydia treatment is warranted.

- Erythromycin should be avoided early postpartum due to elevated risk of hypertrophic pyloric stenosis in the infant.

Medications

- AMOXICILLIN   (*Larotid, Amoxil*)
    - AAP = Maternal Medication Usually Compatible with Breastfeeding
    - LRC = L1
    - RID = 1%
    - Pregnancy = B

- ◦ Comment: Amoxicillin is a popular oral penicillin used for otitis media and many other pediatric/ adult infections. In one group of six mothers who received 1 gm oral doses, the concentration of amoxicillin in breastmilk ranged from 0.68 to 1.3 mg/L of milk (average= 0.9 mg/L). Peak levels occurred at four to five hours. Milk/plasma ratios at one, two and three hours were 0.014, 0.013, and 0.043. Less than 0.95% of the maternal dose is secreted into milk. No harmful effects have been reported.

- **AZITHROMYCIN** (*Zithromax*)
    - ◦ AAP = Not reviewed
    - ◦ LRC = L2
    - ◦ RID = 5.9%
    - ◦ Pregnancy = B
    - ◦ Comment: Azithromycin belongs to the erythromycin family. It has an extremely long half-life, particularly in tissues. Azithromycin is concentrated for long periods in phagocytes, which are known to be present in human milk. In one study of a patient who received 1 gm initially followed by 500 mg doses each at 24 hour intervals, the concentration of azithromycin in breastmilk varied from 0.64 mg/L (initially) to 2.8 mg/L on day three. The predicted dose of azithromycin received by the infant would be approximately 0.4 mg/kg/day. This would suggest that the level of azithromycin ingested by a breastfeeding infant is not clinically relevant.

- **DOXYCYCLINE** (*Doxychel, Vibramycin, Periostat*)
    - ◦ AAP = Not reviewed
    - ◦ LRC = L3
    - ◦ RID = 4.2-13.3%
    - ◦ Pregnancy = D
    - ◦ Comment: Doxycycline is a long half-life tetracycline antibiotic. In a study of 15 subjects, the average doxycycline level in milk was 0.77 mg/L following a 200 mg oral dose. One oral dose of 100 mg was administered 24 hours later, and the breastmilk levels were 0.380 mg/L. Following a dose of 100 mg daily in 10 mothers, doxycycline levels in milk on day two averaged 0.82 mg/L (range 0.37-1.24 mg/L) at three hours after the dose, and 0.46 mg/L (range 0.3-0.91 mg/L) 24 hours after the dose. The relative infant dose in an infant would be < 6% of the maternal weight-adjusted dosage. Following a single dose of 100 mg in three women or 200 mg in three women, peak milk levels occurred between two and four hours following the dose. The average "peak" milk levels were 0.96 mg/L (100 mg dose) or 1.8 mg/L (200 mg dose). After repeated dosing for five days, milk levels averaged 3.6 mg/L at doses of 100 mg twice daily. In a study of 13 women receiving 100-200 mg doses of doxycycline, peak levels in milk were 0.6 mg/L (n=3 @100 mg dose) and 1.1 mg/L (n=11 @ 200 mg dose).

        Tetracyclines administered orally to infants are known to bind in teeth, producing discoloration and inhibiting bone growth, although doxycycline and oxytetracycline stain teeth the least severe. Although most tetracyclines secreted into milk are generally bound to calcium, thus inhibiting their absorption, doxycycline is the least bound (20%) and may be better absorbed in a breastfeeding infant than the older tetracyclines. While the absolute absorption of older tetracyclines may be dramatically reduced by calcium salts, the newer doxycycline and minocycline analogs bind less and their overall absorption, while slowed, may be significantly higher than earlier versions.

- ERYTHROMYCIN   (*E-Mycin, Ery-Tab, Eryc, Ilosone*)
  - ◦ AAP = Maternal Medication Usually Compatible with Breastfeeding
  - ◦ LRC = L2
  - ◦ RID = 1.4-1.7%
  - ◦ Pregnancy = B
  - ◦ Comment: Erythromycin is an older, narrow-spectrum antibiotic. In one study of patients receiving 400 mg three times daily, milk levels varied from 0.4 to 1.6 mg/L. Doses as high as 2 gm per day produced milk levels of 1.6 to 3.2 mg/L. One case of hypertrophic pyloric stenosis apparently linked to erythromycin administration has been reported. In a study of two to three patients who received a single 500 oral dose, milk levels at four hours ranged from 0.9 to 1.4 mg/L, with a milk/plasma ratio of 0.92. Newer macrolide-like antibiotics (azithromycin) may preclude the use of erythromycin. A recent and large study now suggests a strong positive correlation between the use of erythromycin in breastfeeding mothers and infantile hypertrophic pyloric stenosis in newborns.

Clinical Tips

Recommended treatment includes either Azithromycin or Doxycycline. Azithromycin as a single dose of 1 gm orally is preferred due to its ease of compliance and its documented efficacy. Doxycycline 100 mgs twice daily for seven days may also be used, though azithromycin may be a better choice for breastfeeding mothers. Doxycycline is generic, much cheaper, and is an effective alternative. Another alternative treatment is erythromycin base 500 mg four times daily or Erthromycin ethylsuccinate (EES) 800mgs four times daily for seven days. Erythromycin formulations are less efficacious and are limited by nausea and vomiting as frequent side effects. In addition, it is well known that erythromycin may increase the risk of hypertropic pyloric stenosis in infants less than six weeks of age. Azithromycin is recommended instead.

Ofloxacin (300 mg PO BID for seven days) has similar efficacy as either azithromycin or doxycycline, but is more expensive and has no advantage over azithromycin. Patients should be instructed to refrain from sexual intercourse for seven days after treatment, and partners should be referred for treatment.

Treatment in pregnant patients includes azithromycin (1 gram orally once), amoxicillin 500 mg TID for seven days, or erythromycin base 500 mg four times daily for seven days. Doxycycline should not be used in pregnant patients.

It is recommended that pregnant women be retested three weeks or after treatment to assure eradication of infection. Most treatment failures are likely to result from incomplete couple therapy. Abstinence of both partners is recommended for seven days after a single dose or a seven day treatment regiem.

Suggested Reading

Baud, D., Regan, L., & Greub, G. (2008). Emerging role of Chlamydia and Chlamydia-like organisms in adverse pregnancy outcomes. *Curr Opin Infect Dis, 21*(1), 70-76.

Drury, N. E., Dyer, J. P., Breitenfeldt, N., Adamson, A. S., & Harrison, G. S. (2004). Management of acute epididymitis: are European guidelines being followed? *Eur Urol, 46*(4), 522-524; discussion 524-525.

Geisler, W. M. (2007). Management of uncomplicated Chlamydia trachomatis infections in adolescents and adults: evidence reviewed for the 2006 Centers for Disease Control and Prevention sexually transmitted diseases treatment guidelines. *Clin Infect Dis, 44 Suppl 3*, S77-83.

Miller, K. E. (2006). Diagnosis and treatment of Chlamydia trachomatis infection. *Am Fam Physician, 73*(8), 1411-1416.

MMWR. (2006). Sexually transmitted diseases treatment guidelines. MMWR, 55(RR11), 1-94.

Peipert, J. F. (2003). Clinical practice. Genital chlamydial infections. *N Engl J Med, 349*(25), 2424-2430.

Ross, J. D. (2003). Pelvic inflammatory disease: how should it be managed? *Curr Opin Infect Dis, 16*(1), 37-41.

Scholes, D., Grothaus, L., McClure, J., Reid, R., Fishman, P., Sisk, C., et al. (2006). A randomized trial of strategies to increase chlamydia screening in young women. *Prev Med, 43*(4), 343-350.

Senn, L., Hammerschlag, M. R., & Greub, G. (2005). Therapeutic approaches to Chlamydia infections. *Expert Opin Pharmacother, 6*(13), 2281-2290.

Trigg, B. G., Kerndt, P. R., & Aynalem, G. (2008). Sexually transmitted infections and pelvic inflammatory disease in women. *Med Clin North Am, 92*(5), 1083-1113.

Cholelithiasis

Principles of Therapy

Cholelithiasisis (gall stones) is a common difficulty for women, especially during pregnancy and the early postpartum period and in women over 40. Sex hormones are theorized to be implicated in physiologic changes to the biliary tract and bile acid synthesis. Progesterone appears to delay gallbladder emptying. Gallstones also appear to have a genetic predisposition, and both obesity and rapid weight loss may predispose to disease. Other diseases, such as diabetes, and medications, such as oral contraceptives and clofibrate, increase risk. Symptoms are most frequently midepigastric or right upper quadrant pain, which may be severe and develops hours after a meal and lasts one to two hours. Nausea and vomiting may occur as well.

Treatment options for gallstones depend on the particular situation and the extent of the disease. Often surgical intervention is pursued, but in some cases medical therapy or dissolution of gallstones may be undertaken. Acute care often involves the use of anti-emetics and pain medication.

Treatment

- Bile acid therapy for select patients with mild symptoms.

- Extracorporeal shock-wave lithotripsy may be successful for some patient populations.

- Cholecystectomy is often the treatment of choice and can be performed using laparoscopic techniques with minimal interruption to the breastfeeding dyad.

Medications

- CHENODEOXYCHOLIC ACID (Chenodal)
    ◦ AAP = Not reviewed
    ◦ LRC = L4
    ◦ RID =
    ◦ Pregnancy = X
    ◦ Comment = Chenodiol is the non-proprietary name for chenodeoxycholic acid, a naturally occurring human bile acid. As a bile acid, it is highly absorbable from the GI tract and approximately 80% is absorbed by the liver first pass. Because of the potential hepatoxicity of chenodiol, poor response rates in some subgroups of chenodiol-treated patients, and an increased rate of a need for cholecystectomy in other chenodiol-treated subgroups, chenodiol is not an appropriate treatment for many patients with gallstones. Chenodeoxycholic acid should be reserved for carefully selected patients, and treatment must be accompanied by systematic monitoring for liver function alterations. No data are available on its transfer into human milk, but it is unlikely due to the high first-pass uptake by the maternal liver.

- KETOROLAC (*Toradol, Acular*)
  - ○ AAP = Maternal Medication Usually Compatible with Breastfeeding
  - ○ LRC = L2
  - ○ RID = 0.2%
  - ○ Pregnancy = C in first and second trimesters
  - ○ Comment: Ketorolac is a popular, nonsteroidal analgesic. Although previously used in labor and delivery, its use has subsequently been contraindicated because it is believed to adversely effect fetal circulation and inhibit uterine contractions, thus increasing the risk of hemorrhage.

    In a study of ten lactating women who received 10 mg orally four times daily, milk levels of ketorolac were not detectable in four of the subjects. In the six remaining patients, the concentration of ketorolac in milk two hours after a dose ranged from 5.2 to 7.3 µg/L on day one and 5.9 to 7.9 µg/L on day two. In most patients, the breastmilk level was never above 5 µg/L. The maximum daily dose an infant could absorb (maternal dose = 40 mg/day) would range from 3.16 to 7.9 µg/day assuming a milk volume of 400 mL or 1000 mL. An infant would therefore receive less than 0.2% of the daily maternal dose. (Please note, the original paper contained a misprint on the daily intake of ketorolac (mg instead of µg).

- SIMVASTATIN (*Zocor*)
  - ○ AAP = Not reviewed
  - ○ LRC = L3
  - ○ RID =
  - ○ Pregnancy = X
  - ○ Comment: Simvastatin is an HMG-CoA reductase inhibitor that reduces the production of cholesterol in the liver. Like lovastatin, simvastatin reduces blood cholesterol levels. Others in this family are known to be secreted into human and rodent milk, but no data are available on simvastatin. It is likely that milk levels will be low because less than 5% of simvastatin reaches the plasma, most being removed first-pass by the liver.

    Atherosclerosis is a chronic process. Discontinuation of lipid-lowering drugs during pregnancy and lactation should have little to no impact on the outcome of long-term therapy of primary hypercholesterolemia. Cholesterol and other products of cholesterol biosynthesis are essential components for fetal and neonatal development, and the use of cholesterol-lowering drugs would not be advisable under any circumstances. Simvastatin has been shown to reduce the incidence of cholelithiasis.

- URSODIOL (*Actigall*)
  - ○ AAP = Not reviewed
  - ○ LRC = L3
  - ○ RID =
  - ○ Pregnancy = B
  - ○ Comment: Ursodiol (ursodeoxycholic acid) is a bile salt found in small amounts in humans that is used to dissolve cholesterol gallstones. It is almost completely absorbed orally via the portal circulation and is extracted almost completely by the liver. Ursodiol suppresses hepatic synthesis and excretion of cholesterol. Following extraction by the liver, it is conjugated with glycine or taurine

and is re-secreted into the hepatic bile duct. Only trace amounts are found in the plasma, and it is not likely significant amounts would be present in milk. While no breastfeeding data are available, only small amounts of bile salts are known to be present in milk. With the low levels of ursodiol in the maternal plasma, it is not likely that clinically relevant amounts would enter milk.

Clinical Tips

The primary treatment for cholelithiasis is still cholecystectomy. Cholecystectomy is curative and minimizes the concern for recurrent disease. With current laparoscopic techniques, this may often be performed in an outpatient setting with only minimal impact on the lactating dyad. For acute pain, NSAIDS, such as diclofenac or perhaps ketorolac, are preferred. Avoid most opiates which may inhibit the sphincter of odi and reduce gall bladder emptying. Meperidine is preferred for severe pain although it is a poor choice in breastfeeding mothers.

Medical therapy aimed at dissolution may be started with bile acid therapy. This is most likely successful in patients with normal gallbladder function, small stones (< 1cm), minimal calcification, and mild symptoms. Chenodeoxycholic acid and ursodeoxycholic acid have been used. Dissolution rates of 50-60% have been found with optimal results in those with small "buoyant" stones (suggesting high cholesterol content). Statins may also be of use in treatment of cholesterol gallstones, though the benefit of this compared to dissolution therapy alone is unclear.

Direct contact dissolution performed by either puncture into the gallbladder or via catheterization during ERCP with application of a solvent has also been attempted. The most commonly used solvent is Methyl tert-butyl ether (MTBE). Complications due to the solvent may occur and the risk of recurrent gallstones remains. Often oral bile acid therapy is recommended in conjunction to these procedures.

Extracorporeal shock-wave lithotripsy, either using ultrasound or fluoroscopic guidance, is another potential treatment option. Again, the therapy is most successful in patients with mild symptoms, normal gallbladder function, stones < 2 cm, three or fewer stones, and stones that are radiolucent. Obese patients are not good candidates for lithotripsy treatment, and pregnancy is an exclusion criteria. Success rates are lower with more than one stone, and complications are common. Some degree of biliary colic related to passage of stone fragments commonly occurs. Most patients will require analgesia or anesthesia. A more recent study suggested that 33% of patients undergoing lithotripsy required cholecystectomy at a later time for recurrent disease.

Surgical therapy is frequently performed for cholelithiasis and is commonly the treatment of choice. Cholecystectomy is curative and minimizes the concern for recurrent disease. With current laparoscopic techniques, this may often be performed in an outpatient setting with only minimal impact on the lactating dyad.

Chenodeoxycholic acid (Chenodiol) is presently approved by the FDA for dissolution of gallstones in patients in whom elective surgery is not advised.

Suggested Reading

Adamek HE, Rochlitz C, Von Bubnoff AC, Schilling D, Riemann JF. Predictions and associations of cholecystectomy in patients with cholecystolithiasis treated with extracorporeal shock wave lithotripsy. *Dig Dis Sci 2004*;49(11-12):1938-42.

Garcia G, Young HS. Biliary extracorporeal shock-wave lithotripsy. *Gastroenterol Clin North Am* (1991);20:201-8.

Janowitz P, Schumacher KA, Swobonik W, Kratzer W, Tudyka J, Wechsler JG. Transhepatic topical dissolution of gallbladder stones with MTBE and EDTA. Results, side effects and correlation with CT imaging. *Dig Dis Sci.* 1993;38 (11):2121-9.

Rubin RA, Kowalski TE, Khandelwal M, Malet PF. Ursodiol for hepatobiliary disorders. *Ann Intern Med.* (1994);121:207-18.

Tazuma S, Kajiyama G, Yamashita G, Miura H, Kajihara T, Hattori Y, Miyake H, Nishioka T, Hyogo H, Sumani Y, Yasumiba S, Ochi H, Matsumoto T, Abe A, Adachi K, Omata F, Ueno F, Sugata F, Ohguri S, Shibata H, Kokubu S. A combination therapy with simvastatin and ursodeoxycholic acid is more effective for cholesterol gallstone dissolution than ursodeoxycholic monotherapy. *J Clin Gastroenterol* (1998);26:287-91.

Conjunctivitis, Bacterial/Viral

Principles of Therapy

Conjunctivitis is the most common eye disorder. It may be acute or chronic and accounts for 30% of eye complaints in the US. Acute bacterial conjunctivitis is characterized by an abrupt onset of conjunctival hyperemia (redness), mucopurulent discharge, a foreign body sensation, and crusting of lids at early morning. Most cases are due to staphylococcal or streptococcal infections. Neonatal conjunctivitis may, in addition, be due to gonococci (*Ophthalmia neonatorum*) or *Chlamydia trachomatis*. Bacterial conjunctivitis is usually unilateral, while viral conjunctivitis is usually bilateral. Viral conjunctivitis is usually due to infections from adenovirus type three, four and seven. Other more severe viral infections occur, but are rare, and include varicella zoster and herpes simplex. While viral conjunctivitis often produces a watery discharge, it is easily distinguished from the mucopurulent discharge characteristically seen in bacterial infections.

Treatment

- Stop contact lens use.

- Bacterial conjunctivitis is usually self-limiting in two to five days, but can be treated with ophthalmic antibiotics.

- Ophthalmic antibiotics include fluoroquinolone (ciprofloxacin, levofloxacin, etc.), azithromycin ophthalmic solution, sulfonamide drops (trimethoprim + polymmyxin B or sulfacetamide).

- Gonococcal conjunctivitis should be treated with ceftriaxone 1 g IM.

- Viral conjunctivitis usually resolves in 10-21 days, but ophthalmic lubricants may help reduce symptoms.

- Never use ophthalmic drops that contain steroids in either of these infectious syndromes.

Medications

- AZITHROMYCIN   (*Zithromax*)
  - AAP = Not reviewed
  - LRC = L2
  - RID = 5.9%
  - Pregnancy = B
  - Comment: In one study of a patient who received 1 gm orally initially, followed by 500 mg doses each at 24 hour intervals, the concentration of azithromycin in breastmilk varied from 0.64 mg/L (initially) to 2.8 mg/L on day three. The predicted dose of azithromycin received by the infant

would be approximately 0.4 mg/kg/day. This would suggest that the level of azithromycin ingested by a breastfeeding infant is not clinically relevant. Levels of azithromycin in milk following the ophthalmic use is unknown, but probably is minimal to nil.

- **AZITHROMYCIN OPHTHALMIC DROPS** (*AzaSite*)
  - AAP = Not reviewed
  - LRC = L2
  - RID = 5.8%
  - Pregnancy = B
  - Comment: In one study of a patient who received 1 gm orally initially, followed by 500 mg doses each at 24 hour intervals, the concentration of azithromycin in breastmilk varied from 0.64 mg/L (initially) to 2.8 mg/L on day three. The predicted dose of azithromycin received by the infant would be approximately 0.4 mg/kg/day. This would suggest that the level of azithromycin ingested by a breastfeeding infant is not clinically relevant. Levels of azithromycin in milk following the ophthalmic use is unknown, but probably is minimal to nil.

- **CEFTRIAXONE** (*Rocephin*)
  - AAP = Maternal Medication Usually Compatible with Breastfeeding
  - LRC = L2
  - RID = 4.1-4.2%
  - Pregnancy = B
  - Comment: Ceftriaxone is a very popular third-generation broad-spectrum cephalosporin antibiotic. Small amounts are transferred into milk (3-4% of maternal serum level). Following a 1 gm IM dose, breastmilk levels were approximately 0.5-0.7 mg/L at between four to eight hours. The estimated mean milk levels at steady state were 3-4 mg/L. Another source indicates that following a 2 g/d dose and at steady state, approximately 4.4% of the dose penetrates into milk. In this study, the maximum breastmilk concentration was 7.89 mg/L after prolonged therapy (seven days). Poor oral absorption of ceftriaxone would further limit systemic absorption by the infant. Even at this high dose, no adverse effects were noted in the infant. Ceftriaxone levels in breastmilk are probably too low to be clinically relevant, except for changes in GI flora.

- **CIPROFLOXACIN OPHTHALMIC DROPS** (*Ciloxan*)
  - AAP = Maternal Medication Usually Compatible with Breastfeeding
  - LRC = L3
  - RID =
  - Pregnancy = C
  - Comment: Levels secreted into breastmilk (2.26 to 3.79 mg/L) are somewhat conflicting. They vary from the low to moderate range to levels that are higher than maternal serum up to 12 hours after a dose. In one study of 10 women who received 750 mg orally every 12 hours, milk levels of ciprofloxacin ranged from 3.79 mg/L at two hours postdose to 0.02 mg/L at 24 hours. As the absolute dose presented to the nursing mother is minimal, ophthalmic formulations would not be contraindicated in breastfeeding mothers.

- **ERYTHROMYCIN** (*E-Mycin, Ery-Tab, Eryc, Ilosone*)
  - AAP = Maternal Medication Usually Compatible with Breastfeeding

- ○ LRC = L2
- ○ RID = 1.4-1.7%
- ○ Pregnancy = B
- ○ Comment: Erythromycin is an older, narrow-spectrum antibiotic. In one study of patients receiving orally 400 mg three times daily, milk levels varied from 0.4 to 1.6 mg/L. Doses as high as 2 gm per day produced milk levels of 1.6 to 3.2 mg/L. In a study of two to three patients who received a single 500 oral dose, milk levels at four hours ranged from 0.9 to 1.4 mg/L, with a milk/plasma ratio of 0.92. Newer macrolide-like antibiotics (azithromycin) may preclude the use of erythromycin. A recent and large study now suggests a strong positive correlation between the use of erythromycin in breastfeeding mothers and infantile hypertrophic pyloric stenosis in newborns.

- LEVOFLOXACIN OPHTHALMIC DROPS   (*Quixin*)
  - ○ AAP = Not reviewed
  - ○ LRC = L3
  - ○ RID =
  - ○ Pregnancy = C
  - ○ Comment: In one case report of a mother receiving 500 mg/day, the 24 hour average milk level was reported to be approximately 5 μg/mL. The half-life of levofloxacin in milk was estimated to be seven hours, which would result in undetectable amounts in milk after 48 hours. The authors report the average milk level reported was 5 μg/mL. Using these data, the relative infant dose would range from 10.5% to 17% following oral administration. Observe the infant for changes in gut flora, candida overgrowth, or diarrhea. Maternal use of Levofloxacin ophthalmic drops is unlikely to cause effects in the infant.

- OFLOXACIN   (*Ocuflox*)
  - ○ AAP = Maternal Medication Usually Compatible with Breastfeeding
  - ○ LRC = L2
  - ○ RID = 3.1%
  - ○ Pregnancy = C
  - ○ Comment: Ofloxacin is a typical fluoroquinolone antimicrobial. Breastmilk concentrations are reported equal to maternal plasma levels. In one study in lactating women who received 400 mg oral doses twice daily, drug concentrations in breastmilk averaged 0.05-2.41 mg/L in milk (24 hours and two hours postdose, respectively). The drug was still detectable in milk 24 hours after a dose. The fluoroquinolones are becoming more popular in pediatrics due to recent studies and reviews showing their safe use. It is very unlikely that arthropathy would ensue following the dose received via milk. The only probable risk is a change in gut flora, diarrhea, and a remote risk of overgrowth of *Clostridium difficile*. Ofloxacin levels in breastmilk are consistently lower (37%) than ciprofloxacin. If a fluoroquinolone is required, ofloxacin, levofloxacin, or norfloxacin drops are probably the better choices for breastfeeding mothers.

Clinical Tips

Hyperacute bacterial conjunctivitis is a severe, sight-threatening infection that warrants immediate care. It is characterized by copious yellow-green purulent discharge of abrupt onset. Symptoms also include redness, irritation, tenderness, lid swelling, and conjunctival chemosis (edema). The most frequent causes of hyperacute bacterial conjunctivitis are *N. gonorrhoeae* and *Neisseria meningitidis*. Gonococcal infections occur most commonly in newborns (five days postpartum) and young adults (sexually active). All patients with severe symptoms should be treated with systemic antibiotics supplemented by topical ocular antibiotics and saline. The systemic agent of choice is ceftriaxone (Rocephin), due to the prevalence of resistance of *N. gonorrhoeae,* although a two-week course of systemic erythromycin is effective for gonococcal infections.

Acute bacterial conjunctivitis typically presents with irritation, burning, excessive tearing, and usually a mucopurulent discharge. Eye matting on awakening, conjunctival swelling, and mild eyelid edema may be noted. The most common pathogens are *S. pneumoniae*, *H. influenzae,* and *Staphylococcus aureus*. Topical preparations suitable for these milder infections include erythromycin ointment, ciprofloxacin, ofloxacin, or gatifloxacin drops, or trimethoprim-polymyxin B (Polytrim). While the aminoglycosides can be used in some cases, they do not cover gram-positive species as well, including staphylococcus and streptococcus.

For gonococcal conjunctivitis, systemic antibiotics are recommended, and include ceftriaxone 1 gm intramuscularly once. For infants, ceftriaxone 25-50 mg/kg intravenously or intramuscularly once is recommended.

For chlamydial conjunctivitis, erythromycin base (50 mg/kg/day) divided into four doses daily for 14 days is recommended. While these are the present recommendations, azithromycin could potentially be substituted for erythromycin and reduce the risk of pyloric stenosis known to occur in neonates following erythromycin use.

For maternal conjunctivitis, the Fluoroquinolones, which include ciprofloxacin, levofloxacin, ofloxacin, and norfloxacin (Chibroxin), are becoming more popular and are very effective, particularly in those patients hypersensitive to erythromycins or penicillins. However, they are not effective for MRSA conjunctivitis. Although they are not cleared for pediatric use, the amount of maternal absorption following maternal use (via ocular administration) is minimal and would produce exceedingly low levels in milk, probably undetectable. Due to cost, these agents should probably be reserved for resistant cases that have documented sensitivity studies showing efficacy of these agents. Gentamycin and tobramycin are probably unsuitable, due to major resistance in streptococcal strains. Polymyxin B only covers gram-negative organisms, so it is relatively ineffective when used alone.

The ophthalmic use of chloramphenicol, while effective, has been associated with subsequent cases of aplastic anemia and thus should be avoided.

Viral Conjunctivitis:

Viral conjunctivitis is usually due to infections from adenovirus type three or seven. There are no real treatments for this syndrome, other than warm eye compresses and lubricant eye drops. Adenoviral infections generally resolve in 10-21 days. Infections due to herpes simplex and varicella zoster should be considered emergency situations and probably require a referral to an ophthalmologist for immediate treatment with antivirals. NEVER use steroids in viral infections of the eye.

Suggested Reading

Epling, J., & Smucny, J. (2005). Bacterial conjunctivitis. In: *Clinical Evidence*. London: BMJ Publishing Group.

Mandal, R., Banerjee, A. R., Biswas, M. C., Mondal, A., Kundu, P. K., & Sasmal, N. K. (2008). Clinicobacteriological study of chronic dacryocystitis in adults. *J Indian Med Assoc, 106*(5), 296-298.

Rietveld, R. P., ter Riet, G., Bindels, P. J., Schellevis, F. G., & van Weert, H. C. (2007). Do general practitioners adhere to the guideline on infectious conjunctivitis? Results of the Second Dutch National Survey of General Practice. *BMC Fam Pract, 8*, 54.

Sheikh, A., Hurwitz, B., & Cave, J. (2000). Antibiotics versus placebo for acute bacterial conjunctivitis. . *Cochrane Database of Systematic Reviews* (1).

Shields, S. R. (2000). Managing eye disease in primary care. Part 2. How to recognize and treat common eye problems. *Postgrad Med, 108*(5), 83-86, 91-86.

Yetman, R. J., & Coody, D. K. (1997). Conjunctivitis: a practice guideline. *J Pediatr Health Care, 11*(5), 238-241.

Contraception

Principles of Therapy

It is generally recognized that most women who breastfeed exclusively enter a period of lactational amenorrhea. During this time, potential for ovulation is reduced. Conception rates during lactational amenorrhea vary over time since delivery. During the first six months post-partum, in the exclusively breastfeeding woman experiencing amenorrhea, the chances of conception are approximately 0.5 to 2%. For this effectiveness, supplementation should be avoided and the longest nighttime feeding interval should be no longer than six hours, with eight or greater feedings daily. Over the next six months, chances for conception increase, though some reduction in fertility is preserved while amenorrhea persists. In mothers providing exclusive breastmilk for their young infants, but who are separated from the infants and, therefore, using milk expression, the effectiveness of lactational amenorrhea method (LAM) may be slightly decreased, with an anticipated pregnancy rate of about 5% at six months. Some contraceptives when used injudiciously can seriously impact breastmilk production and reduce the growth rate of the infant. This most often occurs with estrogen-containing products. For this reason, it is well known that during the first six to eight weeks postpartum, oral contraceptives containing estrogens should be strongly discouraged. Many authorities agree that breastfeeding women should avoid estrogen-containing products throughout breastfeeding. Progestin-only products are generally preferred for breastfeeding mothers, as they have consistently been found to produce fewer effects on breastmilk production.

Treatment

- Lactational amenorrhea effectiveness is 98% during initial first six months of exclusive breastfeeding if amenorrhea persists.

- Provide easy availability to alternate contraception once LAM is no longer applicable.

- Non-hormonal options do not impact lactation but barrier methods may lack desired efficacy once fertility resumes.

- Ideally, defer beginning hormonal contraceptive options until after lactation is well established (six week postpartum visit).

- Progesterone-only contraceptive options may, but are less likely, to negatively impact milk production.

- If estrogen containing (combination) contraception is chosen, use lowest estrogen dosage appropriate and instruct mother to monitor milk supply.

Contraceptive Types

Barrier Contraceptives

Barrier methods of contraception, such as diaphragms and condoms, have no impact on milk production, and though they offer reduced efficacy compared to many alternatives, they may be satisfactory during lactation due to the relative reduction in fertility afforded by lactation. Barrier methods may require the use of vaginal lubricants during lactation due to the vaginal atrophy frequently experienced by recently postpartum and lactating women. The following table suggests the efficacy expected in the "typical" user, not specific for lactating women. Failure rates for typical use of condom, diaphragm, and contraceptive sponge are similiar at approximately 15%. The use of spermicide only, female condom, cervical cap, withdrawal, and rhythm methods are somewhat less effective. Symptom-based fertility monitoring may be more challenging during the postpartum period due to the variability of return to fertility during lactation.

Method	"Typical" Use Efficacy
Spermicide	79%
Male Condom	85%
Female Condom	85%
Diaphragm	
Cervical Cap	82%
Rhythm method	

Mechanical Contraceptives (IUD)

Mechanical methods of contraception may or may not have hormonal effects that could be pertinent to lactation. Those that are non-hormonal do not impact milk supply. A major disadvantage to the intrauterine device or IUD is that it requires insertion and removal by a healthcare provider. Some older information suggests that there may be a slight increased risk of uterine perforation upon insertion of the IUD in lactating women, though this risk is quite small and should not dissuade IUD use in otherwise good candidates for this contraceptive option. Currently, available alternative IUD's may be the non-hormonal copper containing type or the hormonal progesterone containing type. Progesterone doses in the IUD are low and are felt to exert a local effect on the endometrial lining which minimizes vaginal bleeding. To what extent these progesterone IUD's result in blood levels which could impact lactation has not been well investigated, but is speculated to be less than that of other progesterone contraceptive methods. Effectiveness of the IUD for contraception is approximately 97%. IUD's are typically placed at six weeks postpartum or later due to an increased risk of IUD expulsion when placed in the early postpartum period.

Medications

- LEVONORGESTREL   (*Seasonale, Mirena IUD*)
    - AAP = Maternal Medication Usually Compatible with Breastfeeding
    - LRC = L2
    - RID =

- ○ Pregnancy = X
- ○ Comment: Levonorgestrel (LNG) is the active progestin in Norplant and Mirena. Norplant is a contraceptive method that involves placing six match-size, flexible capsules under the skin of a woman's upper arm. These release a low dose of synthetic progestin continuously for up to five years. Mirena is a levonorgestrel-releasing intrauterine (IUD) contraceptive that delivers 20 µg/day of levonorgestrel directly into the uterus and protects against pregnancy for up to five full years. The contraceptive effect of Mirena is mainly based on the local effects of levonorgestrel in the uterine cavity.

From several studies, levonorgestrel appears to produce limited, if any, effect on milk volume or quality. One report of 120 women with implants at five to six weeks postpartum showed no change in lactation. The level of progestin in the infant is approximately 10% that of maternal circulation. In a study of nine women who were taking levonorgestrel oral minipills (30 µg daily) and 10 women who were using the subdermal implants from 4-15 weeks postpartum, no significant differences in infant follicle stimulating hormone (FSH), luteinizing hormone (LH), or testosterone levels in urine were noted when compared to controls. These results suggest that the sexual development of children exposed via milk to trace levels of LNG is normal.

The plasma concentration of levonorgestrel produced by Mirena is even lower than those produced by LNG contraceptive implants and with oral contraceptives. Because Mirena produces even lower plasma levels of this progestin, it is probably less likely to affect milk production than oral or implantable forms of progestins.

In a recent study of 163 and 157 women who received Mirena intrauterine systems or a Copper T380A intrauterine device, respectively, no change in breastfeeding rate, infant growth, or infant development was noted over 12 months in either the LNG-containing insert or the copper insert. Only approximately 0.1% of the serum dose of LNG has been reported to transfer via milk to infants. Increased endometrial copper concentrations have been noted in a study of 95 breastfeeding mothers with copper intrauterine devices, but no change was noted in serum or milk copper concentrations.

The data from the levonorgestrel-only intrauterine devices suggest minimal to no effect on breastfeeding.

The Seasonale extended-cycle oral contraceptive contains both levonorgestrel and ethinyl estradiol. It is used continuously for a three month period followed by withdrawal and menstruation. Due to its estrogen content, caution is recommended in breastfeeding mothers due to potential reduced milk supply.

Progestin-Only Containing Contraceptives

Progestin-only contraceptives are generally preferred in breastfeeding women over combination hormonal contraceptives containing estrogen. Depending on the particular contraceptive, these methods are also highly efficacious. Often progestin-only contraceptives result in irregular menstruation in non-lactating women. In lactating women, however, amenorrhea is a frequent occurrence, and the woman should be counseled about this anticipated result. The fall in progesterone that occurs after delivery is important in establishment of the mother's milk supply. Theoretically, initiating progestin contraception in the first few days after delivery could theoretically interfere with this natural process and result in poor milk supply. To date, there has been inadequate research done regarding the potential impact of early initiation of progestin contraception to provide sufficient scientific guidance. Information from those studies that have been done looking at early initiation of progesterone-only contraception do not document problems with poor milk supply or infant growth, but have been done in largely mixed feeding populations. It is prudent to begin these forms of contraception four to six weeks after delivery or later, unless circumstances require earlier use. This would be unlikely if exclusive breastfeeding is anticipated. Progestin-only contraception is available as a daily pill, injectable medication, implantable device, vaginal ring (not presently available in US), and in IUD's. Injectable and implantable devices have the benefit of improved efficacy and less reliance on user compliance, but are less easily reversible should concerns about milk supply develop. Theoretically, norethindrone-containing oral contraceptives may have some potential peripheral conversion to estrogen that levonorgestrel pills lack; however, no clinical difference has been noted with regard to lactation. Another potential concern has been the exposure of the nursing infant to hormones. Though progestins have been detected in breastmilk of mothers using these contraceptive methods, adverse outcomes have not been found in the nursing infant.

Medications

- ETONOGESTREL IMPLANT   (*Implanon*)
    - ◦ AAP = Not reviewed
    - ◦ LRC = L2
    - ◦ RID =
    - ◦ Pregnancy = X
    - ◦ Comment: Implanon is a slow release single-rod contraceptive implant. It consists of a non-biodegradable rod, measuring 40 mm in length and 2 mm in diameter, which releases, on average, 40 μg/day of etonogestrel over a three year period of use. Etonogestrel is the biologically active metabolite of desogestrel and has both high progestational activity and low intrinsic androgenicity. Implanon does not contain estrogen, making it suitable for women who do not tolerate or are advised not to use estrogens. Small amounts of progestins are known to pass into milk, but long-term follow-up of children whose mothers used hormonal contraceptives while breastfeeding has shown no deleterious effects on infants. Like other progestogen-only contraceptives, the use of Implanon is associated with irregular menstrual bleeding and sometimes absence of bleeding. Counseling is required to ensure women make informed choices. Of the contraceptives, progestin-only contraceptives are generally preferred as they produce fewer changes in milk production compared to estrogen-containing products. This product is probably quite safe for use in breastfeeding mothers, although all mothers should be counseled to observe for changes in milk production.

- MEDROXYPROGESTERONE   (*Provera, Depo-Provera, Cycrin*)
    - ◦ AAP = Maternal Medication Usually Compatible with Breastfeeding
    - ◦ LRC = L1
    - ◦ RID =
    - ◦ Pregnancy = X
    - ◦ Comment: Depo Medroxyprogesterone (DMPA) is a synthetic progestin compound. It is used orally for amenorrhea, dysmenorrhea, uterine bleeding, and infertility. It is used intramuscularly for contraception. Due to its poor oral bioavailability, it is seldom used orally.

    Saxena has reported that the average concentration in milk is 1.03 μg/L. Koetswang reported average milk levels of 0.97 μg/L. In a series of huge studies, the World Health Organization reviewed the developmental skills of children and their weight gain following exposure to progestin-only contraceptives during lactation. These studies documented that no adverse effects on overall development or rate of growth were notable. Further, they suggested there is no apparent reason to deny lactating women the use of progestin-only contraceptives, preferably after six weeks postpartum.

The use of Depo-Provera in breastfeeding women is common, but will probably always be somewhat controversial. Depo Provera has been documented to significantly elevate prolactin levels in breastfeeding mothers and increase milk production in some mothers.

It is well known, but undocumented, that estrogens may suppress milk production. With progestins, it has been suggested that some women may experience a decline in milk production or arrested early production following an injection of DMPA, particularly when the progestin is used early postpartum (12-48 hours). At present, there are no published data to support this, nor is the relative incidence of this untoward effect known. Therefore, in some instances, it might be advisable to recommend treatment with oral progestin-only contraceptives postpartum rather than DMPA, so that women who experience reduced milk supply can easily withdraw from the medication without significant loss of breastmilk supply. Progestins should be avoided early postnatally, and perhaps longer.

- NORETHINDRONE   (*Aygestin, Norlutate, Micronor, NOR-Q.D.*)
  - ◦ AAP = Not reviewed
  - ◦ LRC = L1
  - ◦ RID =
  - ◦ Pregnancy = X
  - ◦ Comment: Norethindrone is a typical synthetic progestational agent that is used for oral contraception and other endocrine functions. It produces a dose-dependent suppression of lactation at higher doses, although somewhat minimal at lower doses. It may reduce lactose content and reduce overall milk volume and nitrogen/protein content, resulting in lower infant weight gain, although these effects are unlikely if doses are kept low. Progestin-only mini pills are preferred oral contraceptives in breastfeeding mothers.

    However, recent reports claim that Micronor can be associated with decreased breastmilk production. In a report of 13 women taking Micronor who presented with poor milk production, 10 women experienced an increase in lactation upon withdrawl of Micronor. While norethindrone birth control pills are considered ideal for most breastfeeding mothers, some women retain sensitivity to these products and may suffer from reduced milk production. Each and every breastfeeding mother should be individually counseled about the possible reduction in milk synthesis following the use of this product.

Estrogen-Containing Combination Contraceptives

Estrogen-containing contraceptives are not recommended as an initial choice for breastfeeding women due to the possible negative impact on milk supply. This effect is more pronounced with higher estrogen levels. Many commercially advertised "low dose" estrogen containing birth control pills are available with estrogen doses ranging from 20 to 35 µg of estrogen. If a breastfeeding woman chooses an estrogen-containing contraceptive, theoretically the lower estrogen dose should have the least impact on milk supply. A 20 µg pill would be the best available oral option. Many different progestins are available in combination oral contraceptives. The impact of the different progestins on lactation has not been well studied. Most research has focused only on the different estrogen amounts available in different pills. Various progestins have slightly different side effect profiles, so differences in effect on lactation are possible. Drosperinone is a progestin, which has a spironolactone-like effect. Though this may be beneficial for the side effect profile of this oral contraceptive in general, there is a small theoretic risk that this could impact milk supply, though scientific investigation in this regard has not been done. Additionally, there are rare concerns regarding electrolyte changes with elevated potassium levels in women using other specific medications.

All estrogen containing contraceptives have an increased risk of thromboembolism relative to no contraception. Estrogen-containing contraceptives should not be used in women with known contraindications, such as prior history of thromboembolism, current pregnancy, migraines with focal neurologic signs, coronary artery disease, and cerebral vascular disease. Additionally, estrogen-containing contraception is not recommended in women over age 35 who smoke, have hypertension, vascular disease, or obesity.

Estrogen-containing oral contraceptive pills contain varying amounts of ethinyl estradiol, in addition to one of several different progestin compounds. These products have slightly different combinations and doses designed to give various different formulations slightly different side effect profiles. The impact of various different combinations on the lactating mother-baby dyad has not been well researched. Reduction in milk supply seems to at least be related to the amount of estrogen contained in the contraceptive. Therefore, theoretically the lowest estrogen dose available would be expected to be least detrimental to milk supply, though some effect would still be expected. If this method is chosen, begin the lowest estrogen dose available after milk supply has been well established, and counsel the patient about the potential for reduction in milk supply and discontinuation of the pills if milk volume reduction is noted.

A transdermal patch is available which delivers both an estrogen and progestin. The patch is changed weekly for three weeks and then remains off the forth week during which time withdrawal bleeding ensues. It is felt that this formuation has somewhat higher peak estrogen levels, which would likely make this a less desirable option for a breastfeeding mother, and higher levels would be more likely to adversely impact supply. Additionally, there may be a slight increase in the risk of clotting complications with this method, though the overall risk remains quite low.

A vaginal delivery method for estrogen and a progestin is available as a vaginal ring. This device is self-inserted by the woman, remains in the vagina for three weeks, and is then removed with withdrawal bleeding following removal. The absorbed estrogen dosage with this formulation is felt to be quite low. This option may be similar or even preferable to a 20 microgram estrogen pill in a breastfeeding mother who chooses a combination contraceptive option after counseling. There is currently no available research to substantiate the best estrogen-containing option during breastfeeding, and future research in this area is needed.

Medications

- ETONOGESTREL + ETHINYL ESTRADIOL   (*NuvaRing*)
  - AAP = Not reviewed
  - LRC = L3
  - RID =
  - Pregnancy = X
  - Comment: NuvaRing is a slow release vaginal ring which releases on average 0.120 mg/day of etonogestrel and 0.015 mg/day of ethinyl estradiol over a three week period of use. Etonogestrel is the biologically active metabolite of desogestrel and has both high progestational activity with low intrinsic androgenicity. The bioavailability of ethinyl estradiol when administered intravaginally

is approximately 55.6%, which is comparable to when it is administered orally. Small amounts of estrogens and progestins are known to pass into milk, but long-term follow-up of children whose mothers used combination hormonal contraceptives while breastfeeding has shown no deleterious effects on infants. Estrogen-containing contraceptives may interfere with milk production by decreasing the quantity and quality of milk production.

- NORELGESTROMIN + ETHINYL ESTRADIOL   (*Ortho Evra*)
  - AAP = Not reviewed
  - LRC = L3
  - RID =
  - Pregnancy =
  - Comment: Ortho Evra is a new combination progestin and estrogen-containing patch. It delivers approximately 150 μg/day norelgestromin and 20 μg/d ethinyl estradiol to the plasma compartment of the female. Small amounts of estrogens and progestins are known to pass into milk, but long-term follow-up of children whose mothers used combination hormonal contraceptives while breastfeeding has shown no deleterious effects on infants. Estrogen-containing contraceptives may interfere with milk production by decreasing the quantity and quality of milk production.

Post-Coital Contraception

Post-coital contraception is also known as the "morning after" pill or emergency contraception. For this to provide optimal effectiveness in preventing pregnancy, it should be initiated as soon as possible, but within 72 hours of unprotected intercourse. Some studies suggest moderate effectiveness even when the initial dosage is given up to 120 hours after intercourse. The progesterone-only form described below is slightly more efficacious and is less likely to negatively impact lactation.

- LEVONORGESTREL + ETHINYL ESTRADIOL   (*Preven*)
  - AAP = Not reviewed
  - LRC = L3
  - RID =
  - Pregnancy = X
  - Comment: Levonorgestrel and ethinyl estradiol (Preven) can be used as an emergency contraceptive. It is believed to act by preventing ovulation or fertilization by altering tubal transport of sperm and/or ova. It may partially inhibit implantation by altering the endometrium. For more details on each ingredient, see their individual monographs.

    Preven is an emergency contraceptive that can be used to prevent pregnancy following unprotected intercourse or a known or suspected contraceptive failure. It is not effective if the woman is already pregnant or once the process of implantation has begun. Each tablet contains 0.25 mg levonorgestrel and 0.05 mg ethinyl estradiol. They should not be used in known or suspected pregnancy, or in patients with pulmonary edema, ischemic heart disease, deep vein thrombosis, etc. The initial treatment of two tablets should be administered as soon as possible, but within 72 hours of unprotected intercourse. This is followed by the second dose of two tablets 12 hours later.

- LEVONORGESTREL (*Plan B*)
  - ◦ AAP = Not reviewed
  - ◦ LRC = L2
  - ◦ RID =
  - ◦ Pregnancy = X
  - ◦ Comment: Levonorgestrel is a progestin that can be used as an emergency contraceptive. It is believed to act by preventing ovulation or fertilization by altering tubal transport of sperm and/or ova. It may partially inhibit implantation by altering the endometrium. For more details, see detailed monograph on levonorgestrel.

    Plan B is an emergency contraceptive that can be used to prevent pregnancy following unprotected intercourse or a known or suspected contraceptive failure. It is not effective if the woman is already pregnant or once the process of implantation has begun. To obtain maximal efficacy, the first tablet should be taken as soon as possible within 72 hours of intercourse. The second tablet should be taken 12 hours later.

    A study of 12 breastfeeding mothers showed levonorgestrel peak concentrations in plasma at one to four hours postdose, and in milk two to four hours postdose after a 1.5 mg dose of levonorgestrel. Estimated infant exposure to the drug was 1.6 μg on the day of the dose, 0.3 μg the day after, and 0.2 μg on the third day. Therefore, nursing mothers who use relatively high doses of levonorgestrel are recommended to discontinue nursing for at least eight hours postdose. They can resume feeding within 24 hours.

Clinical Tips

It is now well known that estrogen-containing birth control products can seriously reduce breastmilk production and should be avoided in breastfeeding women. Most authorities agree, including the World Health Organization, that breastfeeding women should avoid estrogen-containing products throughout breastfeeding. Estrogens significantly reduce lactose and protein production in the alveolar epithelial cells that produce milk, hence milk volume and protein content may be reduced in many patients.

While numerous forms of birth control medications exist, the most important consideration is the presence of estrogen, regardless of the form. Rings, gels, and even patches containing estrogen produce clinical ranges in the plasma of the user; hence, they may suppress milk production just as oral tablet formulations. These would not be easily reversible if a decrease in milk production were to occur. During the early postpartum period (after six weeks), progestin-only products are strongly recommended. If the patient is non-compliant, then the injectable medroxyprogesterone may be used. However, there are reports suggesting that even with Depo-Provera, some patients may have reduced milk supply, particularly if used before breastfeeding is well established (particularly the first week postpartum). For this reason, a preliminary trial of low-dose oral progestin-only products (norethindrone 0.35 mg, norgestrel 0.075 mg) is suggested. If the mother's milk supply is sustained following use of these products, then the repository form of medroxyprogesterone (Depo-Provera), the implantable levonorgestrel (Implanon) system or the levonorgesterel IUD (Mirena) could probably be used safely. Frequently reported break-through bleeding experienced by the non-lactating woman using progestin-only products is much less common in the postpartum period of breastfeeding mothers. Numerous studies show that the amount of progestin/estrogen transferred via milk to the infant is low and would not be expected to have an effect on the breastfed infant.

Suggested Reading

Academy of Breastfeeding Medicine Committee. (2006). ABM clinical protocol #13: contraception during breastfeeding. *Breastfeed Med, 1*(1), 43-51.

Erdahl, K. J., & Holten, K. B. (2006). Emergency contraception care. *J Fam Pract, 55*(12), 1073-1075.

Guilbert, E., Boroditsky, R., Black, A., Kives, S., Leboeuf, M., Mirosh, M., et al. (2007). Canadian Consensus Guideline on Continuous and Extended Hormonal Contraception, 2007. *J Obstet Gynaecol Can, 29*(7 Suppl 2), S1-32.

Isley, M. M., & Edelman, A. (2007). Contraceptive implants: an overview and update. *Obstet Gynecol Clin North Am, 34*(1), 73-90.

Peterson, H. B., & Curtis, K. M. (2005). Clinical practice. Long-acting methods of contraception. *N Engl J Med, 353*(20), 2169-2175.

Rowlands, S. (2009). New technologies in contraception. *BJOG, 116*(2), 230-239.

Spencer, A. L., Bonnema, R., & McNamara, M. C. (2009). Helping women choose appropriate hormonal contraception: update on risks, benefits, and indications. *Am J Med, 122*(6), 497-506.

Cough

Principles of Therapy

Cough is one of the most common complaints presented to physicians in the USA, accounting for 3.6% of all office visits. Cough is generally characterized by duration and etiology. The cough reflex is generally stimulated by activation of the receptors located in the tracheobronchial tree, the upper airway, and in other areas, such as the sinuses, pleura, pericardium, esophagus, and other sites. The four most common causes are: postnasal drip due to allergies, cough-variant asthma, gastroesophageal reflux, and postinfectious pulmonary infections. Occasionally, acute cough can result from inflammation and mild bronchospasm of the airways. Chronic, persistent cough should always be considered abnormal. Chronic persistent cough often occurs in smokers, asthmatics, and patients with chronic obstructive pulmonary disorder. Persistent, hacking cough can also occur following the use of drugs, such as the ACE inhibitors, beta-blockers, L-dopa, environmental chemicals, or in cardiac disease. Treatment requires an accurate determination of etiology. Removal of offending agents, such as ACE inhibitors, environmental chemicals, and allergens in the case of asthmatics, may be required in those select patients. Treatment of infectious conditions may be required in those with infected sinuses. Acute cough, particularly in cases of influenza, may require the temporary use of opioids, such as codeine or dextromethorphan.

Treatment

- Determination of etiology first.

- Removal of offending agents, such as ACE inhibitors, environmental chemicals, and allergens in the case of asthmatics, may be required in those select patients.

- Treatment of postnasal drip.

- Treatment of gastroesophageal drip or nasal congestion.

- Treatment of infectious conditions may be required in those with infected sinuses.

- Sore or irritated throats may respond to topical preparations, such as OTC lozenges, honey, and other soothing products.

- Acute cough, particularly in cases of influenza, may require the temporary use of opioids, such as codeine or dextromethorphan.

Medications

- BECLOMETHASONE   (*Vanceril, Beclovent, Beconase*)
    - AAP = Not reviewed
    - LRC = L2
    - RID =
    - Pregnancy = C
    - Comment: Beclomethasone is a potent steroid that is generally used via inhalation in asthma or via intranasal administration for allergic rhinitis. Due to its potency, only very small doses are generally used; therefore, minimal plasma levels are attained. Intranasal absorption is generally minimal. Due to small doses administered, absorption into maternal plasma is extremely small. Therefore, it is unlikely that these doses would produce clinical significance in a breastfeeding infant. See corticosteroids.

- CODEINE   (*Empirin #3 # 4, Tylenol # 3 # 4*)
    - AAP = Maternal Medication Usually Compatible with Breastfeeding
    - LRC = L3
    - RID = 8.1%
    - Pregnancy = C
    - Comment: Codeine is considered a mild opiate analgesic whose action is probably due to its metabolism to small amounts (about 7%) of morphine. The amount of codeine secreted into milk is low and dose dependent. Infant response is higher during the neonatal period (first or second week). Four cases of neonatal apnea have been reported following administration of 60 mg codeine every four to six hours to breastfeeding mothers, although codeine was not detected in serum of the infants tested. Apnea resolved after discontinuation of maternal codeine. Tylenol # 3 tablets contain 30 mg and Tylenol #4 tablets contain 60 mg of codeine in the USA.

      In a study of seven mothers consuming 60 mg codeine, codeine and morphine levels were studied in breastmilk of 17 samples, and neonatal plasma of 24 samples from 11 healthy, term neonates. Milk codeine levels ranged from 33.8 to 314 µg/L 20 to 240 minutes after codeine; morphine levels ranged from 1.9 to 20.5 µg/L. Infant plasma samples one to four hours after feeding had codeine levels ranging from <0.8 to 4.5 µg/L; morphine ranged from <0.5 to 2.2 µg/L. The authors suggest that moderate codeine use during breastfeeding (< or = four 60 mg doses) is probably safe.

      In a recent report, an infant death was reported following the use of codeine 30 mg (initially two tablets every 12 hours, reduced to half that dose from day two to two weeks because of maternal somnolence and constipation) in a mother. Codeine levels in milk were reported to be 87 µg/L, while the average reported milk levels in most mothers range from 1.9 to 20.5 µg/L at doses of 60 mg every six hours. Genotype analysis of this specific mother indicated that she was an ultra-rapid metabolizer of codeine. This genotype (which is very rare) leads to increased formation of morphine from codeine.

      Ultimately, each infant's response to exposure to codeine should be independently determined. In the vast majority of mothers, codeine taken in moderation should be safe for their breastfed infant. However, any report of overt somnolence, apnea, poor feeding, or grey skin should be reported to the physician and could be associated with exposure to codeine.

- DEXTROMETHORPHAN   (*DM, Benylin, Delsym, Pertussin, Robitussin DM*)
    - AAP = Not reviewed
    - LRC = L1
    - RID =
    - Pregnancy = C
    - Comment: Dextromethorphan is a weak antitussive commonly used in infants and adults. It is a congener of codeine and appears to elevate the cough threshold in the brain. It does not have addictive, analgesic, or sedative actions, and it does not produce respiratory depression at normal doses. It is the safest of the antitussives and is routinely used in children and infants. No data on its transfer to human milk are available. It is very unlikely that enough would transfer via milk to provide clinically significant levels in a breastfed infant.

- FLUTICASONE   (*Flonase, Flovent, Cutivate, Veramyst*)
    - AAP = Not reviewed
    - LRC = L3
    - RID =
    - Pregnancy = C
    - Comment: Fluticasone is a typical steroid primarily used intranasally for allergic rhinitis and intrapulmonary for asthma. Intranasal form is called Flonase or Veramyst, inhaled form is Flovent. When instilled intranasally, the absolute bioavailability is less than 2%, so virtually none of the dose is absorbed systemically. Oral absorption following inhaled fluticasone is approximately 30%, although almost instant first-pass absorption virtually eliminates plasma levels of fluticasone. Peak plasma levels following inhalation of 880 µg is only 0.1 to 1.0 nanogram/mL. Adrenocortical suppression following oral or even systemic absorption at normal doses is extremely rare due to limited plasma levels. Plasma levels are not detectable when using suggested doses. Although fluticasone is secreted into milk of rodents, the dose used was many times higher than found under normal conditions. With the above limited oral and systemic bioavailability and rapid first-pass uptake by the liver, it is not likely that milk levels will be clinically relevant, even with rather high doses.

Clinical Tips

Treatment of cough depends solely on the etiology of the syndrome. Protocols are based on the anatomy and distribution of the cough (anatomic diagnostic protocol). Acute severe cough of infectious etiology is generally treated with antimicrobials and antitussives, such as dextromethorphan or codeine. Of course, infections of viral etiology are only treated occasionally and with similar antitussives. Cough of inflammatory origin, such as in asthmatics, is generally treated with inhaled steroids and beta-2 agonists, such as albuterol (see asthma). Maternal plasma levels of these agents are generally far too low to produce clinically relevant milk levels. Cough following postnasal drip of allergic etiology is best treated with intranasal steroids or non-sedating antihistamines. Coughs due to gastroesophageal reflux are managed with lifestyle changes, including eating a high protein low fat diet, avoiding eating for two hours prior to lying down, elevating the head of the bed, using prokinetic drugs, such as metoclopramide, or acid blocking drugs, such as famotidine, nizatidine, or omeprazole. Regardless of the etiology, the best antitussives still contain codeine or hydrocodone. Dextromethorphan is the least effective.

Suggested Reading

Chung, K. F., McGarvey, L., & Widdicombe, J. (2006). American College of Chest Physicians' cough guidelines. *Lancet, 367*(9515), 981-982.

Chung, K. F., & Widdicombe, J. (2009). The 2008 Fifth International Cough Symposium: mechanisms and treatment. *Pulm Pharmacol Ther, 22*(2), 57-58.

Dettmar, P. W., Strugala, V., Fathi, H., Dettmar, H. J., Wright, C., & Morice, A. H. (2009). The online Cough Clinic: developing guideline-based diagnosis and advice. *Eur Respir J, 34*(4), 819-824.

Dettmar, P. W., Strugala, V., Fathi, H., Dettmar, H. J., Wright, C., & Morice, A. H. (2009). The online Cough Clinic: developing guideline-based diagnosis and advice. *Eur Respir J, 34*(4), 819-824.

Hampton, T. (2006). New guidelines released for managing cough. *JAMA, 295*(7), 746-747.

Irwin, R. S. (2006). Introduction to the diagnosis and management of cough: ACCP evidence-based clinical practice guidelines. *Chest, 129*(1 Suppl), 25S-27S.

McCrory, D. C., & Lewis, S. Z. (2006). Methodology and grading of the evidence for the diagnosis and management of cough: ACCP evidence-based clinical practice guidelines. *Chest, 129*(1 Suppl), 28S-32S.

Deep Vein Thrombosis /
Pulmonary Embolism

Principles of Therapy

Venous thromboembolism is a common cause of morbidity and mortality in hospitalized patients. Deep vein thromboembolism almost invariably starts in the lower limbs and ultimately may detach to cause pulmonary embolism. Consequently, prevention of pulmonary embolism is achieved by preventing deep vein thromboembolism (DVT). Pulmonary embolism is more common in the postpartum period. Patient factors that predispose to thromboembolic disorders include age over 40, pregnancy, puerperium, recent surgery, orthopedic trauma, immobility, artificial heart valves or atrial fibrillation, and marked obesity. Many hereditary thrombophilia disorders can also now be detected which predispose to thromboembolism. Diagnosis of DVT can be confirmed using a lower extremity doppler study, but usually presents as extreme pain, tenderness, and swelling following periods of prolonged immobility, such as following surgery or confinement in an airplane. Pulmonay embolus frequently occurs without clinical evidence of DVT.

Diagnosis of PE can be confirmed by using spiral computed tomography (CT). Depending on available technology, a ventilation – perfusion (V/Q) scan using technetium may be performed instead. Breastfeeding may be restricted for a brief period of time after this study (see section on radioactive procedures). Pharmacotherapy of DVT / PE has long included the use of heparin and the vitamin K antagonist (warfarin). However, the newer low molecular weight heparins have significant advantages (longer half-lives, more stable kinetics, fewer bleeds).

Prevention of DVT / PE during hospitalization, especially for planned major surgery is a frequent patient safety goal. The only recommendation for low risk patients is early ambulation. Many patients, however will be at moderate or high risk. For these patients, DVT prophylaxis is typically initiated pre-operatively with mechanical methods (compression stockings and /or pneumatic compression devices). Additional prophylactic anticoagulation using heparin or low molecular weight heparin may be used depending on the patients risk category. Mechanical methods are employed throughout the surgery and post-operative period. Once post-operative bleeding has been ruled out, use of post-operative prophylactic anticoagulation for moderate and high risk patients is typically continued throughout the hospitalization and until the patient is fully ambulatory. Combination of mechanical and medical therapy appears to provide improved risk reduction in at risk populations which have been studied. Patients with known thrombophilia, malignancy, or orthopedic procedures are at greastest risk.

Treatment

•   Prevention of DVT/PE with early ambulation and appropriate prophylaxis for surgical patients.

•   Low molecular weight heparin: enoxaparin, arteparin, certoparin, parneparin, dalteparin.

- Heparin, unfractionated.

- Warfarin.

Medications

- DALTEPARIN SODIUM (*Fragmin, Low Molecular Weight Heparin*)
  - AAP = Not reviewed
  - LRC = L2
  - RID = 15.54%
  - Pregnancy = B
  - Comment: Dalteparin is a low molecular weight polysaccharide fragment of heparin used clinically as an anticoagulant. In a study of two patients who received 5000-10,000 IU of dalteparin, none was found in human milk.

    In another study of 15 post-cesarean patients early postpartum (mean= 5.7 days), blood and milk levels of dalteparin were determined three to four hours post-treatment. Following subcutaneous doses of 2500 IU, maternal plasma levels averaged 0.074 to 0.308 IU/mL. Breastmilk levels of dalteparin ranged from <0.005 to 0.037 IU/mL of milk. The milk/plasma ratio ranged from 0.025 to 0.224. Using these data, an infant ingesting 150 mL/kg/day would ingest approximately 5.5 IU/kg/day. Due to the polysaccharide nature of this product, oral absorption is unlikely. Further, because this study was done early postpartum, it is possible that the levels in 'mature' milk would be lower. The authors suggest that "it appears highly unlikely that puerperal thromboprophylaxis with LMWH has any clinically relevant effect on the nursing infant." Although the RID appears high, it would be largely unabsorbable.

- ENOXAPARIN (*Lovenox, Low Molecular Weight Heparin*)
  - AAP = Not reviewed
  - LRC = L3
  - RID =
  - Pregnancy = B
  - Comment: Enoxaparin is a low molecular weight fraction of heparin used clinically as an anticoagulant. In a study of 12 women receiving 20-40 mg of enoxaparin daily for up to five days postpartum for venous pathology (n= 4) or cesarean section (n= 8), no change in anti-Xa activity was noted in the breastfed infants. Because it is a peptide fragment of heparin, its molecular weight is large (2000-8000 daltons). The size alone would largely preclude its entry into human milk at levels clinically relevant. Due to minimal oral bioavailability, any present in milk would not be orally absorbed by the infant. A similar compound, dalteparin, has been studied and milk levels are extremely low as well. See dalteparin.

- FONDAPARINUX SODIUM (*Arixtra*)
  - AAP = Not reviewed
  - LRC = L3
  - RID =
  - Pregnancy = B

- ○ Comment: Fondaparinux sodium is a synthetic pentasaccharide and is used for treatment and prophylaxis of deep vein thrombosis. Fondaparinux sodium causes antithrombin III-mediated inhibition of factor Xa, thus interrupting the coagulation cascade and prohibiting thrombus development. As a pentasaccharide, it would not be orally bioavailable in an infant, nor would it likely enter the milk compartment due to its structure. No data are available on the transmission of fondaparinux sodium to a nursing infant, but based on the kinetic profile, it is highly unlikely that it would be passed to the infant.

- HEPARIN   (*Heparin*)
  - ○ AAP = Not reviewed
  - ○ LRC = L1
  - ○ RID =
  - ○ Pregnancy = C
  - ○ Comment: Heparin is a large protein molecule. It is used SC, IM, and IV because it is not absorbed orally in mother or infant. Due to its high molecular weight (range= 12,000-15,000 daltons), it is unlikely any would transfer into breastmilk. Any that did enter the milk would be rapidly destroyed in the gastric contents of the infant.

- WARFARIN   (*Coumadin, Panwarfin*)
  - ○ AAP = Maternal Medication Usually Compatible with Breastfeeding
  - ○ LRC = L2
  - ○ RID =
  - ○ Pregnancy = X
  - ○ Comment: Warfarin is a potent anticoagulant. Warfarin is highly protein bound in the maternal circulation and, therefore, very little is secreted into human milk. Very small and insignificant amounts are secreted into milk, but it depends to some degree on the dose administered. In one study of two patients who were anticoagulated with warfarin, no warfarin was detected in the infant's serum, nor were changes in coagulation detectable. In another study of 13 mothers, less than 0.08 μmol per liter (25 ng/mL) was detected in milk, and no warfarin was detected in the infants' plasma.

    According to these authors, maternal warfarin apparently poses little risk to a nursing infant, and thus far has not produced bleeding anomalies in breastfed infants. Other anticoagulants, such as phenindione, should be avoided. Observe infant for bleeding, such as excessive bruising or reddish petechia (spots). While the risks in breastfeeding premature infants (which are more susceptible to intracranial bleeding) is still low, oral supplementation with vitamin K1 will preclude any chance of hemorrhage. Even modest doses of Vitamin K1 counteract high doses of warfarin.

Clinical Tips

Treatment of DVT primarily rests on the use of anticoagulants, such as the heparin derivatives, particularly the low molecular weight heparins (enoxaparin, dalteparin). Because of the risk of thrombocytopenia with heparin, the LMW heparins are now preferred. Because of their large molecular weights, heparin and its low molecular weight derivatives, enoxaparin and dalteparin, transfer only marginally into human milk and are not orally bioavailable. Fondaparinux is a suitable alternative to heparin when co-administered with warfarin. Warfarin derivatives do cross the placenta and are relatively contraindicated during pregnancy. Potential side effects of concern with heparin use include heparin-induced osteoporosis and heparin-induced thrombocytopenia in the mother. Heparin-induced osteoporosis usually follows courses of therapy lasting seven weeks or longer. Low molecular weight heparin has a longer half-life, and regional anesthetics should be avoided for 12 to 24 hours after administration, depending on dosage. Duration of therapy after initial treatment for DVT / PE depends on the particulars of the clinical situation, but typically therapy is continued for three to six months after the acute event. Certain situations may dictate prolonging therapy outside of this time frame.

Suggested Reading

Alikhan, R., & Spyropoulos, A. C. (2008). Epidemiology of venous thromboembolism in cardiorespiratory and infectious disease. *Am J Med, 121*(11), 935-942.

Clark, P. (2008). Maternal venous thrombosis. *Eur J Obstet Gynecol Reprod Biol, 139*(1), 3-10.

Crowther, M. A., & Cook, D. J. (2008). Preventing venous thromboembolism in critically ill patients. *Semin Thromb Hemost, 34*(5), 469-474.

Duhl, A. J., Paidas, M. J., Ural, S. H., Branch, W., Casele, H., Cox-Gill, J., et al. (2007). Antithrombotic therapy and pregnancy: consensus report and recommendations for prevention and treatment of venous thromboembolism and adverse pregnancy outcomes. *Am J Obstet Gynecol, 197*(5), 457. E451-421.

Ko, R., Mazur, J. E., Pastis, N. J., Chang, E., Sahn, S. A., & Boylan, A. M. (2008). Common problems in critically ill obstetric patients, with an emphasis on pharmacotherapy. *Am J Med Sci, 335*(1), 65-70.

Marik, P. E., & Plante, L. A. (2008). Venous thromboembolic disease and pregnancy. *N Engl J Med, 359*(19), 2025-2033.

Nelson, S. M., & Greer, I. A. (2007). Thromboembolic events in pregnancy: pharmacological prophylaxis and treatment. *Expert Opin Pharmacother, 8*(17), 2917-2931.

Righini, M., Perrier, A., De Moerloose, P., & Bounameaux, H. (2008). D-Dimer for venous thromboembolism diagnosis: 20 years later. *J Thromb Haemost, 6*(7), 1059-1071.

Rosenberg, V. A., & Lockwood, C. J. (2007). Thromboembolism in pregnancy. *Obstet Gynecol Clin North Am, 34*(3), 4841-4500.

Snow, V., Qaseem, A., Barry, P., & et. al. (2007). Management of venous thromboembolism: A Clinical Practice Guideline from the American College of Physicians and the American Academy of Family Physicians. *Ann Intern Med, 146*, 204-210.

Wakefield, T. W., Caprini, J., & Comerota, A. J. (2008). Thromboembolic diseases. *Curr Probl Surg, 45*(12).

Diabetes Mellitus

Principles of Therapy

Diabetes mellitus (DM) is a heterogenous group of disorders characterized by abnormal insulin secretion and abnormal lipid and carbohydrate metabolism. It is also the most common endocrine disorder affecting women in pregnancy. In Type 1 DM, the pancreas fails to make and secrete insulin, thus these patients require exogenous insulin. In Type 2 DM, while insulin is present, the peripheral cells become insulin resistant. Over 90% of diabetics have non-insulin dependent diabetes (NIDDM), while 5-10% have insulin-dependent diabetes (IDDM). The hallmark of IDDM is the loss of the pancreatic beta cells and their source of insulin. Exogenous insulin repletion is the only source of treatment. In IDDM mothers, exogenous insulin does not transfer into human milk; its molecular weight is simply too large to permit entry into the milk compartment. Hence, insulin treatment in IDDM patients is not a contraindication to breastfeeding. But the vast majority of patients are NIDDM who may require oral antidiabetic agents. Unfortunately, the number of oral antidiabetic medications that have been studied in breastfeeding mothers is limited. Gestational diabetes requiring medication is usually treated with insulin and will not require extended therapy beyond pregnancy unless the underlying problem was truly undiagnosed pre-existing diabetes. However, approximately 50% of women with gestational diabetes will go on to develop overt diabetes within 20 years. All infants of diabetic mothers, regardless of type, are at increased risk of hypoglycemia at birth, and glucose testing of the infant within 30 minutes of birth is recommended.

Treatment

- In insulin-dependent DM, exogenous insulin supplementation is required.

- In gestational diabetes, most, but not all cases are controlled with diet and/or exogenous insulin. Maternal treatment is unlikely required after delivery, but later life risk of diabetes is increased.

- In NIDDM, oral medications, including metformin, sulfonylureas and thiazolidinediones, are required.

- Dietary modification required, especially limitations of sugar and carbohydrate intake.

- Infants of all diabetic mothers are at risk for hypoglycemia at birth.

Medications

- ACARBOSE   (*Precose, Prandase*)
  - AAP = Not reviewed
  - LRC = L3

- ○ RID =
- ○ Pregnancy = B
- ○ Comment: Acarbose is an oral alpha-glucosidase inhibitor used to reduce the absorption of carbohydrates in the management of Type II (NIDDM) diabetics. The reduction of carbohydrate absorption reduces the rapid rise in glucose following a meal; hence, glycosylated hemoglobin (Hemoglobin A1C) levels are reduced. Acarbose is less than 2% bioavailable as an intact molecule. No data are available on the transfer of acarbose into human milk, but with a bioavailability of less than 2%, it is very unlikely any would reach the milk compartment or be orally absorbed by the infant.

- **CHLORPROPAMIDE** (*Diabinese*)
  - ○ AAP = Not reviewed
  - ○ LRC = L3
  - ○ RID = 10.5%
  - ○ Pregnancy = C
  - ○ Comment: Chlorpropamide stimulates the secretion of insulin in some patients. Following one 500 mg dose, the concentration of chlorpropamide in milk after five hours was approximately 5 mg/L of milk. It may cause hypoglycemia in infants, although effects are largely unknown and unreported. It is a poor choice for breastfeeding mothers.

- **GLYBURIDE** (*Micronase, Diabeta, Glynase, Glucovance, Metaglip*)
  - ○ AAP = Not reviewed
  - ○ LRC = L2
  - ○ RID =
  - ○ Pregnancy = B
  - ○ Comment: Glyburide is a "second generation" sulfonylurea agent useful in the treatment of non insulin-dependent (Type II) diabetes mellitus. It belongs to the sulfonylurea family (tolbutamide, glipizide) of hypoglycemic agents, of which glyburide is one of the most potent. Glyburide apparently stimulates insulin secretion, thus reducing plasma glucose. In a study of six mothers who received a single dose (5 mg) and two mothers who received a single dose of 10 mg glyburide, all breastmilk samples were below the limit of detection of 0.005 µg/mL. In a group of five mothers who received daily doses of glyburide (non micronized 5 mg) or glipizide (immediate-release 5 mg), neither glyburide or glipizide were detectable in milk. Infant plasma glucose levels were normal. The product Glucovance contains metformin and glyburide.

- **GLIPIZIDE** (*Glucotrol XL, Glucotrol*)
  - ○ AAP = Not reviewed
  - ○ LRC = L3
  - ○ RID =
  - ○ Pregnancy = C
  - ○ Comment: Glipizide is a potent hypoglycemic agent that belongs to sulfonylurea family. It is formulated in regular and extended release formulations, and it is used only for non insulin-dependent (Type II) diabetes. Thus the half-life and time-to-peak depends on the formulation used. It reduces glucose levels by stimulating insulin secretion from the pancreas. In a group of five

mothers who received daily doses of glyburide (non micronized 5 mg) or glipizide (immediate-release 5 mg), neither glyburide or glipizide were detectable in milk. Detection limit for glipizide was 0.08 μg/mL. Infant plasma glucose levels were normal. The product METAGLIP contains Glipizide and metformin.

- INSULIN   (*Humulin*)
  - AAP = Not reviewed
  - LRC = L1
  - RID =
  - Pregnancy = B
  - Comment: Insulin is a large peptide that is not secreted into milk. Even if secreted, it would be destroyed in the infant's GI tract leading to minimal or no absorption.

- METFORMIN   (*Glucophage, Glucovance*)
  - AAP = Not reviewed
  - LRC = L1
  - RID = 0.3-0.7%
  - Pregnancy = B
  - Comment: Metformin belongs to the biguanide family and is used to reduce glucose levels in non-insulin dependent diabetics. Oral bioavailability is only 50%. In a study of seven women taking metformin (median dose 1500 mg/d), the mean milk-to-plasma ratio (AUC) for metformin was 0.35. The mean average concentration in milk over the dose interval was 0.27 mg/L. The absolute infant dose averaged 0.04 mg/kg/d, and the mean relative infant dose was 0.28%. Metformin was present in very low or undetectable concentrations in the plasma of four of the infants who were studied. No health problems were found in the six infants who were evaluated. In a recent study of five women consuming an average dose of 500 mg twice daily, the mean peak and trough metformin concentrations in breastmilk were 0.42 mg/L (range 0.38-0.46 mg/L) and 0.39 mg/L (range 0.31-0.52 mg/L), respectively. The average milk/serum ratio was 0.63 (range 0.36-1.00) and the estimated relative infant dose was 0.65% (range 0.43-1.08%). Blood glucose concentrations in three infants were normal, ranging from 47-77 mg/dL. The mothers reported no side effects were noted in the breastfed infants. Metformin is also used to treat polycystic ovary syndrome. In one study of 61 nursing infants whose mothers were taking a median of 2.55 g/day throughout pregnancy and lactation, the growth, motor, and social development of the infants were recorded to be normal. The authors concluded that metformin was safe and effective during lactation in the first six months of an infant's life.

    The new product Glucovance contains metformin and glyburide. The new product METAGLIP contains Glipizide and metformin.

- TOLBUTAMIDE   (*Oramide, Orinase*)
  - AAP = Maternal Medication Usually Compatible with Breastfeeding
  - LRC = L3
  - RID = 0.02%
  - Pregnancy = C

  ◦ Comment: Tolbutamide is a short-acting sulfonylurea used to stimulate insulin secretion in type II diabetics. Only low levels are secreted into breastmilk. Following a dose of 500 mg twice daily, milk levels in two patients were 3 and 18 μg/L, respectively. Maternal serum levels averaged 35 and 45 μg/L. Observe infant closely for jaundice and hypoglycemia.

Clinical Tips

Insulin, due to its large molecular weight (>6000), does not enter milk in clinically relevant amounts, so it can be readily used in breastfeeding mothers with IDDM. Of the sulfonylureas, tolbutamide and chlorpropamide are presently poor choices for breastfeeding mothers and are seldom used today. The levels of these two sulfonylureas in breastmilk are quite small, and probably subclinical, but are not necessarily ideal for pregnancy or breastfeeding.

The newer second-generation sulfonylureas (e.g., glipizide, glimepiride, glyburide) are poorly studied in breastfeeding mothers, but levels in milk reported thus far are exceedingly low. They are probably compatible with breastfeeding with close observation of the infant blood glucose levels. No reports of hypoglycemic infants have been found. Metformin transfer into human milk is poor. In a study of seven women receiving 1500 mg daily, the average milk concentration was only 0.27 mg/L. The absolute infant dose from breastmilk averaged 0.04 mg/kg/day and the mean relative infant dose was only 0.28% of the maternal dose. Metformin levels in the plasma of the studied infants were very low or undetectable. It is unlikely the amount transferred to an infant would be clinically relevant. Metformin, glipizide, and glyburide are probably compatible with breastfeeding.

Of these hypoglycemic agents, metformin has a number of benefits and is often a first choice drug in women with polycystic ovary disease and now NIDDM. Its use in women with polycystic ovary syndrome is common and growing, and this has increased its use in pregnant and postpartum breastfeeding women. The fact that it induces weight loss in many patients is advantageous. The newer thiazolidinediones, such as rosiglitazone (Avandia) and pioglitazone (Actos), have yet to be studied in breastfeeding mothers, but maternal plasma levels are quite low, and their protein binding is very high (> 99%), thus milk levels would probably be quite low, although this is only theoretical.

The alpha-glucosidate inhibitors, such as acarbose (Precose) and miglitol (Glyset), act by slowing the absorption of carbohydrates in the intestine. Interestingly, they are poorly bioavailable and stay in the gut. It is not at all likely they would ever transfer into milk and produce effects in an infant, but this has yet to be studied in breastfeeding mothers.

A risk-vs-benefit assessment may assist the clinician prior to the use of oral hypoglycemic agents in breastfeeding mothers. It is important to remember that gestational diabetics often revert to normal soon after delivery, suggesting that a few months of insulin therapy or metformin, if it works, would be ideal for continuing breastfeeding.

In pregnant patients, glyburide and glipizide have little or no transfer across the placenta. Metform and rosiglitazone readily transfer, although they have no reported complications. While human data are limited, there are no data that suggest metformin, rosiglitazone, glipizide, or glyburide are teratogenic. Glyburide and metformin are ideal candidates for gestational diabetes, although they are not always successful in producing optimal glucose control.

Suggested Reading

Bentley-Lewis, R., Levkoff, S., Stuebe, A., & Seely, E. W. (2008). Gestational diabetes mellitus: postpartum opportunities for the diagnosis and prevention of type 2 diabetes mellitus. *Nat Clin Pract Endocrinol Metab, 4*(10), 552-558.

Cypryk, K., Kosiński, M., Kamińska, P., Kozdraj, T., & Lewiński, A. (2008). Diabetes control and pregnancy outcomes in women with type 1 diabetes treated during pregnancy with continuous subcutaneous insulin infusion or multiple daily insulin injections. *Pol Arch Med Wewn, 118*(6), 339-344.

Feig, D. S., Briggs, G. G., & Koren, G. (2007). Oral antidiabetic agents in pregnancy and lactation: a paradigm shift? *Ann Pharmacother, 41*(7), 1174-1180.

Khandelwal, M. (2008). GDM: postpartum management to reduce long-term risks. *Curr Diab Rep, 8*(4), 287-293.

Levine, J. P. (2008). Type 2 diabetes among women: clinical considerations for pharmacological management to achieve glycemic control and reduce cardiovascular risk. *J Womens Health (Larchmt), 17*(2), 249-260.

Theodoraki, A., & Baldeweg, S. E. (2008). Gestational diabetes mellitus. *Br J Hosp Med (Lond), 69*(10), 562-567.

Drug and Substance Abuse

Principles of Therapy

The treatment of drug abuse obviously varies according to the class of drug used. Opiates, such as heroin, morphine, codeine, hydrocodone, and oxycodone, are the most frequent opioids abused. Other classes of drugs of abuse include ethanol, cocaine, amphetamines, marijuana, etc. The treatment of these various conditions is far beyond the scope of this text; however, below are many of the medications commonly recommended for therapy of these varied conditions. When treating breastfeeding mothers for addictive conditions, the clinician must always take into consideration the relative risk of the medication, the physical and mental state of the mother, her ability to care for and protect the infant, and the risk to the infant from breastmilk exposure to these various drugs. It is not always necessary to discontinue breastfeeding, but this is a decision that should be left largely up to the physician and team managing the patient.

Treatment

- Psychosocial treatments

- Drug counseling programs

- Alterations of lifestyle

- Medications

Medications

- ACAMPROSATE (*Campral*)
    - AAP = Not reviewed
    - LRC = L3
    - RID =
    - Pregnancy = C
    - Comment: Acamprosate is a medication used for ethanol dependency. Its mechanism of action is not fully known; however, it does increase levels of GABA and decrease levels of glutamate. During use, it reduces alcohol intake without the disulfram-like effects. There are no data available on the transfer of acamprosate to human milk. It is not a sedative and is not additive, and its oral absorption is minimal. Due to the relatively low molecular weight and the lack of protein binding, transfer could be possible. In addition, alcohol-dependent mothers may not be a good risk for breastfeeding. However, this drug poses a minimal risk to infants.

- BUPRENORPHINE   (*Buprenex, Subutex*)
  - AAP = Not reviewed
  - LRC = L2
  - RID   = 1.9%
  - Pregnancy = C
  - Comment: Buprenorphine is a potent, long-acting narcotic agonist and antagonist and may be useful as a replacement for methadone treatment in addicts. It is also recently approved for the treatment of opiate dependence. Its elimination half-life varies from paper to paper, but new recent sublingual studies suggests it ranges from 23-30 hours.

    In one patient who received 4 mg/day to facilitate withdrawal from other opiates, the amount of buprenorphine transferred via milk was only 3.28 µg/day, an amount that was clinically insignificant. No symptoms were noted in this breastfed infant. In another study of continuous epidural bupivacaine and buprenorphine in post-cesarean women for three days, it was suggested that buprenorphine may suppress the production of milk (and infant weight gain), although this was not absolutely clear.

    In another study of one patient on buprenorphine maintenance for seven months, and who received 8 mg daily sublingually over four days, milk levels of buprenorphine and norbuprenorphine ranged from 1.0 to 14.7 ng/mL and 0.6 to 6.3 ng/mL, respectively. Plasma concentrations of both analytes ranged from 0.2 to 20.1 ng/mL (buprenorphine) and 1.2 to 4.4 ng/mL (norbuprenorphine) over four days of study. Using peak levels only, the concentration of buprenorphine and norbuprenorphine were 1.47 and 0.63 µg/100 mL of breastmilk, respectively. Assuming an intake of 150 mL/kg/day, the authors estimated the daily dose would be less than 10 µg for a 4 kg infant, a dose that is probably far subclinical.

- BUPRENORPHINE + NALOXONE   (*Suboxone*)
  - AAP = Not reviewed
  - LRC = L3
  - RID =
  - Pregnancy = C
  - Comment: Suboxone is a sublingual tablet that contains a partial opioid agonist (buprenorphine) and an opioid antagonist (naloxone) in a 4:1 (buprenorphine: naloxone) ratio. Buprenorphine reduces the patients' craving for opioids, and naloxone discourages the use of other opioids by blocking the opiate receptor. Naloxone is poorly absorbed orally, and buprenorphine is only 31% absorbed. It is unlikely breastmilk levels will be significant. See individual monographs on these two drugs.

- METHADONE   (*Dolophine*)
  - AAP = Maternal Medication Usually Compatible with Breastfeeding
  - LRC = L3
  - RID   = 1.9-6.5%
  - Pregnancy = C
  - Comment: Methadone is a potent and very long-acting opiate analgesic. It is primarily used to prevent withdrawal in opiate addiction. In one study of 10 women receiving methadone 10-80 mg/day, the average milk/plasma ratio was 0.83. Due to the variable doses used, the milk concentrations ranged from 0.05 mg/L in one patient receiving 10 mg/day, to 0.57 mg/L in a patient receiving

80 mg/day. One infant death has been reported in a breastfeeding mother receiving maintenance methadone therapy, although it is not clear that the only source of methadone to this infant was from breastmilk.

In a more recent study of 12 breastfeeding women on methadone maintenance doses ranging from 20-80 mg/day, the mean concentration of methadone in plasma and milk was 311 (207-416) μg/L and 116 (72-160) μg/L, respectively, yielding a mean M/P ratio of 0.44 (0.24-0.64). The mean absolute oral dose to infant was 17.4 (10.8-24) μg/kg/day. This equates to a mean of 2.79% of the maternal dose per day. In this study, 64% of the infants exhibited neonatal abstinence syndrome requiring treatment.

In two women receiving 30 mg twice daily and another who received 73 mg of methadone once daily, the average breastmilk methadone concentrations was 0.169 mg/L and 0.132 mg/L, respectively. The milk/plasma ratios were 1.215 and 0.661, respectively. While the infant of the second mother died at 3½ months of SIDS, it was apparently not due to methadone, as none was present in the infant's plasma, and the infant was significantly supplemented with formula.

In an excellent study of eight mother/infant pairs ingesting from 40 to 105 mg/day methadone, the average (AUC) concentration of R-methadone and S-methadone enantiomers varied from 42-259 μg/L and 26-126 μg/L, respectively. The relative infant dose was estimated to be 2.8% of the maternal dose. Interestingly, there was little difference in methadone milk levels in immature and mature milk.

Most studies thus far show that only small amounts of methadone pass into breastmilk despite doses as high as 105 mg/day. In fact, neonatal abstinence syndromes are well known to occur in breastfeeding infants following delivery. In one study, 58% of infants developed neonatal abstinence syndrome while still breastfeeding. However, some methadone is undoubtedly transferred via milk, and abrupt cessation of breastfeeding during high dose therapy has resulted in neonatal abstinence in some infants.

In a recent study of eight methadone-maintained lactating women (dose: 50-105 mg/day), the concentration of methadone in milk was low (range: 2-462 ng/mL) and, interestingly, was not related to maternal dose. Maternal plasma levels rose over a four week period postpartum to reach a high at 30 days. Median milk/plasma ratios ranged from 0.22 to 0.92. The average amount of methadone ingestible by the infant was estimated to be < 0.2mg/day at day 30 postpartum. Infant plasma levels of methadone ranged from 2.2 to 8.1 ng/mL. Again, there was no correlation between maternal dose and infant plasma level. There were no significant neurobehavioral changes noted.

In summary, the dose of R plus S methadone transferred via milk is largely dose dependent, but generally averages less than 2.8% of the maternal dose. This is significantly less than the conventional cut-off value of 10% of the maternal dose corrected for weight. However, the amount in milk is insufficient to prevent neonatal withdrawal syndrome. The Academy of Pediatrics recently placed methadone in the "approved" category for breastfeeding women.

- NALTREXONE   (*ReVia*)
  - AAP = Not reviewed
  - LRC = L1
  - RID = 1.4%
  - Pregnancy = C
  - Comment: Naltrexone is a long acting narcotic antagonist similar in structure to Naloxone. Orally absorbed, it has been clinically used in addicts to prevent the action of injected heroin. It occupies

and competes with all opioid medications for the opiate receptor. When used in addicts, it can induce rapid and long lasting withdrawal symptoms. Although the half-life appears brief, the duration of antagonism is long lasting (24-72 hours). Naltrexone is quite lipid soluble, has a high pKa, and transfers into the brain easily (brain/plasma ratio= 0.81). It is readily metabolized to 6-beta-naltrexol (active) and two minor metabolites. The activity of naltrexone is believed to be mainly due to parent and 6-beta-naltrexol.

In a study of one patient (60 kg) receiving 50 mg/day, the average concentration of naltrexone and 6-beta-naltrexol in milk were 1.7 and 46 μg/L. The milk/plasma ratios of naltrexone and 6-beta-naltrexol were 1.9 and 3.4, respectively. The absolute infant dose was 0.26 and 6.86 μg/kg/day, respectively. The relative infant dose was 0.06 and 1.0% (range= 0.86-1.06%). The infant was reported to have achieved all expected milestones and showed no drug-related side effects. Naltrexone was undetectable in the infant's plasma, and levels of 6-beta-naltrexol were only marginally detectable at 1.1 μg/L.

Clinical Tips

Patients with drug abusing conditions often have numerous co-morbid psychiatric conditions, including conduct and personality disorders; schizohrenic, manic, and bipolar disorders; depressive disorders; post-traumatic stress; and other anxiety disorders. All must be treated effectively before drug abuse can be altered.

Opiate Dependence: It is now generally agreed that opiate dependence is best treated with a number of interventions, including the use of the opiate agonist, methadone. Prolonged oral treatment with methadone (methadone maintenance therapy) is now well known to reduce illicit opiate use, the transmission of many STD infections, and criminal activity, all of which are risk factors for a breastfeeding infant. The use of methadone in breastfeeding mothers has been approved by the Academy of Pediatrics for some years now, although there are still concerns about the dose used. In the last decade, the dose of methadone has risen enormously, as it has become well known that the higher the dose, the less effect exogenous heroin has. Thus, larger doses are now used to completely block the effect of heroin and effectively reduce the need or desire to use illicit heroin. The data in breastfeeding mothers are clear, methadone levels in milk are quite low (2.8% of maternal dose) and are easily tolerated by breastfeeding infants. It is true that at higher maternal doses, the infant may develop some degree of dependence on methadone, but this has not proven to be a problem, other than mild withdrawal rarely reported in the infant. While postpartum withdrawal in infants born of mothers who used methadone during gestation is common, withdrawal of infants exposed only to breastmilk heroin is exceedingly rare. Because levels of methadone in breastmilk are so low, infants suffering from withdrawal almost invariably require treatment with exogenous opiates to reduce symptoms. There is simply too little methadone in milk to reduce their withdrawal symptoms.

New data now suggests that buprenorphine is also quite effective. Buprenorphine, a partial opiate agonist, is becoming more popular due to the fact that withdrawal symptoms are less severe than with methadone. Buprenorphine has been studied in breastfeeding mothers and levels in milk are exceedingly low. Levels in one study suggest the infant would only receive nanograms of buprenorphine daily.

The use of narcotic antagonists in breastfeeding mothers should be used with great care. They should not be used in the infant early postnatally unless the infant is toxic. The use of narcotic antagonists in newborns may induce an immediate withdrawal, which could be more problematic than the slow withdrawal otherwise seen.

Alcohol Dependence: Alcohol readily transfers into human milk, and breastfeeding infants can receive significant doses if maternal use is significant. In general, levels in milk are subclinical until the maternal plasma levels rise. Excessive use may lead to drowsiness, deep sleep, weakness, and decreased linear growth rate in infants. Ethanol is a potent inhibitor of oxytocin release and can suppress milk letdown; hence, the amount of milk released to the infant can be severely reduced. The old theory that beer increases milk production is absolutely wrong, it severely reduces milk let down. Another study reported one infant that developed pseudo-Cushing syndrome as a result of exposure to alcohol in breastmilk. The mother consumed at least fifty 12 ounce beers weekly, in addition to other concentrated alcoholic beverages.

While the abuse of alcohol may be problematic, the social use of low doses of alcohol, such as one or two drinks, does not normally produce maternal plasma levels high enough to impact the breastfeeding infant. In these situations, a brief interruption of approximately two hours per drink consumed virtually removes any transfer of drug into milk.

Suggested Reading

Haber, P. S., Demirkol, A., Lange, K., & Murnion, B. (2009). Management of injecting drug users admitted to hospital. *Lancet, 374*(9697), 1284-1293.

Hays, J. T., Ebbert, J. O., & Sood, A. (2009). Treating tobacco dependence in light of the 2008 US Department of Health and Human Services clinical practice guideline. *Mayo Clin Proc, 84*(8), 730-735; quiz 735-736.

Lin, K. W., & Finnell, V. W. (2009). Screening for illicit drug use. *Am Fam Physician, 80*(6), 629.

Mattick, R. P., Breen, C., Kimber, J., & Davoli, M. (2003). Methadone maintenance therapy versus no opioid replacement therapy for opioid dependence. *The Cochrane Database of Systematic Reviews,* (2).

Mayet, S., Farrell, M., Ferri, M., & et al. (2004). Psychosocial treatment for opiate abuse and dependence. *Cochrane Database of Systematic Reviews, 4.*

Walker, L., Brown, P., Beeching, N. J., & Beadsworth, M. B. (2009). Managing alcohol withdrawal syndromes: the place of guidelines. *Br J Hosp Med (Lond), 70*(8), 444-445, 448-449.

Endometriosis

Principles of Therapy

Endometriosis is defined as the presence of ectopic endometrial epithelium, glands and stroma, most commonly in the pelvic peritoneum. It occurs in approximately 7-10% of women. It is predominately associated with infertility, adnexal masses, dysmenorrhea, dysparunia, and pelvic pain. There appears to be a familial association, and it is also more common in women with anomalies of the genital tract. The diagnosis can only be confirmed by surgical evaluation with direct visualization (such as laparoscopy), but it is frequently made presumptively based on clinical features. Severity of observed endometrial lesions correlates poorly with degree of pain.

Endometriosis is typically improved and quiescent during pregnancy. During the period of lactational amenorrhea, the emergence of recurrent endometriosis would be unexpected as endometrial atrophy would be anticipated. Once menstrual cycles have resumed, however, recurrent symptoms would be possible. Treatment options focus on agents that result in endometrial thinning. In situations where pursuing pregnancy is not an immeadiate goal, typically initial agents include estrogen containing oral contraceptive pills or progestational agents. NSAIDS may frequently be employed as well. Other treatment options which are used in women failing to respond to the previously mentioned therapies include danazol and gonadotropin releasing hormone (GnRH) agonists.

Treatment

- Symptoms and disease may be suppressed during lactational amenorrhea.

- Oral contraceptives, NSAIDS or progestin agents would be initial therapy.

- During lactation, progestins may be preferred therapy if symptoms recur, as they would be expected to have the least adverse impact on the breastfeeding dyad.

- Danazol and GnRH agonists are used for disease unresponsive to other therapies.

- Surgical therapy is used for ablation of endometriotic lesions unresponsive to medical therapy, confirmation of diagnosis, or evaluation of infertility.

Medications

- DANAZOL   (*Danocrine*)
  - AAP = Not reviewed
  - LRC = L5
  - RID =

- Pregnancy = X
- Comment: Danazol suppresses the pituitary-ovarian axis by inhibiting output of pituitary and hypothalamic hormones. It also appears to inhibit the synthesis of sex steroids and provides antiestrogenic effects. It is primarily used for treating endometriosis. Due to its effect on pituitary hormones and its androgenic effects, it may reduce the rate of breastmilk production, although this has not been documented. No data on its transfer to human milk are available. Danazol has been associated with masculinization of the female fetus and should never be used in pregnant women.

- ETONOGESTREL IMPLANT   (*Implanon*)
  - AAP = Not reviewed
  - LRC = L2
  - RID =
  - Pregnancy = X
  - Comment: Implanon is a slow release single-rod contraceptive implant. It consists of a non-biodegradable rod measuring 40 mm in length and 2 mm in diameter which releases on average 40 μg/day of etonogestrel over a three year period of use. Etonogestrel is the biologically active metabolite of desogestrel and has both high progestational activity and low intrinsic androgenicity. Implanon does not contain estrogen, making it suitable for women who do not tolerate or are advised to not use estrogens. Small amounts of progestins are known to pass into milk, but long-term follow-up of children whose mothers used hormonal contraceptives while breastfeeding has shown no deleterious effects on infants. Like other progestogen-only contraceptives, the use of Implanon is associated with irregular menstrual bleeding and sometimes absence of bleeding. Counseling is required to ensure women make informed choices. Of the contraceptives, progestin-only contraceptives are generally preferred as they produce fewer changes in milk production compared to estrogen-containing products. This product is probably quite safe for use in breastfeeding mothers, although all mothers should be counseled to observe for changes in milk production.

- GOSERELIN ACETATE IMPLANT   (*Zoladex*)
  - AAP = Not reviewed
  - LRC = L3
  - RID =
  - Pregnancy = X
  - Comment: Goserelin is a synthetic decapeptide analogue of luteinizing hormone releasing factor. It acts as a potent inhibitor of pituitary gonadotropin secretion. Following initial administration in males, goserelin causes an initial increase in serum luteinizing hormone (LH) and follicle stimulating hormone (FSH) levels. Chronic administration of goserelin leads to sustained suppression of pituitary gonadotropins and serum levels testosterone in males. In females, a down-regulation of the pituitary gland following chronic exposure leads to suppression of gonadotropin secretion and a decrease in serum estradiol to levels consistent with the menopausal state. Serum LH and FSH are suppressed to follicular phase levels within four weeks. No data are available on its transfer into human milk, but due to its structure and molecular weight, it is very unlikely to enter milk or to be orally bioavailable in the infant.

- LEUPROLIDE ACETATE   (*Lupron, Viadur*)
  - AAP = Not reviewed

- ○ LRC = L5
- ○ RID =
- ○ Pregnancy = X
- ○ Comment: Leuprolide is a synthetic nonapeptide analog of naturally occurring gonadotropin-releasing hormone with greater potency than the naturally occurring hormone. After initial stimulation, it inhibits gonadotropin release from the pituitary and after sustained use, suppresses ovarian and testicular hormone synthesis (two to four weeks). Almost complete suppression of estrogen, progesterone, and testosterone result. Although Lupron is contraindicated in pregnant women, no reported birth defects have been reported in humans. It is commonly used prior to fertilization, but should never be used during pregnancy.

  It is not known whether leuprolide transfers into human milk, but due to its nonapeptide structure, it is not likely that its transfer would be extensive. In addition, animal studies have found that it has zero oral bioavailability; therefore, it is unlikely it would be orally bioavailable in the human infant if ingested via milk. Its effect on lactation is unknown, but it could suppress lactation particularly early postpartum. Lupron would reduce estrogen and progestin levels to menopausal ranges, which may or may not suppress lactation, depending on the duration of lactation. Interestingly, several studies show no change in prolactin levels, although these were not in lactating women. One study of a hyperprolactinemic patient showed significant suppression of prolactin, which is the reason for my L5 risk categorization. It is of no risk to the breastfed infant, only to milk production.

- **MEDROXYPROGESTERONE**   (*Provera, Depo-Provera, Cycrin*)
  - ○ AAP = Maternal Medication Usually Compatible with Breastfeeding
  - ○ LRC = L1
  - ○ RID =
  - ○ Pregnancy = X
  - ○ Comment: Depo Medroxyprogesterone (DMPA) is a synthetic progestin compound. It is used orally for amenorrhea, dysmenorrhea, uterine bleeding, and infertility. It is used intramuscularly for contraception. Due to its poor oral bioavailability, it is seldom used orally.

    Saxena has reported that the average concentration in milk is 1.03 µg/L. Koetsawang reported average milk levels of 0.97 µg/L. In a series of huge studies, the World Health Organization reviewed the developmental skills of children and their weight gain following exposure to progestin-only contraceptives during lactation. These studies documented that no adverse effects on overall development or rate of growth were notable. Further, they suggested there is no apparent reason to deny lactating women the use of progestin-only contraceptives, preferably after six weeks postpartum.

    There have been consistent and controversial studies suggesting that males exposed to early postnatal progestins have higher feminine scores. However, Ehrhardt's studies have provided convincing data that males exposed to early progestins were no different than controls. A number of other short and long-term studies available on development of children have found no differences with control groups.

    Interestingly, an excellent study of the transfer of DMPA into breastfed infants has been published. In this study of 13 breastfeeding women who received 150 mg injections of DMPA on day 43 and again on day 127 postpartum, urine and plasma collections in infants (n= 22) from day 38 to day 137 were collected. Urinary follicle stimulating hormone (FSH), luteinizing hormone (LH), unconjugated testosterone, unconjugated cortisol, medroxyprogesterone and metabolites were measured. No differences (from untreated controls) were found in LH, FSH, or unconjugated testosterone urine levels in the infants. Urine cortisol levels were not altered from those of control infants. Medroxyprogesterone or its metabolites were at no time detected in any of the infant urine samples. The data conclude that only small trace amounts of MPA are transferred to breastfeeding infants and that these amounts are not expected to have any influence on breastfeeding infants. In support of this, using calculations based on MPA levels in the blood of DMPA users and a plasma to milk MPA ratio, Benagiano and Fraser suggest that the actual amounts of MPA in the infant's system is probably at or below trace levels. Koetsewant states that the small amount of MPA present in milk is unlikely to have any significant clinical adverse effects on the infant. A long-term follow-up study by Jimenez found no changes in growth, development, and health status in 128 breast-fed infants at 4.5 years of age. DMPA mothers lactated significantly longer than controls in this study. The use of Depo-Provera in breastfeeding women is common, but will probably always be somewhat controversial. Depo Provera has been documented to significantly elevate prolactin levels in breastfeeding mothers and to increase milk production in some mothers.

It is well known that estrogens suppress milk production. With progestins, it has been suggested that some women may experience a decline in milk production or arrested early production, following an injection of DMPA, particularly when the progestin is used early postpartum (12-48 hours). At present, there are no published data to support this, nor is the relative incidence of this untoward effect known. Therefore, in some instances, it might be advisable to recommend treatment with oral progestin-only contraceptives postpartum rather than DMPA, so that women who experience reduced milk supply could easily withdraw from the medication without significant loss of breastmilk supply. Progestins should be avoided early postnatally, and perhaps longer.

- NAPROXEN   (*Anaprox, Naprosyn, Aleve*)
  - AAP = Maternal Medication Usually Compatible with Breastfeeding
  - LRC = L3
  - RID = 3.3%
  - Pregnancy = C
  - Comment: Naproxen is a popular NSAID analgesic. In a study done at steady state in one mother consuming 375 mg twice daily, milk levels ranged from 1.76-2.37 mg/L at four hours. Total naproxen excretion in the infant's urine was only 0.26% of the maternal dose. Although the amount of naproxen transferred via milk is minimal, one should use with caution in nursing mothers because of its long half-life and its effect on infant cardiovascular system, kidneys, and GI tract. However, its short term use postpartum or infrequent or occasional use would not necessarily be incompatible with breastfeeding. One case of prolonged bleeding, hemorrhage, and acute anemia has been reported in a seven-day-old infant. The relative infant dose on a weight-adjusted maternal daily dose would probably be less than 3.3%.

- NORETHINDRONE   (*Aygestin, Norlutate, Micronor, NOR-Q.D.*)
  - AAP = Not reviewed
  - LRC = L1
  - RID =
  - Pregnancy = X

- ○ Comment: Norethindrone is a typical synthetic progestational agent that is used for oral contraception and other endocrine functions. It is believed to be secreted into breastmilk in small amounts. It produces a dose-dependent suppression of lactation at higher doses, although somewhat minimal at lower doses. It may reduce lactose content and reduce overall milk volume and nitrogen/protein content, resulting in lower infant weight gain, although these effects are unlikely if doses are kept low. Progestin-only mini pills are preferred oral contraceptives in breastfeeding mothers.

  However, recent reports claim that Micronor can be associated with decreased breastmilk production. In a report of 13 women taking Micronor who presented with poor milk production, 10 women experienced an increase in lactation upon withdrawl of Micronor. While norethindrone birth control pill are considered ideal for most breastfeeding mothers, some women retain sensitivity to these products and may suffer from reduced milk production. Each and every breastfeeding mother should be individually counselled about the possible reduction in milk synthesis following the use of this product.

Clinical Tips

Endometriosis is a clinically diffucult condition to treat. While symptoms can be managed, it is generally not considered curable. Low dose oral contraceptives without estrogen may be safely used in breastfeeding mothers. NSAIDS, such as naproxen, have been found useful in controlling endometriosis-associated pain and may be safely used for brief periods of up to one to two weeks in breastfeeding mothers. Progestogens, oral or injectable, are generally effective and reduce endometriosis-associated pain significantly. Various randomized controlled trials suggest that progestins are relatively equivalent to leuprolide in reducing endometriosis-associated pain, with a lesser impact on bone mineralization. Estrogen-containing products should be avoided as estrogens tend to suppress milk production in breastfeeding mothers, and they may predispose the endometrial tissue to grow and increase symptoms.

While gonatropin releasing hormone analogs (GnRH) have been found effective in reducing endometrial pain, they have numerous side effects which must be balanaced against their use. GnRH analogs (e.g., Goserelin) act as potent inhibitors of pituitary gonadotropin secretion, which after chronic use lead to a decrease in serum estradiol to levels consistent with the postmenopausal state, and would be expected to lead to a reduction of ovarian size and function, reduction in the size of the uterus and mammary gland, as well as a regression of sex hormone-responsive tumors, if present. The use of these products is not consistent with continued lactation, and they should be avoided in breastfeeding mothers. Hot flashes, vaginitis, headache, and demineralization of bone are major complications of their use.

Suggested Reading

ACOG Committee on Practice Bulletins-Gynecology. (2000). ACOG practice bulletin. Medical management of endometriosis. Number 11, December 1999. Clinical management guidelines for obstetrician-gynecologists. Int J Gynaecol Obstet, 71(2), 183-196.

Mezo G., Manea M. (2009). Luteinizing hormone-releasing hormone antagonists. *Expert Opin Ther Pat. 19*(12):1771-85. Review.

Howard F.M. (2009). Endometriosis and mechanisms of pelvic pain. *J Minim Invasive Gynecol. 16*(5):540-50. Review.

Quinn M. (2009). Endometriosis: the elusive epiphenomenon. *J Obstet Gynaecol. 29*(7):590-3. Review.

Jarrell J.F., Vilos G.A., Allaire C., et al. (2005). SOGC Clinical Practice Guidelines. Consensus Guidelines for the Management of Chronic Pelvic Pain. *J Obstet Gynaecol Can 27*:781-801

Mounsey A.L., Wilgus A., Slawson D.C. (2006). Diagnosis and management of endometriosis. *Am Fam Physician74*:594-600

Fever

Principles of Therapy

Fever is a common manifestation of numerous medical conditions, both serious and minor. Fever is generally protective, and only in rare conditions is treatment actually required. There are multiple causes of hyperthermia which include infectious disease (particularly pneumonia, *clostridium difficile*, colitis, sinusitis, cytomegalovirus, herpes simplex virus, hepatitis, etc.), chemicals (such as salicylates, anticholinergics, stimulants, anesthetics), dehydration, elevated environmental temperatures, excessive body wrapping, excessive exercise, head trauma, malignancies, hyperthyroidism, etc. Fever is in many instances beneficial in that it stimulates the immune system and accelerates the destruction of viruses, bacteria, and some malignancies. The relationship between excessive fever and brain damage is weak, and most data suggest otherwise. Treatment of fever solely depends on determining the etiology of the syndrome, whether infectious, chemical, or environmental. Appropriate treatment of fever in a breastfeeding woman will depend on treatment of the specific underlying instigating cause.

Treatment

- Appropriate treatment of fever in a breastfeeding woman will depend on treatment of the specific underlying etiology

- Antipyretics, including ibuprofen, acetaminophen, naproxen, aspirin (rarely), dantrolene, etc.

- Whole body cooling

Medications

- ACETAMINOPHEN   (*Tempra, Tylenol, Paracetamol*)
    - AAP = Maternal Medication Usually Compatible with Breastfeeding
    - LRC = L1
    - RID = 8.8-24.2%
    - Pregnancy = B
    - Comment: Only small amounts are secreted into breastmilk and are considered too small to be hazardous. In a study of 11 mothers who received 650 mg of acetaminophen orally, the highest milk levels reported were from 10-15 mg/L. The milk/plasma ratio was 1.08. In another study of three patients who received a single 500 mg oral dose, the reported milk and plasma concentrations of acetaminophen was 4.2 mg/L and 5.6 mg/L, respectively. The milk/plasma ratio was 0.76. The maximum observed concentration in milk was 4.4 mg/L. In another study of women who ingested 1000 mg acetaminophen, milk levels averaged 6.1 mg/L and provided an average dose of 0.92 mg/kg/d, according to the authors. There seems to be wide variation in the milk concentrations in these studies, but the relative infant dose is probably less than 6.4% of the maternal dose.

This is significantly less than the pediatric therapeutic dose. Acetaminophen is compatible with breastfeeding.

- ASPIRIN   (*Anacin, Aspergum, Empirin, Genprin, Arthritis Foundation Pain Reliever, Ecotrin*)
  - ○ AAP = Drugs associated with significant side effects and should be given with caution
  - ○ LRC = L3
  - ○ RID   = 2.5 - 10.8%
  - ○ Pregnancy = C during first and second trimester
  - ○ Comment: Only small amounts are secreted into breastmilk. Few harmful effects have been reported. In one study, salicylic acid (active metabolite of Aspirin) penetrated poorly into milk (dose =454 mg ASA), with peak levels of only 1.12 to 1.60 µg/mL, whereas peak plasma levels were 33 to 43.4 µg/mL.

    In another study of a rheumatoid arthritis patient who received 4 gm/day aspirin, none was detectable in her milk (<5 mg/100cc). Extremely high doses in the mother could potentially produce slight bleeding in the infant. Because aspirin is implicated in Reye syndrome, it is a poor choice of analgesic to use in breastfeeding mothers. However, in rheumatic fever patients, it is still one of the anti-inflammatory drugs of choice and a risk-vs-benefit assessment must be done in this case.

    In a study of a patient consuming aspirin chronically, salicylate concentrations in milk peaked at three hours at a concentration of 10 mg/L following a maternal dose of 975 mg. Maternal plasma levels peaked at 2.25 hours at 108 mg/L. The milk/plasma ratio was reported to be 0.08.

    In a study of eight women following the use of 1 gram oral doses of aspirin, average milk levels of salicylic acid (active metabolite of aspirin) were 2.4 mg/L at three hours. The metabolite salicyluric acid, reached a peak of 10.2 mg/L at nine hours. Averaging total salicylates and salicyluric acid metabolites, the author suggests the relative infant dose would be 9.4% of the maternal dose.

    While the direct use of aspirin in infants and children is certainly implicated in Reye syndrome, the use of the 82 mg/day dose in breastfeeding mothers is unlikely to increase the risk of this syndrome. Unfortunately, we do not at present know of any dose-response relationship between aspirin and Reye syndrome. Therefore, the use of aspirin in breastfeeding mothers is questionable, but the risk is probably quite low. See ibuprofen or acetaminophen as better choices. Never use these products if the infant has a viral syndrome.

- DANTROLENE   (*Dantrium*)
  - ○ AAP = Not reviewed
  - ○ LRC = L4
  - ○ RID   = 7.9%
  - ○ Pregnancy = C
  - ○ Comment: Dantrolene produces a direct skeletal muscle relaxation and is indicated for spasticity resulting from upper motor neuron disorders, such as multiple sclerosis, cerebral palsy, etc. It is not indicated for rheumatic disorders or musculoskeletal trauma.

    In one study, a mother received IV dantrolene (160 mg) for symptoms of malignant hyperthermia after the umbilical cord was clamped just after the delivery of her baby. Concentrations of dantrolene in breastmilk ranged from 1.2 mg/L on day 2 to 0.05 mg/L on day four. The relative infant dose is calculated at 7.88% of the maternal dose. The highest concentration in breastmilk was detected 36 hours after the first IV bolus of dantrolene. Based on the elimination half-life determined in this study (9.02 hours), the authors suggest that breastfeeding is safe two days after discontinuation of IV dantrolene administration in the mother. The infant should be monitored for nausea, vomiting, fatigue, and muscle weakness, which are all known side effects of therapeutic doses in adults.

- IBUPROFEN   (*Advil, Nuprin, Motrin, Pediaprofen*)
    ○ AAP = Maternal Medication Usually Compatible with Breastfeeding
    ○ LRC = L1
    ○ RID = 0.1-0.7%
    ○ Pregnancy = B in first and second trimester
    ○ Comment: Ibuprofen is a nonsteroidal anti-inflammatory analgesic. It is frequently used for fever in infants. Ibuprofen enters milk only in very low levels (less than 0.6% of maternal dose). Even large doses produce very small milk levels. In one patient receiving 400 mg twice daily, milk levels were less than 0.5 mg/L.

      In another study of 12 women who received 400 mg doses every six hours for a total of five doses, all breastmilk levels of ibuprofen were less than 1.0 mg/L, the lower limit of the assay. Data in these studies document that no measurable concentrations of ibuprofen are detected in breastmilk following the above doses. Ibuprofen is presently popular for therapy of fever in infants. Current recommended dose in children is 5-10 mg/kg every six hours. Ibuprofen is an ideal analgesic for breastfeeding mothers.

Clinical Tips

Non-drug therapies of fever include hydration, removing of excess clothing, avoidance of exercise, removal from excessive environmental temperatures, and bathing in lukewarm water (not ice water or alcohol). Cooling blankets may be used in an inpatient setting. Topical alcohol is absorbed through the skin, can induce a chemical pneumonitis or ketosis, and should not be used. Acetaminophen is an ideal antipyretic when administered in proper doses. Except in rare circumstances with severe hepatotoxicity, normal therapeutic doses appear to be very safe. Doses in adults are 325 – 650 mg every three to four hours. Ibuprofen has become very popular as an antipyretic. Therapeutic doses of ibuprofen produce a more rapid fall in temperature and a longer duration (five to eight hours) than with acetaminophen. This effect is more evident upon initial use and may not sustain itself after repeated use. Ibuprofen is the safest NSAID for use in breastfeeding mothers, as milk levels are very small. Ibuprofen should not be used in patients with gastric ulcers, nor in a mother in her third trimester (closure of ductus arteriosus), and only cautiously in asthmatic patients. Although aspirin levels in milk are low, the fear of Reye syndrome precludes their use in pediatrics.

Dipyrone is an antipyretic from the pyrazolone nonsteroidal anti-inflammatory family. Because of the risk of agranulocytosis, it is no longer used in the US, but it is still used in other countries. There is no evidence that it is more effective than ibuprofen, and it is only used in life-threatening hyperthermia unresponsive to other drugs. While it is unlikely to enter milk in clinically relevant amounts, it should not be used in breastfeeding mothers.

Suggested Reading

Goodman, E. L. (2000). Practice guidelines for evaluating new fever in critically ill adult patients. *Clin Infect Dis, 30*(1), 234.

Kayman, H. (2003). Management of fever: making evidence-based decisions. *Clin Pediatr (Phila), 42*(5), 383-392.

Osborne, L., Snyder, M., Villecco, D., Jacob, A., Pyle, S., & Crum-Cianflone, N. (2008). Evidence-based anesthesia: fever of unknown origin in parturients and neuraxial anesthesia. *Aana J, 76*(3), 221-226.

Thompson, H. J., Kirkness, C. J., Mitchell, P. H., & Webb, D. J. (2007). Fever management practices of neuroscience nurses: national and regional perspectives. *J Neurosci Nurs, 39*(3), 151-162.

Zuckermann, J., Moreira, L. B., Stoll, P., Moreira, L. M., Kuchenbecker, R. S., & Polanczyk, C. A. (2008). Compliance with a critical pathway for the management of febrile neutropenia and impact on clinical outcomes. *Ann Hematol, 87*(2), 139-145.

Gastroesophageal Reflux Disease

Principles of Therapy

Gastroesophageal reflux disease (GERD) is the most common disorder of the esophagus and is most commonly associated with a significant relaxation of the lower esophageal sphincter. GERD arises following recurrent regurgitation of gastric acids past the lower esophageal sphincter and into the lower esophagus. The major determinant of esophageal symptoms and damage is prolonged contact of refluxed gastric acid with the lower esophageal epithelium. Symptoms occur most often at night when the patient is recumbent and include hyperacidity, burping, and severe chest pain similar but distinct from those with a heart attack. Gastric acids can easily pass the lower esophageal sphincter and enter the esophagus while the patient is horizontal. Medical therapy alleviates many of the symptoms, but GERD should be considered a chronic condition, especially in patients with inflammatory esophagitis. Treatment consists of the use of antacids, acid blocking agents, and occasionally the prokinetic drugs (metoclopramide).

Treatment

- Lifestyle modifications, such as smoking cessation, weight loss, elevation of the head of the bed, avoidance of certain foods, such as coffee, alcohol, fatty or spicy foods, etc.

- Antacids.

- Antisecretory medications, such as the proton pump inhibitors (PPI) and histamine H2 receptor blockers.

- PPI's should be administered 30 minutes prior to breakfast for optimal results.

Medications

- ESOMEPRAZOLE   (*Nexium*)
    - AAP = Not reviewed
    - LRC = L2
    - RID =
    - Pregnancy = C
    - Comment: Esomeprazole is just the L isomer of omeprazole (Prilosec) and is essentially identical to Prilosec. See omeprazole for breastfeeding recommendations.

- FAMOTIDINE   (*Pepcid, Axid-AR, Pepcid-AC*)
    - AAP = Not reviewed
    - LRC = L1

- ◦ RID = 1.9%
- ◦ Pregnancy = B
- ◦ Comment: Famotidine is a typical Histamine-2 antagonist that reduces stomach acid secretion. In one study of eight lactating women receiving a 40 mg/day dose, the peak concentration in breastmilk was 72 µg/L and occurred at six hours postdose. The milk/plasma ratios were 0.41, 1.78, and 1.33 at 2, 6, and 24 hours, respectively. These levels are apparently much lower than other histamine H-2 antagonists (ranitidine, cimetidine) and make it a preferred choice.

- LANSOPRAZOLE   (*Prevacid, Prevpac, Prevacid NapraPak*)
  - ◦ AAP = Not reviewed
  - ◦ LRC = L3
  - ◦ RID =
  - ◦ Pregnancy = B
  - ◦ Comment: Lansoprazole is a proton pump inhibitor that suppresses the release of acid protons from the parietal cells in the stomach, effectively raising the pH of the stomach. Structurally similar to omeprazole, it is very unstable in stomach acid, and to a large degree, it is denatured by acidity of the infant's stomach. A new study shows milk levels of omeprazole are minimal (see omeprazole), and it is likely milk levels of lansoprazole are small as well. Although there are no studies of lansoprazole in breastfeeding mothers, transfer to milk and its oral absorption (via milk) is likely to be minimal in a breastfed infant.

- NIZATIDINE   (*Axid*)
  - ◦ AAP = Not reviewed
  - ◦ LRC = L2
  - ◦ RID = 0.5%
  - ◦ Pregnancy = B
  - ◦ Comment: Nizatidine is an antisecretory, histamine-2 antagonist that reduces stomach acid secretion. In one study of five lactating women using a dose of 150 mg, milk levels of nizatidine were directly proportional to circulating maternal serum levels, yet were very low. Over a 12 hour period, 96 µg (less than 0.1% of dose) was secreted into the milk. No effects on infants have been reported.

- OMEPRAZOLE   (*Prilosec*)
  - ◦ AAP = Not reviewed
  - ◦ LRC = L2
  - ◦ RID = 1.1%
  - ◦ Pregnancy = C
  - ◦ Comment: Omeprazole is a potent inhibitor of gastric acid secretion. In a study of one patient receiving 20 mg omeprazole daily, the maternal serum concentration was negligible until 90 minutes after ingestion, and then reached 950 nM at 240 minutes. The breastmilk concentration of omeprazole began to rise minimally at 90 minutes after ingestion and peaked after 180 minutes at only 58 nM, or less than 7% of the highest serum level. This would indicate a maximum dose of 3 µg/kg/day in a breastfed infant. Omeprazole milk levels were essentially flat over four hours of observation. Omeprazole is extremely acid labile with a half-life of 10 minutes at pH values below four. Virtually all omeprazole ingested via milk would probably be destroyed in the stomach of the infant prior to absorption.

- **PANTOPRAZOLE** (*Protonix*)
  - AAP = Not reviewed
  - LRC = L1
  - RID = 1%
  - Pregnancy = B
  - Comment: Pantoprazole is a proton-pump inhibitor similar to omeprazole (Prilosec). The pharmaceutical manufacturer reports 0.02% of an administered dose is excreted into milk. In a 61.6 kg patient who received a single 40 mg tablet, pantoprazole levels in milk were undetectable, except at two hours(0.036 mg/L) and four hours (0.024 mg/L) after administration. The pantoprazole levels in milk were estimated to be only 2.8% of the maternal plasma levels (AUC), so the M/P ratio is extraordinarily low. Using the highest concentration achieved, the relative infant dose would only be 0.95%. The daily dose would be many times lower than this, as the milk levels were undetectable at five hours. As with all the proton-pump inhibitors, pantoprazole is completely unstable in an acid milieu, and when presented in milk, it would be largely destroyed before absorption.

- **RABEPRAZOLE** (*Aciphex*)
  - AAP = Not reviewed
  - LRC = L3
  - RID =
  - Pregnancy = B
  - Comment: Rabeprazole is an antisecretory proton pump inhibitor similar to omeprazole (Prilosec). Rodent studies suggest a high milk/plasma ratio, but as we know, these do not correlate well with humans. No data are available in humans. Further, rabeprazole is only 52% bioavailable in adults when enteric coated due to its instability in gastric acids. As presented in milk, it would be virtually destroyed in the infant's stomach prior to absorption.

- **RANITIDINE** (*Zantac*)
  - AAP = Not reviewed
  - LRC = L2
  - RID = 1.3-4.6%
  - Pregnancy = B
  - Comment: Ranitidine is a prototypic histamine-2 blocker used to reduce acid secretion in the stomach. It has been widely used in pediatrics without significant side effects, primarily for gastroesophageal reflux (GER). Following a dose of 150 mg for four doses, concentrations in breastmilk were 0.72, 2.6, and 1.5 mg/L at 1.5, 5.5, and 12 hours, respectively. The milk/serum ratios varied from 6.81, 8.44, to 23.77 at 1.5, 5.5, and 12 hours, respectively. Although the milk/plasma ratios are quite high, using these data, an infant would ingest at most 0.4 mg/kg/d. This amount is quite small considering the pediatric dose currently recommended is 2-4 mg/kg/24 hours. See nizatidine or famotidine for alternatives.

- **SUCRALFATE** (*Carafate*)
  - AAP = Not reviewed
  - LRC = L2

- RID = 1.9%
- Pregnancy = B
- Comment: Sucralfate is a sucrose aluminum complex used for stomach ulcers. When administered orally, sucralfate forms a complex that physically covers stomach ulcers. Less than 5% is absorbed orally. At these plasma levels, it is very unlikely to penetrate into breastmilk.

Clinical Tips

Initial therapy of mild GERD is comprised of antacids or the H2 receptor blockers (e.g., famotidine, ranitidine). Of the antacids, Gaviscon (alginic acids and antacids) is quite popular, as it floats on the stomach contents, thus covering the lower esophageal sphincter. However, in more difficult cases of erosive esophagitis, the H2 blockers are poorly effective. Famotidine and nizatidine produce only minimal levels in breastmilk and are probably preferred over ranitidine. However, ranitidine levels in breastmilk are probably too low to produce a clinical effect.

In more severe cases of GERD, one of the many proton pump inhibitors (PPI) is preferred. Of the many PPIs, omeprazole or its congener, esomeprazole, are probably preferred, as so little is reportedly present in milk. Further, any omeprazole present in milk would be instantly destroyed in the infant's stomach prior to absorption. Esomeprazole (Nexium) is the active ingredient of omeprazole (Prilosec) and should be safe for use in breastfeeding mothers. Sucralfate is the aluminum salt of sucrose octasulfate. It acts topically, binding to acid, pepsin, and bile on the stomach or esophageal lining. None would be expected to enter milk.

Suggested Reading

Ali, R. A., & Egan, L. J. (2007). Gastroesophageal reflux disease in pregnancy. *Best Pract Res Clin Gastroenterol, 21*(5), 793-806.

Ford, A. C., & Moayyedi, P. (2008). Current guidelines for dyspepsia management. *Dig Dis, 26*(3), 225-230.

Jian, R., Hassani, Z., El Kebir, S., & Barthelemy, P. (2007). Management of gastro-esophageal reflux disease in primary care. Results from an observational study of 2,474 patients (AO). *Gastroenterol Clin Biol, 31*(1), 72-77.

Nava-Ocampo, A. A., Velázquez-Armenta, E. Y., Han, J. Y., & Koren, G. (2006). Use of proton pump inhibitors during pregnancy and breastfeeding. *Can Fam Physician, 52*, 853-854.

Thukral, C., & Wolf, J. L. (2006). Therapy insight: drugs for gastrointestinal disorders in pregnant women. *Nat Clin Pract Gastroenterol Hepatol, 3*(5), 256-266.

Vakil, N., Malfertheiner, P., Salis, G., Flook, N., & Hongo, M. (2008). An international primary care survey of GERD terminology and guidelines. *Dig Dis, 26*(3), 231-236.

Wang, C., & Hunt, R. H. (2008). Medical management of gastroesophageal reflux disease. *Gastroenterol Clin North Am, 37*(4), 879-899, ix.

Giardiasis

Principles of Therapy

Giardiasis is an infection of the small intestine caused by Giardia lamblia, a flagellated protozoan, and occurs with an estimated prevalence of 3-9% depending on the country. The infection is found worldwide, especially in children where sanitation conditions are poor. *Giardia lamblia* attaches to the intestinal brush border, especially in the duodenum. The incubation period is one to two weeks post exposure. Risks are higher for patients with HIV, gastrectomies, lower gastric acidity, and immunodeficiencies. Symptoms in adults may be acute or chronic, usually mild, and consist of nausea, flatulence, epigastric pain, abdominal cramps, malodorous stools, and diarrhea. Acute diarrhea due to giardiasis can be differentiated from other intestinal infections by the lack of blood or mucous in the stools, presence of upper abdominal cramping, distention, and malodorous stools. Contamination often occurs during camping trips and among children or workers at day care centers. Contamination can also occur through sexual activity, including potential oral-fecal contamination.

Treatment

- Drug of choice: Metronidazole (250 mg TID for five days).

- Pediatric dosing of metronidazole is 15 mg/kg/day for five days.

- Tinidazole (2 gm oral dose) is an option, single dose. Generally only recommended for metronidazole-resistant species.

- Furazolidone (100 mg four times daily for 7-10 days) is a poorer choice due to nauea and vomiting.

- Quinacrine (100 mg TID for five days).

- Nitazoxanide (Alinia) is an alternate choice.

Medications

- ALBENDAZOLE   (*Albenza*)
    - AAP = Not reviewed
    - LRC = L3
    - RID =
    - Pregnancy = C
    - Comment: Albendazole is a broad-spectrum anthelmintic used for treating intestinal parasite infections. It is virtually unabsorbed (<5%) orally and would be unlikely to harm an infant even if present in milk. It is often used to treat common parasitic infections in pediatric patients all over the world.

- FURAZOLIDONE   (*Furoxone*)
  - AAP = Not reviewed
  - LRC = L2
  - RID =
  - Pregnancy = C
  - Comment: Furazolidone belongs to the nitrofurantoin family of antibiotics (see nitrofurantoin). It has a broad-spectrum of activity against gram-positive and gram-negative enteric organisms including cholera, but is generally used for giardiasis. Following an oral dose, furazolidone is poorly absorbed (<5%) and is largely inactivated in the gut. Concentrations transferred to milk are unreported, but the total amounts would be exceedingly low due to the low maternal plasma levels attained by this product. Due to poor oral absorption, systemic absorption in a breastfeeding infant would likely be minimal. Caution should be observed in early postpartum newborns.

- TINIDAZOLE   (*Tindamax*)
  - AAP = Drugs whose effect on nursing infants is unknown but may be of concern
  - LRC = L2
  - RID = 12.2%
  - Pregnancy = C
  - Comment: Tinidazole is an antimicrobial agent that is sometimes used for the treatment of anaerobic infections and protozoal infections, such as intestinal amebiasis, Giardia, and trichomoniasis. It is similar to metronidazole. Tinidazole is highly lipophilic and passes membranes easily attaining high concentrations in virtually all body tissues. Concentrations in saliva and bile are equivalent to that of the plasma compartment. In a study of 24 women who received a single IV infusion immediately postpartum of 500 mg, aliquots of milk and serum were collected at 12, 24, 48, 72, and 96 hours after the injection. At 48 and 72 hours, fore and hind milk samples were also taken, whereas at 12 and 24 hours only mixed milk samples were collected. Milk levels at 12 and 24 hours were 5.8 and 3.5 mg/L, respectively. Serum levels at 12 and 24 hours averaged 6.1 and 3.7 mg/L, respectively. The milk/serum ratios at 12 and 24 hours were 0.94 and 0.95, respectively, further suggesting the high lipid solubility of this product. At 48 and 72 hours, the fore milk levels were 1.28 and 0.32 mg/L, respectively. Hind milk levels at these same times were 1.2 and 0.3, respectively. At 96 hours only trace amounts were present in milk and none in serum. Another study of five women taking a dose of 1600 mg IV, reported milk-to-plasma ratios of between 0.62 and 1.39. After 72 hours, the majority of the milk samples were below 0.5 µg/mL. The authors, therefore, concluded that breastfeeding should be withheld for 72 hours after a 1600 mg IV dose of tinidazole.

    Please be aware that the studies above were done using IV tinidazole, not the oral formulation recommended for giardia infections. Orally, levels would be much lower than intravenous studies.

- METRONIDAZOLE   (*Flagyl, Metizol, Trikacide, Protostat, Noritate*)
  - AAP = Drugs whose effect on nursing infants is unknown but may be of concern
  - LRC = L2
  - RID = 12.6-13.5%
  - Pregnancy = B
  - Comment: Metronidazole is indicated in the treatment of vaginitis due to Trichomonas Vaginalis and various anaerobic bacterial infections, including Giardiasis, H. Pylori, B. Fragilis, and

Gardnerella vaginalis. Metronidazole has become the treatment of choice for pediatric giardiasis (AAP). Metronidazole absorption is time and dose dependent and also depends on the route of administration (oral vs. vaginal). Following a 2 gm oral dose, milk levels were reported to peak at 50-57 mg/L at two hours. Milk levels after 12 hours were approximately 19 mg/L, and at 24 hours were approximately 10 mg/L. The average drug concentration reported in milk at two, eight, 12, and 12-24 hours was 45.8, 27.9, 19.1, and 12.6 mg/L, respectively. If breastfeeding were to continue uninterrupted, an infant would consume 21.8 mg via breastmilk. With a 12 hour discontinuation, an infant would consume only 9.8 mg. In a group of 12 nursing mothers receiving 400 mg three times daily, the mean milk/plasma ratio was 0.91. The mean milk metronidazole concentration was 15.5 mg/L. Infant plasma metronidazole levels ranged from 1.27 to 2.41 µg/mL. No adverse effects were attributable to metronidazole therapy in these infants. In another study in patients receiving 600 and 1200 mg daily, the average milk metronidazole concentration was 5.7 and 14.4 mg/L, respectively. The plasma levels of metronidazole (two hours) at the 600 mg/d dose were 5 µg/mL (mother) and 0.8 µg/mL (infant). At the 1200 mg/d dose (two hours), plasma levels were 12.5 µg/mL (mother) and 2.4 µg/mL (infant). The authors estimated the daily metronidazole dose received by the infant at 3.0 mg/kg, with 500 mL milk intake per day, which is well below the advocated 10-20 mg/kg recommended therapeutic dose for infants.

It is true that the relative infant dose via milk is moderately high depending on the dose and timing. Infants whose mothers ingest 1.2 gm/d will receive approximately 13.5% or less of the maternal dose or approximately 2.3 mg/kg/day. Bennett has calculated the relative infant dose from 11.7% to as high as 24% of the maternal dose. Heisterberg found metronidazole levels in infant plasma to be 16% and 19% of the maternal plasma levels following doses of 600 mg/d and 1200 mg/d. While these levels seem significant, it is still pertinent to remember that metronidazole is a commonly used drug in premature neonates, infants, and children, and 2.3 mg/kg/d is still much less than the therapeutic dose used in infants/children (7.5-30 mg/kg/d). Thus far, virtually no adverse effects have been reported.

Clinical Tips

The treatment of adult giardiasis as recommended by the World Health Organization is metronidazole in a dose of 250 mg TID for five days. Oral tinidazole is sometimes recommended for metronidazole-resistant giardiasis. In some cases, furazolidone (100 mg QID X 7 days) can be used. Metronidazole entry into breastmilk has been well studied and is moderate and dose dependent. Metronidazole concentrations in milk vary widely from 9.9% to 13% of the maternal dose at doses of 0.6 g/d to 1.2 g/d. No untoward effects have been reported in breastfed infants in numerous studies. Metronidazole, just as in patients, may impart a metallic taste to milk. Some infants reject milk for this reason.

Albendazole is also useful and is a potent antiparisiticide.

Suggested Reading

Buret, A. G. (2008). Pathophysiology of enteric infections with Giardia duodenalius. *Parasite, 15*(3), 261-265.

Escobedo, A. A., & Cimerman, S. (2007). Giardiasis: a pharmacotherapy review. *Expert Opin Pharmacother, 8*(12), 1885-1902.

Jones, J. L., Schulkin, J., & Maguire, J. H. (2005). Therapy for common parasitic diseases in pregnancy in the United States: a review and a survey of obstetrician/gynecologists' level of knowledge about these diseases. *Obstet Gynecol Surv, 60*(6), 386-393.

Kiser, J. D., Paulson, C. P., & Brown, C. (2008). Clinical inquiries. What's the most effective treatment for giardiasis? *J Fam Pract, 57*(4), 270-272.

ten Hove, R., Schuurman, T., Kooistra, M., Moller, L., van Lieshout, L., & Verweij, J. J. (2007). Detection of diarrhoea-causing protozoa in general practice patients in The Netherlands by multiplex real-time PCR. *Clin Microbiol Infect, 13*(10), 1001-1007.

Yoder, J. S., & Beach, M. J. (2007). Giardiasis surveillance--United States, 2003-2005. *MMWR Surveill Summ, 56*(7), 11-18.

Glaucoma

Principles of Therapy

Glaucoma is a group of ocular diseases that have in common an optic neuropathy that causes visual loss. Elevated intraocular pressure is the most important and only modifiable risk factor for glaucoma. Treatment for the various types of glaucoma are specific, and the essential diagnosis of the mechanism of glaucoma is required. Acute (angle-closure) glaucoma occurs most commonly in older patients with acute onset pain, profound visual loss, red eye, steamy cornea, and dilated pupil. Primary acute angle-closure glaucoma is almost always associated with pupillary dilation from setting in a darkened environment, at times of stress, from pharmacologic mydriasis during eye examinations, or from systemic anticholinergic medications (atropine-like). Open-angle glaucoma, on the other hand, has an insidious onset, generally in older age groups. Symptoms are minimal, if present at all, with gradual loss of peripheral vision over a period of years. In open-angle glaucoma, the intraocular pressure is consistently elevated. Over months and years, this ultimately results in optic atrophy with loss of vision. In the USA, it is estimated that 1-2% of people over 40 have glaucoma. About 90% are open-angle glaucoma. Unfortunately, breastfeeding studies of the agents used to treat glaucoma are poor and few. The medications below are primarily used to reduce intraocular pressures by one of several mechanisms.

Treatment

- The medications below are primarily used to reduce intraocular pressures by one of several mechanisms.

- For closed-angle glaucoma, immediate surgery is usually performed to alleviate the increased pressure.

- For open-angle glaucoma, various medications can be used to decrease the production of aqueous humor. These include prostaglandins, beta-blockers, alpha-agonists, and carbonic anhydrase inhibitors. Surgery and laser treatments can also be used to facilitate drainage of the aqueous humor.

- We unfortunately do not have much data concerning these drugs in breastfeeding mothers. However, because these drugs are applied locally in the eye and absorption is local, the systemic absorption and plasma levels are exceeding low. Thus the risk to breastfed infants is probably quite low.

Medications

- ACETAZOLAMIDE   (*Dazamide, Diamox*)
    - AAP = Maternal Medication Usually Compatible with Breastfeeding
    - LRC = L2
    - RID = 2.2%

- Pregnancy = C
- Comment: Acetazolamide is a carbonic anhydrase inhibitor dissimilar to other thiazide diuretics. In a patient receiving 500 mg of acetazolamide twice daily, acetazolamide concentrations in milk were 1.3 to 2.1 mg/L, while the maternal plasma levels ranged from 5.2-6.4 mg/L. Plasma concentrations in exposed infants were 0.2 to 0.6 µg/mL 2-12 hours after breastfeeding. These amounts are unlikely to cause adverse effects in the infant.

- BETAXOLOL   (*Kerlone, Betoptic*)
  - AAP = Not reviewed
  - LRC = L3
  - RID =
  - Pregnancy = C
  - Comment: Betaxolol is a long-acting, cardioselective beta blocker primarily used for glaucoma, but can be used orally for hypertension. One report by the manufacturer reports side effects which occurred in one nursing infant. Many in this family readily transfer into human milk (see atenolol, acebutolol), others do so poorly (propranolol, metoprolol). Betaxolol, when use ophthalmically, is apparently poorly absorbed systemically, as no evidence of beta blockade can be found in patients following its use ophthalmically. When used orally, one set of authors suggest a milk/plasma ratio of 3.0, and another suggest a milk/plasma ratio of 2.5-3.0. These data suggests some may actually reach the milk compartment.

- BRIMONIDINE   (*Alphagan*)
  - AAP = Not reviewed
  - LRC = L3
  - RID =
  - Pregnancy = B
  - Comment: Brimonidine is an alpha adrenergic receptor antagonist used to reduce intraocular pressure in open-angle glaucoma by reducing aqueous humor production and increasing uveoscleral outflow. No data are available on its transfer into human milk. If used in breastfeeding mothers, observe the infant closely for alpha adrenergic blockage, although this is unlikely.

- BIMATOPROST   (*Lumigan*)
  - AAP = Not reviewed
  - LRC = L3
  - RID =
  - Pregnancy = C
  - Comment: Bimatoprost is used in open-angle glaucoma or ocular hypertension to reduce intraocular pressure. No breastfeeding data are available. However, after intraocular administration, plasma levels peak at 10 minutes, then fall rapidly to undetectable levels within 1.5 hours. Combined with low plasma levels and high protein binding, it is unlikely this product will produce measurable levels in human milk.

- CARTEOLOL   (*Cartrol*)
  - AAP = Not reviewed

- LRC = L3
- RID =
- Pregnancy = C
- Comment: Carteolol is a typical beta-blocker used for hypertension. Carteolol is reported to be excreted in breastmilk of lactating animals. No data are available on human milk.

- **DORZOLAMIDE** (*Trusopt*)
  - AAP = Not reviewed
  - LRC = L3
  - RID =
  - Pregnancy = C
  - Comment: Dorzolamide is a carbonic anhydrase inhibitor used to treat interocular hypertension, open-angle glaucoma, etc. It is a unique formulation that exerts its effects directly in the eye. No data are available on its transfer into human milk. However, this product would be only slightly absorbed by the mother. This agent is stored for long periods in the red blood cells, although plasma levels are exceedingly low. Milk levels will probably be low to undetectable.

- **LATANOPROST** (*Xalatan*)
  - AAP = Not reviewed
  - LRC = L3
  - RID =
  - Pregnancy = C
  - Comment: Latanoprost is a prostaglandin F2-alpha analogue used for the treatment of ocular hypertension and glaucoma. One drop used daily is usually effective. No data are available on the transfer of this product into human milk, but it is unlikely. Prostaglandins are by nature rapidly metabolized. Plasma levels are barely detectable, and then only for one hour after use. Combined with the short half-life, minimal plasma levels, and poor oral bioavailability, untoward effects via milk are unlikely.

- **LEVOBUNOLOL** (*Bunolol*)
  - AAP = Not reviewed
  - LRC = L3
  - RID =
  - Pregnancy = C
  - Comment: Levobunolol is a typical beta blocker used ophthalmically for treatment of glaucoma. Some absorption has been reported, with resultant bradycardia in adult patients. No data on transfer to human milk are available.

- **PILOCARPINE** (*Isopto Carpine, Pilocar, Akarpine, Ocusert Pilo*)
  - AAP = Not reviewed
  - LRC = L3
  - RID =

- ◦ Pregnancy = C
- ◦ Comment: Pilocarpine is a direct acting cholinergic agent used primarily in the eyes for treatment of open-angle glaucoma. The ophthalmic dose is approximately 1 mg or less per day, while the oral adult dose is approximately 15-30 mg daily. It is not known if pilocarpine enters milk, but it probably does in low levels due to its minimal plasma level. It is not likely that an infant would receive a clinical dose via milk, but this is presently unknown. Side effects would largely include diarrhea, gastric upset, excessive salivation, and other typical cholinergic symptoms.

- **TIMOLOL**   (*Blocadren*)
  - ◦ AAP = Maternal Medication Usually Compatible with Breastfeeding
  - ◦ LRC = L2
  - ◦ RID = 1.1%
  - ◦ Pregnancy = C
  - ◦ Comment: Timolol is a beta blocker used for treating hypertension and glaucoma. It is secreted into milk. Following a dose of 5 mg three times daily, milk levels averaged 15.9 µg/L. Both oral and ophthalmic drops produce modest levels in milk. Breastmilk levels following ophthalmic use of 0.5% timolol drops was 5.6 µg/L at 1.5 hours after the dose. Untoward effects on infants have not been reported. These levels are probably too small to be clinically relevant.

Clinical Tips

The first-line treatment for glaucoma is generally the prostaglandin analog products (bimatoprost, latanoprost, travoprost). Second-line therapy is generally with the beta blockers.

Although no data are available, latanoprost (Xalatan) could probably be useful in breastfeeding mothers, as its plasma half-life (17 minutes) is extremely brief, and its poor systemic bioavailability is unlikely to produce clinically relevant levels in milk. A topical prostaglandin, latanoprost in a single daily application effectively lowers intraocular pressure for 24 hours. It is generally well tolerated with few systemic side effects. The major ocular side effects are increased pigmentation of the iris, particularly in hazel-colored irises, and possible worsening of uveitis. A new prostaglandin F2-alpha analogue, travoprost (Travatan) with ocular hypotensive activity also produces minimal plasma levels and has a brief half-life of less than 30 minutes. While the manufacturer suggests it is present in rodent milk, no human data are available. It is not likely to be orally bioavailable in an infant.

The topical beta-blockers, timolol, levobunolol, and betaxolol, are effective ocular hypotensives and work by decreasing the production of aqueous humor. Systemic absorption via absorption by the nasal mucosa is known and can be reduced by digital occlusion of the nasolacrimal drainage system for several minutes following installation of the drops. Reported side effects associated with topical beta-blockers include bronchospasm and shortness of breath, depression, fatigue, confusion, impotence, hair loss, heart failure, and bradycardia. Several studies of timolol show no effect on nursing infants. Betaxolol may be a lesser choice following one report of side effects in a nursing infant.

Oral carbonic anhydrase inhibitors (e.g., acetazolamide, methazolamide, brinzolamide) are effective in lowering intraocular pressure IOP. However, their side effects include anorexia, depression, kidney stones, fatigue, abnormalities in serum electrolytes, and blood dyscrasias, which often limit their usefulness. They are probably not suitable for long-term use in breastfeeding mothers, but are probably of little risk to a breastfeeding infant.

Other agents, such as the organophosphates, which include echothiophate, have not been studied in breastfeeding women, but should be used with caution as they irreversibly inhibit acetylcholine esterase and can produce systemic effects.

Suggested Reading

Alm, A., Grierson, I., & Shields, M. B. (2008). Side effects associated with prostaglandin analog therapy. *Surv Ophthalmol, 53*(Suppl 1), S93-105.

Boland, M. V., Quigley, H. A., & Lehmann, H. P. (2008). The impact of risk calculation on treatment recommendations made by glaucoma specialists in cases of ocular hypertension. *J Glaucoma, 17*(8), 631-638.

Coleman, A. L., Mosaed, S., & Kamal, D. (2005). Medical therapy in pregnancy. *J Glaucoma, 14*(5), 414-416.

Goldberg, L. D. (2002). Clinical guidelines for the treatment of glaucoma. *Manag Care, 11*(11 Suppl), 16-24.

Kwon, Y. H., Fingert, J. H., Kuehn, M. H., & Alward, W. L. (2009). Primary open-angle glaucoma. *N Engl J Med, 360*(11), 1113-1124.

McColl, E. (2005). I just want the protocol, doctor! *Qual Saf Health Care, 14*(3), 155.

Sloan, F. A., Brown, D. S., Carlisle, E. S., Picone, G. A., & Lee, P. P. (2004). Monitoring visual status: why patients do or do not comply with practice guidelines. *Health Serv Res, 39*(5), 1429-1448.

Gonorrhea

Principles of Therapy

Gonorrhea is an acute infectious disease of the epithelium of the urethra, cervix, rectum, pharynx, or eyes due to infection with *N. gonorrhoeae*. The cervix is the most common mucosal site of infection. *N. gonorrhoeae* is identified in discharges as pairs or clumps of gram-negative diplococci. The disease is spread by sexual contact. Women are often asymptomatic carriers of the organisms for weeks or months and may only be identified by tracing sexual partners. In men, the incubation period is 2-14 days. Onset is marked by mild discomfort in the urethra, dysuria, and purulent discharge. In women, symptoms usually begin 7-21 days after infection. Symptoms are generally mild and include dysuria, frequency, and vaginal discharge. Often women may be asymptomatic until symptoms of pelvic inflammatory disease are present. Treatment of gonorrhea has become more complicated due to the high frequency of concurrent infection with *Chlamydia trachomatis* in some populations. Depending on the frequency of coinfection in the particular population, it may be more cost effective to treat for presumed coinfection with chlamydia than screen for the disease. An additional concern is the increasing resistance of *N. gonorrhoeae* to penicillins. *N. gonorrhoeae* resistance to fluoroquinolone antibiotics has also been sporadically reported, though this is presently rare (< 0.05%) in the United States. There are numerous treatment regimens available, and the clinician must choose according to sensitivity and allergies of patient and sensitivity of the organism.

Treatment

* CDC-recommended first-line treatment is with ceftriaxone (125 mg IM single dose) or cefixime (Suprax) 400 mg orally in single dose.

* Unless Chlamydia infection has been ruled out, patients with gonorrhea require empiric treatment for chlamydia.

* Spectinomycin 2 gm IM once. (Not currently available in US market)

* Cefoxitin 2 gm IM plus probenecid 1 gm orally.

* Cefotaxime 50 mg IM once.

* Ceftizoxime 50 mg IM once.

* Azithromycin 2 gm orally once for treatment of gonorrhea. The 1 gm oral dose is for treatment of chlamydia.

* Fluoroquinolones are no longer recommended.

* Sexual partners need to be evaluated; men are often asymptomatic carriers of gonorrhea and will re-infect their treated partners, as well as spread infection to other partners.

Medications

- AZITHROMYCIN (*Zithromax*)
  - AAP = Not reviewed
  - LRC = L2
  - RID = 5.9%
  - Pregnancy = B
  - Comment: Azithromycin belongs to the erythromycin family. It has an extremely long half-life, particularly in tissues. Azithromycin is concentrated for long periods in phagocytes, which are known to be present in human milk. In one study of a patient who received 1 gm initially followed by 500 mg doses each at 24 hour intervals, the concentration of azithromycin in breastmilk varied from 0.64 mg/L (initially) to 2.8 mg/L on day three. The predicted dose of azithromycin received by the infant would be approximately 0.4 mg/kg/day. This would suggest that the level of azithromycin ingested by a breastfeeding infant is not clinically relevant.

- CEFIXIME (*Suprax*)
  - AAP = Not reviewed
  - LRC = L2
  - RID =
  - Pregnancy = B
  - Comment: Cefixime is an oral, third-generation cephalosporin used in treating infections. It is poorly absorbed (30-50%) by the oral route. It is secreted to a limited degree in the milk, although in one study of a mother receiving 100 mg, it was undetected in the milk from one to six hours after the dose.

- CEFOTAXIME (*Claforan*)
  - AAP = Maternal Medication Usually Compatible with Breastfeeding
  - LRC = L2
  - RID = 0.3%
  - Pregnancy = B
  - Comment: Cefotaxime is poorly absorbed orally and is only used via IV or IM administration. Milk levels following a 1000 mg IV maternal dose were 0.26 mg/L at one hour, 0.32 mg/L at two hours, and 0.30 mg/L at three hours. No effect on infant or lactation were noted. Milk/serum ratio at three hours was 0.160. In a group of two to three patients receiving 1000 mg IV, none to trace amounts were found in milk after six hours.

- CEFOXITIN (*Mefoxin*)
  - AAP = Maternal Medication Usually Compatible with Breastfeeding
  - LRC = L1
  - RID = 0.1-0.3%
  - Pregnancy = B
  - Comment: Cefoxitin is a cephalosporin antibiotic with a spectrum similar to the second generation family. It is transferred into human milk in very low levels. In a study of 18 women receiving 2000-

4000 mg doses, only one breastmilk sample contained cefoxitin (0.9 mg/L); all the rest were too low to be detected. In another study of two to three women who received 1000 mg IV, only trace amounts were reported in milk over six hours. In a group of five women who received an IM injection of 2000 mg, the highest milk levels were reported at four hours after dose. The maternal plasma levels varied from 22.5 at two hours to 77.6 µg/mL at four hours. Maternal milk levels ranged from <0.25 to 0.65 mg/L. Observe for changes in gut flora.

- CEFTIZOXIME   (*Cefizox, Baxam*)
  - ○ AAP = Not reviewed
  - ○ LRC = L1
  - ○ RID = 0.3-0.6%
  - ○ Pregnancy = B
  - ○ Comment: Ceftizoxime is a third generation cephalosporin used for many infections, similar to ceftriaxone and others. In a study of 18 patients who received 1 gm IV daily, milk levels of ceftizoxime averaged 0.52 mg/L. The maximum reported concentration was 2.38 mg/L. In studies of five and seven women (1 gm IV), milk levels averaged 0.43 and 0.54 mg/L. In a study of six women who received 1 gm IV, milk levels of 0.25 mg/L were reported at one hour postdose. In four good studies, Ceftizoxime produced only negligible levels in milk. The relative infant dose is only 0.55%. Observe for changes in gut flora and diarrhea.

- CEFTRIAXONE   (*Rocephin*)
  - ○ AAP = Maternal Medication Usually Compatible with Breastfeeding
  - ○ LRC = L2
  - ○ RID = 4.1-4.2%
  - ○ Pregnancy = B
  - ○ Comment: Ceftriaxone is a very popular third-generation broad-spectrum cephalosporin antibiotic. Small amounts are transferred into milk (3-4% of maternal serum level). Following a 1 gm IM dose, breastmilk levels were approximately 0.5-0.7 mg/L at between four to eight hours. The estimated mean milk levels at steady state were 3-4 mg/L. Another source indicates that following a 2 g/d dose and at steady state, approximately 4.4% of dose penetrates into milk. In this study, the maximum breastmilk concentration was 7.89 mg/L after prolonged therapy (seven days). Poor oral absorption of ceftriaxone would further limit systemic absorption by the infant. The half-life of ceftriaxone in human milk varies from 12.8 to 17.3 hours (longer than maternal serum). Even at this high dose, no adverse effects were noted in the infant. Ceftriaxone levels in breastmilk are probably too low to be clinically relevant, except for changes in GI flora. Ceftriaxone is commonly used in neonates.

Clinical Tips

Recommended therapy for gonorrhea in a breastfeeding woman is ceftriaxone 125 mg IM. Secondary choices include spectinomycin (2 gm IM once only for use in pregnant patients allergic to beta-lactams), doxycycline (not in pregnant women) (100 mg BID for seven days), or azithromycin (2 gm single dose). Although the risks of doxycycline are remote, azithromycin therapy may be a better choice in breastfeeding patients. Azithromycin levels in milk are very low. The fluoroquinolones were previously recommended for gonorrhea, but are no longer recommended due to resistance world-wide. Cefixime 400 mgs orally can also be substituted for ceftriaxone IM. Cefixime has a slightly lower clinical cure rate of approximately 97% compared to the 99% or better cure rate with ceftriaxone. A 2 gram single oral dose of Azithromycin is an effective alternative treatment for both gonorrhea and chlamydia (1 gram orally), but it is expensive and may include possible gastrointestinal side effects. As with treatment for chlamydia, patients with gonorrhea should be instructed to refer their sexual partners for therapy and should refrain from intercourse until after treatment has been given.

Suggested Reading

CDC. (2007). Update to CDC's sexually transmitted diseases treatment guidelines, 2006: fluoroquinolones no longer recommended for treatment of gonococcal infections. *MMWR Morb Mortal Wkly Rep, 56*(14), 332-336.

Donders, G. G. (2006). Management of genital infections in pregnant women. *Curr Opin Infect Dis, 19*(1), 55-61.

Farhi, D., Hotz, C., Poupet, H., Gerhardt, P., Morand, P., Poyart, C., et al. (2009). Neisseria gonorrhoeae antibiotic resistance in Paris, 2005 to 2007: implications for treatment guidelines. *Acta Derm Venereol, 89*(5), 484-487.

Kropp, R. Y., Latham-Carmanico, C., Steben, M., Wong, T., & Duarte-Franco, E. (2007). What's new in management of sexually transmitted infections? Canadian Guidelines on Sexually Transmitted Infections, 2006 Edition. *Can Fam Physician, 53*(10), 1739-1741.

Trigg, B. G., Kerndt, P. R., & Aynalem, G. (2008). Sexually transmitted infections and pelvic inflammatory disease in women. *Med Clin North Am, 92*(5), 1083-1113, x.

Workowski, K. A., Berman, S. M., & Douglas, J. M. J. (2008). Emerging antimicrobial resistance in Neisseria gonorrhoeae: urgent need to strengthen prevention strategies. *Ann Intern Med, 148*(8), 606-613.

Headache, Migraine

Principles of Therapy

Classic migraine headache is a lateralized throbbing headache that occurs episodically. It is three times more common in females than males, and occurs in 18% of adult women. The symptoms of migraine vary enormously between patients, and the classification is largely based on the headache's characteristics and associated symptoms. Two major varieties of migraine have been described and are the migraine with aura (classic migraine) or the migraine without aura (common migraine). The aura is a focal neurologic symptom that often precedes the attack and may consist of visual hallucinations, such as stars, sparks, light flashes, and luminous hallucinations (scintillating scotomas).

The etiology of migraine is obscure, although it is no longer considered a vascular-based phenomenon (vasoconstriction followed by vasodilation). Nausea occurs in 90% of patients, as well as photophobia, phonophobia, and blurred vision. Treatment of migraine is either to prevent the acute episode or to prevent future attacks (prophylactic). Acute therapies include mild opioids, ergot alkaloids, antiemetics, sedatives, caffeine adjuvant compound, and serotonin agonists. Prophylactic therapies include beta-blockers, calcium channel blockers, antidepressants, serotonin antagonists, and anticonvulsants. In patients with mild to moderate pain, therapy includes the use of analgesics, acetaminophen, mild sedatives, or NSAIDs. If treatment fails, sumatriptan or transnasal butorphanol may be required. Ergot alkaloids should be absolutely avoided in breastfeeding mothers during the first six months postpartum and during pregnancy.

Treatment

- Some migraine patients respond to mild analgesics, such as NSAIDS and acetaminophen.

- Triptans (sumatriptan, zolmitriptan, eletriptan, etc.) are widely used as first-line treatment due to their efficacy and safety profile.

- Hyperbaric oxygen may be effective.

- Dihydroergotamine is efficacious, but has more side effects.

- Acute use of metoclopramide is commonly used in emergency rooms.

- Antiemetics (prochlorperazine) are helpful in relieving nausea and vomiting.

- Opioids are efficacious, but should be avoided.

- For prophylaxis of migraine attacks, many options exist, including topiramate, beta blockers, and tricyclic antidepressants.

- Avoid sildenafil (Viagra), as it has a high propensity to induce migraines.

- Oral contraceptives are no longer believed associated with increased risk of migraine.

Medications

- ACETAMINOPHEN   (*Tempra, Tylenol, Paracetamol*)
  - AAP = Maternal Medication Usually Compatible with Breastfeeding
  - LRC = L1
  - RID = 8.8-24.2%
  - Pregnancy = B
  - Comment: Only small amounts are secreted into breastmilk and are considered too small to be hazardous. In a study of 11 mothers who received 650 mg of acetaminophen orally, the highest milk levels reported were from 10-15 mg/L. The milk/plasma ratio was 1.08. In another study of three patients who received a single 500 mg oral dose, the reported milk and plasma concentrations of acetaminophen was 4.2 mg/L and 5.6 mg/L, respectively. The milk/plasma ratio was 0.76. The maximum observed concentration in milk was 4.4 mg/L. In another study of women who ingested 1000 mg acetaminophen, milk levels averaged 6.1 mg/L and provided an average dose of 0.92 mg/kg/d according to the authors. There seems to be wide variation in the milk concentrations in these studies, but the relative infant dose is probably less than 6.4% of the maternal dose. This is significantly less than the pediatric therapeutic dose. Acetaminophen is compatible with breastfeeding.

- AMITRIPTYLINE   (*Elavil, Endep*)
  - AAP = Drugs whose effect on nursing infants is unknown but may be of concern
  - LRC = L2
  - RID = 1.9-2.8%
  - Pregnancy = C
  - Comment: Amitriptyline and its active metabolite, nortriptyline, are secreted into breastmilk in small amounts. In one report of a mother taking 100 mg/day of amitriptyline, milk levels of amitriptyline and nortriptyline (active metabolite) averaged 143 µg/L and 55.5 µg/L, respectively; maternal serum levels averaged 112 µg/L and 72.5 µg/L, respectively. No drug was detected in the infant's serum. From these data, an infant would consume approximately 21.5 µg/kg/day, a dose that is unlikely to be clinically relevant. In another study following a maternal dose of 25 mg/day, the amitriptyline and nortriptyline (active metabolite) levels in milk were 30 µg/L and <30 µg/L, respectively. In the same study when the dosage was 75 mg/day, milk levels of amitriptyline and nortriptyline averaged 88 µg/L and 69 µg/L, respectively. Both drugs were essentially undetectable in the infant's serum. Therefore, the authors estimated that a nursing infant would receive less than 0.1 mg/day.

    In another mother taking 175 mg/day, amitriptyline levels in the mother's milk were the same as in her serum on day one (24-27 µg/mL), but milk levels decreased to 54% of the serum concentration on days 2-26. Milk concentrations of nortriptyline were 74% of that in the mother's serum (87 ng/mL). Thus the authors reported the absolute infant dose as 35 µg/kg, 80 times lower than the mother's dose. Neither compound could be detected in the infant's serum on day 26, nor were there any signs of sedation or other adverse effects.

- BUTALBITAL COMPOUND   (*Fioricet, Fiorinal, Bancap, Two-Dyne*)
  - AAP = Not reviewed
  - LRC = L3
  - RID =
  - Pregnancy = C
  - Comment: Mild analgesic with acetaminophen (325 mg) or aspirin, caffeine (40 mg), and butalbital (50 mg). Butalbital is a mild, short-acting barbiturate that probably transfers into breastmilk to a limited degree, although it is unreported. No data are available on the transfer of butalbital to breastmilk, but it is likely minimal.

- DICLOFENAC   (*Cataflam, Voltaren*)
  - AAP = Not reviewed
  - LRC = L2
  - RID = 1.05%
  - Pregnancy = B topical/ C oral
  - Comment: Diclofenac is a typical nonsteroidal analgesic (NSAID). Voltaren is a sustained release product, whereas Cataflam is an immediate release product. In one study of six postpartum mothers receiving three 50 mg doses on day one, followed by two 50 mg doses on day two, the levels of diclofenac in breastmilk were approximately 5 ng/mL of milk, although the limit of detection was reported as <19 ng/mL. In another patient on long-term treatment with diclofenac, milk levels of 0.1 μg/mL milk were reported, which would amount to 0.015 mg/kg/d ingested. These amounts are probably far too low to affect an infant.

- IBUPROFEN   (*Advil, Nuprin, Motrin, Pediaprofen*)
  - AAP = Maternal Medication Usually Compatible with Breastfeeding
  - LRC = L1
  - RID = 0.1-0.7%
  - Pregnancy = B in first and second trimester
  - Comment: Ibuprofen is a nonsteroidal anti-inflammatory analgesic. It is frequently used for fever in infants. Ibuprofen enters milk only in very low levels (less than 0.6% of maternal dose). Even large doses produce very small milk levels. In one patient receiving 400 mg twice daily, milk levels were less than 0.5 mg/L.

    In another study of 12 women who received 400 mg doses every six hours for a total of five doses, all breastmilk levels of ibuprofen were less than 1.0 mg/L, the lower limit of the assay. Data in these studies document that no measurable concentrations of ibuprofen are detected in breastmilk following the above doses. Ibuprofen is presently popular for therapy of fever in infants. Current recommended dose in children is 5-10 mg/kg every six hours. Ibuprofen is an ideal analgesic for breastfeeding mothers.

- KETOROLAC   (*Toradol, Acular*)
  - AAP = Maternal Medication Usually Compatible with Breastfeeding
  - LRC = L2
  - RID = 0.2%

- Pregnancy = C in first and second trimesters
- Comment: Ketorolac is a popular, nonsteroidal analgesic. Although previously used in labor and delivery, its use has subsequently been contraindicated because it is believed to adversely effect fetal circulation and inhibit uterine contractions, thus increasing the risk of hemorrhage.

  In a study of ten lactating women who received 10 mg orally four times daily, milk levels of ketorolac were not detectable in four of the subjects. In the six remaining patients, the concentration of ketorolac in milk two hours after a dose ranged from 5.2 to 7.3 μg/L on day one and 5.9 to 7.9 μg/L on day two. In most patients, the breastmilk level was never above 5 μg/L. The maximum daily dose an infant could absorb (maternal dose = 40 mg/day) would range from 3.16 to 7.9 μg/day, assuming a milk volume of 400 mL or 1000 mL. An infant would, therefore, receive less than 0.2% of the daily maternal dose. (Please note, the original paper contained a misprint on the daily intake of ketorolac [mg instead of μg].)

- METOCLOPRAMIDE   (*Reglan*)
  - AAP = Drugs whose effect on nursing infants is unknown but may be of concern
  - LRC = L2
  - RID = 4.7-14.3%
  - Pregnancy = B
  - Comment: Metoclopramide has multiple functions, but is primarily used for increasing the lower esophageal sphincter tone in gastroesophageal reflux in patients with reduced gastric tone. In breastfeeding, it is sometimes used in lactating women to stimulate prolactin release from the pituitary and enhance breastmilk production. Since 1981, a number of publications have documented major increases in breastmilk production following the use of metoclopramide, domperidone, or sulpiride. With metoclopramide, the increase in serum prolactin and breastmilk production appears dose-related, up to a dose of 15 mg three times daily. Many studies show 66 to 100% increases in milk production, depending on the degree of breastmilk supply in the mother prior to therapy and maybe her initial prolactin levels. Doses of 15 mg/day were found ineffective, whereas doses of 30-45 mg/day were most effective. In most studies, major increases in prolactin were observed, such as from 125 ng/mL to 172 ng/mL in one patient.

    In Kauppila's study, the concentration of metoclopramide in milk was consistently higher than the maternal serum levels. The peak occurred at two to three hours after administration of the medication. During the late puerperium, the concentration of metoclopramide in the milk varied from 20 to 125 μg/L, which was less than the 28 to 157 μg/L noted during the early puerperium. The authors estimated the daily dose to infant to vary from 6 to 24 μg/kg/day during the early puerperium and from 1 to 13 μg/kg/day during the late phase. These doses are minimal compared to those used for therapy of reflux in pediatric patients (0.1 to 0.5 mg/kg/day). In these studies, only one of five infants studied had detectable blood levels of metoclopramide; hence, no accumulation or side effects were observed. While plasma prolactin levels in the newborns were comparable to those in the mothers prior to treatment, Kauppila found slight increases in prolactin levels in four of seven newborns following treatment with metoclopramide, although a more recent study did not find such changes. However, prolactin levels are highly variable and subject to diurnal rhythm, thus timing is essential in measuring prolactin levels and could account for this inconsistency.

    In another study of 23 women with premature infants, milk production increased from 93 mL/day to 197 mL/day between the first and seventh day of therapy with 30 mg/day. Prolactin levels, although varied, increased from 18.1 to 121.8 ng/mL. While basal prolactin levels were elevated significantly, metoclopramide seems to blunt the rapid rise of prolactin when milk was expressed. Nevertheless, milk production was still elevated.

Gupta studied 32 mothers with inadequate milk supply. Following a dose of 10 mg three times daily, a 66-100% increase in milk supply was noted. Of twelve cases of complete lactation failure, eight responded to treatment in an average of three to four days after starting therapy. In this study, 87.5% of the total 32 cases responded to metoclopramide therapy with greater milk production. No untoward effects were noted in the infants. Side effects, such as gastric cramping and diarrhea, limit the compliance of some patients, but are rare. Further, it is often found that upon rapid discontinuation of the medication, the supply of milk may, in some instances, reduce significantly. Tapering of the dose is generally recommended, and one possible regimen is to decrease the dose by 10 mg per week. Long-term use of this medication (>four weeks) may be accompanied by increased side effects, such as depression in the mother, although some patients have used it successfully for months. Another dopamine antagonist, Domperidone, due to minimal side effects, is a preferred choice, but is, unfortunately, not available in the USA, other than in compounding pharmacies.

Two recent cases of serotonin-like reactions (agitation, dysarthria, diaphoresis, and extrapyramidal movement disorder) have been reported when metoclopramide was used in patients receiving sertraline or venlafaxine.

- METOPROLOL (*Toprol-XL, Lopressor*)
  - ○ AAP = Maternal Medication Usually Compatible with Breastfeeding
  - ○ LRC = L3
  - ○ RID = 1.4%
  - ○ Pregnancy = C
  - ○ Comment: At low doses, metoprolol is a very cardioselective beta-1 blocker, and it is used for hypertension, angina, and tachyarrhythmias. In a study of three women four to six months postpartum who received 100 mg twice daily for four days, the peak concentration of metoprolol ranged from 0.38 to 2.58 µmol/L, whereas the maternal plasma levels ranged from 0.1 to 0.97 µmol/L. The mean milk/plasma ratio was 3.0. Assuming ingestion of 75 mL of milk at each feeding and the maximum concentration of 2.58 µmol/L, an infant would ingest approximately 0.05 mg metoprolol at the first feeding and considerably less at subsequent feedings. In another study of nine women receiving 50-100 mg twice daily, the maternal plasma and milk concentrations ranged from 4-556 nmol/L and 19-1690 nmol/L, respectively. Using these data, the authors calculated an average milk concentration throughout the day as 280 µg/L of milk. This dose is 20-40 times less than a typical clinical dose. The milk/plasma ratio in these studies averaged 3.72.

    Although the milk/plasma ratios for this drug are, in general high, the maternal plasma levels are quite small, so the absolute amount transferred to the infant are quite small. Although these levels are probably too low to be clinically relevant, clinicians should use metoprolol under close supervision.

- NAPROXEN (*Anaprox, Naprosyn, Aleve*)
  - ○ AAP = Maternal Medication Usually Compatible with Breastfeeding
  - ○ LRC = L3
  - ○ RID = 3.3%
  - ○ Pregnancy = C

- ○ Comment: Naproxen is a popular NSAID analgesic. In a study done at steady state in one mother consuming 375 mg twice daily, milk levels ranged from 1.76-2.37 mg/L at four hours. Total naproxen excretion in the infant's urine was only 0.26% of the maternal dose. Although the amount of naproxen transferred via milk is minimal, one should use with caution in nursing mothers because of its long half-life and its effect on the infant's cardiovascular system, kidneys, and GI tract. However, its short term use postpartum, or infrequent or occasional use, would not necessarily be incompatible with breastfeeding. One case of prolonged bleeding, hemorrhage, and acute anemia has been reported in a seven-day-old infant. The relative infant dose on a weight-adjusted maternal daily dose would probably be less than 3.3%.

- NIFEDIPINE   (*Adalat, Procardia*)
  - ○ AAP = Maternal Medication Usually Compatible with Breastfeeding
  - ○ LRC = L2
  - ○ RID = 2.3-3.4%
  - ○ Pregnancy = C
  - ○ Comment: Nifedipine is an effective antihypertensive. It belongs to the calcium channel blocker family of drugs. Two studies indicate that nifedipine is transferred to breastmilk in varying, but generally low levels. In one study in which the dose was varied from 10-30 mg three times daily, the highest concentration (53.35 µg/L) was measured at one hour after a 30 mg dose. Other levels reported were 16.35 µg/L 60 minutes after a 20 mg dose and 12.89 µg/L 30 minutes after a 10 mg dose. The milk levels fell linearly with the milk half-lives estimated to be 1.4 hours for the 10 mg dose, 3.1 hours for the 20 dose, and 2.4 hours for the 30 mg dose. The milk concentration measured eight hours following a 30 mg dose was 4.93 µg/L. In this study, using the highest concentration found and a daily intake of 150 mL/kg of human milk, the amount of nifedipine intake would only be 8 µg/kg/day (less than 1.8% of the therapeutic pediatric dose). The authors conclude that the amount ingested via breastmilk poses little risk to an infant. In another study, concentrations of nifedipine in human milk one to eight hours after 10 mg doses varied from <1 to 10.3 µg/L (median 3.5 µg/L) in six of 11 patients. In this study, milk levels three days after discontinuing medication ranged from <1 to 9.4 µg/L. The authors concluded the exposure to nifedipine through breastmilk is not significant. In a study by Penny and Lewis, following a maternal dose of 20 mg nifedipine daily for 10 days, peak breastmilk levels at one hour were 46 µg/L. The corresponding maternal serum level was 43 µg/L. From these data, the authors suggest a daily intake for an infant would be approximately 6.45 µg/kg/day.

- NORTRIPTYLINE   (*Aventyl, Pamelor*)
  - ○ AAP = Drugs whose effect on nursing infants is unknown but may be of concern
  - ○ LRC = L2
  - ○ RID = 1.7-3.1%
  - ○ Pregnancy = D
  - ○ Comment: Nortriptyline (NT) is a tricyclic antidepressant and is the active metabolite of amitriptyline (Elavil). In one patient receiving 125 mg of nortriptyline at bedtime, milk concentrations of NT averaged 180 µg/L after six to seven days of administration. Based on these concentrations, the authors estimate the average daily infant exposure would be 27 µg/kg/d. The relative dose in milk would be 1.5% of the maternal dose. Several other authors have been unable to detect NT in maternal milk nor the serum of infants after prolonged exposure. So far, no untoward effects have been noted.

A pooled analysis of 35 studies, with an average dose of 78 mg/day, reported a detectable level of nortriptyline in the breastmilk in only one patient, with a concentration of 230 ng/mL. The authors suggest that breastfeeding infants exposed to nortriptyline are unlikely to develop detectable concentrations in plasma. Therefore, breastfeeding during nortriptyline therapy is not contraindicated.

- PROPRANOLOL   (*Inderal*)
  - AAP = Maternal Medication Usually Compatible with Breastfeeding
  - LRC = L2
  - RID = 0.3-0.5%
  - Pregnancy = C
  - Comment: Propranolol is a popular beta blocker used in treating hypertension, cardiac arrhythmia, migraine headache, and numerous other syndromes. In general, the maternal plasma levels are exceedingly low; hence, the milk levels are low as well. Milk/plasma ratios are generally less than one. In one study of three patients, the average milk concentration was only 35.4 µg/L after multiple dosing intervals. The milk/plasma ratio varied from 0.33 to 1.65. Using these data, the authors suggest that an infant would receive only 70 µg/L of milk per day, which is <0.1% of the maternal dose.

    In another study of a patient receiving 20 mg twice daily, milk levels varied from 4 to 20 µg/L, with an estimated average dose to infant of 3 µg/day. In another patient receiving 40 mg four times daily, the peak concentration occurred at three hours after dosing. Milk levels varied from 0-9 µg/L. After a 30 day regimen of 240 mg/day propranolol, the predose and postdose concentration in breastmilk was 26 and 64 µg/L, respectively. No symptoms or signs of beta blockade were noted in this infant. The above amounts in milk would likely be clinically insignificant. Long-term exposure has not been studied and caution is urged. Of the beta blocker family, propranolol is probably preferred in lactating women. Use with great caution, if at all, in mothers or infants with asthma.

- SUMATRIPTAN SUCCINATE   (*Imitrex*)
  - AAP = Maternal Medication Usually Compatible with Breastfeeding
  - LRC = L3
  - RID = 3.5-15.3%
  - Pregnancy = C
  - Comment: Sumatriptan is a 5-HT (Serotonin) receptor agonist and a highly effective new drug for the treatment of migraine headache. It is not an analgesic, rather it produces a rapid vasoconstriction in various regions of the brain, thus temporarily reducing the cause of migraines. In one study using five lactating women, each were given 6 mg subcutaneous injections and samples were drawn for analysis over eight hours. The highest breastmilk levels were 87.2 µg/L at 2.6 hours postdose and rapidly disappeared over the next six hours. The mean total recovery of sumatriptan in milk over the eight hour duration was only 14.4 µg. On a weight-adjusted basis, this concentration in milk corresponded to a mean infant exposure of only 3.5% of the maternal dose. Further, assuming an oral bioavailability of only 14%, the weight-adjusted dose an infant would absorb would be approximately 0.49% of the maternal dose. The authors suggest that continued breastfeeding following sumatriptan use would not pose a significant risk to a nursing infant.

The maternal plasma half-life is 1.3 hours; the milk half-life is 2.2 hours. Although the milk/plasma ratio was 4.9 (indicating significant concentrating mechanisms in milk), the absolute maternal plasma levels were small; hence, the absolute milk concentrations were low.

- TOPIRAMATE   (*Topamax*)
    - ○ AAP = Not reviewed
    - ○ LRC = L3
    - ○ RID = 24.5%
    - ○ Pregnancy = C
    - ○ Comment: Topiramate is an anticonvulsant used in controlling refractory partial seizures. In a group of two women receiving topiramate (150-200 mg/day) at three weeks postpartum, the mean milk/plasma ratio was 0.86 (range=0.67-1.1). The concentration of topiramate in milk averaged 7.9 uM (range= 1.6 to 13.7). The weight normalized relative infant dose (RID), assuming a milk intake of 150 mL/kg/d, was 3-23% of the maternal dose/day. The absolute infant dose was 0.1 to 0.7 mg/kg/day. The plasma concentrations of topiramate in two infants were 1.4 and 1.6 uM, respectively. The plasma level in another infant was undetectable. The plasma concentrations in the two infants were 10-20% of the maternal plasma level. At four weeks, the milk/plasma ratio had dropped to 0.69 and plasma levels in the infant were <0.9 uM and 2.1 uM, respectively.

    Topiramate has become increasingly popular due to its fewer adverse side effects. Due to the fact that the plasma levels found in breastfeeding infants were significantly less than in maternal plasma, the risk of using this product in breastfeeding mothers is probably acceptable. Close observation for sedation is advised.

- VALPROIC ACID   (*Depakene, Depakote*)
    - ○ AAP = Maternal Medication Usually Compatible with Breastfeeding
    - ○ LRC = L2
    - ○ RID = 1.4-1.7%
    - ○ Pregnancy = D
    - ○ Comment: Valproic acid is a popular anticonvulsant used in grand mal, petit mal, myoclonic, and temporal lobe seizures. In a study of 16 patients receiving 300-2400 mg/d, valproic acid concentrations ranged from 0.4 to 3.9 mg/L (mean=1.9 mg/L). The milk/plasma ratio averaged 0.05. In a study of one patient receiving 250 mg twice daily, milk levels ranged from 0.18 to 0.47 mg/L. The milk/plasma ratio ranged from 0.01 to 0.02. Alexander reports milk levels of 5.1 mg/L following a larger dose of up to 1600 mg/d.

    In another study of six women receiving 9.5 to 31 mg/kg/d valproic acid, milk levels averaged 1.4 mg/L, while serum levels averaged 45.1 mg/L. The average milk/serum ratio was 0.027.

    Most authors agree that the amount of valproic acid transferring to the infant via milk is low. Breastfeeding would appear safe. However, the infant may need monitoring for liver and platelet changes.

- VERAPAMIL   (*Calan, Isoptin, Covera-HS*)
    - ○ AAP = Maternal Medication Usually Compatible with Breastfeeding
    - ○ LRC = L2
    - ○ RID = 0.2%

- ○ Pregnancy = C
- ○ Comment: Verapamil is a typical calcium channel blocker used as an antihypertensive. It is secreted into milk, but in very low levels, which are highly controversial. Anderson reports that in one patient receiving 80 mg three times daily, the average steady-state concentrations of verapamil and norverapamil in milk were 25.8 and 8.8 μg/L, respectively. The respective maternal plasma level was 42.9 μg/L. The milk/plasma ratio for verapamil was 0.60. No verapamil was detected in the infant's plasma. Inoue reports that in one patient receiving 80 mg four times daily, the milk level peaked at 300 μg/L at approximately 14 hours. These levels are considerably higher than the aforementioned. In another study of a mother receiving 240 mg daily, the concentrations in milk were never higher than 40 μg/L. See bepridil, diltiazem, nifedipine as alternates. From these three studies, the relative infant dose would vary from 0.15%, 0.98%, and 0.18%, respectively. Regardless of the variability, the relative amount transferred to the infant is still quite small. Lastly, calcium channel blockers are not very effective in the treatment of migraine headaches.

Clinical Tips

Numerous therapies for migraine attacks are available. The choice depends on the severity and frequency of attack, the presence of other conditions (pregnancy, breastfeeding), and patient acceptance. Initial therapy generally starts with oral analgesics; NSAIDs, such as ibuprofen or naproxen; or caffeine adjuvant compounds (Fiorinal). Ibuprofen, due to low milk levels, is an ideal NSAID. Naproxen, when used infrequently, is also useful in some patients. Caffeine adjuvant compounds, such as butalbital compound (Fiorinal, Fioricet), may work in some patients if used sparingly. Recently, diclofenac has been approved for treatment of migraine. Non-pharmacologic treatments include cold gel pack to head, constant temporal artery pressure, hyperbaric oxygen treatment, and even oxygen treatment via mask.

More severe headaches may require oral, intranasal, or subcutaneous sumatriptan. Studies show that milk levels of sumatriptan are quite low, and its oral bioavailability is low (10-15%). Numerous other triptans (almotriptan, eletriptan, rizatriptan, naratriptan, etc.) are available, but have not yet been studied in breastfeeding mothers. Their enhanced oral bioavailability should probably preclude their use in breastfeeding mothers.

For long-term prophylaxis, propranolol or metoprolol are ideal beta-blockers and have been used in many breastfeeding mothers. Although other beta-blockers have been used (nadolol, atenolol), these have been associated with side effects in infants. Beta-blockers should not be used in patients with low energy levels, depression, congestive heart failure, or asthma. Observe the infant for typical beta-blocker side effects, including hypoglycemia, hypotension, weakness, and apnea, although these are unlikely.

Tricyclic antidepressants (TCAs) have been used for many years. Amitriptyline has medium to high efficacy and is particularly useful for patients with sleep disturbances (insomnia). Side effects of TCAs are common and include dry mouth, constipation, blurred vision, and sedation. However, their poor penetration into milk makes them ideal candidates for chronic pain, including migraine.

The anticonvulsant valproic acid is a highly effective treatment for migraines. It is primarily used in a sustained release formulation (divalproex), and plasma levels are maintained as high as 120 μg/mL. It can be safely used in patients with other co-morbid states, such as asthma, diabetes, depression, and Raynaud's phenomena - conditions that are usually contraindications to the use of beta-blockers. The anticonvulsant topiramate has become increasingly popular for the acute treatment of migraine. While its relative infant dose is high, short-term use would probably be acceptable.

The ergotamine alkaloids (DHE-45, Cafergot, etc.) are contraindicated in breastfeeding mothers due to their suppression of prolactin. However, this is not an absolute contraindication, as breastfeeding becomes less dependent on prolactin at four to six months, and occasional doses later on may not overtly suppress lactation. The limited amount transferred via milk and the poor oral bioavailability of the ergot alkaloids would limit their clinical effect on an older infant. Recently, the use of intravenous metoclopramide in emergency departments suggests it may be effective alone in treatment of migraine. This use is yet unapproved, but would certainly not be contraindicated in breastfeeding mothers.

Suggested Reading

Bigal, M. E., & Lipton, R. B. (2008). Excessive acute migraine medication use and migraine progression. *Neurology, 71*(22), 1821-1828.

De Klippel, N., Jansen, J. P., & Carlos, J. S. (2008). Survey to evaluate diagnosis and management of headache in primary care: Headache Management Pattern programme. *Curr Med Res Opin, 24*(12), 3413-3422.

Firnhaber, J. M., & Rickett, K. (2009). Clinical inquiries. What are the best prophylactic drugs for migraine? *J Fam Pract, 58*(11), 608-610.

Lipton, R. B., Bigal, M. E., Diamond, M., Freitag, F., Reed, M. L., & Stewart, W. F. (2007). Migraine prevalence, disease burden, and the need for preventive therapy. *Neurology, 68*(5), 343-349.

Marcus, D. A. (2008). Managing headache during pregnancy and lactation. *Expert Rev Neurother, 8*(3), 385-395.

Scharfman, H. E., & MacLusky, N. J. (2008). Estrogen-growth factor interactions and their contributions to neurological disorders. *Headache, 48*(Suppl 2), S77-89.

Silberstein, S., Loder, E., Diamond, S., Reed, M. L., Bigal, M. E., & Lipton, R. B. (2007). Probable migraine in the United States: results of the American Migraine Prevalence and Prevention (AMPP) study. *Cephalalgia, 27*(3), 220-234.

Sun-Edelstein, C., Bigal, M. E., & Rapoport, A. M. (2009). Chronic migraine and medication overuse headache: clarifying the current International Headache Society classification criteria. *Cephalalgia, 29*(4), 445-452.

Zeeberg, P., Olesen, J., & Jensen, R. (2009). Medication overuse headache and chronic migraine in a specialized headache centre: field-testing proposed new appendix criteria. *Cephalalgia, 29*(2), 214-220.

Headache, Tension

Principles of Therapy

Headache is such a common term and can occur for so many reasons that it is difficult to properly evaluate. Although underlying pathology, such as brain tumor, is very uncommon, it is important to remember that over 33% of brain tumor patients present with headache. The choice of therapy largely depends on frequency, intensity, site, and preexisting conditions (pregnancy, breastfeeding, etc.) in the patient. For the purpose of this category, migraine is presented in its own section. Tension headaches are extremely common and usually due to tension in the scalp or cervical muscles. The pain is usually bilateral and commonly described as pressure, squeezing, throbbing, or pounding.

Treatment

- Over-the-counter analgesics are first-line treatment, such as acetaminophen, naproxen, and ibuprofen.

- Have the patient document the details of their headaches when they occur.

- For chronic headaches, tricyclic antidepressants and SSRIs have been shown to be effective.

Medications

- ACETAMINOPHEN (*Tempra, Tylenol, Paracetamol*)
  - AAP = Maternal Medication Usually Compatible with Breastfeeding
  - LRC = L1
  - RID = 8.8-24.2%
  - Pregnancy = B
  - Comment: Only small amounts are secreted into breastmilk and are considered too small to be hazardous. In a study of 11 mothers who received 650 mg of acetaminophen orally, the highest milk levels reported were from 10-15 mg/L. The milk/plasma ratio was 1.08. In another study of three patients who received a single 500 mg oral dose, the reported milk and plasma concentrations of acetaminophen was 4.2 mg/L and 5.6 mg/L, respectively. The milk/plasma ratio was 0.76. The maximum observed concentration in milk was 4.4 mg/L. In another study of women who ingested 1000 mg acetaminophen, milk levels averaged 6.1 mg/L and provided an average dose of 0.92 mg/kg/d according to the authors. There seems to be wide variation in the milk concentrations in these studies, but the relative infant dose is probably less than 6.4% of the maternal dose. This is significantly less than the pediatric therapeutic dose. Acetaminophen is compatible with breastfeeding.

- CODEINE   (*Empirin #3 # 4, Tylenol # 3 # 4*)
    - AAP = Maternal Medication Usually Compatible with Breastfeeding
    - LRC = L3
    - RID   = 8.1%
    - Pregnancy = C
    - Comment: Codeine is considered a mild opiate analgesic, whose action is probably due to its metabolism to small amounts (about 7%) of morphine. The amount of codeine secreted into milk is low and dose dependent. Infant response is higher during the neonatal period (first or second week). Four cases of neonatal apnea have been reported following administration of 60 mg codeine every four to six hours to breastfeeding mothers, although codeine was not detected in serum of the infants tested. Apnea resolved after discontinuation of maternal codeine. Tylenol # 3 tablets contain 30 mg and Tylenol #4 tablets contain 60 mg of codeine in the USA.

      In another study, following a dose of 60 mg, milk concentrations averaged 140 µg/L of milk, with a peak of 455 µg/L at one hour. Following 12 doses in 48 hours, the authors estimate the dose of codeine in milk (2000 mL milk) was 0.7 mg. There are few reported side effects following codeine doses of 30 mg, and it is believed to produce only minimal side effects in newborns. In a study of seven mothers, codeine and morphine levels were studied in breastmilk of 17 samples and neonatal plasma of 24 samples from 11 healthy, term neonates. Milk codeine levels ranged from 33.8 to 314 µg/L 20 to 240 minutes after ingestion of codeine; morphine levels ranged from 1.9 to 20.5 µg/L. Infant plasma samples one to four hours after feeding had codeine levels ranging from <0.8 to 4.5 µg/L; morphine ranged from <0.5 to 2.2 µg/L. The authors suggest that moderate codeine use during breastfeeding (< or = four 60 mg doses) is probably safe.

      In a recent report, an infant death was reported following the use of codeine (initially two tablets every 12 hours, reduced to half that dose from day two to two weeks because of maternal somnolence and constipation) in a mother. Codeine levels in milk were reported to be 87 µg/L, while the average reported milk levels in most mothers range from 1.9 to 20.5 µg/L at doses of 60 mg every six hours. Genotype analysis of this specific mother indicated that she was an ultra-rapid metabolizer of codeine. This genotype (which is very rare) leads to increased formation of morphine from codeine.

      Ultimately, each infant's response to exposure to codeine should be independently determined. In the vast majority of mothers, codeine taken in moderation should be safe for their breastfed infant. However, any report of overt somnolence, apnea, poor feeding, or gray skin should be reported to the physician and could be associated with exposure to codeine.

- IBUPROFEN   (*Advil, Nuprin, Motrin, Pediaprofen*)
    - AAP = Maternal Medication Usually Compatible with Breastfeeding
    - LRC = L1
    - RID   = 0.1-0.7%
    - Pregnancy = B in first and second trimester
    - Comment: Ibuprofen is a nonsteroidal anti-inflammatory analgesic. It is frequently used for fever in infants. Ibuprofen enters milk only in very low levels (less than 0.6% of maternal dose). Even large doses produce very small milk levels. In one patient receiving 400 mg twice daily, milk levels were less than 0.5 mg/L. In another study of twelve women who received 400 mg doses every six hours for a total of five doses, all breastmilk levels of ibuprofen were less than 1.0 mg/L, the lower limit of the assay. Data in these studies document that no measurable concentrations of ibuprofen

are detected in breastmilk following the above doses. Ibuprofen is presently popular for therapy of fever in infants. Current recommended dose in children is 5-10 mg/kg every six hours. Ibuprofen is an ideal analgesic for breastfeeding mothers.

- HYDROCODONE   (*Lortab, Vicodin*)
  - ○ AAP = Not reviewed
  - ○ LRC = L3
  - ○ RID = 3.1-3.7%
  - ○ Pregnancy = B
  - ○ Comment: Hydrocodone is a narcotic analgesic and antitussive structurally related to codeine although somewhat more potent. It is commonly used in breastfeeding mothers throughout the USA. In a study of two breastfeeding women taking hydrocodone for various periods, patient one received a total of 63,525 μg (998.8 μg/kg) over 86.5 hours. Patient two, received 9075 μg (123.5 μg/kg) over 36 hours.

    In patient one, the AUC of the drug concentration in milk was 4946.1 μg/L.hr and an average milk concentration of 57.2 μg/L. The authors estimate the relative infant dose at 3.1%. In patient two, the AUC of the drug concentration in milk was 735.6 μg/L.hr and an average milk concentration of 20.4 μg/L. The authors estimate the relative infant dose at 3.7%. This paper concluded that high doses of hydrocodone in mothers who are nursing newborn or premature infants can be concerning. Mothers should be advised to watch for sedation and appropriate weight gain in their infants.

- METOCLOPRAMIDE   (*Reglan*)
  - ○ AAP = Drugs whose effect on nursing infants is unknown but may be of concern
  - ○ LRC = L2
  - ○ RID = 4.7-14.3%
  - ○ Pregnancy = B
  - ○ Comment: Metoclopramide has multiple functions, but is primarily used for increasing the lower esophageal sphincter tone in gastroesophageal reflux in patients with reduced gastric tone. For migraine and tension headache, it has proven more effective than meperidine when administered IV (10 mg). In breastfeeding, it is sometimes used in lactating women to stimulate prolactin release from the pituitary and enhance breastmilk production. Since 1981, a number of publications have documented major increases in breastmilk production following the use of metoclopramide, domperidone, or sulpiride. Metoclopramide is commonly used in breastfeeding women and is not contraindicated, although maternal depression is a common complication.

- NAPROXEN   (*Anaprox, Naprosyn, Aleve*)
  - ○ AAP = Maternal Medication Usually Compatible with Breastfeeding
  - ○ LRC = L3
  - ○ RID = 3.3%
  - ○ Pregnancy = C
  - ○ Comment: Naproxen is a popular NSAID analgesic. In a study done at steady state in one mother consuming 375 mg twice daily, milk levels ranged from 1.76-2.37 mg/L at four hours. Total naproxen excretion in the infant's urine was only 0.26% of the maternal dose. Although the amount

of naproxen transferred via milk is minimal, one should use with caution in nursing mothers because of its long half-life and its effect on the infant's cardiovascular system, kidneys, and GI tract. However, its short term use postpartum or infrequent or occasional use would not necessarily be incompatible with breastfeeding. One case of prolonged bleeding, hemorrhage, and acute anemia has been reported in a seven-day-old infant. The relative infant dose on a weight-adjusted maternal daily dose would probably be less than 3.3%.

Clinical Tips

Acetaminophen, particularly early postpartum, is the ideal choice for analgesia. It does not affect clotting, nor does it transfer to the infant in clinically relevant doses. Ibuprofen is an ideal analgesic as well for breastfeeding mothers because the milk levels are so low, its half-life is short, and it is cleared for use in pediatric patients. It has been commonly used in postpartum women with minimal side effects for quite some time. Intravenous metoclopramide (Reglan) has been found more effective than meperidine in one study. Its use in emergency departments for migraine headache is well known.

While using opiates for headaches is not always advisable, codeine is not contraindicated in breastfeeding women. It and hydrocodone are the most common analgesics used for postpartum pain management. While naproxen is not definitely contraindicated, its use should be limited to infrequent and brief periods.

Suggested Reading

Cady, R. K., Dodick, D. W., Levine, H. L., Schreiber, C. P., Eross, E. J., Setzen, M., et al. (2005). Sinus headache: a neurology, otolaryngology, allergy, and primary care consensus on diagnosis and treatment. *Mayo Clin Proc, 80*(7), 908-916.

Johnson, C. J. (2004). Headache in women. *Prim Care, 31*(2), 417-428, viii.

Leone, M., Filippini, G., D'Amico, D., Farinotti, M., & Bussone, G. (1994). Assessment of International Headache Society diagnostic criteria: a reliability study. *Cephalalgia, 14*(4), 280-284.

Marcus, D. A. (2008). Managing headache during pregnancy and lactation. *Expert Rev Neurother, 8*(3), 385-395.

Menon, R., & Bushnell, C. D. (2008). Headache and pregnancy. *Neurologist, 14*(2), 108-119.

Wynkoop, T., McCoy, K., & Dean, R. S. (1996). Diagnostic agreement in the classification of headache using Ad Hoc Committee and IHS criteria. *Int J Neurosci, 85*(3-4), 285-290.

Heart Failure

Principles of Therapy

Also called congestive heart failure, right/left heart failure, ventricular failure, or chronic heart failure, this syndrome is characterized by a marked inability to pump enough blood to supply oxygen needs to tissues. At any one time, three million Americans are affected by this syndrome.

Chronic congestive heart failure results from various etiologies, including valvular heart disease, hypertension, ischemic heart disease, peri-partum cardiomyopathy, and primarily myocardial diseases. Presenting symptoms include dyspnea, fatigue, edema, pulmonary venous hypertension, and decreased cardiac output. The classic enlargement of the heart is pathognomic of impending pump failure. CHF can result from insufficient coronary blood flow, myocardial infarct, increasing scar tissue, high blood pressure, rheumatic heart disease and valvular dysfunction, primary cardiomyopathy (perhaps viral), and endocarditis/myocarditis. As the cardiac output decreases, the heart swells in size to compensate. As the swelling increases, contractility of the myocardium begins to fail.

Therapeutic options include diuretics, digitalis, beta-blockers (rarely), calcium channel blockers, nitrate vasodilators, antiarrhythmic drugs, and other antihypertensives. The objective of pharmacotherapy is to improve cardiac output, reduce fluid overload, reduce hypertension, reduce peripheral resistance, and increase exercise tolerance.

Peripartum cardiomyopathy (PPCM) is a particular form of heart failure which may occur at a time during which women may be breastfeeding. It is defined as heart failure which occurs during the last month of pregnancy or first five months after delivery in the absence of other know causes of heart failure or heart disease. Left ventricular dysfunction with an ejection fraction of < 45% is also required to meet the diagnostic criteria. Heart failure occurring earlier in pregnancy does not meet this definition and is usually related to underlying cardiac conditions. Women with underlying cardiac disease will frequently become more symptomatic earlier in pregnancy as a result of the hemodynamic alterations of pregnancy.

Treatment of peripartum cardiomyopathy is similar to the treatment of heart failure due to the other etiologies discussed above and focuses on medications to optimize cardiac performance, control arrhythmias, and improve long term outcome. Due to the hypercoagulable state during the peripartum period, the use of anticoagulants with an ejection fraction of < 30% should be an additional component of therapy. A small percentage (4 to 7%) of women with peripartum cardiomyopathy may require cardiac transplantation. Of those women who survive and do not require transplantation, women with peripartum cardiomyopathy may recover cardiac function usually over the initial six months after diagnosis. This recovery was less likely to be seen in women with an ejection fraction of < 30%.

The risk of subsequent pregnancy in women with prior peripartum cardiomyopathy (or prior cardiomyopathy from other etiologies) is poorly researched but is high. It appears that those women who recover with higher left ventricular function do better than those with more severe persistent ventricular function. Even women who recover ventricular function after PPCM will likely have recurrent ventricular dysfunction with subsequent pregnancy, and they should, therefore, be counseled regarding these risks and monitored.

Treatment

- Fluid and sodium restriction.

- Diuretics.

- Digoxin.

- ACE or angiotensin receptor blockers (ARB).

- Beta blockers rarely (not useful during acute phase).

- Exercise training.

- Implantable cardioverter-defibrillator.

- Cardiac transplantation.

Medications

- ATENOLOL   (*Tenoretic, Tenormin*)
  - AAP = Drugs associated with significant side effects and should be given with caution
  - LRC = L3
  - RID = 6.6%
  - Pregnancy = D
  - Comment: Atenolol is a potent cardio-selective beta-blocker. Data conflict on the secretion of atenolol into breastmilk. One author reports an incident of significant bradycardia, cyanosis, low body temperature, and low blood pressure in the breastfeeding infant of a mother consuming 100 mg atenolol daily, while a number of others have failed to detect plasma levels in the neonate or untoward side effects.

    In another study, women taking 50-100 mg/day were found to have M/P ratios of 1.5-6.8. However, even with high M/P ratios, the calculated intake per day (at peak levels) for a breastfeeding infant would only be 0.13 mg. In a study by White, breastmilk levels in one patient were 0.7, 1.2 and 1.8 mg/L of milk at doses of 25, 50 and 100 mg daily, respectively. In another study, the estimated daily intake for an infant receiving 500 mL milk per day would be 0.3 mg. In these five patients who received 100 mg daily, the mean milk concentration of atenolol was 630 µg/L. In a study by Kulas, the amount of atenolol transferred into milk varied from 0.66 mg/L with a maternal dose of 25 mg, 1.2 mg/L with a maternal dose of 50 mg, and 1.7 mg/L with a maternal dose of 100 mg per day. Although atenolol is approved by the AAP, some caution is recommended due to the milk/plasma ratios and the reported problem with one infant.

- BENAZEPRIL HCL   (*Lotensin, Lotrel*)
  - AAP = Not reviewed
  - LRC = L2
  - RID = 0.00005%
  - Pregnancy = C during first trimester

- Comment: Benazepril belongs to the ACE inhibitor family. Oral absorption is rather poor (37%). The active component (benazeprilat) reaches a peak at approximately two hours after ingestion. In a patient receiving 20 mg daily for three days, milk levels averaged 0.15 ng/L. Thus the levels in milk are almost unmeasurable. The manufacturer suggests a newborn infant ingesting only breastmilk would receive less than 0.1% of the mg/kg maternal dose of benazepril and benazeprilat.

- CANDESARTAN   (*Atacand*)
  - AAP = Not reviewed
  - LRC = L3
  - RID =
  - Pregnancy = C in first trimester
  - Comment: Candesartan is a specific blocker of the receptor site (AT1) for angiotensin II. It is typically used as an antihypertensive similar to the ACE inhibitor family. No data are available on the use of the angiontensin receptor blockers.

- CAPTOPRIL   (*Capoten*)
  - AAP = Maternal Medication Usually Compatible with Breastfeeding
  - LRC = L2
  - RID = 0.02%
  - Pregnancy = C in first trimester
  - Comment: Captopril is a typical angiotensin converting enzyme inhibitor (ACE) used to reduce hypertension. Small amounts are secreted (4.7 µg/L milk). In one report of 12 women treated with 100 mg three times daily, maternal serum levels averaged 713 µg/L, while breastmilk levels averaged 4.7 µg/L at 3.8 hours after administration. Data from this study suggest that an infant would ingest approximately 0.02% of the free captopril consumed by its mother (300mg) on a daily basis. No adverse effects have been reported in this study. Use with care in mothers with premature infants.

- CARVEDILOL   (*Coreg*)
  - AAP = Not reviewed
  - LRC = L3
  - RID =
  - Pregnancy = C
  - Comment: Carvedilol is a nonselective beta-adrenergic blocking agent (and partial alpha-1 blocking activity) with high lipid solubility and no intrinsic sympathomimetic activity. There are no data available on the transfer of this drug into human milk. However, due to its high lipid solubility, some may transfer. As with any beta-blocker, some caution is recommended until milk levels are reported.

- DIGOXIN   (*Lanoxin, Lanoxicaps*)
  - AAP = Maternal Medication Usually Compatible with Breastfeeding
  - LRC = L2
  - RID = 2.7-2.8%
  - Pregnancy = C

- Comment: Digoxin is a cardiac stimulant used primarily to strengthen the contractile process. In one mother receiving 0.25 mg digoxin daily, the amount found in breastmilk ranged from 0.96 to 0.61 µg/L at four and six hours postdose, respectively. Mean peak breastmilk levels varied from 0.78 µg/L in one patient to 0.41 µg/L in another. Plasma levels in the infants were undetectable. In another study of five women receiving digoxin therapy, the average breastmilk concentration was 0.64 µg/L. From these studies, it is apparent that a breastfeeding infant would receive less than 1 µg/day of digoxin, too low to be clinically relevant. The small amounts secreted into breastmilk have not produced problems in nursing infants.

- **DOPAMINE-DOBUTAMINE** (*Intropin*)
  - AAP = Not reviewed
  - LRC = L2
  - RID =
  - Pregnancy = C
  - Comment: Dopamine and dobutamine are catecholamine pressor agents used in shock and severe hypotension. They are rapidly destroyed in the GI tract and are only used IV. It is not known if they transfer into human milk, but the half-life is so short they would not last long. Dopamine, while in the plasma, significantly (>60%) inhibits prolactin secretion and would likely inhibit lactation while being used.

- **ENALAPRIL MALEATE** (*Vasotec*)
  - AAP = Maternal Medication Usually Compatible with Breastfeeding
  - LRC = L2
  - RID = 0.2%
  - Pregnancy = C in first trimester
  - Comment: Enalapril maleate is an ACE inhibitor used as an antihypertensive. Upon absorption, it is rapidly metabolized by the adult liver to enalaprilat, the biologically active metabolite. In one study of five lactating mothers who received a single 20 mg dose, the mean maximum milk concentration of enalapril and enalaprilat was only 1.74 µg/L and 1.72 µg/L, respectively. The author suggests that an infant consuming 850 mL of milk daily would ingest less than 2 µg of enalaprilat daily. The milk/plasma ratios for enalapril and enalaprilat averaged 0.013 and 0.025, respectively. In a study by Rush of a patient receiving 10 mg/day, the total amount of enalapril and enalaprilat measured in milk during the 24 hour period was 81.9 ng and 36.1 ng, respectively, or 1.44 µg/L and 0.63 µg/L of milk, respectively.

- **FUROSEMIDE** (*Lasix*)
  - AAP = Not reviewed
  - LRC = L3
  - RID =
  - Pregnancy = C
  - Comment: Furosemide is a potent loop diuretic with a rather short duration of action. Furosemide is frequently used in neonates in pediatric units, so pediatric use is common. The oral bioavailability of furosemide in newborns is exceedingly poor and very high oral doses are required (1-4 mg/kg BID). It is very unlikely the amount transferred into human milk would produce any effects in a nursing infant, although its maternal use could suppress lactation.

- HYDRALAZINE (*Apresoline*)
  - AAP = Maternal Medication Usually Compatible with Breastfeeding
  - LRC = L2
  - RID = 1.2%
  - Pregnancy = C
  - Comment: Hydralazine is a popular antihypertensive used for severe pre-eclampsia and gestational and postpartum hypertension. In a study of one breastfeeding mother receiving 50 mg three times daily, the concentrations of hydralazine in breastmilk at 0.5 and two hours after administration was 762, and 792 nmol/L, respectively. The respective maternal serum levels were 1525, and 580 nmol/L at the aforementioned times. From these data, an infant consuming 1000 mL of milk would consume only 0.17 mg of hydralazine - an amount too small to be clinically relevant.

- IRBESARTAN (*Avapro*)
  - AAP = Not reviewed
  - LRC = L3
  - RID =
  - Pregnancy = C in first trimester
  - Comment: Irbesartan is an angiotensin-II receptor antagonist used as an antihypertensive. No data are available on the use of the angiontensin receptor blockers in breastfeeding women.

- LISINOPRIL (*Prinivil, Zestril*)
  - AAP = Not reviewed
  - LRC = L3
  - RID =
  - Pregnancy = C in first trimester
  - Comment: Lisinopril is a typical long-acting ACE inhibitor used as an antihypertensive. No breastfeeding data are available on this product.

- LOSARTAN (*Cozaar, Hyzaar*)
  - AAP = Not reviewed
  - LRC = L3
  - RID =
  - Pregnancy = C in first trimester
  - Comment: Losartan is a new ACE-like antihypertensive. Rather than inhibiting the enzyme that makes angiotensin, such as the ACE inhibitor family, this medication selectively blocks the ACE receptor site, preventing attachment of angiotensin II. No data are available on its transfer to human milk. Although it penetrates the CNS significantly, its high protein binding would probably reduce its ability to enter milk. This product is only intended for those few individuals who cannot take ACE inhibitors. No data on transfer into human milk are available. The trade name Hyzaar contains losartan plus hydrochlorothiazide.

- **METOPROLOL**   (*Toprol-XL, Lopressor*)
  - AAP = Maternal Medication Usually Compatible with Breastfeeding
  - LRC = L3
  - RID = 1.4%
  - Pregnancy = C
  - Comment: At low doses, metoprolol is a very cardioselective beta-1 blocker used for the treatment of hypertension, angina, and tachyarrhythmias. In a study of three women four to six months postpartum who received 100 mg twice daily for four days, the peak concentration of metoprolol ranged from 0.38 to 2.58 μmol/L, whereas the maternal plasma levels ranged from 0.1 to 0.97 μmol/L. Assuming ingestion of 75 mL of milk at each feeding and the maximum concentration of 2.58 μmol/L, an infant would ingest approximately 0.05 mg metoprolol at the first feeding and considerably less at subsequent feedings. In another study of nine women receiving 50-100 mg twice daily, the maternal plasma and milk concentrations ranged from 4-556 nmol/L and 19-1690 nmol/L, respectively. Using these data, the authors calculated an average milk concentration throughout the day as 280 μg/L of milk. This dose is 20-40 times less than a typical clinical dose. These levels are probably too low to be clinically relevant.

- **NIFEDIPINE**   (*Adalat, Procardia*)
  - AAP = Maternal Medication Usually Compatible with Breastfeeding
  - LRC = L2
  - RID = 2.3-3.4%
  - Pregnancy = C
  - Comment: Nifedipine is an effective antihypertensive. It belongs to the calcium channel blocker family of drugs. Two studies indicate that nifedipine is transferred to breastmilk in varying, but generally low levels. In one study in which the dose was varied from 10-30 mg three times daily, the highest concentration (53.35 μg/L) was measured at one hour after a 30 mg dose. Other levels reported were 16.35 μg/L 60 minutes after a 20 mg dose and 12.89 μg/L 30 minutes after a 10 mg dose. The milk concentration measured eight hours following a 30 mg dose was 4.93 μg/L. In this study, using the highest concentration found and a daily intake of 150 mL/kg of human milk, the amount of nifedipine intake would only be 8 μg/kg/day (less than 1.8% of the therapeutic pediatric dose). The authors conclude that the amount ingested via breastmilk poses little risk to an infant. In another study, concentrations of nifedipine in human milk one to eight hours after 10 mg doses varied from <1 to 10.3 μg/L (median 3.5 μg/L) in 6 of 11 patients. The authors concluded the exposure to nifedipine through breastmilk is not significant. In a study by Penny and Lewis, following a maternal dose of 20 mg nifedipine daily for ten days, peak breastmilk levels at one hour were 46 μg/L. The corresponding maternal serum level was 43 μg/L. From these data, the authors suggest a daily intake for an infant would be approximately 6.45 μg/kg/day.

- **NIMODIPINE**   (*Nimotop*)
  - AAP = Not reviewed
  - LRC = L2
  - RID = 0.04%
  - Pregnancy = C

- Comment: Nimodipine is a calcium channel blocker, although it is primarily used in preventing cerebral artery spasm and improving cerebral blood flow. In one study of a patient three days postpartum who received 60 mg every four hours for one week, breastmilk levels paralleled maternal serum levels with a milk/plasma ratio of approximately 0.33. The highest milk concentration reported was approximately 3.5 µg/L, while the maternal plasma was approximately 16 µg/L. In another study, a 36-year-old mother received a total dose of 46 mg IV over 24 hours. Nimodipine concentration in milk was much lower than in maternal serum, with a milk/serum ratio of 0.06 to 0.15. Assuming a daily milk intake of 150 mg/kg, an infant would ingest approximately 0.063 to 0.705 µg/kg/day or 0.008 to 0.092% of the weight-adjusted dose administered to the mother.

- NITRENDIPINE   (*Baypress*)
  - AAP = Not reviewed
  - LRC = L2
  - RID = 0.1%
  - Pregnancy =
  - Comment: Nitrendipine is a typical calcium channel antihypertensive. In a group of three breastfeeding mothers who received 20 mg/d for five days, nitrendipine was excreted in breastmilk at peak concentrations ranging from 4.3 to 6.5 µg/L one to two hours after acute dosing, while its inactive pyridine metabolite ranged from 6.9 to 11.9 µg/L. On the fourth day of continuous dosing, average concentrations of nitrendipine from 24 hour collections of the milk were 1.1 to 3.8 µg/L. Thus nitrendipine and its metabolite are excreted in very low concentrations in human breastmilk. Based on a maternal dose of 20 mg daily, a newborn infant would ingest an average of 1.7 µg/d of nitrendipine, or a relative dose of 0.1%.

- QUINAPRIL   (*Accupril, Accuretic*)
  - AAP = Not reviewed
  - LRC = L2
  - RID = 1.6%
  - Pregnancy = C in first trimester
  - Comment: Quinapril is an angiotensin converting enzyme inhibitor (ACE) used as an antihypertensive. Accuretic products also contain the diuretic hydrochlorothiazide. Once in the plasma compartment, quinapril is rapidly converted to quinaprilat, the active metabolite. In a study of six women who received 20 mg/d, the milk/plasma ratio for quinapril was 0.12. Quinapril was not detected in milk after four hours. No quinaprilat (metabolite) was detected in any of the milk samples. The estimated dose of quinapril that would be received by the infant was 1.6% of the maternal dose, adjusted for respective weights.

- RAMIPRIL   (*Altace*)
  - AAP = Not reviewed
  - LRC = L3
  - RID = 0.3%
  - Pregnancy = C in first trimester
  - Comment: Ramipril is rapidly metabolized to ramiprilat, which is a potent ACE inhibitor with a long half-life. It is used in hypertension. ACE inhibitors can cause increased fetal and neonatal morbidity

and should not be used in pregnant women. Ingestion of a single 10 mg oral dose produced an undetectable level in breastmilk.

- SPIRONOLACTONE (*Aldactone*)
  - AAP = Maternal Medication Usually Compatible with Breastfeeding
  - LRC = L2
  - RID = 4.3%
  - Pregnancy = D
  - Comment: Spironolactone is metabolized to canrenone, which is known to be secreted into breastmilk. In one mother receiving 25 mg of spironolactone, at two hours postdose, the maternal serum and milk concentrations of canrenone were 144 and 104 µg/L, respectively. At 14.5 hours, the corresponding values for serum and milk were 92 and 47 µg/L, respectively. Milk/plasma ratios varied from 0.51 at 14.5 hours to 0.72 at two hours.

- VERAPAMIL (*Calan, Isoptin, Covera-HS*)
  - AAP = Maternal Medication Usually Compatible with Breastfeeding
  - LRC = L2
  - RID = 0.2%
  - Pregnancy = C
  - Comment: Verapamil is a typical calcium channel blocker used as an antihypertensive. It is secreted into milk, but in very low levels, which are highly controversial. Anderson reports that in one patient receiving 80 mg three times daily, the average steady-state concentrations of verapamil and norverapamil in milk were 25.8 and 8.8 µg/L, respectively. The respective maternal plasma level was 42.9 µg/L. The milk/plasma ratio for verapamil was 0.60. No verapamil was detected in the infant's plasma. Inoue reports that in one patient receiving 80 mg four times daily, the milk level peaked at 300 µg/L at approximately 14 hours. These levels are considerably higher than the aforementioned. In another study of a mother receiving 240 mg daily, the concentrations in milk were never higher than 40 µg/L. From these three studies, the relative infant dose would vary from 0.15%, 0.98%, and 0.18%, respectively.

Clinical Tips

Treatment of early stage heart failure offers the best chance at long-term survival. At this time, loop diuretics and ACE inhibitors have the best record. Diuretics include furosemide, bumetanide, or torsemide. Of the loop diuretics, furosemide is generally recommended in breastfeeding patients, rather than bumetanide, because it is poorly bioavailable in the infant. Bumetanide is not absolutely contraindicated in breastfeeding mothers, rather we have no breastmilk data on this product as of yet. Thiazide diuretics should be avoided during pregnancy.

Angiotensin receptor blockers provide more effective blockade of the renin-angiotensin system than do ACE inhibitors, decrease mortality similar in degree to that of ACE inhibitors, have fewer side effects than ACE inhibitors, and may be useful in individuals bothered by persistent ACE-induced cough. Unfortunately, we do not have breastfeeding data for any of the angiotensin receptor blockers, and they should be used cautiously until we have more data on this class of medications. ACE inhibitors and ARB's are contraindicated during pregnancy, particularly the second and third trimesters.

The combination of spironolactone along with an ACE inhibitor may provide some added benefit as recent studies suggest significant benefit of a potassium-sparing diuretic in congestive heart failure (CHF) patients.

ACE inhibitors, particularly captopril, have been found to greatly reduce morbidity in these patients, and experts agree that 50-75% of CHF patients should receive ACE inhibitors. Although other ACE inhibitors are probably fine, captopril is ideal due to its low milk levels and studies that show it significantly reduces morbidity in patients with congestive heart failure. Again, caution is urged in neonates, as they have poor control of their blood pressure and cases of hypotension have been reported in mothers ingesting ACE inhibitors prior to delivery. After several weeks postpartum and in full term, stable infants, the use of ACE inhibitors in breastfeeding mothers is less hazardous. As of yet, the only potassium-sparing diuretic studied in breastfeeding mothers has been spironolactone. Only 0.2% of the maternal dose transfers to the infant, and its use is approved by the AAP. At present, we do not have data on amiloride or triamterene. The use of ACE inhibitors with potassium-sparing diuretics is somewhat risky, as elevated serum potassium levels may result. Potassium-sparing diuretics should probably be used cautiously or not at all in patients taking ACE inhibitors.

The use of calcium channel blockers (CCB) in CHF is controversial and, in general, is not recommended, as they tend to worsen the syndrome. These include nifedipine, diltiazem, and verapamil. Newer CCBs, such as amlodipine (Norvasc), may reduce death rate in some subgroups, but the effect seems minimal. No data on its use in breastfeeding mothers are available.

Previously, the use of beta-blockers in CHF was discouraged, as they were believed to reduce the pumping action of the heart (ionotropy). New data seems to suggest that certain beta-blockers may have significant benefits to heart failure patients. Some of the beta-blockers now recommended include atenolol, carvedilol (Coreg), metoprolol (Lopressor), and bisoprolol (Zebeta). Of this family, atenolol has been associated with hypotension in breastfed infants, but this may be rare. Many patients have breastfed using this beta-blocker without problems, but some caution is recommended. At present, metoprolol is the only beta-blocker that is known to pass poorly to breastfed infants, have minimal side effects in breastfed infants, and be rated usually compatible by the AAP. At present, we do not have breastfeeding data on carvedilol or bisoprolol. However, the use of beta-blockers in CHF patients must be approached cautiously because beta-blockers reduce pumping action and worsening of heart failure may occur. Fatigue, lethargy, exacerbation of asthma, sexual dysfunction, and other side effects are common with their use. In breastfed infants, severe hypotension has been reported (although rarely) in patients consuming atenolol and acebutolol, so caution is recommended with these two agents.

Digoxin, although only moderately efficacious, is still the recommended inotropic agent of choice. It has been shown to improve symptoms, enhance exercise capacity, improve patients' quality of life and clinical status, and reduce hospitalization rates. Hydralazine can be used, but it is often poorly efficacious. Dopamine and dobutamine are not orally bioavailable to the infant and can be used if needed. For other antiarrhythmic agents, see 'Cardiac Antiarrhythmias'.

Suggested Reading

Braithwaite, R. S., Concato, J., Chang, C. C., Roberts, M. S., & Justice, A. C. (2007). A framework for tailoring clinical guidelines to comorbidity at the point of care. *Arch Intern Med, 167*(21), 2361-2365.

Collins, S. P., Lindsell, C. J., Naftilan, A. J., Peacock, W. F., Diercks, D., Hiestand, B., et al. (2009). Low-risk acute heart failure patients: external validation of the Society of Chest Pain Center's recommendations. *Crit Pathw Cardiol, 8*(3), 99-103.

Donlan, S. M., Quattromani, E., Pang, P. S., & Gheorghiade, M. (2009). Therapy for acute heart failure syndromes. *Curr Cardiol Rep, 11*(3), 192-201.

Howlett, J. G. (2008). Current treatment options for early management in acute decompensated heart failure. *Can J Cardiol, 24 Suppl B*, 9B-14B.

Jessup, M., Abraham, W. T., Casey, D. E., Feldman, A. M., Francis, G. S., Ganiats, T. G., et al. (2009). 2009 focused update: ACCF/AHA Guidelines for the Diagnosis and Management of Heart Failure in Adults: a report of the American College of Cardiology Foundation/American Heart Association Task Force on Practice Guidelines: developed in collaboration with the International Society for Heart and Lung Transplantation. *Circulation, 119*(14), 1977-2016.

Mehra, M. R., Rockman, H. A., & Greenberg, B. H. (2008). Highlights of the 2007 Scientific Meeting of the Heart Failure Society of America: Washington, DC, September 16-19, 2007. *J Am Coll Cardiol, 51*(3), 320-327.

Peters-Klimm, F., Muller-Tasch, T., Remppis, A., Szecsenyi, J., & Schellberg, D. (2008). Improved guideline adherence to pharmacotherapy of chronic systolic heart failure in general practice--results from a cluster-randomized controlled trial of implementation of a clinical practice guideline. *J Eval Clin Pract, 14*(5), 823-829.

Peters-Klimm, F., Muller-Tasch, T., Schellberg, D., Remppis, A., Barth, A., Holzapfel, N., et al. (2008). Guideline adherence for pharmacotherapy of chronic systolic heart failure in general practice: a closer look on evidence-based therapy. *Clin Res Cardiol, 97*(4), 244-252.

Remme, W. J. (2007). Filling the gap between guidelines and clinical practice in heart failure treatment: still a far cry from reality. *Eur J Heart Fail, 9*(12), 1143-1145.

Stork, S., Hense, H. W., Zentgraf, C., Uebelacker, I., Jahns, R., Ertl, G., et al. (2008). Pharmacotherapy according to treatment guidelines is associated with lower mortality in a community-based sample of patients with chronic heart failure: a prospective cohort study. *Eur J Heart Fail, 10*(12), 1236-1245.

Toth-Pal, E., Wardh, I., Strender, L. E., & Nilsson, G. (2008). A guideline-based computerised decision support system (CDSS) to influence general practitioners management of chronic heart failure. *Inform Prim Care, 16*(1), 29-39.

Trupp, R. J., & Abraham, W. T. (2009). American College of Cardiology/American Heart Association 2009 clinical guidelines for the diagnosis and management of heart failure in adults: update and clinical implications. *Pol Arch Med Wewn, 119*(7-8), 436-438.

Yancy, C. W., Fonarow, G. C., Albert, N. M., Curtis, A. B., Stough, W. G., Gheorghiade, M., et al. (2009). Influence of patient age and sex on delivery of guideline-recommended heart failure care in the outpatient cardiology practice setting: findings from IMPROVE HF. *Am Heart J, 157*(4), 754-762 e752.

Hepatitis A

Principles of Therapy

Hepatitis A is a relatively common viral infection that typically presents in adults with acute jaundice. Approximately one-third of cases of acute hepatitis are caused by this infection. The disease is generally self-limiting in people who have a healthy liver; fulminant hepatitis can occur but is rare. Hepatitis A is typically fecal-oral spread often related to poor sanitation or poor hygiene techniques. Other risk factors may include household contact with a person known to have hepatitis A. Travel to endemic areas or epidemic outbreaks due to contaminated uncooked food or water may also be implicated in this infection. The incubation period may be from 15 to 50 days. Hepatitis A infection is usually a self-limited infection, with fewer than 20% of patients requiring hospitalization. Treatment is usually supportive, consisting of intravenous hydration. No chronic carrier state exists, and fatal outcomes related to this disease are rare (2/1,000). Perinatal transmission or transmission via breastfeeding have not been documented. Careful hygiene should be effective in preventing tranmission to the breastfed infant. Treatment options available to prevent hepatitis A include immune globulin and inactivated hepatitis A vaccination. Immune globulin is most effective when given within 72 hours of exposure, but may provide benefit given within six days. Fortunately, infants are seldom affected by Hepatitis A.

Treatment

- Supportive treatment, including intravenous fluids for dehydrated patients, antiemetics, diphenhydramine for itching, and cholestyramine for binding bile acids.

- Avoid hepatotoxic agents, including alcohol and acetaminophen.

- Patients must avoid handling food while actively infected.

- BayGam is most efficacious when given before or soon after exposure to Hepatitis A. It should not be used in patients with symptoms.

Medications

- IMMUNE GLOBULIN (HUMAN) (*BayGam, IG, IGIM, Gamma Globulin, IgG*)
    - AAP = Not reviewed
    - LRC = L1
    - RID =
    - Pregnancy = C
    - Comment: IGGs enter milk in small to negligible amounts. In two patients who received IVIG during the colostral period (400-500 and 600-700 mg/kg monthly), colostrum levels of IgG and

IgM were only slightly higher or within the normal range. There are no known risks to the use of immune globulin in breastfeeding mothers or their infants. Any present in milk is unlikely to be systemically absorbed orally by the infant. It is considered safe for use in breastfeeding mothers by the World Health Organization.

- HEPATITIS A VACCINE   (*Havrix*)
  - ◦ AAP = Not reviewed
  - ◦ LRC = L2
  - ◦ RID =
  - ◦ Pregnancy = C
  - ◦ Comment: Hepatitis A vaccine is an inactivated, noninfectious viral vaccination for Hepatitis A. Although there are no specific data on the use of Hepatitis A vaccine in breastfeeding women, it can be used in pregnant women after 14 weeks and in children two years of age and older. There is little likelihood that Hepatitis A vaccinations in breastfeeding women would cause untoward effects in breastfed infants.

Clinical Tips

Good personal hygiene should be protective against spreading hepatitis A. Post-exposure prophylaxis is indicated for household and sexual contacts of those recently exposed to a person infected with hepatitis A unless the exposed person has been vaccinated at least one month prior. Hepatitis A immune globulin (IG) is a dose of 0.02 ml/kg and can generally be administered for up to two weeks after exposure. Breastfeeding women who are otherwise candidates for either immune globulin or vaccination should be given treatment. It is unclear if the potential exposure of a breastfed infant to an infected mother would warrant treatment of the infant, providing meticulous hygiene and adequate sanitation exist. In infants, the syndrome is either asymptomatic or causes only mild nonspecific symptoms. Current therapy recommended following exposure to Hepatitis A is an injection of gamma globulin. A majority of the population is immune to Hepatitis A due to prior exposure. Fulminant hepatitis A infection is rare in children, and a carrier state is unknown. Unless the mother is jaundiced and acutely ill, breastfeeding can continue without interruption. Proper hygiene should be stressed. Pruritus can be treated with diphenhydramine 50 mg every six hours and cholestyramine 4 grams twice daily.

Suggested Reading

Campos-Outcalt, D. (2006). Are you up to date with new immunization recommendations? *J Fam Pract, 55*(3), 232-234.

CDC, Workowski, K. A., & Berman, S. M. (2006). Sexually transmitted diseases treatment guidelines, 2006. *MMWR Recomm Rep, 55*(RR-11), 1-94.

Degertekin, B., & Lok, A. S. (2009). Update on viral hepatitis: 2008. *Curr Opin Gastroenterol, 25*(3), 180-5.

Haun, L., Kwan, N., & Hollier, L. M. (2007). Viral infections in pregnancy. *Minerva Ginecol, 59*(2), 159-174.

Steele, M., Cochrane, A., Wakefield, C., Stain, A. M., Ling, S., Blanchette, V., et al. (2009). Hepatitis A and B immunization for individuals with inherited bleeding disorders. *Haemophilia, 15*(2), 437-447.

Hepatitis B

Principles of Therapy

Hepatitis B (HBV) is caused by a DNA virus. Three principal antigens exist which are useful for testing for infection: hepatitis B surface antigen (HbsAg), hepatitis B core antigen (HBcAg), and hepatitis B e antigen (HbeAg). Presence of HbeAg indicates higher probability of inefectivity. Approximately 40-45% of hepatitis in the United States is related to hepatitis B. Hepatitis B is spread through sexual contacts (semen, saliva, blood) and exposure to infected blood such as occurs with blood transfusion or shared needles with intravenous drug use. Acute HBV infection carries a mortality of about 1% and a long incubation period of 50-180 days. Chronic HBV infection occurs in 1-15% of cases and can lead to further transmission of the infection, as well as chronic liver disease, potentially leading to cirrhosis and hepatocellular carcinoma. Diagnosis of chronic HBV infection is made based on a persistently postive test for HbsAg. Perinatal transmission of hepatitis B without treatment ranges from 10 to 85%, depending on timing of infection and e antigen status. Those with a positive e antigen and infection in the third trimester of pregnancy are at greatest risk. Transmission via household contact and close postnatal contact has also been reported. Hepatitis B DNA has been found in colostrum; however, with the use of HBV immunoprophylaxis for hepatitis B mothers, breastfeeding does not appear to increase the risk of infection in the infant. Chronic HBV infection occurs in 90% of infected newborns who are at especially high risk for chronic liver disease. Immune globulin and vaccination are recommended for all potentially exposed infants. No adequate treatment is available for hepatitis B infection once acute infection occurs. Care again focuses on supportive measures. Chronic HBV infection has been treated with interferon alpha-2b with approximately 25-40% efficacy. Options available to prevent hepatitis B infection include hepatitis B immune globulin and inactivated hepatitis B vaccination. Routine screening of all pregnant women and routine vaccination of all newborns is recommended.

Treatment

- Supportive treatment for acute infections.

- Infants of breastfeeding mothers infected with Hepatitis B should receive the Hepatitis B immune globulin and Hepatitis B vaccination within 12 hours of birth.

- Some patients who are chronically infected require treatment; medications include interferon-alpha, lamivudine, and telbivudine.

Medications

- ADEFOVIR DIPIVOXIL   (*Hepsera*)
  - AAP = Not reviewed
  - LRC = L4

- ○ RID =
- ○ Pregnancy = C
- ○ Comment: Adefovir inhibits hepatitis B virus replication. No data are available on the transfer of adefovir into human milk, yet based on the kinetic profile (low protein binding and moderate oral bioavailability), it is likely the drug would cross into the milk compartment to some degree. Because this drug is potentially toxic to a rapidly growing infant and because it is used over long periods of time, it is not recommended for use in lactating mothers at this time.

- **INTERFERON ALFA-2b** (*PegIntron*)
  - ○ AAP = Not reviewed
  - ○ LRC = L3
  - ○ RID =
  - ○ Pregnancy =
  - ○ Comment: Peginterferon alfa-2b is a pegylated form of the antiviral drug interferon alfa-2b. Pegylation confirs protection against enzymatic degradation systemically. It is indicated for the treatment of hepatitis C. While we have no data on its use in breastfeeding mothers, other data on interferons (alfa and beta) suggest they do not readily enter milk, and milk levels will be exceedingly low. When combined with ribavirin, breastfeeding is not recommended. Ribavirin is extremely teratogentic, do not use in pregnant women.

- **PEGINTERFERON ALFA-2a** (*Pegasys*)
  - ○ AAP = Not reviewed
  - ○ LRC = L3
  - ○ RID =
  - ○ Pregnancy = C
  - ○ Comment: Peginterferon alfa-2a is a pegylated form of the antiviral drug interferon alfa-2a. Pegylation confirs protection against enzymatic degradation systemically. It is indicated for the treatment of hepatitis B and C. While we have no data on its use in breastfeeding mothers, other data on interferons (alfa and beta) suggest they do not readily enter milk, and milk levels will be exceedingly low. Life-threatening or fatal neuropsychiatric reactions may manifest in patients receiving therapy with peginterferon alfa-2a and include suicide, suicidal ideation, homicidal ideation, depression, relapse of drug addiction, and drug overdose. This product should be used with extreme caution in patients who report a history of depression. Neuropsychiatric adverse events observed with alpha interferon treatment include aggressive behavior, psychoses, hallucinations, bipolar disorders, and mania. When combined with ribavirin, breastfeeding is not recommended. Ribavirin is extremely teratogentic, do not use in pregnant women.

- **HEPATITIS B IMMUNE GLOBULIN** (*H-BIG, HEP-B-Gammagee, Hyperhep*)
  - ○ AAP =
  - ○ LRC = L2
  - ○ RID =
  - ○ Pregnancy = C
  - ○ Comment: HBIG is a sterile solution of immunoglobulin (10-18% protein) containing a high titer of antibody to hepatitis B surface antigen. It is most commonly used as prophylaxis therapy for

infants born to hepatitis B surface antigen positive mothers. The carrier state can be prevented in about 75% of such infections in newborns given HBIG immediately after birth. HBIG is generally administered to infants from HBsAg positive mothers who wish to breastfeed. The prophylactic dose for newborns is 0.5 mL IM (thigh) as soon after birth as possible, preferably within one hour. The infant should also be immunized with Hepatitis B vaccine (0.5 mL IM) within 12 hours of birth (use separate site), and again at one and six months.

- HEPATITIS B VACCINE   (*Heptavax-B, Energix-B, Recombivax HB*)
  - AAP = Not reviewed
  - LRC = L2
  - RID =
  - Pregnancy = C
  - Comment: Hepatitis B vaccine is an inactivated non-infectious hepatitis B surface antigen vaccine. It can be used in pediatric patients at birth. No data are available on its use in breastfeeding mothers, but it is unlikely to produce untoward effects on a breastfeeding infant. Hepatitis B vaccination is approximately 80-95% effective in preventing acute hepatitis B infections. It requires at least three immunizations, and the immunity lasts about five to seven years. In infants born of HB surface antigen positive mothers, the American Academy of Pediatrics recommends hepatitis B vaccine (along with HBIG) should be administered to the infant within 1-12 hours of birth (0.5 mL IM) and again at one and six months. If so administered, breastfeeding poses no additional risk for acquisition of HBV by the infant.

- LAMIVUDINE   (*Epivir-HBV, 3TC*)
  - AAP = Not reviewed
  - LRC = L2
  - RID = 4.3%
  - Pregnancy = C
  - Comment: Lamivudine is a synthetic nucleoside analogue antiviral used for the treatment of Hepatitis B or HIV infections. It is presently in numerous other combination products (Combivir, Ziagen, etc.). In a study of 20 women receiving either 300 mg once daily or 150 mg twice daily one week postpartum, the mean breastmilk concentration was 1.22 mg/L (range= 0.5-6.09) or 0.183 mg/kg/day. This is significantly less than the clinical dose normally administered to infants (4-8 mg/kg/d). The authors suggested that the amount ingested via breastmilk was negligible relative to therapeutic dosing and would not provide adequate antiretroviral drug concentrations for a neonate. In another study of 18 women receiving antiretroviral treatment for HIV infections, median lamivudine concentrations in maternal serum, breastmilk, and the infant's serum was 678 ng/mL, 1828 ng/mL and 28 ng/mL, respectively. The median milk/serum ratio was 3.34 for lamivudine. The median infant concentration of lamivudine (28 ng/mL) was 5% of the inhibitory concentration (50%), which is 550 ng/mL. These data suggests that the serum levels of lamivudine attained in the infant are probably too low to produce side effects in the infant, and certainly too low to treat HIV effectively.

- TELBIVUDINE   (*Tyzeka*)
  - AAP = Not reviewed

- ○ LRC = L4
- ○ RID =
- ○ Pregnancy = B
- ○ Comment: Telbivudine is a thymidine nucleoside analog that inhibits reverse transcriptase and DNA polymerase in hepatitis B virus infections. It does not inhibit human cellular polymerase. Telbivudine is used in adults with chronic hepatitis B that have evidence of either increased liver function tests or an active infection. It is considered safe in pregnancy, but is very lipid soluble. Therefore, its transfer into milk may be likely, but is probably not clinically relevant. However, this product is intended for chronic use, and exposing an infant to a potential hepatotoxin such as this over a prolonged period is not justified.

- • TENOFOVIR DISOPROXIL FUMARATE (*Viread*)
  - ○ AAP = Not reviewed
  - ○ LRC = L3
  - ○ RID = 0.4%
  - ○ Pregnancy = B
  - ○ Comment: Tenofovir is used in the management of HIV and hepatitis B infections. It interferes with the viral RNA dependent DNA polymerase, inhibiting viral replication. In a recent study in two Rhesus macaques monkeys, and following a subcutaneous dose of 30 mg/kg tenofovir, peak plasma levels were reported to be 18.3 and 30.3 μg/mL. Peak levels in milk were reported to be 0.808 and 0.610 μg/mL. The AUC levels were 68.9 and 12.8 μg.h/mL for plasma and milk in one animal and 56.2 and 12.1 μg.h/mL for plasma and milk in the second animal. Using this peak data, the relative infant dose would only be 0.4% of the maternal dose. In addition, the oral bioavailability of tenofovir (non-salt form) is negligible (5%). Thus the overall risk to a breastfeeding infant would probably be low.

Clinical Tips

In mothers positive for hepatitis B surface antigen, the infant can breastfeed provided hepatitis immune globulin (HBIG 0.5 mL IM) and hepatitis B vaccination are given within 12 hours of birth. Breastfeeding does not need to be withheld until the immune globulin is administered. If the mothers Hepatitis B status is unknown, she should be tested immediately. If the mother tests positive for hepatitis B antigen, Hepatitis B Immune Globulin (HBIG) should be administered to the infant within seven days of birth (preferably the same day). For the treatment of chronic Hepatitis B infections in breastfeeding patients, long-term interferon alpha 2b (5 million units/day for four months) treatments may be required. Lamivudine has been documented to reduce the risk of disease progression and hepatocellular carcinoma and is now approved by the FDA for treatment of adults with chronic hepatitis B. Levels of lamivudine in milk are reportedly low. Tenofovir has documented efficacy and apparently produces low levels in milk. Telbivudine (Tyzeka), emtricitabine, and entecavir have all been approved for treatment of chronic hepatitis B. Nothing is known about their transfer into human milk. Interferon Alpha N3 has been studied in one patient, and its levels in milk were unchanged following huge doses, suggesting these agents may not readily pass into milk. Other studies with interferon beta suggest levels in milk are low to nil. The transfer of many of these agents into milk is believed low due to their large molecular weight. However, long-term exposure of the infant to low doses of these rather hazardous compounds may not be justified in breastfeeding mothers. When ribavirin is added to this regimen, pregnancy must be checked and avoided with at least two forms of contraception.

Suggested Reading

Alazawi, W., & Foster, G. R. (2008). Advances in the diagnosis and treatment of hepatitis B. *Curr Opin Infect Dis, 21*(5), 508-515.

Degertekin, B., & Lok, A. S. (2007). When to start and stop hepatitis B treatment: can one set of criteria apply to all patients regardless of age at infection? *Ann Intern Med, 147*(1), 62-64.

Dienstag, J. L. (2008). Hepatitis B virus infection. *N Engl J Med, 359*(14), 1486-1500.

Kennedy, P. T., Lee, H. C., Jeyalingam, L., Malik, R., Karayiannis, P., Muir, D., et al. (2008). NICE guidelines and a treatment algorithm for the management of chronic hepatitis B: a review of 12 years experience in west London. *Antivir Ther, 13*(8), 1067-1076.

Lai, C. L., & Yuen, M. F. (2007). The natural history and treatment of chronic hepatitis B: a critical evaluation of standard treatment criteria and end points. *Ann Intern Med, 147*(1), 58-61.

McMahon, B. J. (2008). Implementing evidenced-based practice guidelines for the management of chronic hepatitis B virus infection. *Am J Med, 121*(12 Suppl), S45-52.

Papatheodoridis, G. V., & Deutsch, M. (2008). Resistance issues in treating chronic hepatitis B. *Future Microbiol, 3*, 525-538.

Quan, D. J. (2008). Pharmacotherapy of hepatitis B infection: a brief review. *Nephrol Nurs J, 35*(5), 507-510.

Thomas, H. C. (2007). Best practice in the treatment of chronic hepatitis B: a summary of the European Viral Hepatitis Educational Initiative (EVHEI). *J Hepatol, 47*(4), 588-597.

Tong, M. J., Hsien, C., Hsu, L., Sun, H. E., & Blatt, L. M. (2008). Treatment recommendations for chronic hepatitis B: an evaluation of current guidelines based on a natural history study in the United States. *Hepatology, 48*(4), 1070-1078.

Hepatitis C

Principles of Therapy

Hepatitis C is a single-stranded RNA virus. Currently hepatitis C accounts for approximately 20% of acute hepatitis in the US. Approximately 60% -80% of those with acute hepatitis C will develop chronic hepatitis C (HCV), and 20%- 30% of these will develop cirrhosis or chronic active disease. Risk factors for transmission are similar to those for hepatitis B, primarily being transmitted by blood borne exposure. Sexual transmission appears to be significantly less effective than with hepatitis B. Only 15% of spouses without other risk factors have infection. Vertical transmission from mother to fetus occurs in 2-8% of cases and is dependent on viral titer. Prolonged membrane rupture and internal fetal monitoring may also increase vertical transmission. Co-infection with HIV greatly increases vertical transmission and HIV testing should be performed in pregnant women with hepatitis C. Unlike hepatitis A or B, antibodies are not effective in preventing hepatitis C. No immune globulin or vaccination is presently available to prevent this infection. Anti-HCV and HCV-RNA have been detected in human milk. In a small study of 14 patients with HCV-RNA positive serum, only two had HCV-RNA positive breastmilk. Another small study of 15 HCV infected mothers who were HCV-RNA positive found that HCV-RNA was present in colostral samples, though none of the 11 breastfed infants had HCV infection at one year of life. Breastfeeding in the scenario of maternal hepatitis C has not been documented to cause transmission to the infant in those patients which have been studied. In a study of 7,698 parturient women screened for anti-HCV antibodies, 53 were positive and of these 31 were HCV-RNA positive. Three of the 54 (5.6%) children born to these mothers became HCV-RNA positive during follow-up, and all of these were from HCV-RNA positive mothers, though breastfeeding was not evaluated. Another study from this same group in Japan found that in seven infected infants, the mothers had significantly higher HCV-RNA titers.

Present data do not suggest a difference in transmission at one year of life between breastfed and formula fed infants, suggesting that transmission of this infection via breastmilk is unlikely. The CDC and AAP consider maternal hepatitis C to be compatible with breastfeeding. In situations with a high maternal viral load, use of artificial infant formula or banked milk, if available, may be a consideration. In another study of asymptomatic HCV positive mothers, two of 87 infants (2.3%) became infected during follow-up. Two additional infected infants were born to women with chronic HCV infection. In all four of these cases, the mother's HCV-RNA titers were $> 5.0 \times 10^6$. Again, in these studies, breastfeeding was not felt to be a risk factor, but rather familial contact with the person with the high HCV-RNA titers. Treatment for chronic HCV infection with interferon therapy is associated with improvement in 28 to 46% of patients. Relapse rates, however, are as high as 50% within six months of completing therapy.

Treatment

- Vaccination against hepatitis A and hepatitis B.

- Peginterferon and ribavirin.

Medications

- INTERFERON ALFA-2b (PegIntron)
  - AAP = Not reviewed
  - LRC = L3
  - RID =
  - Pregnancy = C
  - Comment: Peginterferon alfa-2b is a pegylated form of the antiviral drug interferon alfa-2b. Pegylation confirs protection against enzymatic degradation systemically. It is indicated for the treatment of hepatitis C. While we have no data on its use in breastfeeding mothers, other data on interferons (alfa and beta) suggest they do not readily enter milk, and milk levels will be exceedingly low. When combined with ribavirin, breastfeeding is not recommended. Ribavirin is extremely teratogentic, do not use in pregnant women.

- PEGINTERFERON ALFA-2a (*Pegasys*)
  - AAP = Not reviewed
  - LRC = L3
  - RID =
  - Pregnancy = C
  - Comment: Peginterferon alfa-2a is a pegylated form of the antiviral drug interferon alfa-2a. Pegylation confirs protection against enzymatic degradation systemically. It is indicated for the treatment of hepatitis B and C. While we have no data on its use in breastfeeding mothers, other data on interferons (alfa and beta) suggest they do not readily enter milk, and milk levels will be exceedingly low. Life-threatening or fatal neuropsychiatric reactions may manifest in patients receiving therapy with peginterferon alfa-2a and include suicide, suicidal ideation, homicidal ideation, depression, relapse of drug addiction, and drug overdose. This product should be used with extreme caution in patients who report a history of depression. Neuropsychiatric adverse events observed with alpha interferon treatment include aggressive behavior, psychoses, hallucinations, bipolar disorders, and mania. When combined with ribavirin, breastfeeding is not recommended. Ribavirin is extremely teratogentic, do not use in pregnant women.

- RIBAVIRIN (*Virazole*, *Rebetol*)
  - AAP = Not reviewed
  - LRC = L4
  - RID =
  - Pregnancy = X
  - Comment: While ribavirin has been used acutely in respiratory syncytial virus infections in infants without major complications, its current use in breastfeeding patients for treatment of hepatitis C infections when combined with interferon alfa (Rebetron) for periods up to one year may be more problematic, as high concentrations of ribavirin could accumulate in the breastfed infant. No data are available on its transfer to human milk, but it is probably low, and its oral bioavailability is low as well. However, ribavirin concentrates in peripheral tissues and in the red blood cells in high concentrations over time (Vd= 802). Its elimination half-life at steady state averages 298 hours, which reflects slow elimination from non-plasma compartments. Red cell concentrations on average

are 60 fold higher than plasma levels and may account for the occasional hemolytic anemia. It is likely the acute exposure of a breastfed infant would produce minimal side effects. However, chronic exposure over 6-12 months may be more risky, so caution is recommended.

- RIBAVIRIN + INTERFERON ALFA-2B   (*Rebetron*)
  - ○ AAP = Not reviewed
  - ○ LRC = L4
  - ○ RID =
  - ○ Pregnancy = X
  - ○ Comment: Rebetron is a combination product containing the antiviral Ribavirin and the immunomodulator drug called interferon alfa-2b. This new combination product is indicated for the long-term treatment of hepatitis C. The typical dose for an individual <75 kg consists of 1000 mg ribavirin daily in divided doses and three million units of interferon three times weekly.

    Ribavirin is a synthetic nucleoside used as an antiviral agent and is effective in a wide variety of viral infections. It has heretofore been used acutely in respiratory syncytial virus infections in infants without major complications. However, its current use in breastfeeding patients for treatment of hepatitis C infections, when combined with interferon alfa (Rebetron), for periods up to one year may be more problematic, as high concentrations of ribavirin could accumulate in the breastfed infant over time. No data are available on its transfer to human milk, but it is probably low, and its oral bioavailability is low as well. However, ribavirin concentrates in peripheral tissues and in the red blood cells in high concentrations over time (Vd= 802). Its elimination half-life at steady state averages 298 hours, which reflects slow elimination from non-plasma compartments. Red cell concentrations on average are 60 fold higher than plasma levels and may account for the occasional hemolytic anemia. It is likely the acute exposure of a breastfed infant would produce minimal side effects. However, chronic exposure over 12 months may be more risky, so caution is recommended.

    Very little is known about the secretion of interferons in human milk, although some interferons are known to be secreted normally and may contribute to the antiviral properties of human milk. However, interferons are large in molecular weight (16-28,000 daltons), which would limit their transfer into human milk. Following treatment with a massive dose of 30 million units IV of interferon alpha in a breastfeeding patient, the amount of interferon alpha transferred into human milk was 894, 1004, 1551, 1507, 788, 721 IU at 0 (baseline), two, four, eight, 12, and 24 hours, respectively. Hence, even following a massive dose, no change in breastmilk levels were noted. One thousand international units is roughly equivalent to 500 nanograms of interferon. So it is unlikely that the interferon in Rebetron would transfer to milk or the infant in amounts clinically relevant.

    Rebetron is extremely dangerous to a fetus and is extremely teratogenic at doses even 1/20th of the above therapeutic doses. Pregnancy must be strictly avoided if this product is used in either the male or female partner. Due to the long half-life of this product, pregnancy should be avoided for at least six months following use.

Clinical Tips

Hepatitis C virus (HCV) is a blood-borne virus that is almost entirely transmitted by direct percutaneous exposures to blood. Infants are at highest risk at delivery, following exposure to maternal blood. At present, there is no evidence of mother-to-infant transmission of HCV during breastfeeding. According to the CDC and the AAP, materal HCV infection is not a contraindication to breastfeeding, even in viremic patients. Good hygiene and avoidance of direct exposure to infected blood appears prudent.

Pharmacologic treatment is not a cure, but only reduces liver damage, as indicated by reduced biochemical and histological markers of disease, such as cirrhosis and liver failure. Combination Peginterferon 2b and ribavirin are now the treatment of choice. The transfer of ribavirin into human milk is probably low, but it could build up in red blood cells over time. We do not know if it is safe to use over a prolonged period. While the use of peginterferon 2b has not been studied in breastfeeding mothers, we know that other versions of interferons (alpha and beta) are not transferred into human milk appreciably. Interferons in general are of minimum or no risk to a breastfed infant. Further investigation in this area is needed. Some authorities recommend that the mother who is HCV positive temporarily refrain from breastfeeding with cracked or bleeding nipples.

Suggested Reading

Agarwal, K., Cross, T. J., & Gore, C. (2007). Chronic hepatitis C. *BMJ, 334*(7584), 54-55.

Bhola, K., & McGuire, W. (2007). Does avoidance of breast feeding reduce mother-to-infant transmission of hepatitis C virus infection? *Arch Dis Child, 92*(4), 365-366.

Clark, E. C., Yawn, B. P., Galliher, J. M., Temte, J. L., & Hickner, J. (2005). Hepatitis C identification and management by family physicians. *Fam Med, 37*(9), 644-649.

Cullen, W., O'Leary, M., Langton, D., Stanley, J., Kelly, Y., & Bury, G. (2005). Guidelines for the management of hepatitis C in general practice: a semi-qualitative interview survey of GPs' views regarding content and implementation. *Ir J Med Sci, 174*(3), 32-37.

King, L. A., Le Strat, Y., Meffre, C., Delarocque-Astagneau, E., & Desenclos, J. C. (2009). Assessment and proposal of a new combination of screening criteria for hepatitis C in France. *Eur J Public Health, 19*(5), 527-533.

Maheshwari, A., Ray, S., & Thuluvath, P. J. (2008). Acute hepatitis C. *Lancet, 372*(9635), 321-332.

Mast, E. E. (2004). Mother-to-infant hepatitis C virus transmission and breastfeeding. *Adv Exp Med Biol, 554*, 211-216.

Patel, K., Muir, A. J., & McHutchison, J. G. (2006). Diagnosis and treatment of chronic hepatitis C infection. *BMJ, 332*(7548), 1013-1017.

Poynard, T., Yuen, M. F., Ratziu, V., & Lai, C. L. (2003). Viral hepatitis C. *Lancet, 362*(9401), 2095-2100.

Shiraki, K., Ohto, H., Inaba, N., Fujisawa, T., Tajiri, H., Kanzaki, S., et al. (2008). Guidelines for care of pregnant women carrying hepatitis C virus and their infants. *Pediatr Int, 50*(1), 138-140.

Vento, S., Cainelli, F., & Temesgen, Z. (2008). Perspectives in therapy for hepatitis C. *Expert Opin Investig Drugs, 17*(11), 1635-1639.

Zeuzem, S., Nelson, D. R., & Marcellin, P. (2008). Dynamic evolution of therapy for chronic hepatitis C: how will novel agents be incorporated into the standard of care? *Antivir Ther, 13*(6), 747-760.

Herpes Simplex

Principles of Therapy

Cutaneous herpes simplex virus infection is an incurable DNA viral infection that causes enlarging of infected epithelial cells, followed by nuclear degeneration and lysing of the cellular membrane. Some fuse to form the multinucleated giant cells typical of this infection. HSV-1 (gingivostomatitis) is most commonly found in the oropharynx, while HSV-2 (herpes genitalis) is most commonly associated with genital infections. Cross-over from this rule occurs, however, making specific HSV typing clinically rarely important. Diagnosis is best made using newer more sensitive methods, such as PCR and hybridization techniques performed on specimens taken from suspected lesions. Samples should be taken from unroofed lesions. Serologic testing for HSV 1 and HSV 2 cannot determine the location of the infection due to the above mentioned cross-over. History and visualization of the suspected lesions remains important in making the correct initial diagnosis. The prevalence of HSV 2 antibodies in US women has been reported to have increased to 26%, though most of these women do not have a known diagnosis of genital herpes. HSV 1 seropositivity occurs in 67% of US women. Paired serologic samples taken two to three weeks apart would be needed to diagnose the specific acute infection and are, therefore, not clinically helpful in guiding treatment. Genital HSV is usually acquired by sexual contact with a primary incubation period of 2-14 days and a duration of up to 21 days. Recurrent episodes typically last five to seven days. Symptoms include fever, myalgia, inguinal adenopathy, and bilateral vesicles, followed by tender ulcers on the vulva and extensive cervicitis. The lesions are often multiple, vesicular or ulcerated, and excruciatingly painful. Atypical appearances are common, so PCR testing of visible lesions, even if uncharacteristic in appearance, is indicated. Systemic symptoms are typically restricted to primary infections. Treatment of the initial episode reduces the duration of symptoms. Recurrent episodes are frequently preceded by prodromal symptoms, which may be described as pain or tingling in the area prior to appearance of vulvar lesions. Treatment of recurrent episodes should be begun during prodrome or the first 24 hours after symptoms begin in order to be effective. Daily suppressive treatment can be given for patients with frequent outbreaks (six or more outbreaks yearly). Suppressive therapy prevents most (80%) of recurrences. Antiviral medications do not eradicate the disease, but are rather used for clinical benefit. Topical therapy for HSV is not effective and its use is, therefore, discouraged.

Treatment

- Varies, primary outbreaks typically treated for seven to ten days while recurrences are treated for three to five days.

- Acyclovir, 400 mg orally three times daily Famciclovir, 250 mg orally three times daily (initial), 125 mg orally twice daily (recurrence) Valacyclovir, 1 gm orally twice daily (initial) or once daily (recurrence) or 500 mg orally twice daily (recurrence).

- Topical acyclovir (Zovirax) not recommended.

- Docosanol (Abreva) five times daily until healed.

- Penciclovir (Denavir) every two hours while awake.

- Suppressive therapy: Acyclovir 400 mg twice daily, Famiciclovir 250mg twice daily or Valacyclovir 500mg to 1 gm daily.

Medications

- ACYCLOVIR   (*Zovirax*)
  - AAP = Maternal Medication Usually Compatible with Breastfeeding
  - LRC = L2
  - RID = 1.1-1.5%
  - Pregnancy = B
  - Comment: Acyclovir is converted by herpes simplex and varicella zoster virus to acyclovir triphosphate, which interferes with viral HSV DNA polymerase. It is currently cleared for use in HSV infections, Varicella-Zoster, and under certain instances, such as cytomegalovirus and Epstein-Barr infections. There is virtually no percutaneous absorption following topical application, and plasma levels are undetectable. The pharmacokinetics in children are similar to adults. Acyclovir levels in breastmilk are reported to be 0.6 to 4.1 times the maternal plasma levels. Maximum ingested dose was calculated to be 1500 µg/day, assuming 750 mL milk intake. This level produced no overt side effects in one infant. In a study by Meyer, a patient receiving 200 mg five times daily produced breastmilk concentrations averaging 1.06 mg/L. Using these data, an infant would ingest less than 1 mg acyclovir daily. In another study, doses of 800 mg five times daily produced milk levels that ranged from 4.16 to 5.81 mg/L (total estimated infant ingestion per day = 0.73 mg/kg/day).

    Topical therapy on lesions other than the nipple is probably safe, but mothers with lesions on or close to the nipple should not breastfeed. Toxicities associated with acyclovir are few and usually minor. Acyclovir therapy in neonatal units is common and produces few toxicities. Calculated intake by the infant would be less than 0.87 mg/kg/d.

- FAMCICLOVIR   (*Famvir*)
  - AAP = Not reviewed
  - LRC = L2
  - RID =
  - Pregnancy = B
  - Comment: Famciclovir is an antiviral used in the treatment of uncomplicated herpes zoster infection (shingles) and genital herpes. It is rapidly metabolized to the active metabolite, penciclovir. Although similar to Acyclovir, no data are available on levels in human milk. Oral bioavailability of famciclovir (77%) is much better than acyclovir (15-30%). Studies with rodents suggest that the milk/plasma ratio is greater than 1.0. Because famciclovir provides few advantages over acyclovir, at this point acyclovir would probably be preferred in a nursing mother, although the side-effect profile is still minimal with this product.

- VALACYCLOVIR   (*Valtrex*)
  - AAP = Not reviewed
  - LRC = L1
  - RID = 4.7%

- Pregnancy = B
- Comment: Valacyclovir is a prodrug that is rapidly metabolized in the plasma to acyclovir. In a study of five women who received 500 mg twice daily for seven days after delivery, the median peak acyclovir concentration in breastmilk was 4.2 mg/L at four hours, while the average concentration (AUC) was 2.24 mg/L if 12 hour dosing intervals were used. Thus the relative infant dose would be 4.7% of the weight-normalized maternal dose. The ratio of milk/serum ratio was highest four hours after the initial dose at 3.4 and reached steady state ratio at 1.85. Valacyclovir is rapidly converted to acyclovir, which transfers into breastmilk. However, the amount of acyclovir in breastmilk after valacyclovir administration is considerably less than that used in therapeutic dosing of neonates.

Clinical Tips

The usefulness of acyclovir is largely determined by when it is used. If oral acyclovir is started early in the prodromal stage of infection, it may reduce the duration of shedding and time to healing by one-third. Treatment depends on if the infection is an initial symptomatic episode or a recurrence.

First episodes are treated with oral acyclovir 400 mg three times daily for seven to ten days or possibly longer if new lesions persist. Alternatively, famciclovir 250 mg three times daily or valacyclovir 1 gm twice daily may be used for a similar duration. Acyclovir is less expensive than other treatment options, but requires more frequent dosing than valacyclovir. Recurrences are usually treated for five days. Acyclovir at similar doses as for first episode disease can be used or a dose of 800 mgs twice daily can be given. Famciclovir 125 mg twice daily or valacyclovir 500 mg twice daily for five days are alternatives. Acyclovir is reasonably effective in suppressing recurrence if suppressive doses of 400 mg twice daily are maintained. Alternative suppressive therapies include famciclovir 250mg twice daily or valacyclovir 500 mg or 1000 mg once daily. Suppressive therapy during breastfeeding may be less desirable than episodic treatment based on symptoms, but would depend on the specific clinical situation. Valacyclovir is an ester of acyclovir, which has improved oral absorption. Famcyclovir also has improved oral absorption. Perinatal infections with HSV are risky for the infant. While the primary mode of transmission to the infant is believed to be via the birth canal, transmission via contact with oropharyngeal and cutaneous lesions has been reported. Postnatally acquired infections can be equally lethal to those acquired during labor. A number of cases of herpes transmission via milk are reported. Caregivers should be urged to use strict cleanliness when providing care to the infant. Lesions directly on the breast should be covered prior to nursing. Lesions directly on the areola or nipple should preclude breastfeeding and/or using pumped milk from the affected breast. Valcyclovir is frequently used due to its improved compliance with therapy, as it does not require as frequent dosing.

Suggested Reading

Gupta, R., Warren, T., & Wald, A. (2007). Genital herpes. *Lancet., 370*(9605), 2127-2137.

Kimberlin, D. W., & Rouse, D. J. (2004). Clinical practice. Genital herpes. *N Engl J Med, 350*(19), 1970-1977.

Kriebs, J. M. (2008). Understanding herpes simplex virus: transmission, diagnosis, and considerations in pregnancy management. *J Midwifery Womens Health, 53*(3), 202-208.

Kropp, R. Y., Latham-Carmanico, C., Steben, M., Wong, T., & Duarte-Franco, E. (2007). What's new in management of sexually transmitted infections? Canadian Guidelines on Sexually Transmitted Infections, 2006 Edition. *Can Fam Physician, 53*(10), 1739-1741.

Nicholson, M. (2008). Herpes simplex is not an "ordinary" STI. *J Fam Health Care, 18*(1), 30.

Urato, A. C. (2009). Maternal and neonatal herpes simplex virus infections. *N Engl J Med, 361*(27), 2678; author reply 2679.rdinary" STI. *J Fam Health Care, 18*(1), 30.

Human Papilloma Virus

Principles of Therapy

There are multiple different human papilloma virus types that cause warts. More than 40 different HPV types can cause infections of the genital tract. Prevalence of HPV infection depends on the population studied, but a study of college women suggested a HPV prevalence rate of approximately 26%. Over 50% of women in that study were positive for HPV at some point. HPV can lead to either cervical dysplasia, genital warts, or both, in addition to other less common problems. High risk oncogenic HPV types include HPV 16 and 18, which can cause high grade cervical lesions, which may then lead to cervical cancer. HPV types 6 and 11 are more commonly associated with low grade cervical lesions and condylomata. Though cervical dysplasia and condlyomata can be treated, the HPV cannot be eradicated and vigilant long term follow-up is needed to detect recurrences. In compliant patients, mild cervical dysplasia (low grade squamous intraepithelial dysplasia) can be followed, as many cases will spontaneously regress. Treatment is indicated for suspected non-compliance, or persistent, progressive, or more advanced dysplasia, depending on the particular senario. Cervical dysplasia treatment usually involves a destructive procedure, such as cryotherapy or a loop electrosurgical excision procedure often referred to as a LEEP. These procedures would not commonly involve medications impacting the breastfeeding dyad. Cryotherapy can usually be performed in the office setting without medication. Occasionally, a paracervical block with lidocaine will be used for pain control for an office LEEP procedure. In other circumstances, general anesthetic may be indicated for a day surgical procedure for a LEEP in an apprehensive or otherwise complicated patient. Please refer to section on cervical dysplasia / cancer for further information regarding cervical disease.

Condylomata may resolve spontaneously in 20-30% of affected women, usually during the initial few months. External genital warts can be treated by either provider applied therapy or by patient applied therapy. Choice of therapy depends largely on the size, location, and number of lesions, in addition to patient preference. With respect to effectiveness of therapy, there is no single treatment that is superior. Provider applied therapies include trichloroacetic acid (TCA), podophyllin, cryotherapy, interferon, and surgical resection. Patient applied therapies include podofilox and imiquimod. Treatment requires repeated applications in most cases. Complications of therapy include pain and, rarely, scar formation.

Vaccinations against certain viral types of HPV are available and can be considered for administration, preferably prior to the onset of sexual activity and potential viral exposure. HPV vaccination is recommended for females age 9-26. Advisory Committee on Immunization Practices (ACIP) recommend routine vaccination of 11-12 year-old females, with catch up vaccination for those 13-26. It is currently recommended that women who have undergone vaccination still obtain cervical screening. Vaccination is now recommended in adolescent males.

Treatment

- Abnormal pap smears require follow-up depending on the actual findings from the Pap smear and HPV DNA testing. See section on cervical dysplasia / cancer.

- Treatment options for cervical dysplasia would not be expected to interfere with breastfeeding.

- Treatment options for genital warts include topical medical therapies applied by either provider or patient or destructive therapy.

Medications

- IMIQUIMOD 5% (*Aldara*)
  - AAP = Not reviewed
  - LRC = L3
  - RID =
  - Pregnancy = C
  - Comment: Imiquimod is an immune response modifier used for typical, nonhyperkeratotic, nonhypertrophic actinic keratoses on the face or scalp in immunocompetent adults and for the treatment of primary superficial basal cell carcinoma, and external genital and perianal warts/ condyloma acuminata in patients 12 years old or older. Its mechanism may include the induction of cytokines within the lesion, including interferon alfa. Systemic exposure is minimal and depends on the surface area treated. The apparent elimination half-life is much longer following topical application than systemic. The average peak serum level in users was 0.1 ng/mL following application of 12.5 mg to the face, and 3.5 ng/mL when 75 mg was applied to hand or arms. Mean urinary recoveries of imiquimod and metabolites combined were 0.08 and 0.15% of the applied dose following three applications per week for 16 weeks. These data suggests the systemic absorption is probably minimal. Data in breastfeeding mothers is unavailable, but it is probably compatible with breastfeeding as long as the surface area exposed is minimized.

- INTRALESIONAL INTERFERON Alfa-B (*Heberon Alfa R, Intron A*)
  - AAP = Not reviewed
  - LRC =
  - RID =
  - Pregnancy = C
  - Comment: Interferon alpha is a pure clone of a single interferon subspecies with antiviral, antiproliferative, and immunomodulatory activity. The alpha-interferons are active against various malignancies and viral syndromes, such as hairy cell leukemia, melanoma, AIDS-related Kaposi's sarcoma, condyloma acuminata, and chronic hepatitis B and C infection. Other forms of interferons such as the Alfa-2b (Peg-Intron) are also available.

    Very little is known about the secretion of interferons in human milk, although some interferons are known to be secreted normally and may contribute to the antiviral properties of human milk. However, interferons are large in molecular weight (16-28,000 daltons), which would limit their transfer into human milk. Following treatment with a massive dose of 30 million units IV in one breastfeeding patient, the amount of interferon alpha transferred into human milk was 894, 1004, 1551, 1507, 788, 721 units at 0 (baseline), two, four, eight, 12, and 24 hours, respectively. Hence, even following a massive dose, no change in breastmilk levels were noted from baseline. One thousand international units is roughly equivalent to 500 nanograms of interferon.

- The oral absorption of interferons is controversial and believed to be minimal. Interferons are relatively nontoxic unless extraordinarily large doses are administered parenterally. Interferons are sometimes used in infants and children to treat idiopathic thromboplastinemia (ITP) in huge doses.

- PODOFILOX   (Condylox, Podophyllotoxin)
  - AAP = Not reviewed
  - LRC = L3
  - RID =
  - Pregnancy = C
  - Comment: Podofilox (also called Podophyllotoxin) is an antimitotic agent used to treat genital warts and Condyloma acuminatum. Its transcutaneous absorption is minimal. Plasma levels in 52 patients following use of 0.05 mL of 0.5% podofilox solution to external genitalia did not result in detectable serum levels. However, applications of 0.1 to 1.5 mL resulted in plasma levels of 1-17 ng/mL one to two hours post treatment. The drug does not accumulate after multiple treatments. No data on its transfer to human milk are available. It would be advisable to limit the dosage used in breastfeeding women and to wait for a minimum of four hours following application before breastfeeding. The infant should be closely monitored for GI distress. The use of this product in breastfeeding women should be avoided if possible.

- PODOPHYLLIN RESIN 10% - 25%   (*Cascanyl, Pod-Ben-25, Podocon-25*)
  - AAP = Not reviewed
  - LRC = L3
  - RID =
  - Pregnancy = C
  - Comment: Podofilox (also called Podophyllotoxin) is an antimitotic agent used to treat genital warts and Condyloma acuminatum. Its transcutaneous absorption is minimal, plasma levels in 52 patients following use of 0.05 mL of 0.5% podofilox solution to external genitalia did not result in detectable serum levels. No data on its transfer to human milk are available. Limit the dosage used in breastfeeding women, and to wait for a minimum of 4 hours following application before breastfeeding. The infant should be closely monitored for GI distress. The use of this product in breastfeeding women should be avoided if possible.

- TRICHLOROACETIC ACID 80% - 90%
  - AAP = Not reviewed
  - LRC = L3
  - RID =
  - Pregnancy =
  - Comment: Trichloroacdetic acid used topically is poorly absorbed. Its use topically on small areas should not pose a problem to a breastfed infant.

Clinical Tips

Treatment for cervical dysplasia is unlikely to impact lactation. Various procedures are available, which are locally destructive (see cervical dysplasia/cancer).

Treatment of vulvar condylomata, however, may involve the use of topical medications. Condylomata may proliferate during pregnancy and regress spontaneously in the postpartum period. Treatment may be given during pregnancy, and cesarean delivery is rarely recommended unless the genital warts are obstructive. Persistent or newly occurring condylomata in the postpartum period would indicate treatment. Cryotherapy of condylomata would not impact the breastfed infant and is easily done, inexpensive, and effective in 63-88% of cases. Treatment may be painful, and repeat therapy may be necessary. Surgical resection of condylomata can also be performed in the office setting under local anesthesia in some circumstances. Again, this would have minimal impact on lactation, but can involve pain and scarring as possible consequences. Trichloroacetic acid is a locally caustic agent that induces a chemical cautery effect. Again, treatment requires an office visit, and local extension of this liquid may cause damage to surrounding tissue, but would not impact lactation.

Minimal research has been done regarding the safety of podophyllin, podofilox, and imiquimod during pregnancy and lactation. Podofilox and podophyllin are topical cytotoxic agents, which cause arrest of mitosis. The podophyllin resin is frequently compounded with tincture of benzoin at strengths of 10-25%. Podophyllin requires careful application by the physician. Poisoning due to topical podophyllin application can occur. Treatment area should be limited to 10 cm^2. Most sources consider the use of podofilox and especially podophyllin to be contraindicated during pregnancy, as safer alternatives are available, though evidence of teratogenicity is limited. No data specific to lactation exists.

Imiquimod in a topically active immune enhancing drug which stimulates local production of interferon and cytokines. Five randomized trials found complete clearance of genital warts in 51% of patients. Treatment area should be limited to 20 cm^2. It is quite expensive, and the data does not suggest it is much more effective than podofilox or other office procedures. Topical application of imiquimod results in minimal systemic absorption. Animal studies have not suggested imiquimod to be teratogenic, and it is listed as category C for use during pregnancy.

Suggested Reading

Christopoulos, P., Deligeoroglou, E., Papadias, K., & Creatsas, G. (2008). Human papilloma virus: diagnostic, treatment and preventive issues. *Akush Ginekol (Sofiia), 47*(1), 35-38.

De Clercq, E. (2008). Emerging antiviral drugs. *Expert Opin Emerg Drugs, 13*(3), 393-416.

Ho, G.Y. Bierman R., Beardsley, L., Chang, C.J., & Burk, R.D. (1998). Natural history of cervicalvaginal papillomavirus infection in young women. *N Engl J Med,* 338: 423-8.

Kaliaperumal, K. (2008). Recent advances in management of genital ulcer disease and anogenital warts. *Dermatol Ther, 21*(3), 196-204.

Ljubojević, S., Lipozencić, J., Grgec, D. L., Prstacić, R., Skerlev, M., & Mokos, Z. B. (2008). Human papilloma virus associated with genital infection. *Coll Antropol, 32*(3), 989-997.

Ronco, G., & Giorgi Rossi, P. (2008). New paradigms in cervical cancer prevention: opportunities and risks. *BMC Womens Health, 8,* 23.

Hypertension

Principles of Therapy

Non-Puerperal Hypertension: Primary or essential hypertension is of unknown etiology. Generally, increased total peripheral resistance (TPR) or increased cardiac output lead to elevated blood pressure. Target blood pressure should be 140/85 mm Hg for most patients and less for diabetics and others. The choice of antihypertensive largely rests on the primary source of the syndrome, which could include elevated sympathetic output, elevated plasma volume, elevated renin secretions by the kidney, or other etiologies. Therapy is largely guided by the source of pathology, age, and clinical condition of patient. Women with chronic hypertension are at increased risk for delevloping superimposed pre-eclampsia during pregnancy.

Treatment

- Salt restriction initially.

- Methyldopa, labetalol, and hydralazine.

Medications

- BENAZEPRIL HCL   (*Lotensin, Lotrel*)
    - AAP = Not reviewed
    - LRC = L2
    - RID = 0.00005%
    - Pregnancy = C during first trimester
    - Comment: Benazepril belongs to the ACE inhibitor family. Oral absorption is rather poor (37%). The active component (benazeprilat) reaches a peak at approximately two hours after ingestion. In a patient receiving 20 mg daily for three days, milk levels averaged 0.15 ng/L. Peak benazepril levels (Cmax) were 0.92 ng/L. Thus the levels in milk are almost unmeasurable. The manufacturer suggests a newborn infant ingesting only breastmilk would receive less than 0.1% of the mg/kg maternal dose of benazepril and benazeprilat. My calculations suggest much less or a maximum of 0.00005% of the weight-adjusted maternal dose. Lotrel is a combination product containing benazepril and amlodipine, a calcium channel blocker.

- CAPTOPRIL   (*Capoten*)
    - AAP = Maternal Medication Usually Compatible with Breastfeeding
    - LRC = L2
    - RID = 0.02%

- Pregnancy = C in first trimester
- Comment: Captopril is a typical angiotensin converting enzyme inhibitor (ACE) used to reduce hypertension. Small amounts are secreted (4.7 µg/L milk). In one report of 12 women treated with 100 mg three times daily, maternal serum levels averaged 713 µg/L, while breastmilk levels averaged 4.7 µg/L at 3.8 hours after administration. Data from this study suggest that an infant would ingest approximately 0.002% of the free captopril consumed by its mother (300mg) on a daily basis. No adverse effects have been reported in this study. Use with care in mothers with premature infants.

- **ENALAPRIL MALEATE** (*Vasotec*)
  - AAP = Maternal Medication Usually Compatible with Breastfeeding
  - LRC = L2
  - RID = 0.2%
  - Pregnancy = C in first trimester
  - Comment: Enalapril maleate is an ACE inhibitor used as an antihypertensive. Upon absorption, it is rapidly metabolized by the adult liver to enalaprilat, the biologically active metabolite. In one study of five lactating mothers who received a single 20 mg dose, the mean maximum milk concentration of enalapril and enalaprilat was only 1.74 µg/L and 1.72 µg/L, respectively. The author suggests that an infant consuming 850 mL of milk daily would ingest less than 2 µg of enalaprilat daily. The milk/plasma ratios for enalapril and enalaprilat averaged 0.013 and 0.025, respectively. However, this was only a single dose study, and the levels transferred into milk at steady state may be slightly higher. In a study by Rush of a patient receiving 10 mg/day, the total amount of enalapril and enalaprilat measured in milk during the 24 hour period was 81.9 ng and 36.1 ng, respectively, or 1.44 µg/L and 0.63 µg/L of milk, respectively.

- **FUROSEMIDE** (*Lasix*)
  - AAP = Not reviewed
  - LRC = L3
  - RID =
  - Pregnancy = C
  - Comment: Furosemide is a potent loop diuretic with a rather short duration of action. Furosemide has been found in breastmilk, although the levels are unreported. Diuretics, by reducing blood volume, could potentially reduce breastmilk production, although this is largely theoretical. Furosemide is frequently used in neonates in pediatric units, so pediatric use is common. The oral bioavailability of furosemide in newborns is exceedingly poor and very high oral doses are required (1-4mg/kg BID). It is very unlikely the amount transferred into human milk would produce any effects in a nursing infant, although its maternal use could suppress lactation.

- **HYDROCHLOROTHIAZIDE** (*HydroDIURIL, Esidrix, Oretic*)
  - AAP = Maternal Medication Usually Compatible with Breastfeeding
  - LRC = L2
  - RID =
  - Pregnancy = B
  - Comment: Hydrochlorothiazide (HCTZ) is a typical thiazide diuretic. In one study of a mother receiving a 50 mg dose each morning, milk levels were almost 25% of maternal plasma levels. The

dose ingested (assuming milk intake of 600 mL) would be approximately 50 μg/day, a clinically insignificant amount. The concentration of HCTZ in the infant's serum was undetectable (<20 ng/mL). Some authors suggest that HCTZ can produce thrombocytopenia in the nursing infant, although this is remote and unsubstantiated. Thiazide diuretics could potentially reduce milk production by depleting maternal blood volume, although it is seldom observed. Most thiazide diuretics are considered compatible with breastfeeding if doses are kept low.

- HYDRALAZINE   (*Apresoline*)
  - ○ AAP = Maternal Medication Usually Compatible with Breastfeeding
  - ○ LRC = L2
  - ○ RID   = 1.2%
  - ○ Pregnancy = C
  - ○ Comment: Hydralazine is a popular antihypertensive used for severe pre-eclampsia and gestational and postpartum hypertension. In a study of one breastfeeding mother receiving 50 mg three times daily, the concentrations of hydralazine in breastmilk at 0.5 and two hours after administration was 762, and 792 nmol/L, respectively. The respective maternal serum levels were 1525 and 580 nmol/L at the aforementioned times. From these data, an infant consuming 1000 mL of milk would consume only 0.17 mg of hydralazine, an amount too small to be clinically relevant. The published pediatric dose for hydralazine is 0.75 to 1 mg/kg/day.

- LABETALOL   (*Trandate, Normodyne*)
  - ○ AAP = Maternal Medication Usually Compatible with Breastfeeding
  - ○ LRC = L2
  - ○ RID   = 0.2-0.6%
  - ○ Pregnancy = C
  - ○ Comment: Labetalol is a selective beta blocker with moderate lipid solubility that is used as an antihypertensive and for treating angina. In one study of three women receiving 600 mg, 600 mg, or 1200 mg/day, the peak concentration of labetalol in breastmilk was 129, 223, and 662 μg/L, respectively. In only one infant were measurable plasma levels found (18 μg/L) following a maternal dose of 600 mg. Therefore, only small amounts are secreted into human milk.

- METHYLDOPA   (*Aldomet*)
  - ○ AAP = Maternal Medication Usually Compatible with Breastfeeding
  - ○ LRC = L2
  - ○ RID   = 0.1-0.3%
  - ○ Pregnancy = B
  - ○ Comment: Alpha-methyldopa is a centrally acting antihypertensive. It is frequently used to treat hypertension during pregnancy. In a study of two lactating women who received a dose of 500 mg, the maximum breastmilk concentration of methyldopa ranged from 0.2 to 0.66 mg/L. In another patient who received a 1000 mg dose, the maximum concentration in milk was 1.14 mg/L. The milk/plasma ratios varied from 0.19 to 0.34. The authors indicated that if the infant were to ingest 750 mL of milk daily (with a maternal dose = 1000 mg), the maximum daily ingestion would be less than 855 μg or approximately 0.02% of the maternal dose. In another study of seven women who received 0.750-2.0 gm/day of methyldopa, the free methyldopa concentrations in breastmilk

ranged from zero to 0.2 mg/L, while the conjugated metabolite had concentrations of 0.1 to 0.9 mg/L. These studies generally indicate that the levels of methyldopa transferred to a breastfeeding infant would be too low to be clinically relevant. However, gynecomastia and galactorrhea has been reported in one full-term two week old female neonate following seven days of maternal therapy with methyldopa, 250 mg three times daily (TWH, personal communication).

- METOPROLOL   (*Toprol-XL, Lopressor*)

  ○ AAP = Maternal Medication Usually Compatible with Breastfeeding

  ○ LRC = L3

  ○ RID = 1.4%

  ○ Pregnancy = C

  ○ Comment: In a study of three women four to six months postpartum who received 100 mg twice daily for four days, the peak concentration of metoprolol ranged from 0.38 to 2.58 μmol/L, whereas the maternal plasma levels ranged from 0.1 to 0.97 μmol/L. The mean milk/plasma ratio was 3.0. Assuming ingestion of 75 mL of milk at each feeding, and the maximum concentration of 2.58 μmol/L, an infant would ingest approximately 0.05 mg metoprolol at the first feeding and considerably less at subsequent feedings. In another study of nine women receiving 50-100 mg twice daily, the maternal plasma and milk concentrations ranged from 4-556 nmol/L and 19-1690 nmol/L, respectively. Using these data, the authors calculated an average milk concentration throughout the day as 280 μg/L of milk. This dose is 20-40 times less than a typical clinical dose. The milk/plasma ratio in these studies averaged 3.72. Although the milk/plasma ratios for this drug are in general high, the maternal plasma levels are quite small, so the absolute amount transferred to the infant are quite small.

- NIFEDIPINE   (*Adalat, Procardia*)

  ○ AAP = Maternal Medication Usually Compatible with Breastfeeding

  ○ LRC = L2

  ○ RID = 2.3-3.4%

  ○ Pregnancy = C

  ○ Comment: Nifedipine is an effective antihypertensive. It belongs to the calcium channel blocker family of drugs. Two studies indicate that nifedipine is transferred to breastmilk in varying, but generally low levels. In one study in which the dose was varied from 10-30 mg three times daily, the highest concentration (53.35 μg/L) was measured at one hour after a 30 mg dose. Other levels reported were 16.35 μg/L 60 minutes after a 20 mg dose and 12.89 μg/L 30 minutes after a 10 mg dose. The milk levels fell linearly, with the milk half-lives estimated to be 1.4 hours for the 10 mg dose, 3.1 hours for the 20 mg dose, and 2.4 hours for the 30 mg dose. The milk concentration measured eight hours following a 30 mg dose was 4.93 μg/L. In this study, using the highest concentration found and a daily intake of 150 mL/kg of human milk, the amount of nifedipine intake would only be 8 μg/kg/day (less than 1.8% of the therapeutic pediatric dose). The authors conclude that the amount ingested via breastmilk poses little risk to an infant. In another study, concentrations of nifedipine in human milk one to eight hours after 10 mg doses varied from <1 to 10.3 μg/L (median 3.5 μg/L) in six of eleven patients. In this study, milk levels three days after discontinuing medication ranged from <1 to 9.4 μg/L. The authors concluded the exposure to nifedipine through breastmilk is not significant. In a study by Penny and Lewis, following a maternal dose of 20 mg nifedipine daily for 10 days, peak breastmilk levels at one hour were 46 μg/L. The corresponding maternal serum level was 43 µg/L. From these data, the authors suggest a daily intake for an infant would be approximately 6.45 µg/kg/day. Nifedipine has been found clinically useful for nipple vasospasm. Because of the similarity to Raynaud's Phenomenon, sustained release formulations providing 30-60 mg per day are suggested.

- NIMODIPINE (*Nimotop*)
  - ◦ AAP = Not reviewed
  - ◦ LRC = L2
  - ◦ RID = 0.04%
  - ◦ Pregnancy = C
  - ◦ Comment: Nimodipine is a calcium channel blocker, although it is primarily used in preventing cerebral artery spasm and improving cerebral blood flow. Nimodipine is effective in reducing neurologic deficits following subarachnoid hemorrhage, acute stroke, and severe head trauma. It is also useful in prophylaxis of migraine. In one study of a patient three days postpartum who received 60 mg every four hours for one week, breastmilk levels paralleled maternal serum levels with a milk/plasma ratio of approximately 0.33. The highest milk concentration reported was approximately 3.5 µg/L, while the maternal plasma was approximately 16 µg/L. In another study, a 36-year-old mother received a total dose of 46 mg IV over 24 hours. Nimodipine concentration in milk was much lower than in maternal serum, with a milk/serum ratio of 0.06 to 0.15. During IV infusion, nimodipine concentrations in milk raised initially to 2.2 µg/L and stabilized at concentrations between 0.87 and 1.6 µg/L of milk. Assuming a daily milk intake of 150 mg/kg, an infant would ingest approximately 0.063 to 0.705 µg/kg/day or 0.008 to 0.092% of the weight-adjusted dose administered to the mother.

- VERAPAMIL (*Calan, Isoptin, Covera-HS*)
  - ◦ AAP = Maternal Medication Usually Compatible with Breastfeeding
  - ◦ LRC = L2
  - ◦ RID = 0.2%
  - ◦ Pregnancy = C
  - ◦ Comment: Verapamil is a typical calcium channel blocker used as an antihypertensive. It is secreted into milk, but in very low levels, which are highly controversial. Anderson reports that in one patient receiving 80 mg three times daily, the average steady-state concentrations of verapamil and norverapamil in milk were 25.8 and 8.8 µg/L, respectively. The respective maternal plasma level was 42.9 µg/L. The milk/plasma ratio for verapamil was 0.60. No verapamil was detected in the infant's plasma. Inoue reports that in one patient receiving 80 mg four times daily, the milk level peaked at 300 µg/L at approximately 14 hours. These levels are considerably higher than the aforementioned. In another study of a mother receiving 240 mg daily, the concentrations in milk were never higher than 40 µg/L. See bepridil, diltiazem, and nifedipine as alternates. From these three studies, the relative infant dose would vary from 0.15%, 0.98%, and 0.18%, respectively. Regardless of the variability, the relative amount transferred to the infant is still quite small.

Clinical Tips

Initial therapy for non-puerperal hypertension should include dietary changes and modification of lifestyle, such as weight loss for obese patients, smoking cessation, restriction of alcohol and sodium intake, and exercise. If these methods are unsuccessful after three months or the clinical situation otherwise warrants medication, then pharmacologic agents are begun. If the patient is less than 55 years of age or black, ACE inhibitors, angiotension receptor blockers (ARBs), and beta blockers are most effective. Beta-blockers are indicated for younger patients, patients with arrhythmias, angina pectoris, early onset hypertension, and post-MI patients. However, they are no longer indicated as first line therapy for hypertension. Diuretics (thiazides) and ACE inhibitors are primarily indicated for black patients; older, obese, edematous patients; and individuals subject to congestive heart failure. First line management of chronic hypertension during pregnancy will often employ methyldopa or labetalol. If effective, these may be continued during the lactational period.

Of the beta-blocker family, metoprolol or labetalol are very cardioselective and are preferred choices in breastfeeding patients. Atenolol can and has been often used, but at least one case of infant bradycardia and hypotension has been reported. This can occur with any beta-blocker. When using beta-blockers, be observant for bradycardia, hypotension, and apnea, although these are rare with the above agents. The diuretics have been used extensively in breastfeeding women without problem. Several members of the calcium channel blocker family have been studied. Verapamil, nifedipine, and nimodipine produce subclinical milk levels and appear relatively safe to use. Of the ACE inhibitor family, captopril, nimodipine, and enalapril are transferred to milk in very low levels. Nevertheless, neonates are very sensitive to ACE inhibitors, so be cautious of their use the first month postpartum. At this time, none of the Angiotensin receptor blockers (ARBs) have been studied. Hydralazine and methyldopa have been used extensively early postpartum without problem in breastfed infants. Because breastmilk production is dependent on blood supply and pressure, be aware that a drastic reduction in blood pressure may reduce the supply of milk.

Gestational Hypertension: Overall, hypertensive disorders of pregnancy occur in approximately 12-22% of pregnancies. Hypertension during pregnancy may be either chronic hypertension, which continues or is diagnosed during early pregnancy, or gestational hypertension, which is specifically related to pregnancy and includes pre-eclampsia. For the diagnosis of chronic hypertension, the hypertension should be present prior to the 20th week of pregnancy. Women with chronic hypertension diagnosed outside of pregnancy are at increased risk for also developing superimposed pre-eclampsia during pregnancy. Gestational hypertension includes hypertension diagnosed after 20 weeks gestation. Mild hypertension is diagnosed with a BP > 140/90, while severe hypertension is diagnosed with a BP ≥160-180/110. Pre-eclampsia often involves proteinuria and symptoms such as headache, scotomata, or right upper quadrant pain. HELLP syndrome may also occur in pre-eclampsia and is characterized by hemolysis, elevated liver enzymes, and low platelets. The diagnosis of eclampsia is made when a seizure occurs. Pre-eclampsia is most common during labor, but may also occur in the early postpartum period. Bed rest and continued maternal and fetal surveillance may be indicated for management of pre-eclampsia in preterm gestations. At term, management of pre-eclampsia involves delivery. The use of magnesium is often frequently employed in mild pre-eclampsia. Magnesium for seizure prophylaxis and medication to control severe hypertension are indicated in women with severe pre-eclampsia or eclampsia. Management of postpartum pre-eclampsia may also involve magnesium and control of hypertension. Typically antihypertensive medications should be used to treat diastolic BP> 105-110. Hypertension which is diagnosed during pregnancy, but persists past 12 weeks postpartum is then referred to as chronic hypertension.

First line management of chronic hypertension during pregnancy will often employ methyldopa or labetalol. If effective, these may be continued during the lactational period. Hydralazine has a long history of safety and efficacy in pre-eclampsia and postpartum hypertension. Although the ACE inhibitors are quite safe for adult patients, their use during pregnancy is contraindicated due to renal teratology. ACE inhibitors are contraindicated during the second and third trimester of pregnancy due to an association with adverse fetal/neonatal outcomes, including under-developed calvarium, renal failure, oligohydramnios, fetal growth restriction, renal dysgenesis, pulmonary hypoplasia, and fetal and neonatal death.

Older or full term infants (> 1 month) can probably handle the small amounts of antihypertensive agents present in milk. Atenolol is also discouraged for use during pregnancy due to potential concern for fetal growth restriction, though this information is less conclusive. Women with pre-eclampsia will require the use of magnesium sulfate for seizure prophylaxis during the peri-partum period (see seizure disorders). In this setting, treatment of hypertension depends on severity, but frequently will be accomplished by hydralazine or labetalol. Diuretics are rarely useful in the management of pre-eclampsia.

Suggested Reading

Leeman, L., & Fontaine, P. (2008). Hypertensive disorders of pregnancy. *Am Fam Physician, 78*(1), 93-100.

Magee, L., & Sadeghi, S. (2005). Prevention and treatment of postpartum hypertension. *Cochrane Database Syst Rev, 1*, CD004351.

Magee, L. A., & Abdullah, S. (2004). The safety of antihypertensives for treatment of pregnancy hypertension. *Expert Opin Drug Saf, 3*(1), 25-38.

Moghbeli, N., Pare, E., & Webb, G. (2008). Practical assessment of maternal cardiovascular risk in pregnancy. *Congenit Heart Dis, 3*(5), 308-316.

Petursson, H., Getz, L., Sigurdsson, J. A., & Hetlevik, I. (2009). Current European guidelines for management of arterial hypertension: are they adequate for use in primary care? Modelling study based on the Norwegian HUNT 2 population. *BMC Fam Pract, 10*, 70.

Prabhu, M., Palaian, S., Malhotra, A., Ravishankar, P., Bista, D., Almeida, R., et al. (2005). Therapeutic dimensions of ACE inhibitors--a review of literature and clinical trials. *Kathmandu Univ Med J (KUMJ), 3*(3), 296-304.

Qasqas, S. A., McPherson, C., Frishman, W. H., & Elkayam, U. (2004). Cardiovascular pharmacotherapeutic considerations during pregnancy and lactation. *Cardiol Rev, 12*(4), 201-221.

Scuteri, A., Najjar, S. S., Orru, M., Albai, G., Strait, J., Tarasov, K. V., et al. (2009). Age- and gender-specific awareness, treatment, and control of cardiovascular risk factors and subclinical vascular lesions in a founder population: the SardiNIA Study. *Nutr Metab Cardiovasc Dis, 19*(8), 532-541.

Turk, M. W., Tuite, P. K., & Burke, L. E. (2009). Cardiac health: primary prevention of heart disease in women. *Nurs Clin North Am, 44*(3), 315-325.

Hyperthyroidism

Principles of Therapy

Hyperthyroidism is most commonly caused by Graves' disease, accounting for approximately 95% of cases of hyperthyroidism. Other etiologies of thyroitoxicosis include gestational trophoblastic disease, toxic multinodular goiter, subacute thyroiditis, hyperfunctioning thyroid adenoma, struma ovarii, and other extrathyroid sources of thyroid hormone. Graves' disease is one of the most frequent thyroid disorders and is characterized by elevated circulating thyroid hormone, exophthalmos, goiter, and pretibial myxedema. It is known that Graves' disease results from stimulation of the thyroid gland by circulating antibodies to the thyroid stimulating hormone (TSH) receptor, although the mechanism is not completely understood. Once stimulated, the gland creates and releases high levels of thyroid hormones (T4 and/or T3), which are responsible for the symptoms. Therapy of hyperthyroidism requires a complete understanding of the endocrinology of this syndrome and should not be taken lightly. Treatment involves use of antithyroid medications, beta-blockers for treatment of thyroid storm (thyrotoxicosis), and radioactive Iodine for destruction of the gland in some cases.

Postpartum thyroiditis occurs in approximately 5-8% of postpartum women. It may present as either hyperthyroidism or hypothyroidism, carries a high recurrence risk, and may also occur after miscarriage. The diagnosis is further obscured as the symptoms may mimic expected post-partum complaints. Often postpartum thyroiditis does not require treatment. This is usually the case for postpartum thyroitis resulting in hyperthyroidism.

Treatment

- Initially, beta blockers to decrease symptoms/signs, especially in thyroid storm.

- Thioamides: Methimazole or propylthiouracil to decrease thyroid production (PTU also block conversion of T4 to T3).

- Radioactive Iodine-131 ablation, usually requires exogenous thyroid hormone following ablation.

Medications

- METHIMAZOLE   (*Tapazole*)
  - AAP = Maternal Medication Usually Compatible with Breastfeeding
  - LRC = L3
  - RID   = 2.3%
  - Pregnancy = D
  - Comment: Methimazole, carbimazole, and propylthiouracil are used to inhibit the secretion of thyroxine. Carbimazole is metabolized to the active metabolite, methimazole. Levels depend on

maternal dose, but appear too low to produce clinical effect. In one study of a patient receiving 2.5 mg methimazole every 12 hours, the milk/serum ratio was 1.16, and the dose per day was calculated at 16-39 µg methimazole. This was equivalent to 7-16% of the maternal dose. In a study of 35 lactating women receiving 5-20 mg/day of methimazole, no changes in infant thyroid function were noted in any infant, even those at higher doses. Further, studies by Lamberg in 11 women treated with the methimazole derivative carbimazole (5-15 mg daily, equal to 3.3-10 mg methimazole) found all 11 infants had normal thyroid function following maternal treatments. Thus in small maternal doses, methimazole may also be safe for the nursing mother. In a study of a woman with twins who was receiving up to 30 mg carbimazole daily, the average methimazole concentration in milk was 43 µg/L. The average plasma concentrations in the twin infants were 45 and 52 ng/mL, which is below therapeutic range. Methimazole milk concentrations peaked at two to four hours after a carbimazole dose. No changes in thyroid function in these infants were noted. In a large study of over 139 thyrotoxic lactating mothers and their infants, even at methimazole doses of 20 mg/day, no changes in infant TSH, T4, or T3 were noted in over 12 months of study. The authors conclude that both PTU and methimazole can safely be administered during lactation. However, during the first few months of therapy, monitoring of infant thyroid functioning is recommended.

- METOPROLOL   (*Toprol-XL, Lopressor*)
  - ◦ AAP = Maternal Medication Usually Compatible with Breastfeeding
  - ◦ LRC = L3
  - ◦ RID = 1.4%
  - ◦ Pregnancy = C
  - ◦ Comment: In a study of three women four to six months postpartum who received 100 mg twice daily for four days, the peak concentration of metoprolol ranged from 0.38 to 2.58 µmol/L, whereas the maternal plasma levels ranged from 0.1 to 0.97 µmol/L. The mean milk/plasma ratio was 3.0. Assuming ingestion of 75 mL of milk at each feeding and the maximum concentration of 2.58 µmol/L, an infant would ingest approximately 0.05 mg metoprolol at the first feeding and considerably less at subsequent feedings. In another study of nine women receiving 50-100 mg twice daily, the maternal plasma and milk concentrations ranged from 4-556 nmol/L and 19-1690 nmol/L, respectively. Using these data, the authors calculated an average milk concentration throughout the day as 280 µg/L of milk. This dose is 20-40 times less than a typical clinical dose. The milk/plasma ratio in these studies averaged 3.72. Although the milk/plasma ratios for this drug are in general high, the maternal plasma levels are quite small, so the absolute amount transferred to the infant are quite small.

- PROPRANOLOL   (*Inderal*)
  - ◦ AAP = Maternal Medication Usually Compatible with Breastfeeding
  - ◦ LRC = L2
  - ◦ RID = 0.3-0.5%
  - ◦ Pregnancy = C
  - ◦ Comment: Propranolol is a popular beta blocker used in treating hypertension, cardiac arrhythmia, migraine headache, and numerous other syndromes. In general, the maternal plasma levels are exceedingly low; hence, the milk levels are low as well. Milk/plasma ratios are generally less than one. In one study of three patients, the average milk concentration was only 35.4 µg/L after multiple dosing intervals. The milk/plasma ratio varied from 0.33 to 1.65. Using these data, the authors

suggest that an infant would receive only 70 μg/L of milk per day, which is <0.1% of the maternal dose. In another study of a patient receiving 20 mg twice daily, milk levels varied from 4 to 20 μg/L, with an estimated average dose to infant of 3 μg/day. In another patient receiving 40 mg four times daily, the peak concentration occurred at three hours after dosing. Milk levels varied from zero to 9 μg/L. After a 30 day regimen of 240 mg/day propranolol, the predose and postdose concentration in breastmilk was 26 and 64 μg/L, respectively. No symptoms or signs of beta blockade were noted in this infant. The above amounts in milk would likely be clinically insignificant. Long term exposure has not been studied, and caution is urged. Of the beta blocker family, propranolol is probably preferred in lactating women. Use with great caution, if at all, in mothers or infants with asthma.

- PROPYLTHIOURACIL   (*PTU*)
  - ○ AAP = Maternal Medication Usually Compatible with Breastfeeding
  - ○ LRC = L2
  - ○ RID = 1.8%
  - ○ Pregnancy = D
  - ○ Comment: Propylthiouracil reduces the production and secretion of thyroxine by the thyroid gland. Only small amounts are secreted into breastmilk. Reports thus far suggest that levels absorbed by the infant are too low to produce side effects. In one study of nine patients given 400 mg doses, mean serum and milk levels were 7.7 mg/L and 0.7 mg/L, respectively. No changes in infant thyroid have been reported. The FDA recently issued an alert suggesting an increased risk of liver damage, including liver failure and death in adults and children directly consuming PTU.

    While the levels in milk are probably too low to induce liver problems in breastfed infants, the risk to the mother remains. Methimazole may be a suitable alternative. If used, monitor infant thyroid function (T4, TSH) carefully during therapy.

Clinical Tips

Initial therapy is to control the peripheral symptoms of excess thyroid hormone. These symptoms include tachycardia, atrial fibrillation, tremor, loss of body weight, sweating, heat intolerance, and intestinal hyperactivity. Usually 30-60 mg daily of propranolol is sufficient, but doses as high as 480 mg/day have been used. Propranolol has been studied in breastfeeding women and, in most cases, produces no untoward effect on the infant, but watch for hypotension and hypoglycemia. The use of potassium iodide is problematic in breastfeeding mothers. Iodine concentrates in milk (25 fold), and should be avoided if possible in breastfeeding mothers. Iodine transfer to the infant could be significant enough to suppress thyroid function in the neonate. To suppress maternal thyroid function, methimazole or propylthiouracil (PTU) are usually the drugs of choice in breastfeeding mothers. Numerous studies have shown no change in thyroid function in any infant thus far reported. PTU levels in milk are very low.

Recent studies of methimazole suggest it is the preferred choice in most individuals, including breastfeeding mothers. It is preferred because it can be administered once daily, the dose is low, and side effect profile is minimal. In five studies of over 187 hyperthyroid breastfeeding women treated with methimazole with doses as high as 20 mg/day, no changes in thyroid function were noted in any infant. In most infants, methimazole was undetectable in the plasma.

The FDA recently issued an alert suggesting an increased risk of liver damage, including liver failure and death in adults and children directly consuming PTU. While the levels in milk are probably too low to induce liver problems in breastfed infants, the risk to the mother remains. Monitoring for thyroid function and leukocytopenia in the breastfed neonate, while not mandatory, may be prudent. Radioactive ablation of the gland with Iodine-131 is especially dangerous to a breastfed infant. High doses of radioactive Iodine-131 are known to transfer via milk to the infant, and while not enough to destroy an infant's thyroid, they could predispose the infant to thyroid carcinoma in later years. Further, almost 27% of the radioactive I-131 dose is transferred directly into breast tissue of lactating women. Some authors suggest this may increase the risk of breast cancer. Therefore, the U.S. Nuclear Regulatory Commission recommends that the mother discontinue breastfeeding permanently for this infant. We concur and further recommend that the mother discontinue breastfeeding for at least several weeks prior to undergoing radiotherapy ablation for maximum protection of infant and mother. The U.S. Nuclear Regulatory Commission recommendations for use of radioactive materials in breastfeeding women are in the Appendix.

Suggested Reading

Brent, G. A. (2008). Clinical practice. Graves' disease. *N Engl J Med, 358*(24), 2594-2605.

Felz, M. W. (2005). Who should be screened for thyroid disease? *Postgrad Med, 118*(3), 9-10.

Marx, H., Amin, P., & Lazarus, J. H. (2008). Hyperthyroidism and pregnancy. (2008). *BMJ, 336*(7645), 663-667.

Medical Letter, Inc. (2006). Drugs for hypothyroidism and hyperthyroidism. *Treat Guidel Med Lett, 4*(44), 17-24.

Okosieme, O. E., Marx, H., & Lazarus, J. H. (2008). Medical management of thyroid dysfunction in pregnancy and the postpartum. *Expert Opin Pharmacother, 9*(13), 2281-2293.

Rashid, M., & Rashid, M. H. (2007). Obstetric management of thyroid disease. *Obstet Gynecol Surv, 62*(10), 680-688.

Hypothyroidism

Principles of Therapy

Primary hypothyroidism is probably an autoimmune disease, usually occurring as a sequel to Hashimoto's thyroiditis. While it can occur at any age, those at highest risk are the elderly and postmenopausal patients. Ultimately, hypothyroidism commonly results in a shrunken, fibrotic thyroid gland with little function. Secondary hypothyroidism occurs when there is a failure of the hypothalamic-pituitary axis, leading to reduced levels of circulating Thyroid Stimulating Hormone (TSH). The treatment of hypothyroidism is generally replacement of the thyroid hormone levothyroxine (T4), and rarely with liothyronine (T3). It is important to remember that it requires up to six weeks of therapy before steady-state levels of thyroxine are attained. In addition, serum TSH levels in hypothyroid patients reach their nadir within six weeks of beginning treatment. Therefore, thyroid function tests after six weeks are quite reliable in predicting if exogenous levothyroxine therapy is adequate. The nuances in discerning hypothyroid states are enormous and careful laboratory and/or clinical study of the patient by accomplished clinicians or an endocrinologist is important. Iodidine deficiency is associated with goiter and remains a common cause of hypothyroidism in developing countries. Hypothyroidism is more common in women with type 1 diabetes. Some medications, such as lithium, some sulfonamides, thiourea, iodine, bexarotene, and amiodarone, are known to suppress thyroid function.

Postpartum thyroiditis occurs in approximately 5-8% of postpartum women. It may present as either hyperthyroidism or hypothyroidism, carries a high recurrence risk, and may also occur after miscarriage. Of women with postpartum thyroiditis, approximately 44% have hypothyroidism. One study found that 11% of women diagnosed with postpartum thyroiditis went on to have permanent hypothyroidism. The diagnosis is further obscured as the symptoms may mimic expected post-partum complaints. Often postpartum thyroiditis does not require treatment. The decision to treat depends on clinical symptoms and the extent of thyroid function abnormality.

Treatment

- Thyroxine

- Liothyronine

Medications

- LEVOTHYROXINE   *(Synthroid, Levothroid, Unithroid, Eltroxin, Levoxyl, Thyroid, Levoxyl)*
    - AAP = Maternal Medication Usually Compatible with Breastfeeding
    - LRC = L1
    - RID =
    - Pregnancy = A

- ○ Comment: Levothyroxine is also called T4. Most studies indicate that minimal levels of maternal thyroid are transferred into human milk, and further, that the amount secreted is extremely low and insufficient to protect a hypothyroid infant, even while nursing. The amount secreted after supplementing a breastfeeding mother is highly controversial, and numerous reports conflict. Anderson indicates that levothyroxine is not detectable in breastmilk, although others using sophisticated assay methods have shown extremely low levels (4 ng/mL). It is generally recognized that some thyroxine will transfer, but the amount will be extremely low. It is important to remember that supplementation with levothyroxine is designed to bring the mother into a euthyroid state, which is equivalent to the normal breastfeeding female. Hence, the risk of using exogenous thyroxine is no different than in a normal euthyroid mother. Liothyronine (T3) appears to transfer into milk in higher concentrations than levothyroxine (T4), but liothyronine is seldom used in clinical medicine due to its short half-life (<1 day).

- • LIOTHYRONINE   (*Cytomel*)
  - ○ AAP = Not reviewed
  - ○ LRC = L2
  - ○ RID =
  - ○ Pregnancy = A
  - ○ Comment: Liothyronine is also called T3. It is seldom used for thyroid replacement therapy due to its short half-life. It is generally recognized that only minimal levels of thyroid hormones are secreted in human milk, although several studies have shown that hypothyroid conditions only became apparent when breastfeeding was discontinued. Although some studies indicate that breastfeeding may briefly protect hypothyroid infants, it is apparent that the levels of T4 and T3 are too low to provide long-term protection from hypothyroid disease. Levels of T3 reported in milk vary, but in general are around 238 ng/dl and considerably higher than T4 levels. The maximum amount of T3 ingested daily by an infant would be 357 ng/kg/day or approximately 1/10 the minimum requirement. From these studies, it is apparent that only exceedingly low levels of T3 are secreted into human milk and are insufficient to protect an infant from hypothyroidism.

Clinical Tips

Treatment of hypothyroid disorders is generally initiated with synthetic levothyroxine sodium. About 80% of an oral dose of levothyroxine is absorbed in the small intestine, and it has a half-life of approximately seven days. Steady state requires therapy of at least four to six weeks. Synthetic forms of thyroxine are more stable than those derived from animal organs. They are more standardized (potency) and are better absorbed in the GI tract (60-80% bioavailable). Some controversy exists over the equivalency of generic products. Patients and pharmacists are advised to use the same generic product or to at least advise the patient when a change in product is made. There are numerous drug-thyroid interactions, and the reader is advised to ask advice concerning the use of other drugs with thyroid supplements.

Generic thyroid USP or Armour Thyroid are derived from dessicated porcine thyroid glands and contain thyroxine, liothyronine, and bound iodine. These products generally contain slightly higher T3/T4 ratios, which might lead to supratherapeutic levels of T3.

Thyroxine's long half-life of six days permits single-day dosing regimens with minimal day-to-day variability. Liothyronine (T3), due to a short one day half-life, is generally restricted to use in primary hypothyroidism in patients with thyroid cancer undergoing T4 withdrawal for thyroid scanning or ablation. The transfer of levothyroxine into milk is extremely low.

Thyroid function may vary enormously during pregnancy and the postpartum period. Elevated estrogen levels during pregnancy reduce hepatic clearance of thyroid binding globulin, thus leading to reduced free-T4. This change is manifest during pregnancy and may continue early postpartum. Hormonal levels should be re-evaluated at the postpartum visit in patients with known hypothyroidism. Additionally, it is estimated that 5 to 10% of women have evidence of some transient postpartum thyroid dysfunction that typically occurs after the common six week postpartum follow-up visit. It is well known that postpartum hypothyroidism may be associated with low milk production, and this should be investigated in patients with extremely low milk supply.

Suggested Reading

The Hormone Foundation's patient guide to the management of maternal hypothyroidism before, during and after pregnancy. (2007). *J Clin Endocrinol Metab, 92*(8), 2 p following 10A.

Danzi, S., & Klein, I. (2008). Recent considerations in the treatment of hypothyroidism. *Curr Opin Investig Drugs, 9*(4), 357-362.

Hennessey, J. V., & Scherger, J. E. (2007). Evaluating and treating the patient with hypothyroid disease. *J Fam Pract, 56*(8 Suppl Hot Topics), S31-39.

Lucas A., Pizarro E., Granada M.L., Salinas I., Foz M., Sanmarti A. (2000). Postpartum thyroiditis: epidemiology and clinical evolution in a nonselected population. *Thyroid*, 10, 71-77.

Medical Letter, I. (2006). Drugs for hypothyroidism and hyperthyroidism. *Treat Guidel Med Lett, 4*(44), 17-24.

Okosieme, O. E., Marx, H., & Lazarus, J. H. (2008). Medical management of thyroid dysfunction in pregnancy and the postpartum. *Expert Opin Pharmacother, 9*(13), 2281-2293.

Vaidya, B., & Pearce, S. H. (2008). Management of hypothyroidism in adults. *BMJ, 337*, a801.

Infertility

Principles of Therapy

Infertility is defined as the inability to conceive after one year of unprotected intercourse and affects approximately 10-15% of reproductive age couples. Most couples with infertility are sub-fertile, rather than absolutely infertile. Absolute infertility, meaning pregnancy rate of zero despite treatment, includes those individuals with bilateral tubal occlusion, amenorrhea secondary to gonadotropic cell destruction, ovarian or endometrial failure, or absence of sperm. Only approximately 65% of infertility can be ascribed to the female. For female infertility, approximately 40% is related to ovulatory dysfunction, 40% to tubal and pelvic pathology, and 10% due to anatomic disturbances. The most common reason for ovulatory dysfunction is polycystic ovary syndrome (PCOS), which accounts for 70%, while the remaining causes include hypothalamic amenorrhea (10%), hyperprolactinemia (10%), and premature ovarian failure (10%). Additionally, aging plays an important role in infertility and the risk of spontaneous abortion. An elevated day three FSH may be useful in identifying depletion of ovarian reserve.

Treatment protocols are generally aimed at alleviating the core etiology of infertility. This includes progestational agents for treating luteal phase defects, bromocriptine and other such agents for treating hyperprolactinemic conditions, and clomiphene citrate, GnRH, and other gonadotropins for treating ovulatory defects. Additionally, artifical reproductive techniques involving in vitro fertilization, intracytoplasmic sperm injection, and donor egg programs are available. Hypothalamic anovulation may be associated with anorexia, female athlete triad, hypothalamic lesions, and Kallmann's syndrome. Low BMI may be associated, and in that situation dietician intervention, limitation of excessive exercise, and weight gain may assist with achieving pregnancy.

Ovulation induction frequently begins with clomiphene citrate, an orally active medication which has a weak estrogenic effect and modifies the hypothalamic-pituitary axis so that response to estrogen levels is blunted and FSH and LH levels rise. Up to 80% of anovulatory women will ovulate with clomiphene and about 40% will conceive. Patients most likely to fail to ovulate with clomiphene include those with hyperandrogenism, polycystic ovaries, and obesity (insulin resistance). Weight loss plays an important role in the management of infertility in the obese patient. In patients with high androgen levels that fail to respond to clomiphene, the addition of dexamethasone improves ovulation and pregnancy rates. The induction of ovulation with human gonadotropins requires experience and careful patient evaluation as expense and side effects (both frequency and severity) are more common. Various products ranging from human menopausal gonadotropins collected from post-menopausal women to recombinate and purified products are now available. Gonadotropins are inactive orally and require intramuscular injection or subcutaneous administration. Human chorionic gonadotropin (HCG) may be used to simulate the mid-cycle LH surge during therapy to induce ovulation. Bromocriptine and cabergoline are also used in the treatment of infertile women with hyperprolactinemia and occasionally in those without elevated prolactin levels to improve responsiveness to clomiphene. This treatment in the lactating woman would not be advised as it would suppress prolactin production. Diagnosis of hyperprolactinemia would require a preexisting diagnosis as testing during lactation would produce altered results. Metformin also plays a role in the infertility treatment of women with polycystic ovaries and insulin resistance. While the complete therapy of infertility is beyond the scope of this text, several questions are pertinent to breastfeeding women. One, do these agents suppress lactation or transfer into human milk and affect the infant? Secondly, does continued lactation and its coincident amenorrheic state reduce the fertility of the patient? In other words, should an infertile woman continue to breastfeed? The answers to these questions are not known for certain. Each of the agents commonly used in infertility will be described below.

Treatment

- Weight loss in obese patients may improve ovulation.

- Ovulation induction frequently begins with clomiphene citrate so that response to estrogen levels is blunted and FSH and LH levels rise.

- Patients most likely to fail to ovulate with clomiphene include those with hyperandrogenism, polycystic ovaries, and obesity (insulin resistance).

- Metformin improves ovulation and pregnancy rates in women with polycystic ovarian syndrome who fail to conceive on clomiphene alone.

- Patients with hyperprolactinemia will require treatment to reduce prolactin levels, which include bromocriptine or cabergoline, both of which may suppress lactation.

- In patients with high androgen levels that fail to respond to clomiphene, the addition of dexamethasone improves ovulation and pregnancy rates.

- The induction of ovulation with human gonadotropins requires experience and careful patient evaluation as expense and side effects (both frequency and severity) are more common.

- Several questions pertinent to breastfeeding women remain:
  - Do these agents suppress lactation or transfer into human milk and affect the infant?
  - Will continued breastfeeding affect the fertility of the infertile woman?

Medications

- BROMOCRIPTINE MESYLATE (*Parlodel*)
  - AAP = Drugs associated with significant side effects and should be given with caution
  - LRC = L5 (milk suppression)
  - RID =
  - Pregnancy = B
  - Comment: Bromocriptine is an anti-parkinsonian, synthetic ergot alkaloid which inhibits prolactin secretion and, hence, physiologic lactation. Most of the dose of bromocriptine is absorbed first-pass by the liver, leaving less than 6% to remain in the plasma. Maternal serum prolactin levels remain suppressed for up to 14 hours after a single dose. The FDA approved indication for lactation suppression has been withdrawn. It is no longer approved for this purpose due to numerous maternal deaths, seizures, and strokes.

    Observe for transient hypotension or vomiting. It is sometimes used in hyperprolactinemic patients who have continued to breastfeed, although the incidence of maternal side-effects is significant and newer products are preferred. Several studies have shown the possibility of breastfeeding during bromocriptine therapy for pituitary tumors with no untoward effects in infants. Caution is recommended as profound maternal postpartum hypotension has been reported. While bromocriptine is no longer recommended for suppression of lactation, a newer product, cabergoline (Dostinex), is considered much safer for suppression of prolactin production.

- CABERGOLINE   (*Dostinex*)
  - ◦ AAP = Not reviewed
  - ◦ LRC = L4
  - ◦ RID =
  - ◦ Pregnancy = B
  - ◦ Comment: Cabergoline is a long-acting synthetic ergot alkaloid derivative which produces a dopamine agonist effect similar, but much safer than bromocriptine (Parlodel). Cabergoline directly inhibits prolactin secretion by the pituitary. It is primarily indicated for pathological hyperprolactinemia, but in several European studies, it has been used for inhibition of postpartum lactation. The dose regimen used for the inhibition of physiologic lactation is cabergoline 1 mg administered as a single dose on the first day postpartum. For the suppression of established lactation, cabergoline 0.25 mg is taken every 12 hours for two days for a total of 1 mg. Single doses of 1 mg have been found to completely inhibit postpartum lactation. Transfer into human milk is not reported.

    In patients with hyperprolactinemia, it is possible to carefully administered doses to lower the prolactin to safe ranges, but high enough to retain lactation. In such cases, the infant should be observed for potential ergot side effects, if any. In addition, mothers treated with cabergoline early postpartum may, in some cases, recover their milk supply following pumping and extensive breastfeeding.

- CLOMIPHENE   (*Clomid, Serophene, Milophene*)
  - ◦ AAP = Not reviewed
  - ◦ LRC = L3 in late stage lactation
  - ◦ RID =
  - ◦ Pregnancy = X
  - ◦ Comment: Clomiphene appears to stimulate the release of the pituitary gonadotropins, follicle-stimulating hormone (FSH), and luteinizing hormone (LH), which result in development and maturation of the ovarian follicle, ovulation, and subsequent development and function of the corpus luteum. It has both estrogenic and anti-estrogenic effects. LH and FSH peak at five to nine days after completing clomiphene therapy. In a study of 60 postpartum women (one to four days postpartum), clomiphene was effective in totally inhibiting lactation early postnatally and in suppressing established lactation (day four). Only seven of 40 women receiving clomiphene to inhibit lactation had signs of congestion or discomfort. In the 20 women who received clomiphene to suppress established lactation (on day four), a rapid amelioration of breast engorgement and discomfort was produced. After five days of treatment, no signs of lactation were present. In another study of 177 postpartum women, clomiphene was very effective at inhibiting lactation.

    Clomiphene appears to be very effective in suppressing lactation when used up to four days postpartum. However, its efficacy in reducing milk production in women, months after lactation is established, is unknown but believed to be minimal.

- **DEXAMETHASONE**   (*Decadron, AK-Dex, Maxidex*)
  - AAP = Not reviewed
  - LRC = L3
  - RID =
  - Pregnancy = C
  - Comment: Dexamethasone is a long-acting corticosteroid, similar in effect to prednisone, although more potent. Dexamethasone 0.75 mg is equivalent to a 5 mg dose of prednisone. While the elimination half-life is brief, only three to six hours in adults, its metabolic effects last for up to 72 hours. No data are available on the transfer of dexamethasone into human milk. It is likely similar to that of prednisone, which is extremely low. Doses of prednisone as high as 120 mg fail to produce clinically relevant milk levels. This product is commonly used in pediatrics for treating immune syndromes such as arthritis and, particularly, acute onset asthma or other bronchoconstrictive diseases. It is not likely that the amount in milk would produce clinical effects unless used in high doses over prolonged periods.

- **GONADORELIN ACETATE**   (*Lutrepulse*)
  - AAP = Not reviewed
  - LRC = L3
  - RID =
  - Pregnancy = B
  - Comment: Gonadorelin is used for the induction of ovulation in anovulatory women with primary hypothalamic amenorrhea. Gonadorelin is a small decapeptide identical to the physiologic GnRH secreted by the hypothalamus, which stimulates the pituitary release of luteinizing hormone (LH) and to a lesser degree follicle stimulating hormone (FSH). LH and FSH subsequently stimulate the ovary to produce follicles. Gonadorelin plasma half-life is very brief (<2-4 minutes), and it is primarily distributed to the plasma only. Gonadorelin has been detected in human breastmilk at concentrations of 0.1 to 3 ng/mL (adult dose = 20-100 μg), although its oral bioavailability in the infant would be minimal to none.

- **CHORIONIC GONADOTROPIN**   (*A.P.L., Chorex-5, Profasi, Gonic, Pregnyl, Novarel*)
  - AAP = Not reviewed
  - LRC = L3
  - RID =
  - Pregnancy = X
  - Comment: Human chorionic gonadotropin (HCG) is a large polypeptide hormone produced by the human placenta with functions similar to luteinizing hormone (LH). Its function is to stimulate the corpus luteum of the ovary to produce progesterone, thus sustaining pregnancy. During pregnancy, HCG secreted by the placenta maintains the corpus luteum, supporting estrogen and progesterone secretion, and preventing menstruation. It is used for multiple purposes, including pediatric cryptorchidism, male hypogonadism, and ovulatory failure. HCG has no known effect on fat mobilization, appetite, sense of hunger, or body fat distribution. HCG has NOT been found to be effective in treatment of obesity. Due to the large molecular weight (47,000) of HCG, it would be extremely unlikely to penetrate into human milk. Further, it would not be orally bioavailable due to

destruction in the GI tract. Choriogonadotropin alfa (Ovidrel) is a biosynthetic form of the human chorionic gonadotropin.

- LETROZOLE   (*Femara*)
  - ◦ AAP = Not reviewed
  - ◦ LRC = L4
  - ◦ RID =
  - ◦ Pregnancy = D
  - ◦ Comment: Letrozole is an aromatase inhibitor of estrogen synthesis and is used to treat estrogen-receptor positive breast cancer and other syndromes. No data are available on its transfer to human milk, but the levels are probably low. However, it has a very long half-life, which is concerning in a breastfed infant and could lead to higher plasma levels over time. Therefore, the transfer of small amounts of this agent to an infant could seriously impair bone growth or sexual development, and for this reason, it is probably somewhat hazardous to use in a breastfeeding mother.

- MENOTROPINS   (*Pergonal, Humegon, Repronex*)
  - ◦ AAP = Not reviewed
  - ◦ LRC = L3
  - ◦ RID =
  - ◦ Pregnancy = X
  - ◦ Comment: Menotropins is a purified preparation of gonadotropins hormones extracted from the urine of postmenopausal women. It is a biologically standardized form containing equal activity of follicle stimulating hormone (FSH) and luteinizing hormone (LH). Menotropins and human chorionic gonadotropins (see chorionic gonadotropins) are given sequentially to induce ovulation in the anovulatory female. FSH and LH are large molecular weight peptides and would not likely penetrate into human milk. Further, they are unstable in the GI tract, and their oral bioavailability would be minimal to zero, even in an infant.

- METFORMIN   (*Glucophage, Glucovance*)
  - ◦ AAP = Not reviewed
  - ◦ LRC = L1
  - ◦ RID = 0.3-0.7%
  - ◦ Pregnancy = B
  - ◦ Comment: Metformin belongs to the biguanide family and is used to reduce glucose levels in non-insulin dependent diabetics. Oral bioavailability is only 50%. In a study of seven women taking metformin (median dose 1500 mg/d), the mean milk-to-plasma ratio (AUC) for metformin was 0.35. The mean average concentration in milk over the dose interval was 0.27 mg/L. The absolute infant dose averaged 0.04 mg/kg/d, and the mean relative infant dose was 0.28%. Metformin was present in very low or undetectable concentrations in the plasma of four of the infants who were studied. No health problems were found in the six infants who were evaluated. In another study of five subjects, the median milk/plasma ratio (AUC) for metformin was 0.47. The median calculated infant dose was 0.2% of the weight-adjusted maternal dose. None of the infants exposed to their mothers' milk had detectable levels of metformin in their plasma, nor were any side effects noted. In a recent study of five women consuming an average dose of 500 mg twice daily, the mean peak

and trough metformin concentrations in breastmilk were 0.42 mg/L (range 0.38-0.46 mg/L) and 0.39 mg/L (range 0.31-0.52 mg/L), respectively. The average milk/serum ratio was 0.63 (range 0.36-1.00), and the estimated relative infant dose was 0.65% (range 0.43-1.08%). Blood glucose concentrations in three infants were normal, ranging from 47-77 mg/dL. The mothers reported no side effects were noted in the breastfed infants.

Metformin is also used to treat polycystic ovary syndrome. In one study of 61 nursing infants whose mothers were taking a median of 2.55 g/day throughout pregnancy and lactation, the growth, motor, and social development of the infants was recorded to be normal. The authors concluded that metformin was safe and effective during lactation in the first six months of an infant's life.

- TAMOXIFEN   (*Nolvadex*)
  - AAP = Not reviewed
  - LRC = L5
  - RID =
  - Pregnancy = D
  - Comment: Tamoxifen is a nonsteroidal antiestrogen. Tamoxifen is metabolized by the liver and has an elimination half-life of greater than seven days (range 3-21 days). It is well absorbed orally, and the highest tissue concentrations are in the liver (60 fold). It is 99% protein bound and normally reduces plasma prolactin levels significantly (66% after three months). At present, there are no data on its transfer into breastmilk; however, it has been shown to inhibit lactation early postpartum in several studies. In one study, doses of 10-30 mg twice daily early postpartum completely inhibited postpartum engorgement and lactation. In a second study, tamoxifen doses of 10 mg four times daily significantly reduced serum prolactin and inhibited milk production as well. We do not know the effect of tamoxifen on established milk production. This product has a very long half-life, and the active metabolite is concentrated in the plasma (two fold). This drug has all the characteristics that would suggest a concentrating mechanism in breastfed infants over time. Its prominent effect on reducing prolactin levels will inhibit early lactation and may ultimately inhibit established lactation. In this instance, the significant risks to the infant from exposure to tamoxifen probably outweigh the benefits of breastfeeding. Mothers receiving tamoxifen should not breastfeed until we know more about the levels transferred into milk and the plasma/tissue levels found in breastfed infants.

Clinical Tips

Progesterone is commonly used in some infertile patients to produce a secretory state of the endometrium. In most breastfeeding patients, excess progesterone has not been found to suppress lactation nor penetrate to the infant in clinically relevant doses. Estrogens, however, particularly when used early postpartum, can suppress lactation significantly and should be avoided if possible. In some patients, clomiphene (Clomid, Serophene) is the first-line drug of choice for chronic anovulation, luteal phase defects, and unexplained infertility in patients with normal estrogen levels. When used early in lactation, clomiphene has been documented to completely suppress lactation. However, when used several months postpartum, it is believed to have minimal or no effect on milk production. Gonadorelin (Lutrepulse) is used for the induction of ovulation in anovulatory women with primary hypothalamic amenorrhea. Gonadorelin is a small decapeptide identical to the physiologic GnRH secreted by the hypothalamus which stimulates the pituitary release of luteinizing hormone (LH) and to a lesser degree follicle-stimulating hormone (FSH). Gonadorelin has been detected in human breastmilk at concentrations of 0.1 to 3 nanogram/mL (adult dose = 20-100 micrograms), although its oral bioavailability in the infant would be minimal to none. Its ability to suppress lactation is unknown, but unlikely. Menotropins

(Pergonal, Humegon) is a purified mix of urinary gonadotropins from postmenopausal women and produces FSH and LH activity. FSH and LH are large molecular weight proteins and would not penetrate milk, nor likely suppress milk production.

In some infertile patients with hyperprolactinemia, bromocriptine and, more recently, cabergoline (Dostinex) have been used to suppress plasma prolactin levels. While these agents are generally contraindicated in breastfeeding women due to the possibility of suppressing prolactin, they could be safely used by women with prolactin levels greatly exceeding those common in breastfeeding women. Indeed, titrating the dose accordingly to attain levels approximating 200 ng/mL would both reduce symptoms of exgreme hyperprolactinemia and permit successful breastfeeding.

Suggested Reading

Vaccination guidelines for female infertility patients. (2008). *Fertil Steril, 90*(5 Suppl), S169-171.

Farquhar, C. (2009). Do uterine fibroids cause infertility and should they be removed to increase fertility? *BMJ, 338*, b126.

Lamar, C. A., & DeCherney, A. H. (2009). Fertility preservation: state of the science and future research directions. *Fertil Steril, 91*(2), 316-319.

Matzuk, M. M., & Lamb, D. J. (2008). The biology of infertility: research advances and clinical challenges. *Nat Med, 14*(11), 1197-1213.

Practice Committee of American Society for Reproductive Medicine. (2008). Obesity and reproduction: an educational bulletin. *Fertil Steril, 90*(5 Suppl), S21-29.

Thorogood, M., Seed, M., & De Mott, K. (2009). Management of fertility in women with familial hypercholesterolaemia: summary of NICE guidance. *BJOG, 116*(4), 478-479.

Insomnia

Principles of Therapy

Insomnia is a frequent complaint for women in general, but is a normal consideration for the postpartum woman. Normal breastfeeding schedules in the postpartum period include every three hours feedings. Feeding intervals longer than six hours may be associated with an adverse impact on milk supply. In women with poor milk supply, intervals of six hours or more between feedings should be discouraged.

Despite the expected frequent schedules in the early postpartum period, some women may continue breastfeeding for longer durations, and difficulty with persistent insomnia may occur with older infants that have more extended sleep periods. When evaluating insomnia, a detailed history evaluating sleep habits should be obtained. Is the difficulty due to sleep latency (difficulty falling asleep) or frequent or early morning awakening? Sleep schedules, sleep environment, and consumption of caffeine and alcohol should be explored. Healthy sleep habits should be discussed (does the patient read, work, or watch television in bed). Daytime napping should be avoided. Evaluation for sleep apnea should also be explored, especially in patients with PCOS and obesity. Patients should also be asked about symptoms of restless leg syndrome and symptoms which would be suggestive of depression.

Treatment will vary depending on existence of any coexisting conditions (such as sleep apnea and depression). Behavioral therapy, relaxation therapy, or education about healthy sleep habits may be useful.

Treatment

- Cognitive behavioral therapy may be successful. Components include: sleep hygiene education, relaxation therapy, cognitive therapy, stimulus control, sleep restriction.

- Evaluate for coexisting conditions and treat appropriately: sleep apnea, depression, restless leg syndrome.

- Brief courses of medication, but these may have risks associated with sedation and may adversely affect ability to care for infant. (Tricyclic antidepressants, non-tricyclic antidepressants, alpha-2 antagonists, nonbenzodiazepine receptor agonists, other sedative hypnotics, selective melatonin agonists.)

- Long term use of medications should be strictly avoided as patients often become dependent on these agents for sleep.

Medications

- ALPRAZOLAM   (*Xanax*)
    - AAP = Drugs whose effect on nursing infants is unknown but may be of concern

- LRC = L3
- RID = 8.5%
- Pregnancy = D
- Comment: Alprazolam is a prototypic benzodiazepine drug similar to Valium, but is now preferred in many instances because of its shorter half-life. In a study of eight women who received a single oral dose of 0.5 mg, the peak alprazolam level in milk was 3.7 μg/L, which occurred at 1.1 hours; the observed milk/serum ratio (using AUC method) was 0.36. The neonatal dose of alprazolam in breastmilk is low. The author estimates the average between 0.3 to 5 μg/kg per day. While the infants in this study did not breastfeed, these doses would probably be too low to induce a clinical effect.

  In a brief letter, Anderson reports that the manufacturer is aware of withdrawal symptoms in infants following exposure in utero and via breastmilk. In a mother who received 0.5 mg two to three times daily (PO) during pregnancy, a neonatal withdrawal syndrome was evident in the breastfed infant the first week postpartum. These data suggests that the amount of alprazolam in breastmilk is insufficient to prevent a withdrawal syndrome following prenatal exposure. In another case of infant exposure solely via breastmilk, the mother took alprazolam (dosage unspecified) for nine months while breastfeeding and withdrew herself from the medication over a three week period. The mother reported withdrawal symptoms in the infant including irritability, crying, and sleep disturbances.

  The benzodiazepine family, as a rule, are not ideal for breastfeeding mothers due to relatively long half-lives and the development of dependence. However, it is apparent that the shorter-acting benzodiazepines are safest during lactation, provided their use is short-term or intermittent, low dose, and after the first week of life.

- AMITRIPTYLINE (*Elavil, Endep*)
  - AAP = Drugs whose effect on nursing infants is unknown but may be of concern
  - LRC = L2
  - RID = 1.9-2.8%
  - Pregnancy = C
  - Comment: Amitriptyline and its active metabolite, nortriptyline, are secreted into breastmilk in small amounts. In one report of a mother taking 100 mg/day of amitriptyline, milk levels of amitriptyline and nortriptyline (active metabolite) averaged 143 μg/L and 55.5 μg/L, respectively; maternal serum levels averaged 112 μg/L and 72.5 μg/L, respectively. No drug was detected in the infant's serum. From these data, an infant would consume approximately 21.5 μg/kg/day, a dose that is unlikely to be clinically relevant.

    In another study following a maternal dose of 25 mg/day, the amitriptyline and nortriptyline (active metabolite) levels in milk were 30 μg/L and <30 μg/L, respectively. In the same study when the dosage was 75 mg/day, milk levels of amitriptyline and nortriptyline averaged 88 μg/L and 69 μg/L, respectively. Both drugs were essentially undetectable in the infant's serum. Therefore, the authors estimated that a nursing infant would receive less than 0.1 mg/day.

    In another mother taking 175 mg/day, amitriptyline levels in the mother's milk were the same as in her serum on day one (24-27 μg/mL), but milk levels decreased to 54% of the serum concentration on days 2 to 26. Milk concentrations of nortriptyline were 74% of that in the mother's serum (87 ng/mL). Thus the authors reported the absolute infant dose as 35 μg/kg, 80 times lower than the mother's dose. Neither compound could be detected in the infant's serum on day 26, nor were there any signs of sedation or other adverse effects.

- ESZOPICLONE (*Lunesta*)
  - AAP = Not reviewed
  - LRC = L3
  - RID =
  - Pregnancy = C
  - Comment: Eszopiclone is a non-benzodiazepine hypnotic-sedative drug, although they both interact at the same GABA receptor. Used as a nighttime sedative, its transfer into human milk has not yet been reported. However, a derivative which is virtually identical, Zopiclone, has been studied (see zopiclone) and 1.5% of the maternal dose transferred into milk. Therefore, due to the structural similarly, one should expect about 1.5% of eszopiclone to transfer into human milk as well. The use of eszopiclone in mothers with premature infants or newborns, and particularly those with infants subject to apnea, should be avoided. Use in healthy older infants is probably less risky.

- MIRTAZAPINE (*Remeron*)
  - AAP = Not reviewed
  - LRC = L3
  - RID = 1.6-6.3%
  - Pregnancy = C
  - Comment: Mirtazapine is a unique antidepressant structurally dissimilar to the SSRIs, tricyclics, or the monoamine oxidase inhibitors. Mirtazapine has little or no serotonergic-like side effects, fewer anticholinergic side effects than amitriptyline, produces less sexual dysfunction, and has not demonstrated cardiotoxic or seizure potential in a limited number of overdose cases.

    In a study of three women who received 45, 60, and 45 mg/day mirtazapine, the average concentration (AUC) in milk was 77, 75, and 47 μg/L, respectively. The absolute infant dose was 10, 11.3, and 7.1 μg/kg/d, respectively. The relative infant dose was 1.9%, 1.1%, and 1.5% of the weight-normalized maternal dose, respectively. Mirtazapine was below the limit of quantitation in two of the infants and only 1.5 ng/mL in the third infant. The infants were meeting all developmental milestones and were without side effects.

    Another study of eight women taking an average of 38 mg/day showed average milk concentrations of 53 μg/L and 13 μg/L of mirtazapine and its metabolite, respectively. The average absolute infant dose was 495 μg/kg/day, indicating a relative infant dose of 1.9%. The authors of this study suggest that breastfeeding is safe during mirtazapine therapy.

    In another mother who took 22.5 mg/day, milk levels were 130 μg/L four hours after dosing and 61 μg/L ten hours after the dose (foremilk). This suggests the relative infant dose was 3.9-4.4% and 1.8-2.7%, respectively of the weight-adjusted maternal dose at these two times. At 12.5 hours postdose, infant plasma levels were undetectable.

- NEFAZODONE HCL (*Serzone*)
  - AAP = Not reviewed
  - LRC = L4
  - RID = 1.2%
  - Pregnancy = C

- Comment: Nefazodone is an antidepressant similar to trazodone, but structurally dissimilar from the other serotonin reuptake inhibitors. It is rapidly metabolized to three partially active metabolites that have significantly longer half-lives (1.5 to 18 hours).

  In a study of one patient receiving 200 mg in the morning and 100 mg at night, the infant at nine weeks of age (2.1 kg) was admitted for drowsiness, lethargy, failure to thrive, and poor temperature control. The infant was born premature at 27 weeks. The maximum milk concentration of nefazodone was 358 μg/L, while the maternal plasma C_{max} was 1270 μg/L. The concentration of the metabolites was reported to be 83 μg/L for triazoledione, 32 μg/L for HO-Nefazodone, and 18 μg/L for m-Chlorophenylpiperazine. The relative infant dose was calculated to be 0.45% of the weight-adjusted maternal dose. The AUC milk/plasma ratio ranged from 0.02 to 0.27. Unfortunately, no infant plasma samples were taken for analysis.

  Dodd et al. recently reported a M/P ratio of only 0.1 for nefazodone in a patient receiving 200 mg twice daily. This is approximately one-third of the M/P ratio (0.27) reported by Yapp. However, the Yapp study used AUC data over many points and is probably a more accurate reflection of nefazodone transfer into milk during the day.

  This medication should probably not be used in breastfeeding mothers with young infants, premature infants, infants subject to apnea, or other weakened infants.

- RAMELTEON   *(Rozerem)*
  - AAP = Not reviewed
  - LRC = L3
  - RID =
  - Pregnancy = C
  - Comment: Used for insomnia, Ramelteon is a melatonin receptor agonist, and assists in the synchronization of the circadian rhythm and induces sleep. Unlike the benzodiazepines, ramelteon does not bind to the GABA receptors. There have been no studies of levels of ramelteon in human milk. However, probable small amount in milk would only be 1.8% bioavailable. It is unlikely to sedate an infant.

- TEMAZEPAM   *(Restoril)*
  - AAP = Drugs whose effect on nursing infants is unknown but may be of concern
  - LRC = L3
  - RID =
  - Pregnancy = X
  - Comment: Temazepam is a short acting benzodiazepine that belongs to the Valium family and is primarily used as a nighttime sedative. In one study, the milk/plasma ratio varied from <0.09 to <0.63 (mean = 0.18). Temazepam is relatively water soluble and, therefore, partitions poorly into breastmilk. Levels of temazepam were undetectable in the infants studied, although these studies were carried out 15 hours post-dose. Although the study shows low neonatal exposure to temazepam via breastmilk, the infant should be monitored carefully for sleepiness and poor feeding.

- TRAZODONE   *(Desyrel)*
  - AAP = Drugs whose effect on nursing infants is unknown but may be of concern
  - LRC = L2

- ◦ RID = 2.8%
- ◦ Pregnancy = C
- ◦ Comment: Trazodone is an antidepressant whose structure is dissimilar to the tricyclics and to the other antidepressants. In six mothers who received a single 50 mg dose, the milk/plasma ratio averaged 0.14. Peak milk concentrations occurred at two hours and were approximately 110 µg/L (taken from graph) and declined rapidly thereafter. On a weight basis, an adult would receive 0.77 mg/kg whereas a breastfeeding infant, using these data, would consume only 0.005 mg/kg. The authors estimate that about 0.6% of the maternal dose was ingested by the infant over 24 hours.

- ZOLPIDEM TARTRATE   (*Ambien, Ambien CR*)
  - ◦ AAP = Maternal Medication Usually Compatible with Breastfeeding
  - ◦ LRC = L3
  - ◦ RID = 4.7-19.1%
  - ◦ Pregnancy = C
  - ◦ Comment: Zolpidem, although not a benzodiazepine, interacts with the same GABA-BZ receptor site and shares some of the same pharmacologic effects of the benzodiazepine (Valium) family. In a study of five lactating mothers receiving 20 mg daily, the maximum plasma concentration occurred between 1.75 and 3.75 hours and ranged from 90 to 364 µg/L. The authors suggest that the amount of zolpidem recovered in breastmilk three hours after administration ranged between 0.76 and 3.88 µg or 0.004 to 0.019% of the total dose administered. Breastmilk clearance of zolpidem is very rapid and none was detectable (below 0.5 ng/mL) by four to five hours postdose.

    One case of infant sedation and poor appetite related to zolpidem use has been reported following the nightly use of sertraline (100mg) and 10 mg Zolpidem. Upon discontinuation of zolpidem, the infant regained appetite and became more alert.

Clinical Tips

The first and most important treatment regimen is to advise good sleep hygiene. Numerous sources are available for these data. Avoid medications which interfere with sleep, such as caffeine, amphetamines, methylphenidate, and other psychotherapeutic stimulants. Regular and moderate exercise is clearly beneficial.

The use of sedative or hypnotic medications in breastfeeding mothers should be approached with great caution and indication for using these products largely depends of the condition of the breastfed infant. Most of these preparations will pass to some degree into human milk, due to their lipophilicity and neurological activity. Thus all infants may get small doses. The ability of the infant to handle these doses is part of the clinical evaluation. Infants subject to apnea or breathing difficulties should probably not be exposed to mother's milk which contain sedative drugs. Families with reported sudden infant deaths should avoid these medications at all times. Premature or unstable infants may be at higher risk from exposure to these medications. On the other hand, older full term stable infants can probably easily metabolize and adapt to minor exposure to these medications. Thus the decision to use hypnotic sedatives largely depends on the infant's ability to handle the small exposure.

The shorter half-life benzodiazepines, because they suppress the respiratory center less, are probably preferred and include alprazolam and temazepam. Milk levels of these two have been reported and are low. Nefazodone should be avoided due to reports of drowsiness, lethargy, failure to thrive, and poor temperature control in one infant. In patients subject to some depression, mirtazapine may be suitable as a nighttime sedative, as it is an effective antidepressant as well. In patients with chronic pain or migraine headaches, amitriptyline at bedtime may be suitable, as it is both a good sedative and suppresses chronic pain symptoms as well.

Zolpidem levels in milk have been reported to be low. However, in one case an infant was sedated following the nightly use of this product. In mothers with older, more stable infants, it might be suitable. Although we do not have reported milk levels for ramelteon, its poor oral bioavailability would probably limit its effect in a breastfeeding infant. It is probably compatible with breastfeeding.

Contrary to public opinion, melatonin has little or no effect on insomnia in adults. Some evidence suggests it is modestly effective in children. It should probably not be used in breastfeeding mothers at this time.

Suggested Reading

1: Howland RH.(2009). Prescribing psychotropic medications during pregnancy and lactation: principles and guidelines. *J Psychosoc Nurs Ment Health Serv. 47*(5):19-23. Review.

2: Mortola J.F. (1989). The use of psychotropic agents in pregnancy and lactation. *Psychiatr Clin North Am. 12*(1):69-87. Review.

3: Allison S.K. (2004). Psychotropic medication in pregnancy: ethical aspects and clinical management. *J Perinat Neonatal Nurs. 18*(3):194-205. Review.

Inflammatory Bowel Disease

Principles of Therapy

The term 'chronic idiopathic inflammatory bowel disease' includes ulcerative colitis (UC) and Crohn's disease. Ulcerative colitis is a chronic, recurrent disease characterized by mucosal inflammation of the colon only. Ulcerative colitis invariably involves the rectum and proximalpart or all of the colon. Unlike UC, Crohn's disease is a chronic, recurrent transmural inflammatory condition involving any segment of the GI tract from the mouth to anus, the terminal ileum being the most common site. Although these syndromes vary significantly in their presentation, their pharmacotherapy is quite similar and includes the use of aminosalicylates(5-ASA), corticosteroids, immunosuppressants, antibiotics, antidiarrheals, and opioid analgesics.

Treatment

- Crohn's disease: corticosteroids and aminosalicylates effective for acute attacks, infliximab and tacrolimus often effective for severe or refractory cases. 5-ASA compounds are becoming less popular as they do not seem to maintain remission as well as other products.

- Sulfasalazine and olsalazine are less active in Crohn's disease since they must be activated by colonic bacteria. Mesalamine is no longer preferred for maintenance of remission, although this does seem to facilitate tapering of steroid doses. Large doses (4 gm/day) are now recommended in some patients.

- Ulcerative colitis: sulfasalazine or other salicylates, corticosteroids, azathriopine.

Medications

- AZATHIOPRINE   (*Imuran*)
    - AAP = Not reviewed
    - LRC = L3
    - RID = 0.25%
    - Pregnancy = D
    - Comment: Azathioprine is a powerful immunosuppressive agent that is metabolized to 6-Mercaptopurine (6-MP). In two mothers receiving 75 mg azathioprine, the concentration of 6-Mercaptopurine in milk varied from 3.5-4.5 µg/L in one mother and 18 µg/L in the second mother. Both levels were peak milk concentrations at two hours following the dose. The authors conclude that these levels would be too low to produce clinical effects in a breastfed infant. Using these data for 6-MP, an infant would absorb only 0.1% of the weight-adjusted maternal dose, which is probably too low to produce adverse effects in a breastfeeding infant. Plasma levels in treated patients is maintained at 50 ng/mL or higher. One infant continued to breastfeed during therapy and

displayed no immunosuppressive effects. Numerous other studies in more than 18 mothers suggest that azathioprine levels in milk are low. Levels in infants were low to undetectable.

- BUDESONIDE   (*Entocort EC*)
  - AAP = Not reviewed
  - LRC = L1
  - RID = 0.3%
  - Pregnancy = C
  - Comment: Budesonide is a potent corticosteroid used intranasally for allergic rhinitis, inhaled for asthma, and in capsule form for Crohn's disease. Once absorbed systemically, budesonide is a weak systemic steroid and should not be used to replace other steroids. Via inhalation, budesonid levels in milk are exceedingly low, with an RID of < 0.3%. The new oral formulation of budesonide (Entocort EC) is used for Crohn's disease and is placed in special granules that pass the stomach before releasing the drug in controlled-release manner in the duodenum. Portal plasma budesonide has a high clearance rate due to high uptake by the liver. Plasma levels are low and brief, and its ability to suppress normal cortisol levels is about half that of prednisone. Because of its high first-pass clearance, it is rather unlikely to produce high or even measurable levels in milk or be orally bioavailable to a significant degree in breastfeeding infants.

- BALSALAZIDE DISODIUM   (*Colazal*)
  - AAP = Not reviewed
  - LRC = L3
  - RID =
  - Pregnancy = B
  - Comment: Balsalazide is a prodrug that is metabolized to mesalamine (5-aminosalicylic acid). Balsalazide is delivered intact to the colon where it is cleaved by bacterial enzymes to release the active drug mesalamine. The oral absorption of balsalazide is very low. Less than 1% of the parent drug is recovered in the urine. Because it is metabolized to mesalamine, see mesalamine for breastmilk concentrations.

- INFLIXIMAB   (*Remicade*)
  - AAP = Not reviewed
  - LRC = L2
  - RID =
  - Pregnancy = B
  - Comment: Infliximab is a monoclonal antibody to tumor necrosis factor-alpha (TNF-alpha) used to treat Crohn's disease and rheumatoid arthritis. Infliximab is a very large molecular weight antibody and is largely retained in the vascular system. In multiple studies, none was detectable in human milk. Infliximab is probably too large to enter milk in clinically measurable amounts. It would not be orally bioavailable.

- MESALAMINE   (*Asacol, Pentasa, Rowasa, Canasa, Colazal, Lialda*)
  - AAP = Should be given to nursing mothers with caution
  - LRC = L3

- ○ RID = 0.1-8.8%
- ○ Pregnancy = B
- ○ Comment: Mesalamine or Mesalazine (UK) is an anti-inflammatory agent used in ulcerative colitis. Although it contains 5-aminosalicylic acid (5-ASA), the mechanism of action is unknown. Some 5-aminosalicylic acid can be converted into salicylic acid and absorbed, but the amount is very small. Acetyl-5-aminosalicyclic (Acetyl-5-ASA) acid is the common metabolite and has been found in breastmilk. The effect of mesalamine is primarily local on the mucosa of the colon itself. Mesalamine is poorly absorbed from the GI tract. Only 20-30% of a dose is absorbed orally. In one patient receiving 500 mg mesalamine orally three times daily, the concentration of 5-ASA in breastmilk was 0.11 mg/L, and the Acetyl-5-ASA metabolite was 12.4 mg/L of milk. Using these data, the weight-adjusted relative infant dose would be 8.7%. In another patient receiving 1000 mg PO three times daily, milk levels of 5 aminosalicylic acid following seven and 11 days of treatment and five hours following the dose were both 0.1 mg/L, and the milk/plasma ratios were 0.07 and 0.09. Observe for GI changes, such as watery diarrhea in breastfed infants.

- • OLSALAZINE   (*Dipentum*)
  - ○ AAP = Not reviewed
  - ○ LRC = L3
  - ○ RID = 0.9%
  - ○ Pregnancy = C
  - ○ Comment: Olsalazine is converted to 5-aminosalicylic acid (mesalamine:5-ASA) in the gut, which has anti-inflammatory activity in ulcerative colitis. After oral administration, only 2.4% is systemically absorbed, while the majority is metabolized in the GI tract to 5-ASA. 5-ASA is slowly and poorly absorbed. Plasma levels are exceedingly small (1.6-6.2 mmol/L), the half-life very short, and protein binding is very high. In one study of a mother who received a single 500 mg dose of olsalazine, acetylated-5-ASA achieved concentrations of 0.6, 0.86, and 1.24 μmol/L in breastmilk at 10, 14, and 24 hours, respectively. Olsalazine, olsalazine-S, and 5-ASA were undetectable in breastmilk. While clinically significant levels in milk are remote, infants should be closely monitored for gastric changes, such as diarrhea.

- • PREDNISONE-PREDNISOLONE   (*Prednisone, Prednisolone*)
  - ○ AAP = Maternal Medication Usually Compatible with Breastfeeding
  - ○ LRC = L2
  - ○ RID = 1.8-5.3%
  - ○ Pregnancy = C
  - ○ Comment: Small amounts of most corticosteroids are secreted into breastmilk. Following a 10 mg oral dose of prednisone, peak milk levels of prednisolone and prednisone were 1.6 μg/L and 2.67 μg/L, respectively. In a group of ten women who received 10-80 mg/d prednisolone, the milk levels were only 5-25% of the maternal serum levels. In one patient who received 80 mg/day prednisolone, the Cmax at one hour was 317 μg/L. The AUC average milk concentration in this mother was 156 μg/L over six hours. This is significantly less than 2% of the weight-normalized maternal dose. Because this last estimate was only determined over six hours and this dose was administered once each 24 hours, the total daily estimate would be much less than the 2% estimate. In another study of a single patient who received 120 mg prednisone/day, the total combined

steroid levels (prednisone + prednisolone) peaked at two hours. The peak level of combined steroid was 627 µg/L. Assuming the infant received 120 mL of milk every four hours, the total possible ingestion would only be 47 µg/day.

In a group of seven women who received radioactive labeled prednisolone 5 mg, the total recovery per liter of milk during the 48 hours after the dose was 0.14%. With high doses (>40 mg/day), particularly for long periods, steroids could potentially produce problems in infant growth and development, although we have absolutely no data in this area or know which doses would pose problems. Brief applications of high dose steroids are probably not contraindicated as the overall exposure is low. With prolonged high dose therapy, the infant should be closely monitored for growth and development.

- SULFASALAZINE (*Azulfidine*)
  - AAP = Drugs associated with significant side effects and should be given with caution
  - LRC = L3
  - RID = 0.3-1.1%
  - Pregnancy = B
  - Comment: Sulfasalazine is a conjugate of sulfapyridine and 5-Aminosalicylic acid and is used as an anti-inflammatory for ulcerative colitis. Only one-third of the dose is absorbed by the mother. Most stays in the GI tract. Secretion of 5-aminosalicylic acid (active compound) and its inactive metabolite (acetyl -5-ASA) into human milk is very low. In one study of 12 women receiving 1 to 2 grams/day of sulfasalazine, the amount of sulfasalazine in milk in patients receiving 1 gm/day was far less than 1 mg/L and approximately 0.5 to 2 mg/L in those receiving 2 gm/day. In this study, small milk levels were found in only two women. It was estimated by the authors that breastfed infants would receive approximately 0.3 mg/kg/day of sulfapyridine. This very small amount may be regarded as negligible in considering kernicterus because sulfapyridine and sulfadiazine are known to have a poor bilirubin-displacing capacity. Few, if any, adverse effects have been observed in most nursing infants. However, there has been one reported case of toxicity, which may have been an idiosyncratic allergic response. Use with some caution. Mesalamine or other products are probably safer.

- TACROLIMUS (*Prograf, Protopic*)
  - AAP = Not reviewed
  - LRC = L3
  - RID = 0.1-0.5%
  - Pregnancy = C
  - Comment: Tacrolimus is an immunosuppressant formerly known as SK506. It is used to reduce rejection of transplanted organs, including liver and kidney. In one report of 21 mothers who received tacrolimus while pregnant, milk concentrations in colostrum averaged 0.79 ng/mL and varied from 0.3 to 1.9 ng/mL. Maternal doses (PO) ranged from 9.8 to 10.3 mg/day. Milk/blood ratio averaged 0.54. Using these data and an average daily milk intake of 150 mL/kg, the average dose to the infant per day via milk would be <0.1 µg/kg/day. Because the oral bioavailability is poor (<32%), an infant would likely ingest less than 100 ng/kg/day. The usual pediatric dose (PO) for preventing rejection varies from 0.15 to 0.20 mg/kg/day (equivalent to 150,000-200,000 nanograms/kg/day).

In a 32-year-old woman who had taken tacrolimus 0.1 mg/kg/d throughout pregnancy, samples were manually expressed at 0 (trough), 1, 6, 9, 11, and 12 hours after the morning dose. Using AUC data, the mean milk concentration was calculated to be 0.429 ng/mL. From these measurements, the exclusively breastfed infant would ingest, on average, 0.06 µg/kg/d, which corresponds to 0.06% of the mother's weight-normalized dose. Given the low oral bioavailability of tacrolimus, the maximum amount the baby would receive is 0.02% of the mother's weight-adjusted dose. At 2.5 months of age, the infant was developing well, both physically and neurologically.

Clinical Tips

Crohn's Disease: Initial therapy of Crohn's disease is generally with the 5-aminosalicylic acid products (mesalamine), but only those that are specifically activated in the small intestine and do not require colonic bacteria for activation. Mesalamine (5-ASA) is primarily released in the small intestine and is useful for Crohn's disease in that segment of the GI tract. Oral budesonide (Entocort EC), while more effective than mesalamine, has not been found better than conventional oral steroids in producing remission. Azathioprine and its active metabolite, 6-mercaptopurine, have in numerous studies been found effective for inducing remission in Crohn's disease. Myelotoxicity has been found to occur in only about 3% of adult patients treated with azathioprine per year of treatment. Methotrexate, while quite active, has not been found to be more effective than azathioprine. Methotrexate penetrates milk at low levels (2.6 µg/L), but its affinity for gastric mucosa in infants is high and concerning. It is probably not a suitable choice for breastfeeding women long-term.

Infliximab and other TNF inhibitors are profoundly effective in most patients with significant rates of remission, although they may not last longer than a year or more. Infliximab levels in milk are undetectable, and thus it should be a suitable choice for breastfeeding mothers. Other TNF inhibitors include adalimubab (Humira) and certolizumab (Cimzia). While not studied in breastfeeding mothers, their similar IgG structure would suggest their milk levels should be exceedingly low, just as with infliximab. Further, it is unlikely they would be orally bioavailable in the infant.

Ulcerative Colitis: Preparations of 5-ASA are formulated to release the drug at specific sites in the GI tract to intensify efficacy. 5-ASA is a topical agent that has a variety of anti-inflammatory effects. It is used during the active phase of inflammation and during disease inactivity to maintain remission. Newer 5-ASA preparations are generally preferred over sulfasalazine.

Sulfasalazine is bio-converted by bacterial azoreductases in the colon to 5-ASA and sulfapyridine. While the initial dose is 500 mg twice daily, the dose is increased until therapeutic effects are produced, usually around 4-6 grams per day. Sulfasalazine has been associated with male infertility. Olsalazine is converted to two molecules of 5-ASA. Balsalazide (6.75 gm/day) is cleaved by colonic bacteria to deliver mesalamine (2.4 gm/day) to the colon. 5-ASA is virtually unabsorbed, although high doses may induce (although remote) watery diarrhea in some breastfed infants. Recently, the doses of these various preparations have increased up to approximately 6 grams per day. We do not have data in breastfeeding women at these doses. At these doses, caution should be used in breastfeeding mothers. Perhaps salicylate levels should be periodically done in the infant.

Prednisone, both oral and rectal, is a common component of therapy. Numerous studies show that oral prednisone penetrates milk poorly. Rather high doses (40-60 mg/day) do not apparently produce significant levels in milk. However, some caution is due and close monitoring of the infant's growth rate is warranted. With severe UC and Crohn's disease, immunosuppressants may be warranted, particularly 6-MP. We have numerous studies on the use of azathioprine in breastfeeding mothers. Thus far, levels in milk are low, and no complications have been reported. The use of methotrexate in breastfeeding mothers is risky and questionable. Some studies question the efficacy of methotrexate in UC anyway, and it is not a suitable medication to use in breastfeeding women.

In some patients, infliximab (Remicade) has proven effective for moderate to severe ulcerative colitis and is as effective as steroid treatments. Infliximab would be compatible with breastfeeding, as levels have been determined in milk and are low, and it is unabsorbed orally.

Probiotics may in some cases be as effective as mesalamine. Lactobacillus GG has been documented to maintain remission equivalent to mesalamine.

Oral tacrolimus used briefly and at a dose of 0.025 mg/kg (plasma levels= 10-15 ng/mL) was highly effective. It is probably compatible with breastfeeding, due to low milk levels and lower oral bioavailability in the infant.

Suggested Reading

Collins, P., & Rhodes, J. (2006). Ulcerative colitis: diagnosis and management. *BMJ, 333*(7563), 340-343.

Cullen, G., Keegan, D., Mulcahy, H. E., & O'Donoghue, D. P. (2009). A 5-year prospective observational study of the outcomes of international treatment guidelines for Crohn's disease. *Clin Gastroenterol Hepatol, 7*(3), 323-328; quiz 252.

Ferguson, C. B., Mahsud-Dornan, S., & Patterson, R. N. (2008). Inflammatory bowel disease in pregnancy. *BMJ, 337*, a427.

Habal, F. M., & Ravindran, N. C. (2008). Management of inflammatory bowel disease in the pregnant patient. *World J Gastroenterol, 14*(9), 1326-1332.

Kane, S., & Reddy, D. (2006). Guidelines do help change behavior in the management of osteoporosis by gastroenterologists. *Am J Gastroenterol, 101*(8), 1841-1844.

Keller, J., Frederking, D., Layer, P., & Medscape. (2008). The spectrum and treatment of gastrointestinal disorders during pregnancy. *Nat Clin Pract Gastroenterol Hepatol, 5*(8), 430-443.

Kornbluth, A., Hayes, M., Feldman, S., Hunt, M., Fried-Boxt, E., Lichtiger, S., et al. (2006). Do guidelines matter? Implementation of the ACG and AGA osteoporosis screening guidelines in inflammatory bowel disease (IBD) patients who meet the guidelines' criteria. *Am J Gastroenterol, 101*(7), 1546-1550.

Langan, R. C., Gotsch, P. B., Krafczyk, M. A., & Skillinge, D. D. (2007). Ulcerative colitis: diagnosis and treatment. *Am Fam Physician, 76*(9), 1323-1330.

Mottet, C., Juillerat, P., Pittet, V., Gonvers, J. J., Froehlich, F., Vader, J. P., et al. (2007). Pregnancy and breastfeeding in patients with Crohn's disease. *Digestion, 76*(2), 149-160.

Pache, I., Rogler, G., & Felley, C. (2009). TNF-alpha blockers in inflammatory bowel diseases: practical consensus recommendations and a user's guide. *Swiss Med Wkly, 139*(19-20), 278-287.

Roblin, X., & Bonaz, B. (2007). Osteoporosis and inflammatory bowel disease. *Am J Gastroenterol, 102*(1), 209; author reply 209-210.

Sandborn, W. J. (2008). Current directions in IBD therapy: what goals are feasible with biological modifiers? *Gastroenterology, 135*(5), 1442-1447.

Sauk, J., & Kane, S. (2005). The use of medications for inflammatory bowel disease during pregnancy and nursing. *Expert Opin Pharmacother, 6*(11), 1833-1839.

Shah, S. B., & Hanauer, S. B. (2007). Treatment of diarrhea in patients with inflammatory bowel disease: concepts and cautions. *Rev Gastroenterol Disord, 7*(Suppl 3), S3-10.

Shah, S. B., & Hanauer, S. B. (2008). Risks and benefits of the use of concomitant immunosuppressives and biologics in inflammatory bowel disease. *Rev Gastroenterol Disord, 8*(3), 159-168.

Vader, J. P., Froehlich, F., Juillerat, P., Burnand, B., Felley, C., Gonvers, J. J., et al. (2006). Appropriate treatment for Crohn's disease: methodology and summary results of a multidisciplinary international expert panel approach--EPACT. *Digestion, 73*(4), 237-248.

Insufficient Milk Supply

Principles of Therapy

While insufficient milk production is one of the most commonly perceived dysfunctions in breastfeeding, it occurs rarely. Because new mothers often worry that the infant is receiving insufficient volumes of milk, this is almost universally the main reason that many new mothers give for early weaning and for supplementation with formulas. The vast majority of women who wean due to suspected poor supply are incorrect in their perception. Objective evidence for insufficient milk supply should be sought prior to beginning pharmacologic therapy. Further support for the social component regarding milk production is that other cultures often complain more of oversupply, rather than undersupply. Because it is difficult to ascertain how much volume the infant is receiving, even in infants that are gaining and thriving, the mother frequently worries that her supply is insufficient. Prior to assuming insufficient milk production, the clinician must assess a number of critical indicators, such as: 1) the number of stools per day (normally five to ten by the end of the first week), but this varies depending on age of the child, 2) the number of wet diapers per day (at least six to eight), 3) the baby should show no signs of dehydration or hyperbilirubinemia, and 4) the infant is gaining weight along an acceptable growth curve. An insufficient milk supply may predispose to hyperbilirubinemia. The definitive indicator of sufficiency in the early neonatal period is infant weight gain. Specialized infant scales are available to allow pre and post feeding weights in an attempt to quantify the amount of milk received at a nursing.

Treatment

- Objective evidence of insufficient supply should be sought as most mother's perceiving insufficient supply are incorrect in their belief.

- The definitive indicator of sufficiency is infant weight gain.

- Specialized infant scales are available to allow pre and post feeding weights in an attempt to quantify the amount of milk received at a nursing.

- An insufficient milk supply may predispose to hyperbilirubinemia.

Medications

- DOMPERIDONE   (*Motilium, Motilidone*)
    - AAP = Maternal Medication Usually Compatible with Breastfeeding
    - LRC = L1
    - RID = 0.01-0.04%
    - Pregnancy = C

○ Comment: Domperidone (Motilium) is a peripheral dopamine antagonist (similar to Reglan) generally used for controlling nausea and vomiting, dyspepsia, and gastric reflux. It blocks peripheral dopamine receptors in the GI wall and in the CRTZ (nausea center) in the brain stem and is currently used in Canada as an antiemetic. Unlike metoclopramide (Reglan), it does not enter the brain compartment, and it has few CNS effects, such as depression.

It is also known to produce significant increases in prolactin levels and has proven useful as a galactagogue. Serum prolactin levels have been found to increase from 8.1 ng/mL to 124.1 ng/mL in non-lactating women after one 20 mg dose. Concentrations of domperidone reported in milk vary according to dose. But following a dose of 10 mg three times daily, the average concentration in milk was only 2.6 µg/L.

In a study by da Silva, 16 mothers with premature infants and low milk production (mean = 112.8 mL/d in domperidone group; 48.2 mL/d in placebo group) were randomly chosen to receive placebo (n= 9) or domperidone (10 mg TID) (n= 7) for seven days. Milk volume increased from 112.8 to 162.2 mL/d in the domperidone group and 48.2 to 56.1 mL/d in the placebo group. Prolactin levels increased from 12.9 to 119.3 µg/L in the domperidone group and 15.6 to 18.1 µg/L in the placebo group. On day five, the mean domperidone concentration was 6.6 ng/mL in plasma and 1.2 µg/L in breastmilk of the treated group (n= 6). No adverse effects were reported in infants or mothers.

In a new study just released, a group of six breastfeeding women were placed in a double blind randomized crossover trial to compare doses of domperidone. In this trial, mothers were studied in a run-in phase (no drug treatment), 30 mg, or 60 mg domperidone daily doses (10 or 20 mg every eight hours). Milk volume created per hour and plasma prolactin levels were monitored. With milk production, two mothers did not respond to domperidone treatment. Four other mothers showed a significant increase from 8.7 g/hour in the run-in phase to 23.6 g/h for the 30 mg/d dose, to 29.4 g/h for the 60 mg dose. While plasma prolactin levels were increased by domperidone treatment, there was no significant difference between levels at 30 mg and 60 mg doses. Median domperidone concentrations in milk were 0.28 µg/L and 0.49 µg/L for the 30 mg and 60 mg doses, respectively. The mean Relative Infant Dose was 0.012% at 30 mg daily and 0.009% at the 60 mg/day dose.

The usual oral dose for controlling GI distress is 10-20 mg three to four times daily, although for nausea and vomiting the dose can be higher (up to 40 mg). The galactagogue dose is suggested to be 10-20 mg orally three to four times daily. The prior studies clearly suggest that doses of 10-20 mg three to four times daily elevate prolactin levels to levels more than adequate to produce milk. Doses higher than this should be avoided in breastfeeding mothers.

Recently the US FDA issued a warning on this product stating that it could induce arrhythmias in patients. These claims were derived from data many years old where domperidone was used intravenously as an antiemetic during cancer chemotherapy (20 mg stat followed by 10 mg/kg/24 h). Many of these patients were undergoing extensive chemotherapy, were extremely ill, and hypokalemic to begin with. In addition, intravenous domperidone produces plasma levels many times higher than oral use. Thus far, we do not have any recent published data suggesting that domperidone used orally in breastfeeding mothers is arrhythmogenic, although its use in women who are already arrhythmic is not recommended.

- METOCLOPRAMIDE   (*Reglan*)

  ○ AAP = Drugs whose effect on nursing infants is unknown but may be of concern

  ○ LRC = L2

  ○ RID = 4.7-14.3%

- Pregnancy = B
- Comment: Metoclopramide has multiple functions, but is primarily used for increasing the lower esophageal sphincter tone in gastroesophageal reflux in patients with reduced gastric tone. In breastfeeding, it is sometimes used in lactating women to stimulate prolactin release from the pituitary and enhance breastmilk production. Since 1981, a number of publications have documented major increases in breastmilk production following the use of metoclopramide, domperidone, or sulpiride. With metoclopramide, the increase in serum prolactin and breastmilk production appears dose-related up to a dose of 15 mg three times daily. Many studies show 66 to 100% increases in milk production depending on the degree of breastmilk supply in the mother prior to therapy and maybe her initial prolactin levels. Doses of 15 mg/day were found ineffective, whereas doses of 30-45 mg/day were most effective. In most studies, major increases in prolactin were observed, such as from 125 ng/mL to 172 ng/mL in one patient.

In Kauppila's study, the concentration of metoclopramide in milk was consistently higher than the maternal serum levels. The peak occurred at two to three hours after administration of the medication. During the late puerperium, the concentration of metoclopramide in the milk varied from 20 to 125 µg/L, which was less than the 28 to 157 µg/L noted during the early puerperium. The authors estimated the daily dose to infant to vary from 6 to 24 µg/kg/day during the early puerperium and from 1 to 13 µg/kg/day during the late phase. These doses are minimal compared to those used for therapy of reflux in pediatric patients (0.1 to 0.5 mg/kg/day). In these studies, only one of five infants studied had detectable blood levels of metoclopramide; hence, no accumulation or side effects were observed. While plasma prolactin levels in the newborns were comparable to those in the mothers prior to treatment, Kauppila found slight increases in prolactin levels in four of seven newborns following treatment with metoclopramide, although a more recent study did not find such changes. However, prolactin levels are highly variable and subject to diurnal rhythm, thus timing is essential in measuring prolactin levels and could account for this inconsistency.

In another study of 23 women with premature infants, milk production increased from 93 mL/day to 197 mL/day between the first and seventh day of therapy with 30 mg/day. Prolactin levels, although varied, increased from 18.1 to 121.8 ng/mL. While basal prolactin levels were elevated significantly, metoclopramide seems to blunt the rapid rise of prolactin when milk was expressed. Nevertheless, milk production was still elevated.

Gupta studied 32 mothers with inadequate milk supply. Following a dose of 10 mg three times daily, a 66-100% increase in milk supply was noted. Of twelve cases of complete lactation failure, eight responded to treatment in an average of three to four days after starting therapy. In this study, 87.5% of the total 32 cases responded to metoclopramide therapy with greater milk production. No untoward effects were noted in the infants.

In a study of five breastfeeding women who were receiving 30 mg/day, daily milk production increased significantly from 150.9 mL/day to 276.4 mL/day in this group. Infant plasma prolactin levels in breastfed infants were determined as well on the fifth postnatal day and no changes were noted; thus the amount of metoclopramide transferred in milk was not enough to change the infants' prolactin levels.

In a study by Lewis in ten patients who received a single oral dose of 10 mg, the mean maternal plasma and milk levels at two hours was 68.5 ng/mL and 125.7 µg/L, respectively.

Hansen's study showed that 28 women receiving 30 mg/day had no significant increase in milk production as compared to the placebo group. However, this study was initiated within 96 hours of delivery, a time when virtually all mothers would have had exceedingly high plasma prolactin levels anyway. Metoclopramide should not be expected to work as a galactagogue when plasma prolactin levels are high.

It is well recognized that metoclopramide increases a mother's milk supply, but it is exceedingly dose dependent, and yet some mothers simply do not respond. In those mothers who do not respond, Kauppila's work suggests that such patients may already have elevated prolactin levels. In his study, three of the five mothers who did not respond with increased milk production had the highest basal prolactin levels (300-400 ng/mL). Thus it may be advisable to do plasma prolactin levels on under-producing mothers prior to instituting metoclopramide therapy to assess the response prior to treating.

Side effects, such as gastric cramping and diarrhea, limit the compliance of some patients, but are rare. Further, it is often found that upon rapid discontinuation of the medication, the supply of milk may in some instances reduce significantly. Tapering of the dose is generally recommended, and one possible regimen is to decrease the dose by 10 mg per week. Long-term use of this medication (>4 weeks) may be accompanied by increased side effects, such as depression in the mother, although some patients have used it successfully for months. Another dopamine antagonist, Domperidone, due to minimal side effects, is a preferred choice, but is unfortunately not available in the USA other than in compounding pharmacies.

Two recent cases of serotonin-like reactions (agitation, dysarthria, diaphoresis, and extrapyramidal movement disorder) have been reported when metoclopramide was used in patients receiving sertraline or venlafaxine. The FDA has recently warned of symptoms of tardive dyskinesia after three months of exposure.

- SULPIRIDE   (*Dolmatil, Sulparex, Sulpitil*)

  ◦ AAP = Not reviewed
  ◦ LRC = L2
  ◦ RID = 2.7-20.7%
  ◦ Pregnancy =
  ◦ Comment: Sulpiride is a selective dopamine antagonist used as an antidepressant and antipsychotic. Sulpiride is a strong neuroleptic antipsychotic drug; however, several studies using smaller doses have found it to significantly increase prolactin levels and breastmilk production in smaller doses that do not produce overt neuroleptic effects on the mother. In a study with 14 women who received sulpiride (50 mg three times daily), and in a subsequent study with 36 breastfeeding women, Ylikorkala found major increases in prolactin levels and significant, but only moderate, increases in breastmilk production. In a group of 20 women who received 50 mg twice daily, breastmilk samples were drawn two hours after the dose. The concentration of sulpiride in breastmilk ranged from 0.26 to 1.97 mg/L. No effects on breastfed infants were noted. The authors concluded that sulpiride, when administered early in the postpartum period, is useful in promoting initiation of lactation.

In a study by McMurdo, sulpiride was found to be a potent stimulant of maternal plasma prolactin levels. Interestingly, it appears that the prolactin response to sulpiride is not dose-related and reached a maximum at 3-10 mg. Thereafter, further increased doses did not further increase prolactin levels. Sulpiride is not available in the USA.

Clinical Tips

While extremely rare, some women fail to produce sufficient milk for their infant. This may be due to a myriad of problems, including insufficient glandular tissue, breast surgery or reduction, mammoplasty with severing of the ductal tissues near the nipple, anemia, shock, retained placental fragments, or postpartum hemorrhage. Sub-optimal early lactation management is a leading potentially preventable etiology for insufficient milk supply.

Regardless of the cause for low milk supply, continued frequent breastfeeding and, if needed, use of supplemental feeding for the infant until supply increases is indicated. Alternative feeding methods, such as supplemental feeding devices, cup feeding, or finger feeding, instead of the use of a bottle are advocated by some experts. Regardless of feeding method, breast stimulation with manual expression or a pump should be used to stimulate milk supply in these cases. Warm compresses applied to the breasts and relaxation techniques may be of benefit.

Metoclopramide has multiple effects, but is primarily used for increasing the lower esophageal sphincter tone in gastroesophageal reflux in patients with reduced gastric tone. It is sometimes used in lactating women to stimulate prolactin release from the pituitary and enhance breastmilk production. Since 1981, a number of publications have documented major increases in breastmilk production following the use of metoclopramide, domperidone, or sulpiride. All are peripheral dopamine antagonists. With metoclopramide, the increase in serum prolactin and breastmilk production appears dose-related, up to a dose of 15 mg three times daily. Many studies show 66 to 100% increases in milk production, depending on the degree of breastmilk supply in the mother prior to therapy. In another study of 23 women with premature infants, milk production increased from 93 mL/day to 197 mL/day between the first and seventh day of therapy with 30 mg/day. Prolactin levels, although varied, increased from 18.1 to 121.8 ng/mL. Gupta studied 32 mothers with inadequate milk supply. Following a dose of 10 mg three times daily, a 66-100% increase in milk supply was noted. No untoward effects were noted in the infants. Doses of 15 mg/day were found ineffective, whereas doses of 30-45 mg/day were most effective. In most studies, major increases in prolactin were observed, such as 18.1 ng/mL to 121.8 ng/mL after therapy in one study. While it is well recognized that metoclopramide increases milk supply, it is very dose-dependent, and some mothers simply do not respond. Side effects, such as depression, gastric cramping, and diarrhea, limit the compliance of some patients. Further, it is often found that upon discontinuing the medication, the supply of milk reduces rapidly. A slow tapering of the dose over several weeks is generally recommended in those women who respond. Long-term use of this medication (>4 weeks) is not generally recommended, as the incidence of depression and tardive dyskinesia increases. A FDA black box warning regarding this medication was issued in 2007 due to the incidence of tardive dyskinesia. Tardive dyskinesia was reported in 20% of patients taking the medication > three months, and the effect may be permanent in some cases. As postpartum depression carries a high likelihood of recurrence, use of metoclopramide in a mother with prior history of depression provides a relative contraindication. If metoclopramide fails to work within seven days, it is unlikely that longer therapy will be effective.

Domperidone is considered a "peripheral" dopamine antagonist and fails to pass the blood-brain barrier. Due to minimal side effects and superior efficacy, it is considered a better choice, but it is not available in the USA. The usual oral dose for controlling GI distress is 10-20 mg three to four times daily. Recent studies have suggested that doses higher than 10-20 mg three times daily do not increase prolactin levels above the lower dose. The FDA has issued a warning to healthcare providers and breastfeeding women not to use this unapproved drug to increase milk production, as they are concerned about potential health risks.

Sulpiride is a selective dopamine antagonist used as an antidepressant and antipsychotic. Several studies using smaller doses have found it to significantly increase prolactin levels and breastmilk production in smaller doses that do not produce overt neuroleptic effects on the mother. This drug is also not available in the US.

Multiple herbal therapies are touted as benefiting poor milk supply. Scientific evidence supporting the effectiveness of many of these compounds is limited. Concern also exists regarding the relative potency and quality control of herbal products in the United States. Fenugreek in doses of three 600 mg tablets three times daily has been suggested to improve milk supply. In a case-control study of ten exclusively breast pumping women, the increase in milk production was > 20% in five of ten mothers and >100% in three of these. Further study is needed regarding the safety and effectiveness of herbal galactogogues.

Clinicians may consider drawing plasma prolactin levels surrounding breastfeeding to assess response.

Suggested Reading

Amir, L. H. (2006). Breastfeeding--managing 'supply' difficulties. *Aust Fam Physician, 35*(9), 686-689.

Anderson, P. O., & Valdes, V. (1993). Increasing breastmilk supply. *Clin Pharm, 12*(7), 479-480.

Anderson, P. O., & Valdes, V. (2007). A critical review of pharmaceutical galactagogues. *Breastfeed Med, 2*(4), 229-242.

Heinig, M. J., & Ishii, K. D. (2005). Managing your milk supply: going with the flow. *J Hum Lact, 21*(2), 201-202.

Hill, P. D., Aldag, J. C., Zinaman, M., & Chatterton, R. T. (2007). Predictors of preterm infant feeding methods and perceived insufficient milk supply at week 12 postpartum. *J Hum Lact, 23*(1), 32-38; quiz 39-43.

Huang, Y. Y., Lee, J. T., Huang, C. M., & Gau, M. L. (2009). Factors related to maternal perception of milk supply while in the hospital. *J Nurs Res, 17*(3), 179-188.

Marasco, L. (2008). Inside track. Increasing your milk supply with galactogogues. *J Hum Lact, 24*(4), 455-456.

Spatz, D. L. (2004). Ten steps for promoting and protecting breastfeeding for vulnerable infants. *J Perinat Neonatal Nurs, 18*(4), 385-396.

Williams, N. (2002). Supporting the mother coming to terms with persistent insufficient milk supply: the role of the lactation consultant. *J Hum Lact, 18*(3), 262-263.

Intra-Amniotic Infection/Postpartum Endomyometritis

Principles of Therapy

Intra-amniotic infection occurs prior to delivery, whereas postpartum endomyometritis is diagnosed after delivery. Intra-amniotic infection may also be referred to as chorioamnionitis. Endomyometritis may be referred to as endometritis. Both infections are polymicrobial and likely result from ascending vaginal organisms. The incidence of intra-amniotic infection is higher in pre-term pregnancies with preterm labor or premature membrane rupture. At term the incidence is approximately 2- 4%. Intra-amniotic infection has been associated with both adverse maternal and infant outcome (including neurodevelopmental difficulty). Beginning treatment in labor as soon as the diagnosis is suspected is important for the fetus. Diagnosis is usually made based on fever, uterine tenderness, and other associated symptoms, such as leukocytosis, tachycardia or foul smelling / purulent vaginal discharge. Epidural anesthesia obscures the detection of uterine tenderness, and the diagnosis may be made presumptively based on other clinical features during labor in these women.

Approximately 1 in 50 women who give birth vaginally develops a uterine infection; the number is much higher for women who undergo a cesarean section. The use of prophylactic antibiotics pre-operatively for cesarean delivery has been found to decrease the incidence of post-cesarean infection and is recommended. These infections are due to a number of different bacteria usually ascending from normal vaginal flora. Commonly isolated organisms include two or more of the following *Ureaplasma urealyticum, Peptostreptococcus, gardnerella vaginalis, Bacteroides bividus, Group B Streptococcus, Enterococcus, E coli, Proteus, Klebsiella* and others. Chlamydia may be associated with delayed onset endometritis. Risk factors for infection include: cesarean delivery, prolonged labor and early rupture of membranes, multiple vaginal examinations, prolonged internal monitoring during labor, meconium-stained amniotic fluid, and presence of vaginal infections during pregnancy (such as GBS and bacterial vaginosis).

Treatment

- Treatment includes use of antibiotics and delivery of the infant. Antibiotic options include cefotetan, cephtriaxone, cefoxitin, ampicillin + gentamycin.

- Intra-amniotic infection is frequently treated with ampicillin and gentamycin, with anerobic coverage with clindamycin or metronidazole if a cesarean delivery is indicated.

- Treatment for endometritis often includes IV gentamicin plus clindamycin. Ampicillin is often added for additional coverage.

- Cefotetan and cefoxitin also offer broad spectrum coverage for these pathogens.

Medications

- AMPICILLIN   (*Polycillin, Omnipen*)
  - AAP = Not reviewed
  - LRC = L1
  - RID = 0.2-0.5%
  - Pregnancy = B
  - Comment: Low milk/plasma ratios of 0.2 have been reported. In a study by Matsuda of two to three breastfeeding patients who received 500 mg of ampicillin orally, levels in milk peaked at six hours and averaged only 0.14 mg/L of milk. The milk/plasma ratio was reported to be 0.03 at two hours. In a group of nine breastfeeding women sampled at various times and who received doses of 350 mg TID orally, milk concentrations ranged from 0.06 to 0.17 mg/L, with peak milk levels at three to four hours after the dose. Milk/plasma ratios varied between 0.01 and 0.58. The highest reported milk level (1.02 mg/L) was in a patient receiving 700 mg TID. Ampicillin was not detected in the plasma of any infant.

- AMPICILLIN + SULBACTAM   (*Unasyn*)
  - AAP = Not reviewed
  - LRC = L1
  - RID = 0.5-1.5%
  - Pregnancy = B
  - Comment: Small amounts of ampicillin may transfer (1 mg/L). Possible rash, sensitization, diarrhea, or candidiasis could occur, but is unlikely. This drug may alter GI flora. After a dose of 0.5 to 1 gram, sulbactam is secreted into milk at an average concentration of 0.52 μg/mL. This would lead to a maximal dose of 0.7 mg/kg/day in a breastfeeding infant, which equates to less than 1% of the maternal dose. Therefore, untoward effects are unlikely in a breastfeeding infant.

- CEFOTETAN   (*Cefotan*)
  - AAP = Not reviewed
  - LRC = L2
  - RID = 0.2-0.3%
  - Pregnancy = B
  - Comment: Cefotetan is a third generation cephalosporin that is poorly absorbed orally and is only available via IM and IV injection. The drug is distributed into human milk in low concentrations. Following a maternal dose of 1000mg IM every 12 hours in five patients, breastmilk concentrations ranged from 0.29 to 0.59 mg/L. Plasma concentrations were almost 100 times higher. In a group of two to three women who received 1000 mg IV, the maximum average milk level reported was 0.2 mg/L at four hours with a milk/plasma ratio of 0.02.

- CEFOXITIN   (*Mefoxin*)
  - AAP = Maternal Medication Usually Compatible with Breastfeeding
  - LRC = L1

- ◦ RID   = 0.1-0.3%
- ◦ Pregnancy = B
- ◦ Comment: Cefoxitin is a cephalosporin antibiotic with a spectrum similar to the second generation family. It is transferred into human milk in very low levels. In a study of 18 women receiving 2000-4000 mg doses, only one breastmilk sample contained cefoxitin (0.9 mg/L), all the rest were too low to be detected. In another study of two to three women who received 1000 mg IV, only trace amounts were reported in milk over six hours. In a group of five women who received an IM injection of 2000 mg, the highest milk levels were reported at four hours after dose. The maternal plasma levels varied from 22.5 at two hours to 77.6 µg/mL at four hours. Maternal milk levels ranged from <0.25 to 0.65 mg/L. Observe for changes in gut flora.

- **CLINDAMYCIN**   (*Cleocin, Cleocin T*)
  - ◦ AAP = Maternal Medication Usually Compatible with Breastfeeding
  - ◦ LRC = L2
  - ◦ RID   = 1.7%
  - ◦ Pregnancy = B
  - ◦ Comment: Clindamycin is a broad-spectrum antibiotic frequently used for anaerobic infections. In one study of two nursing mothers and following doses of 600 mg IV every six hours, the concentration of clindamycin in breastmilk was 3.1 to 3.8 mg/L at 0.2 to 0.5 hours after dosing. Following oral doses of 300 mg every six hours, the breastmilk levels averaged 1.0 to 1.7 mg/L at 1.5 to seven hours after dosing. In another study of two to three women who received a single oral dose of 150 mg, milk levels averaged 0.9 mg/L at four hours with a milk/plasma ratio of 0.47.

    An alteration of GI flora is possible, even though the dose is low. One case of bloody stools (pseudomembranous colitis) has been associated with clindamycin and gentamicin therapy on day five postpartum, but this is considered rare. In this case, the mother of a newborn infant was given 600 mg IV every six hours. In rare cases, pseudomembranous colitis can appear several weeks later.

    In a study by Steen, in five breastfeeding patients who received 150 mg three times daily for seven days, milk concentrations ranged from <0.5 to 3.1 mg/L, with the majority of levels <0.5 mg/L. There are a number of pediatric clinical uses of clindamycin (anaerobic infections, bacterial endocarditis, pelvic inflammatory disease, and bacterial vaginosis). The current pediatric dosage recommendation is 10-40 mg/kg/day divided every six to eight hours. In a study of 15 women who received 600 mg clindamycin intravenously, levels of clindamycin in milk averaged 1.03 mg/L at two hours following the dose. The amount of clindamycin in milk is unlikely to harm a breastfeeding infant.

- **GENTAMICIN**   (*Garamycin*)
  - ◦ AAP = Maternal Medication Usually Compatible with Breastfeeding
  - ◦ LRC = L2
  - ◦ RID   = 2.1%
  - ◦ Pregnancy = C
  - ◦ Comment: Gentamicin is a narrow spectrum antibiotic generally used for gram negative infections. The oral absorption of gentamicin (<1%) is generally nil with the exception of premature neonates, where small amounts may be absorbed. In one study of 10 women given 80 mg three times daily IM for five days postpartum, milk levels were measured on day four. Gentamicin levels in milk were 0.42, 0.48, 0.49, and 0.41 mg/L at one, three, five, and seven hours, respectively. The milk/plasma

ratios were 0.11 at one hour and 0.44 at seven hours. Plasma gentamicin levels in neonates were small, were found in only five of the ten neonates, and averaged 0.41 μg/mL. The authors estimate that daily ingestion via breastmilk would be 307 μg for a 3.6 kg neonate (normal neonatal dose = 2.5 mg/kg every 12 hours). These amounts would be clinically irrelevant in most infants.

- METRONIDAZOLE   (*Flagyl, Metizol, Trikacide, Protostat, Noritate*)

  ◦ AAP = Drugs whose effect on nursing infants is unknown but may be of concern

  ◦ LRC = L2

  ◦ RID = 12.6-13.5%

  ◦ Pregnancy = B

  ◦ Comment: Metronidazole is indicated in the treatment of vaginitis due to Trichomonas Vaginalis and various anaerobic bacterial infections, including Giardiasis, H. pylori, B. fragilis, and Gardnerella vaginalis. Metronidazole has become the treatment of choice for pediatric giardiasis (AAP). Metronidazole absorption is time and dose dependent and also depends on the route of administration (oral vs. vaginal). Following a 2 gm oral dose, milk levels were reported to peak at 50-57 mg/L at two hours. Milk levels after 12 hours were approximately 19 mg/L, and at 24 hours were approximately 10 mg/L. The average drug concentration reported in milk at 2, 8, 12, and 12-24 hours was 45.8, 27.9, 19.1, and 12.6 mg/L, respectively. If breastfeeding were to continue uninterrupted, an infant would consume 21.8 mg via breastmilk. With a 12 hour discontinuation, an infant would consume only 9.8 mg. In a group of 12 nursing mothers receiving 400 mg three times daily, the mean milk/plasma ratio was 0.91. The mean milk metronidazole concentration was 15.5 mg/L. Infant plasma metronidazole levels ranged from 1.27 to 2.41 μg/mL. No adverse effects were attributable to metronidazole therapy in these infants. In another study in patients receiving 600 and 1200 mg daily, the average milk metronidazole concentration was 5.7 and 14.4 mg/L, respectively. The plasma levels of metronidazole (two hours) at the 600 mg/d dose were 5 μg/mL (mother) and 0.8 μg/mL (infant). At the 1200 mg/d dose (two hours), plasma levels were 12.5 μg/mL (mother) and 2.4 μg/mL (infant). The authors estimated the daily metronidazole dose received by the infant at 3.0 mg/kg with 500 mL milk intake per day, which is well below the advocated 10-20 mg/kg recommended therapeutic dose for infants.

  It is true that the relative infant dose via milk is moderately high depending on the dose and timing. Infants whose mothers ingest 1.2 gm/d will receive approximately 13.5% or less of the maternal dose or approximately 2.3 mg/kg/day. Bennett has calculated the relative infant dose from 11.7% to as high as 24% of the maternal dose. Heisterberg found metronidazole levels in infant plasma to be 16% and 19% of the maternal plasma levels following doses of 600 mg/d and 1200 mg/d. While these levels seem significant, it is still pertinent to remember that metronidazole is a commonly used drug in premature neonates, infants, and children, and 2.3 mg/kg/d is still much less than the therapeutic dose used in infants/children (7.5-30 mg/kg/d). Thus far, virtually no adverse effects have been reported.

INTRAVENOUS STUDIES

  ◦ Metronidazole is approximately 98% bioavailable orally and it is rapidly absorbed. In one study of intravenous kinetics, the authors found peak plasma levels of 28.9 μg/mL in adults following a 500 mg TID dose. In another study of oral and intravenous kinetics, the authors used 400 mg orally, and 500 mg intravenously. Following 400 mg orally, the Cmax at 90 minutes was 17.4 μg/mL. Following 500 mg IV, the Cmax at 90 minutes was 23.6 μg/mL. Reducing the IV dose to 400 mg would have given a plasma level of approximately 18.8 or an amount similar to the oral plasma level attained in the above group(17.4). From these two sets of data, it is apparent that the peak (Cmax) following an intravenous dose is only slightly higher than that obtained following oral administration. In an elegant study of plasma kinetics of oral and IV metronidazole (both 500 mg and 2000 mg), Loft found that the AUC (500 mg dose) for oral and IV treatments was virtually identical (101 vs. 100 µg/mL-h, respectively). The Cmax (taken from graph) for oral and IV treatments were essentially the same. In another study comparing the plasma kinetics following 800 mg doses orally and IV, Bergan found that plasma levels are virtually identical at two to three hours after the dose. Therefore, in a breastfeeding mother receiving IV metronidazole, a brief interruption of breastfeeding for perhaps one to two hours would expose the infant to almost identical levels as obtained from the same dose given orally.

- ° Data from older studies with rats and mice have shown that metronidazole is potentially mutagenic/carcinogenic. Thus far, no studies in humans have found it to be mutagenic. In fact, the opposite seems to be the finding. Roe suggests that metronidazole is 'essentially free of cancer risk or other serious toxic side effects.' Age-gender stratified analysis did not reveal any association between short-term exposure to metronidazole and cancer in humans.

- VANCOMYCIN   (*Vancocin*)
  - ° AAP = Not reviewed
  - ° LRC = L1
  - ° RID = 6.7%
  - ° Pregnancy = C
  - ° Comment: Vancomycin is an antimicrobial agent. Only low levels are secreted into human milk. Milk levels were 12.7 mg/L four hours after infusion in one woman receiving 1 gm every 12 hours for seven days. Its poor absorption from the infant's GI tract would limit its systemic absorption. Low levels in the infant could provide alterations of GI flora.

Clinical Tips

Therapy for intra-amniotic infection includes ampicillin and gentamycin which are begun during labor in order to reduce potential fetal infectious effects, as well as for maternal benefit. If a cesarean is then required, anaerobic coverage is added, usually with clindamycin or occasionally metronidazole.

The first-line treatment for endometritis is gentamycin plus clindamicin (gentamicin 5 mg/kg and clindamycin 2.7 gm IV once daily). Ampicillin is frequently added to this regiem. Breastfeeding mothers with endometritis can often use these medications in the immediate postpartum period. The course of therapy is usually limited to a few days, typically 24 to 48 hours after the patient has defervesced. With the use of broad-spectrum antibiotics, there is a theoretical risk of pseudomembranous colitis, and observation for diarrhea is warranted. Vancomycin may be substituted for ampicillin in penicillin-allergic patients.

Suggested Reading

Costantine, M. M., Rahman, M., Ghulmiyah, L., Byers, B. D., Longo, M., Wen, T., et al. (2008). Timing of perioperative antibiotics for cesarean delivery: a metaanalysis. *Am J Obstet Gynecol, 199*(3), 301 e301-306.

Fahey, J. O. (2008). Clinical management of intra-amniotic infection and chorioamnionitis: a review of the literature. *J Midwifery Womens Health, 53*(3), 227-235.

Faro, S. (2005). Postpartum endometritis. *Clin Perinatol, 32*(3), 803-814.

Gautam, G., Nakao, T., Yusuf, M., & Koike, K. (2009). Prevalence of endometritis during the postpartum period and its impact on subsequent reproductive performance in two Japanese dairy herds. *Anim Reprod Sci, 116*(3-4), 175-187.

Kaimal, A. J., Zlatnik, M. G., Cheng, Y. W., Thiet, M. P., Connatty, E., Creedy, P., et al. (2008). Effect of a change in policy regarding the timing of prophylactic antibiotics on the rate of postcesarean delivery surgical-site infections. *Am J Obstet Gynecol, 199*(3), 310 e311-315.

Mulic-Lutvica, A., & Axelsson, O. (2007). Postpartum ultrasound in women with postpartum endometritis, after cesarean section and after manual evacuation of the placenta. *Acta Obstet Gynecol Scand, 86*(2), 210-217.

Tharpe, N. (2008). Postpregnancy genital tract and wound infections. *J Midwifery Womens Health, 53*(3), 236-246.

Irritable Bowel Syndrome

Principles of Therapy

Irritable bowel syndrome (IBS) is a chronic intestinal disease which typically presents as recurrent abdominal pain, distension, and bowel habit changes not attributed to any known separate disorder. IBS is extremely common and may affect 11-20% of the adult population in industrialized countries. As the exact cause is unknown, successful treatment can often be difficult to achieve and should focus on addressing the patient's primary concern. In accordance with Rome III criteria (2006), IBS involves abdominal pain and bowel habit disturbance, which are not explained by structural or biochemical abnormalities. Thus a detailed history for things which seem to worsen symptoms, evaluation for mood disorders, and ruling out other gastrointestinal diseases are important. The efficacy of many treatment options for this disorder is not established and placebo may be effective.

Dietary changes may be especially useful in patients who can find a precipitating dietary association. Attempting a trial of a lactose-free diet or a diet which avoids foods known to increase gas may be helpful in some situations. These changes should not be problematic for breastfeeding mothers. Other dietary changes which have been proposed include: low gluten diets, avoidance of a high carbohydrate diet, and increase in dietary fiber. Some authorities also suggest the use of synthetic fiber supplements, as they cause less bloating, but still provide the desired fiber effects, such as bulking. This would also be a safe option during lactation. Behavioral therapies have also been suggested for management.

Medications used for IBS are limited by the chronic nature of the condition. Agents that decrease intestinal spasms may be used for short periods, such as anticholinergic medications. Antidepressants have also been found to be useful. Both SSRI and tri-cyclic antidepressants have been studied, and either of these treatment options outperformed placebo. Medication to control diarrhea may be useful in select cases where that symptom is predominant. Anxiolytic medications have been used; however, the chronic nature of this disease makes this a less favorable option. The use of other medications, such as 5-hydroxytryptamine 3 or 4 receptor antagonists and chloride channel activators, have some support; however, rare but serious complications of some of these drugs may occur and limit their usefulness. The use of antibiotics aimed at diminishing gas producing bacteria has also been attempted, though scientific research has not confirmed this effective. Alternative therapies for IBS are common, such as herbal therapies, probiotics, or enzyme supplementation.

Treatment

- Dietary changes: avoid food triggers, lactose-free diet, avoid foods which induce flatulence, low gluten diet, low carbohydrate diet, low fructose diet, high fiber diet.

- Synthetic fiber supplements.

- Limitation of "stressors," behavioral therapy.

- Medications: anti-spasmotics (anticholinergics), SSRI or TCA anti-depressants, anxiotytics (short course < 2 weeks only), other medications.

- If diarrhea prominent symptom: use of anti-diarrheal agent.

- Alternative therapies: herbs, probiotics, enzyme supplements.

Medications:

- ALOSETRON   (*Lotronex*)
  - AAP = Not reviewed
  - LRC = L3
  - RID =
  - Pregnancy = B
  - Comment: Alosetron (Lotronex) is a new 5-HT3 receptor antagonist which is used to control the symptoms of irritable bowel syndrome. No data are available on the transfer of this medication into human milk. While the manufacturer suggests it is present in animal milk, no data are provided. The peak plasma levels (in young women) of this product are quite small, only averaging 9 nanogram/mL following a 1 mg dose. Although the half-life of the parent alosetron is short (1.5 hours), its metabolites have much longer half-lives, although their importance is unknown. Bioavailability is lessened (<25%) when mixed with food. With these data it is unlikely milk levels will be extraordinarily high or that the levels transferred to the infant will be clinically relevant to the infant. However, its use in breastfeeding patients should be approached with caution until we have more clinical experience with this new product.

- AMITRIPTYLINE   (*Elavil, Endep*)
  - AAP = Drugs whose effect on nursing infants is unknown but may be of concern
  - LRC = L2
  - RID = 1.9-2.8%
  - Pregnancy = C
  - Comment: Amitriptyline and its active metabolite, nortriptyline, are secreted into breastmilk in small amounts. In one report of a mother taking 100 mg/day of amitriptyline, milk levels of amitriptyline and nortriptyline (active metabolite) averaged 143 µg/L and 55.5 µg/L, respectively; maternal serum levels averaged 112 µg/L and 72.5 µg/L, respectively. No drug was detected in the infant's serum. From these data, an infant would consume approximately 21.5 µg/kg/day, a dose that is unlikely to be clinically relevant.

    In another study following a maternal dose of 25 mg/day, the amitriptyline and nortriptyline (active metabolite) levels in milk were 30 µg/L and <30 µg/L, respectively. In the same study when the dosage was 75 mg/day, milk levels of amitriptyline and nortriptyline averaged 88 µg/L and 69 µg/L, respectively. Both drugs were essentially undetectable in the infant's serum. Therefore, the authors estimated that a nursing infant would receive less than 0.1 mg/day.

    In another mother taking 175 mg/day, amitriptyline levels in the mother's milk were the same as in her serum on day one (24-27 µg/mL), but milk levels decreased to 54% of the serum concentration on days 2 to 26. Milk concentrations of nortriptyline were 74% of that in the mother's serum (87 ng/mL). Thus the authors reported the absolute infant dose as 35 µg/kg, 80 times lower than the mother's dose. Neither compound could be detected in the infant's serum on day 26, nor were there any signs of sedation or other adverse effects.

- **DESIPRAMINE** *(Pertofrane, Norpramin)*
  - ○ AAP = Drugs whose effect on nursing infants is unknown but may be of concern
  - ○ LRC = L2
  - ○ RID = 0.3-0.9%
  - ○ Pregnancy = C
  - ○ Comment: Desipramine is a prototypic tricyclic antidepressant. In one case report, a mother taking 200 mg of desipramine at bedtime had milk/plasma ratios of 0.4 to 0.9 with milk levels ranging between 17-35 µg/L. Desipramine was not found in the infant's blood, although these levels are probably too low to measure. In another study of a mother consuming 300 mg of desipramine daily, the milk levels were 30% higher than the maternal serum. The milk concentrations of desipramine were reported to be 316 to 328 µg/L, with peak concentrations occurring at four hours post-dose. Assuming an average milk concentration of 280 µg/L, an infant would receive approximately 42 µg/kg/day. No untoward effects have been reported.

- **DICYCLOMINE** *(Bentyl, Antispas, Spasmoject)*
  - ○ AAP = Not reviewed
  - ○ LRC = L4
  - ○ RID = 6.9%
  - ○ Pregnancy = B
  - ○ Comment: Dicyclomine is a tertiary amine antispasmodic. It belongs to the family of anticholinergics, such as atropine and the belladonna alkaloids. It was previously used for infant colic, but due to overdoses and reported apnea, it is seldom recommended for this use. Infants are exceedingly sensitive to anticholinergics, particularly in the neonatal period. Following a dose of 20 mg in a lactating woman, a 12-day-old infant reported severe apnea. The manufacturer reports milk levels of 131 µg/L, with corresponding maternal serum levels of 59 µg/L. The reported milk/plasma level was 2.22.

- **HYOSCYAMINE** *(Anaspaz, Levsin, NuLev)*
  - ○ AAP = Not reviewed
  - ○ LRC = L3
  - ○ RID =
  - ○ Pregnancy = C
  - ○ Comment: Hyoscyamine is an anticholinergic, antisecretory agent that belongs to the belladonna alkaloid family. Its typical effects are to dry secretions, produce constipation, dilate pupils, blur vision, and it may produce urinary retention. Although no exact amounts are listed, hyoscyamine is known to be secreted into breastmilk in trace amounts. Thus far, no untoward effects from breastfeeding while using hyoscyamine have been found. Levsin (hyoscyamine) drops have in the past been used directly in infants for colic, although it is no longer recommended for this use. As with atropine, infants and children are especially sensitive to anticholinergics and their use is discouraged. Atropine is composed of two isomers of hyoscyamine. See atropine. Use with caution.

- IMIPRAMINE   (*Tofranil, Janimine*)
  - AAP = Drugs whose effect on nursing infants is unknown but may be of concern
  - LRC = L2
  - RID = 0.1-4.4%
  - Pregnancy = D
  - Comment: Imipramine is a classic tricyclic antidepressant. Imipramine is metabolized to desipramine, the active metabolite. Milk levels approximate those of maternal serum. In a patient receiving 200 mg daily at bedtime, the milk levels at 1, 9, 10, and 23 hours were 29, 24, 12, and 18 μg/L, respectively. However, in this previous study, the mother was not in a therapeutic range. In a mother with full therapeutic levels, it is suggested that an infant would ingest approximately 0.2 mg/Liter of milk. This represents a dose of only 30 μg/kg/day, far less than the 1.5 mg/kg dose recommended for older children. The long half-life of this medication in infants could, under certain conditions, lead to high plasma levels, although they have not been reported. Although no untoward effects have been reported, the infant should be monitored closely. Therapeutic plasma levels in children 6-12 years are 200-225 ng/mL. Two good reviews of psychotropic drugs in breastfeeding patients are available.

- LOPERAMIDE   (*Imodium, Pepto Diarrhea Control, Maalox Anti-Diarrheal Caplets, Kaopectate II Caplets, Imodium Advanced*)
  - AAP = Maternal Medication Usually Compatible with Breastfeeding
  - LRC = L2
  - RID = 0.03%
  - Pregnancy = B
  - Comment: Loperamide is an antidiarrheal drug. Because it is only minimally absorbed orally (0.3%), only extremely small amounts are secreted into breastmilk. Following a 4 mg oral dose twice daily in six women (early postpartum), milk levels at 12 hours after the following dose averaged 0.18 μg/L, and six hours after the second dose were 0.27 μg/L. A breastfeeding infant consuming 165 mL/kg/day of milk would ingest 2000 times less than the recommended daily dose. It is very unlikely these reported levels in milk (Relative infant dose = 0.03%) would ever produce clinical effects in a breastfed infant.

- LUBIPROSTONE   (*Amitiza*)
  - AAP = Not reviewed
  - LRC = L3
  - RID =
  - Pregnancy = C
  - Comment: Lysine is a naturally occurring amino acid; the average American ingests from 6-10 grams daily. Aside from its use as a supplement in patients with poor nutrition, it is most often used for the treatment of recurrent herpes simplex infections. The clinical efficacy of lysine in herpes infections is highly controversial, with some advocates and many detractors. Upon absorption, most is sequestered in the liver, but blood levels do rise transiently. However, the risk of toxicity is considered quite low in both adults and infants. Rather high doses have been studied in infants as young as four months, with doses from 60 to 1080 mg L-lysine per eight ounces of milk. At the

higher level, 5.18 grams of L-lysine was consumed. Plasma lysine levels varied only with normal limits, while urinary lysine levels were roughly proportional to the amount of supplementation.

Thomas et al. has reported an elegant study of the transfer of radiolabeled L-lysine into numerous compartments, including milk. In a group of five lactating women who received L-lysine (15N-lysine and 13C-lysine [5 mg/kg/each]), milk levels of labeled lysine reached a peak at approximately 150 minutes. Labeled lysine levels in milk were slightly higher with M/P ratios ranging from 1.29 to 1.43. However, the total amount of radiolabeled lysine present in milk was low. Only 0.54% of the administered dose of lysine was secreted into milk proteins. Further, the lysine present in milk was present as protein, not free amino acid.

Therefore, supplementation of breastfeeding mothers with L-lysine will probably not result in significantly elevated levels of free lysine in milk.

- NORTRIPTYLINE   (*Aventyl, Pamelor*)

  ○ AAP = Drugs whose effect on nursing infants is unknown but may be of concern

  ○ LRC = L2

  ○ RID = 1.7-3.1%

  ○ Pregnancy = D

  ○ Comment: Nortriptyline (NT) is a tricyclic antidepressant and is the active metabolite of amitriptyline (Elavil). In one patient receiving 125 mg of nortriptyline at bedtime, milk concentrations of NT averaged 180 µg/L after six to seven days of administration. Based on these concentrations, the authors estimate the average daily infant exposure would be 27 µg/kg/d. The relative dose in milk would be 1.5% of the maternal dose. Several other authors have been unable to detect NT in maternal milk in the serum of infants after prolonged exposure. So far, no untoward effects have been noted.

  A pooled analysis of 35 studies, with an average dose of 78 mg/day, reported a detectable level of nortriptyline in breastmilk in only one patient, with a concentration of 230 ng/mL. The authors suggest that breastfeeding infants exposed to nortriptyline are unlikely to develop detectable concentrations in plasma, and therefore, breastfeeding during nortriptyline therapy is not contraindicated.

Clinical Tips

The primary goals of treatment include the control of the patients' symptoms and the management of of any associated coexisting conditions, such as depression, anxiety, and other psychiatric syndromes. The strategy of treatment is to control the basic symptoms. For the treatment of gastric pain, antispasmodics are generally first line. Dicyclomine and possibly hyoscyamine should be considered, but only carefully in breastfeeding mothers. Peppermint oil has been found useful in some patients. Second-line therapy would include the tricyclic antidepressants, such as amitriptyline, which has rather profound anticholinergic side effects and may be useful beginning at low doses at bedtime. SSRIs, such as fluoxetine, paroxetine or sertraline, have been used and found effective, although clinical trials are few.

In constipatory IBS, the bulk laxative psyllium (Metamucil) is quite effective and requires rather large doses to swell the colon and reduce symptoms of pain and constipation. Other bulk laxatives may be useful as well (FiberCon, Citrucel), but only in this type of IBS.

In diarrheal IBS, antidiarrheal agents, such as loperamide, are considered first-line. Alosetron may be useful, but should be reserved for severe, refractory diarrhea in women with IBS.

Finally, there is no specific or curative treatment for IBS since it is a chronic disorder and often requires changes in lifestyle and control of anxiety sysmptoms. Treatment of symptoms using the above medications and/or bulk laxatives is indicated. Do not use stimulant laxatives. Low-dose tricylcic antidepressants are a worthwhile treatment, safe in breastfeeding mothers, and inexpensive.

Suggested Reading

1: Halpert A.D. (2010). Importance of early diagnosis in patients with irritable bowel syndrome. *Postgrad Med. 122*(2):102-11. Review.

2: Morcos A., Dinan T., Quigley E.M. (2009). Irritable bowel syndrome: role of food in pathogenesis and management. *J Dig Dis. 10*(4):237-46. Review.

3: Dobrek Ł., Thor P.J. (2009). Pathophysiological concepts of functional dyspepsia and irritable bowel syndrome future pharmacotherapy. *Acta Pol Pharm. 66*(5):447-60. Review.

4. Quartero A.O., Meineche-Schmidt V., Muris J., et al. (2005). Bulking agents, antispasmodic and antidepressant medication for the treatment of irritable bowel syndrome. Cochrane Database of Systematic Reviews. Issue 2. Cochrane Review.

5. Lesbros-Pantoflickova D., Michetti P., Fried M., et al. (2004). Meta-analysis: the treatment of irritable bowel syndrome. *Aliment Pharmacol Ther 20*:1253-69.

6. Bijkerk C.J., Muris J.W., Knottnerus J.A., et al. (2004). Systematic review: the roles of different types of fibre in the treatment of irritable bowel syndrome. *Aliment Pharmacol Ther 19*:245-51.

Low Back Pain

Principles of Therapy

Low back pain is exceedingly common, occurring in over 80% of the population. The differential diagnosis is broad and includes disk herniation, degenerative arthritis, and metastatic cancer. Among the many suffers of low back pain, the diagnostic challenge is to discern those few patients who require additional diagnostic work up. In principle, this means identifying those patients whose pain is due to infection, carcinoma, inflammatory back disease, disk herniation, spondylitic syndromes, and leaking aortic aneurysm. Most back pain resolves within several weeks to one month, and early mobilization is generally recommended following the acute attack. Pharmacotherapy is only marginally effective in many of these syndromes and is comprised primarily of nonsteroidal anti-inflammatory medications, steroid injections, and opioids in some patients. A newer therapy using the anticonvulsants, particularly pregabalin, is proving significantly effective in some patients.

Practical considerations regarding low back pain in the breastfeeding mother include factors which may predispose to musculo-skeletal low back pain, such as poor positioning for infant feeding and poor mechanics for lifting/carrying the infant. Discussion regarding these issues should be considered in breastfeeding mothers with low back pain as a new complaint. Prospective studies regarding epidural anesthesia have not supported an association with chronic back pain.

Treatment

- Most back pain resolves within several weeks to one month.

- Early mobilization is generally recommended following the acute attack.

- Medications include:
  - Nonsteroidal anti-inflammatory medications
  - Steroid injections
  - Opioids in rare cases
  - Anticonvulsants, particularly gabapentin or pregabalin, are proving significantly effective in some patients

Medications

- ACETAMINOPHEN   (*Tempra, Tylenol, Paracetamol*)
  - AAP = Maternal Medication Usually Compatible with Breastfeeding

- ○ LRC = L1
- ○ RID = 8.8-24.2%
- ○ Pregnancy = B
- ○ Comment: Only small amounts are secreted into breastmilk and are considered too small to be hazardous. In a study of 11 mothers who received 650 mg of acetaminophen orally, the highest milk levels reported were from 10-15 mg/L. In another study of three patients who received a single 500 mg oral dose, the reported milk and plasma concentrations of acetaminophen were 4.2 mg/L and 5.6 mg/L, respectively. The milk/plasma ratio was 0.76. The maximum observed concentration in milk was 4.4 mg/L. In another study of women who ingested 1000 mg acetaminophen, milk levels averaged 6.1 mg/L and provided an average dose of 0.92 mg/kg/d according to the authors. There seems to be wide variation in the milk concentrations in these studies, but the relative infant dose is probably less than 6.4% of the maternal dose. This is significantly less than the pediatric therapeutic dose. Acetaminophen is compatible with breastfeeding.

- AMITRIPTYLINE (*Elavil, Endep*)
  - ○ AAP = Drugs whose effect on nursing infants is unknown but may be of concern
  - ○ LRC = L2
  - ○ RID = 1.9-2.8%
  - ○ Pregnancy = C
  - ○ Comment: Amitriptyline and its active metabolite, nortriptyline, are secreted into breastmilk in small amounts. In one report of a mother taking 100 mg/day of amitriptyline, milk levels of amitriptyline and nortriptyline (active metabolite) averaged 143 µg/L and 55.5 µg/L, respectively. No drug was detected in the infant's serum. From these data, an infant would consume approximately 21.5 µg/kg/day, a dose that is unlikely to be clinically relevant.

    In another study following a maternal dose of 25 mg/day, the amitriptyline and nortriptyline (active metabolite) levels in milk were 30 µg/L and <30 µg/L, respectively. In the same study when the dosage was 75 mg/day, milk levels of amitriptyline and nortriptyline averaged 88 µg/L and 69 µg/L, respectively. Both drugs were essentially undetectable in the infant's serum. Therefore, the authors estimated that a nursing infant would receive less than 0.1 mg/day.

    In another mother taking 175 mg/day, amitriptyline levels in the mother's milk were the same as in her serum on day one (24-27 µg/mL), but milk levels decreased to 54% of the serum concentration on days 2 to 26. Milk concentrations of nortriptyline were 74% of that in the mother's serum (87 ng/mL). Thus the authors reported the absolute infant dose as 35 µg/kg, 80 times lower than the mother's dose. Neither compound could be detected in the infant's serum on day 26, nor were there any signs of sedation or other adverse effects.

- AMOXAPINE (*Asendin*)
  - ○ AAP = Drugs whose effect on nursing infants is unknown but may be of concern
  - ○ LRC = L2
  - ○ RID = 0.6%
  - ○ Pregnancy = C
  - ○ Comment: Amoxapine and its metabolite are both secreted into breastmilk at relatively low levels. Following a dose of 250 mg/day, milk levels of amoxapine were less than 20 µg/L and 113 µg/L of the active metabolite. Milk levels of the active metabolite varied from 113 to 168 µg/L in two other

milk samples. Maternal serum levels of amoxapine and metabolite at steady state were 97 µg/L and 375 µg/L, respectively.

- **CODEINE** *(Empirin #3 # 4, Tylenol # 3 # 4)*

  ◦ AAP = Maternal Medication Usually Compatible with Breastfeeding
  ◦ LRC = L3
  ◦ RID = 8.1%
  ◦ Pregnancy = C
  ◦ Comment: Codeine is considered a mild opiate analgesic, whose action is probably due to its metabolism to small amounts (about 7%) of morphine. The amount of codeine secreted into milk is low and dose dependent. Infant response is higher during the neonatal period (first or second week). Four cases of neonatal apnea have been reported following administration of 60 mg codeine every four to six hours to breastfeeding mothers, although codeine was not detected in serum of the infants tested. Apnea resolved after discontinuation of maternal codeine.

    In a study of seven mothers, codeine and morphine levels were studied in breastmilk of 17 samples, and neonatal plasma of 24 samples from 11 healthy term neonates. Milk codeine levels ranged from 33.8 to 314 µg/L 20 to 240 minutes after codeine; morphine levels ranged from 1.9 to 20.5 µg/L. Infant plasma samples one to four hours after feeding had codeine levels ranging from <0.8 to 4.5 µg/L; morphine ranged from <0.5 to 2.2 µg/L. The authors suggest that moderate codeine use during breastfeeding (< or = four 60 mg doses) is probably safe.

    In a recent report, an infant death was reported following the use of codeine (initially two tablets every 12 hours, reduced to half that dose from day two to two weeks because of maternal somnolence and constipation) in a mother. Codeine levels in milk were reported to be 87 µg/L, while the average reported milk levels in most mothers range from 1.9 to 20.5 µg/L at doses of 60 mg every six hours. Genotype analysis of this specific mother indicated that she was an ultra-rapid metabolizer of codeine. This genotype (which is very rare) leads to increased formation of morphine from codeine.

    Ultimately, each infant's response to exposure to codeine should be independently determined. In the vast majority of mothers, codeine taken in moderation should be safe for their breastfed infant. However, any report of overt somnolence, apnea, poor feeding, or grey skin should be reported to the physician and could be associated with exposure to codeine.

- **GABAPENTIN** *(Neurontin)*

  ◦ AAP = Not reviewed
  ◦ LRC = L2
  ◦ RID = 6.6%
  ◦ Pregnancy = C
  ◦ Comment: Gabapentin is a newer anticonvulsant used primarily for partial (focal) seizures with or without secondary generalization. It is also used for postherpetic neuralgia or neuropathic pain. Unlike many anticonvulsants, gabapentin is almost completely excreted renally without metabolism, does not induce hepatic enzymes, and is remarkably well tolerated. In a study of one breastfeeding mother who was receiving 1800 mg/d, milk levels were 11.1, 11.3, and 11.0 mg/L at two, four, and eight hours, respectively, following a dose of 600 mg. No adverse effects to gabapentin were noted in the infant. In another patient receiving 2400 mg/d, milk levels were 9.8, 9.0, and 7.2 mg/L at two, four, and eight hours, respectively, after a dose of 800 mg. Using these data, an infant would

consume approximately 3.7% to 6.5% of the weight-adjusted maternal dose per day. No adverse events were noted in these two infants.

In another study of five mother-infant pairs receiving 900-3200 mg gabapentin per day, the mean milk/plasma ratio ranged from 0.7 to 1.3 from two weeks to three months postpartum. At two to three weeks, two of the five infants had detectable concentrations of gabapentin (1.3 and 1.5 μM), and one was undetectable. These levels were far below the normal plasma levels in the mothers (11-45 μM). Assuming a daily milk intake of 150 mL/day/kg, the infant dose of gabapentin was estimated to be 0.2-1.3 mg/kg/day, which is equivalent to 1.3-3.8% of the weight-normalized dose received by the mother. The plasma levels of gabapentin collected after three months of breastfeeding in another infant was 1.9 μM. The authors concluded that the plasma levels measured were low, if at all detectable, in the infants, and no adverse effects were reported in these infants.

- HYDROCODONE   (*Lortab, Vicodin*)
  - ◦ AAP = Not reviewed
  - ◦ LRC = L3
  - ◦ RID = 3.1-3.7%
  - ◦ Pregnancy = B
  - ◦ Comment: Hydrocodone is a narcotic analgesic and antitussive structurally related to codeine although somewhat more potent. It is commonly used in breastfeeding mothers throughout the USA. In a study of two breastfeeding women taking hydrocodone for various periods, patient one received a total of 63,525 μg (998.8 μg/kg) over 86.5 hours. Patient two, received 9075 μg (123.5 μg/kg) over 36 hours.

    In patient one, the AUC of the drug concentration in milk was 4946.1 μg/L.hr and an average milk concentration of 57.2 μg/L. The authors estimate the relative infant dose at 3.1%. In patient two, the AUC of the drug concentration in milk was 735.6 μg/L.hr and an average milk concentration of 20.4 μg/L. The authors estimate the relative infant dose at 3.7%. This paper concluded that high doses of hydrocodone in mothers who are nursing newborn or premature infants can be concerning. Mothers should be advised to watch for sedation and appropriate weight gain in their infants.

- IBUPROFEN   (*Advil, Nuprin, Motrin, Pediaprofen*)
  - ◦ AAP = Maternal Medication Usually Compatible with Breastfeeding
  - ◦ LRC = L1
  - ◦ RID = 0.1-0.7%
  - ◦ Pregnancy = B in first and second trimester
  - ◦ Comment: Ibuprofen is a nonsteroidal anti-inflammatory analgesic. It is frequently used for fever in infants. Ibuprofen enters milk only in very low levels (less than 0.6% of maternal dose). Even large doses produce very small milk levels. In a study of 12 women who received 400 mg doses every six hours for a total of five doses, all breastmilk levels of ibuprofen were less than 1.0 mg/L, the lower limit of the assay. Data in these studies document that no measurable concentrations of ibuprofen are detected in breastmilk following the above doses. Ibuprofen is presently popular for therapy of fever in infants. Current recommended dose in children is 5-10 mg/kg every six hours. Ibuprofen is an ideal analgesic for breastfeeding mothers.

- IMIPRAMINE   (*Tofranil, Janimine*)
  - ◦ AAP = Drugs whose effect on nursing infants is unknown but may be of concern

- ○ LRC = L2
- ○ RID = 0.1-4.4%
- ○ Pregnancy = D
- ○ Comment: Imipramine is a classic tricyclic antidepressant. Imipramine is metabolized to desipramine, the active metabolite. Milk levels approximate those of maternal serum. In a patient receiving 200 mg daily at bedtime, the milk levels at 1, 9, 10, and 23 hours were 29, 24, 12, and 18 μg/L, respectively. However, in this previous study, the mother was not in a therapeutic range. In a mother with full therapeutic levels, it is suggested that an infant would ingest approximately 0.2 mg/L of milk. This represents a dose of only 30 μg/kg/day, far less than the 1.5 mg/kg dose recommended for older children. The long half-life of this medication in infants could, under certain conditions, lead to high plasma levels, although they have not been reported. Although no untoward effects have been reported, the infant should be monitored closely. Therapeutic plasma levels in children 6-12 years are 200-225 ng/mL. Two good reviews of psychotropic drugs in breastfeeding patients are available.

- **METAXALONE** (*Skelaxin*)
  - ○ AAP = Not reviewed
  - ○ LRC = L3
  - ○ RID =
  - ○ Pregnancy =
  - ○ Comment: Metaxalone is a centrally acting sedative used primarily as a muscle relaxant. Its ability to relax skeletal muscle is weak and is probably due to its sedative properties. Hypersensitivity reactions in adults (allergic) have occurred as well as liver toxicity. No data are available on its transfer into breastmilk.

- **NAPROXEN** (*Anaprox, Naprosyn, Aleve*)
  - ○ AAP = Maternal Medication Usually Compatible with Breastfeeding
  - ○ LRC = L3
  - ○ RID = 3.3%
  - ○ Pregnancy = C
  - ○ Comment: Naproxen is a popular NSAID analgesic. In a study done at steady state in one mother consuming 375 mg twice daily, milk levels ranged from 1.76-2.37 mg/L at four hours. Total naproxen excretion in the infant's urine was only 0.26% of the maternal dose. Although the amount of naproxen transferred via milk is minimal, one should use with caution in nursing mothers because of its long half-life and its effect on infant cardiovascular system, kidneys, and GI tract. However, its short term use postpartum or infrequent or occasional use would not necessarily be incompatible with breastfeeding. One case of prolonged bleeding, hemorrhage, and acute anemia has been reported in a seven-day-old infant. The relative infant dose on a weight-adjusted maternal daily dose would probably be less than 3.3%.

- **PREGABALIN** (*Lyrica*)
  - ○ AAP = Not reviewed
  - ○ LRC = L3
  - ○ RID =
  - ○ Pregnancy = C

- ○ Comment: Pregabalin binds to a subunit of voltage gated calcium channels in central nervous system tissues reducing the calcium-dependant release of several neurotransmitters. It is used in the management of neuropathic pain associated with diabetic peripheral neuropathy and postherpetic neuralgia. There are no data available on the transfer of pregabalin into human milk. However, due to the kinetics of the drug, its passage into the milk compartment is probable, and its oral bioavailability to the infant would be high. Therefore, nursing mothers should use caution taking pregabalin while nursing.

- TRAMADOL   (*Ultram, Ultracet*)
  - ○ AAP = Not reviewed
  - ○ LRC = L2
  - ○ RID = 2.9%
  - ○ Pregnancy = C
  - ○ Comment: Tramadol is a new class analgesic that most closely resembles the opiates, although it is not a controlled substance and appears to have reduced addictive potential. It appears to be slightly more potent than codeine. After oral use, its onset of analgesia is within one hour and reaches a peak in two to three hours. Following a single IV 100 mg dose of tramadol, the cumulative excretion in breastmilk within 16 hours was 100 µg of tramadol (0.1% of the maternal dose) and 27 µg of the M1 metabolite.

    In a recent study of 75 mothers who received 100 mg every six hours after cesarean section, milk samples were taken on days two through four postpartum in transitional milk. At steady state, the Milk/Plasma ratio averaged 2.4 for rac-tramadol and 2.8 for rac-O-desmethyltramadol. The estimated absolute and relative infant doses were 112 µg/kg/day and 30 µg/kg/day for rac-tramadol and its desmethyl metabolite. The relative infant dose was 2.24% and 0.64% for rac-tramadol and its desmethyl metabolite, respectively. No significant neurobehavioral adverse effects were noted between controls and exposed infants.

Clinical Tips

Treatment of low back pain is generally palliative at best. For the most part, the NSAIDs are poorly effective, but may be used briefly. Ibuprofen should be preferred, as milk levels are negligible. Naproxen could be used briefly. The use of the tricyclic antidepressants for chronic pain is well documented and is compatible with breastfeeding. Amitriptyline and imipramine have been well studied in breastfeeding women and appear safe in most instances. New studies have shown that the newer anticonvulsants, such as gabapentin and pregabalin, are significantly effective in chronic low back pain and radiculopathy. Although any of the anticonvulsants may be used, such as valproic acid or carbamazepine, the minimal side effect profile of gabapentin makes it a favorite with patients. Although we have limited data on gabapentin use in breastfeeding mothers, its relative safety in humans is encouraging. While skeletal muscle relaxants have been used extensively, most studies find them minimally effective. Codeine and hydrocodone can be used in some patients in acute pain. Long-term therapy is not advised.

Suggested Reading

Burnett, C., & Day, M. (2008). Recent advancements in the treatment of lumbar radicular pain. *Curr Opin Anaesthesiol, 21*(4), 452-456.

Chou, R., Atlas, S. J., Stanos, S. P., & Rosenquist, R. W. (2009). Nonsurgical interventional therapies for low back pain: a review of the evidence for an American Pain Society clinical practice guideline. *Spine (Phila Pa 1976), 34*(10), 1078-1093.

Chou, R., Loeser, J. D., Owens, D. K., Rosenquist, R. W., Atlas, S. J., Baisden, J., et al. (2009). Interventional therapies, surgery, and interdisciplinary rehabilitation for low back pain: an evidence-based clinical practice guideline from the American Pain Society. *Spine (Phila Pa 1976), 34*(10), 1066-1077.

Chou, R., Qaseem, A., Snow, V., Casey, D., Cross, J. T. J., Shekelle, P., et al. (2007). Diagnosis and treatment of low back pain: a joint clinical practice guideline from the American College of Physicians and the American Pain Society. *Ann Intern Med, 147*(7), 478-491.

Cunningham, C. G., Flynn, T. A., Toole, C. M., Ryan, R. G., Gueret, P. W., Bulfin, S., et al. (2008). Working Backs Project--implementing low back pain guidelines. *Occup Med (Lond), 58*(8), 580-583.

Heran, M. K., Smith, A. D., & Legiehn, G. M. (2008). Spinal injection procedures: a review of concepts, controversies, and complications. *Radiol Clin North Am, 46*(3), 487-514.

Hush, J. M. (2008). Clinical management of occupational low back pain in Australia: what is the real picture? *J Occup Rehabil, 18*(4), 375-380.

Manchikanti, L., Singh, V., Helm, S. n., Trescot, A. M., & Hirsch, J. A. (2008). A critical appraisal of 2007 American College of Occupational and Environmental Medicine (ACOEM) Practice Guidelines for Interventional Pain Management: an independent review utilizing AGREE, AMA, IOM, and other criteria. *Pain Physician, 11*(3), 291-310.

Roelofs, P. D., Deyo, R. A., Koes, B. W., Scholten, R. J., & van Tulder, M. W. (2008). Nonsteroidal anti-inflammatory drugs for low back pain: an updated Cochrane review. *Spine (Phila Pa 1976), 33*(16), 1766-1774.

See, S., & Ginzburg, R. (2008). Choosing a skeletal muscle relaxant. *Am Fam Physician, 78*(3), 365-370.

Staal, J. B., de Bie, R., de Vet, H. C., Hildebrandt, J., & Nelemans, P. (2008). Injection therapy for subacute and chronic low-back pain. *Cochrane Database Syst Rev, 3*, CD001824.

Vleeming, A., Albert, H. B., Ostgaard, H. C., Sturesson, B., & Stuge, B. (2008). European guidelines for the diagnosis and treatment of pelvic girdle pain. *Eur Spine J, 17*(6), 794-819.

Lyme Disease

Principles of Therapy

Lyme disease is a systemic illness caused by the spirochete *Borrelia burgdorferi*. *B. burgdorferi* has been isolated from many tissues, including blood, skin, and cerebrospinal fluid. However, culture from the various sites is often inconclusive and a low-yield procedure. The primary mode of transmission is via the deer tick bite. The tick must feed for 72 hours prior to transmission of the spirochetes. The disease is endemic in most of the northeastern USA, Minnesota, Wisconsin, Oregon, and northern California. Over 90% of cases occur in Connecticut, Delaware, Maryland, Massachusetts, Minnesota, New Jersey, New York, Pennsylvania, Rhode Island, and Wisconsin. While common in the northeastern part of the USA, it also occurs commonly in Europe, where it is transmitted by the sheep tick, Ixodes rincus. Within days to weeks following a tick bite, almost 80% of patients will have a red, expanding "bullseye" rash (called erythema migrans) accompanied by general fever, tiredness, headache, stiff neck, muscle aches, and joint pain. If untreated, some patients may develop arthritis, including intermittent episodes of swelling and pain in the large joints; neurologic abnormalities, such as aseptic meningitis, facial palsy, motor and sensory nerve inflammation (radiculoneuritis), and inflammation of the brain (encephalitis); and, rarely, cardiac problems, such as atrioventricular block, acute inflammation of the tissues surrounding the heart (myopericarditis), or enlarged heart (cardiomegaly). The clinical features of Lyme disease can be differentiated into three general stages: early localized, early disseminated, and later chronic infection. Acute infection with a vigorous inflammatory reaction is responsible for the most commonly observed clinical manifestations of Lyme disease. Features such as neurologic deficits and chronic arthritis occur much later and also respond poorly to treatment. It is not certain that live organisms are responsible for these late manifestations. Erythema migrans (erythematous macule or papule), the hallmark of Lyme disease, occurs at the site of the tick bite generally within 3-32 days. While the lesion may be warm, pruritic, and painful, it is often asymptomatic and easily missed. Spirochetes are readily cultured at this stage from the margins of the infection. Treatment largely depends on the stage of infection. Early infections respond effectively to penicillins, erythromycins, tetracyclines, and cephalosporins.

Treatment

- Prophylaxis: one single dose of doxycycline 200 mg after tick bite.

- Doxycycline (100 mg orally twice daily for 10-21 days) is the drug of choice for non-pregnant patients.

- Other antibiotic options include amoxicillin (500 mg three times daily for 14-21 days) and cefuroxime (500 mg orally twice daily for 14-21 days).

- For neurological involvement, IV ceftriaxone, penicillin, or cefotaxime is preferred.

Medications

- AMOXICILLIN (*Larotid, Amoxil*)
  - AAP = Maternal Medication Usually Compatible with Breastfeeding
  - LRC = L1
  - RID = 1%
  - Pregnancy = B
  - Comment: Amoxicillin is a popular oral penicillin used for otitis media and many other pediatric/adult infections. In one group of six mothers who received 1 gm oral doses, the concentration of amoxicillin in breastmilk ranged from 0.68 to 1.3 mg/L of milk (average= 0.9 mg/L). Peak levels occurred at four to five hours. Milk/plasma ratios at one, two, and three hours were 0.014, 0.013, and 0.043. Less than 0.95% of the maternal dose is secreted into milk. No harmful effects have been reported.

- AZITHROMYCIN (*Zithromax*)
  - AAP = Not reviewed
  - LRC = L2
  - RID = 5.9%
  - Pregnancy = B
  - Comment: Azithromycin belongs to the erythromycin family. It has an extremely long half-life, particularly in tissues. Azithromycin is concentrated for long periods in phagocytes, which are known to be present in human milk. In one study of a patient who received 1 gm initially followed by 500 mg doses each at 24 hour intervals, the concentration of azithromycin in breastmilk varied from 0.64 mg/L (initially) to 2.8 mg/L on day three. The predicted dose of azithromycin received by the infant would be approximately 0.4 mg/kg/day. This would suggest that the level of azithromycin ingested by a breastfeeding infant is not clinically relevant. New pediatric formulations of azithromycin have been recently introduced. Pediatric dosing is 10 mg/kg STAT followed by 5 mg/kg per day for up to five days.

- CEFTRIAXONE (*Rocephin*)
  - AAP = Maternal Medication Usually Compatible with Breastfeeding
  - LRC = L2
  - RID = 4.1-4.2%
  - Pregnancy = B
  - Comment: Ceftriaxone is a very popular third-generation broad-spectrum cephalosporin antibiotic. Small amounts are transferred into milk (3-4% of maternal serum level). Following a 1 gm IM dose, breastmilk levels were approximately 0.5-0.7 mg/L at between four to eight hours. The estimated mean milk levels at steady state were 3-4 mg/L. Another source indicates that following a 2 g/d dose and at steady state, approximately 4.4% of dose penetrates into milk. In this study, the maximum breastmilk concentration was 7.89 mg/L after prolonged therapy (seven days). Poor oral absorption of ceftriaxone would further limit systemic absorption by the infant. The half-life of ceftriaxone in human milk varies from 12.8 to 17.3 hours (longer than maternal serum). Even at this high dose, no adverse effects were noted in the infant. Ceftriaxone levels in breastmilk are probably too low to be clinically relevant, except for changes in GI flora. Ceftriaxone is commonly used in neonates.

- CEFUROXIME   (*Ceftin, Zinacef, Kefurox*)
  - ○ AAP = Not reviewed
  - ○ LRC = L2
  - ○ RID = 0.6-2%
  - ○ Pregnancy = B
  - ○ Comment: Cefuroxime is a broad-spectrum second-generation cephalosporin antibiotic that is available orally and IV. The manufacturer states that it is secreted into human milk in small amounts, but the levels are not available.

    In a study of 38 mothers who received cefuroxime, 2.6% reported mild side effects that were not significantly different from controls (9%). Cefuroxime has a very bitter taste. The IV salt form, cefuroxime sodium, is very poorly absorbed orally. Only the axetil salt form is orally bioavailable.

- DOXYCYCLINE   (*Doxychel, Vibramycin, Periostat*)
  - ○ AAP = Not reviewed
  - ○ LRC = L3
  - ○ RID = 4.2-13.3%
  - ○ Pregnancy = D
  - ○ Comment: Doxycycline is a long half-life tetracycline antibiotic. In a study of 15 subjects, the average doxycycline level in milk was 0.77 mg/L following a 200 mg oral dose. One oral dose of 100 mg was administered 24 hours later, and the breastmilk levels were 0.380 mg/L. Following a dose of 100 mg daily in ten mothers, doxycycline levels in milk on day two averaged 0.82 mg/L (range 0.37-1.24 mg/L) at three hours after the dose, and 0.46 mg/L (range 0.3-0.91 mg/L) 24 hours after the dose. The relative infant dose in an infant would be < 6% of the maternal weight-adjusted dosage. Following a single dose of 100 mg in three women or 200 mg in three women, peak milk levels occurred between two and four hours following the dose. The average "peak" milk levels were 0.96 mg/L (100 mg dose) or 1.8 mg/L (200 mg dose). After repeated dosing for five days, milk levels averaged 3.6 mg/L at doses of 100 mg twice daily. In a study of 13 women receiving 100-200 mg doses of doxycycline, peak levels in milk were 0.6 mg/L (n=3 @100 mg dose) and 1.1 mg/L (n=11 @ 200 mg dose).

    Tetracyclines administered orally to infants are known to bind in teeth, producing discoloration and inhibiting bone growth, although doxycycline and oxytetracycline stain teeth the least severe. Although most tetracyclines secreted into milk are generally bound to calcium, thus inhibiting their absorption, doxycycline is the least bound (20%), and may be better absorbed in a breastfeeding infant than the older tetracyclines. While the absolute absorption of older tetracyclines may be dramatically reduced by calcium salts, the newer doxycycline and minocycline analogs bind less and their overall absorption, while slowed, may be significantly higher than earlier versions. Prolonged use (months) could potentially alter GI flora and induce dental staining, although doxycycline produces the least dental staining. Short term use (three-four weeks) is not contraindicated. No harmful effects have yet been reported in breastfeeding infants, but prolonged use (> 4 weeks) is not advised. For prolonged administration, such as for exposure to anthrax, check the CDC website as they have published specific dosing guidelines.

- LYME DISEASE VACCINE   (*LYMErix*)
  - ○ AAP = Not reviewed

- LRC = L2
- RID =
- Pregnancy = C
- Comment: LYMErix is a noninfectious recombinant vaccine containing a lipoprotein from the outer surface of *Borrelia burgdorferi*. The lipoprotein from this causative agent is a single polypeptide chain of 257 amino acids with lipids covalently bonded to the N terminus. No substance of animal origin is used in the manufacturing process. It is primarily indicated for individuals 15-70 years of age. It is very unlikely to enter milk. Officials from the CDC suggest that it is not contraindicated for use in breastfeeding patients.

Clinical Tips

According to the CDC, antibiotic treatment for 3 to 4 weeks with doxycycline or amoxicillin is generally effective in early disease. Treatment protocols for early Lyme disease now consist of Amoxicillin 500 mg three times daily for 14-21 days; Doxycycline 100 mg twice daily for 21 days; cefuroxime axetil 500 mg twice daily for 21 days; or azithromycin 500 mg daily for seven days (less effective than prior regimens, not recommended for initial therapy). Any of the above regimens are useful in breastfeeding women. Amoxicillin, cefuroxime, and azithromycin levels in breastmilk have been measured and are small. Loose stools or candida superinfections in the infant are possible. Doxycycline, while not ideal in breastfeeding mothers and their infants, would not be a major problem when used for only three weeks. The absorption of doxycycline is reduced, though not eliminated, by calcium salts present in milk. For treatment of later manifestations, such as arthritis or neurologic changes, similar antibiotics are used (ceftriaxone, penicillin G, doxycycline), except the doses are higher and more prolonged. Consult a current guide to antimicrobial therapy for further treatment protocols. Breastfeeding mothers can continue to nurse as soon as they are started on treatment.

The Lyme vaccine (LYMErix) is a noninfectious recombinant vaccine containing a lipoprotein from the outer surface of Borrelia burgdorferi. The lipoprotein from this causative agent is a single polypeptide chain of 257 amino acids with lipids covalently bonded to the N terminus. It is primarily indicated for individuals 15-70 years of age. It is very unlikely to enter milk. Officials from the CDC suggest that it is not contraindicated for use in breastfeeding patients.

Suggested Reading

Bratton, R. L., Whiteside, J. W., Hovan, M. J., Engle, R. L., & Edwards, F. D. (2008). Diagnosis and treatment of Lyme disease. *Mayo Clin Proc, 83*(5), 566-571.

Clark, R. P., & Hu, L. T. (2008). Prevention of lyme disease and other tick-borne infections. *Infect Dis Clin North Am, 22*(3), 381-396, vii.

Edlow, J. A. (1999). Lyme disease and related tick-borne illnesses. *Ann Emerg Med, 33*(6), 680-693.

Larkin, J. M. (2008). Lyme disease in children and pregnant women. *Med Health R I, 91*(7), 212.

Mitty, J., & Margolius, D. (2008). Updates and controversies in the treatment of Lyme disease. *Med Health R I, 91*(7), 222-223.

Morey, S. S. (1999). ACIP issues recommendations for Lyme disease vaccine. Advisory Committee on Immunization Practices. *Am Fam Physician, 60*(7), 2171-2172.

Nadelman, R. B., & Wormser, G. P. (1998). Lyme borreliosis. *Lancet, 352*(9127), 557-565.

Stanek, G., & Strle, F. (2003). Lyme borreliosis. *Lancet, 362*(9396), 1639-1647.

Vanousova, D., & Hercogova, J. (2008). Lyme borreliosis treatment. *Dermatol Ther, 21*(2), 101-109.

Walsh, C. A., Mayer, E. W., & Baxi, L. V. (2007). Lyme disease in pregnancy: case report and review of the literature. *Obstet Gynecol Surv, 62*(1), 41-50.

Wormser, G. P. (2006). Clinical practice. Early Lyme disease. *N Engl J Med, 354*(26), 2794-2801.

Malaria

Principles of Therapy

Malaria is one of the oldest reported diseases and has infected more than 500 million humans world-wide. Symptoms include history of exposure in a malaria-endemic area, periodic attacks of chills, fever and sweating, headache, myalgia, splenomegaly, and anemia. Four Plasmodium species cause human malaria: *Plasmodium vivax, P. malariae, P. ovale, and P. falciparum. Plasmodium vivax* and *falciparum* account for most infections. The infective agent is the sporozoite, which is injected into the human by the bite of the mosquito. Treatment is separated into two modalities: prophylaxis treatment to prevent the disease or suppressive treatment to destroy the parasite. Treatment and prophylaxis have become increasingly difficult in recent years due to the spread of drug-resistant species. Resistance to chloroquine, primaquine, and now mefloquine is growing rapidly, and many regions of the world must depend on newer antimalarials for protection. Treating malaria appropriately requires knowledge of the infecting species, the location where the species was acquired, and the geographic patterns of drug resistance. Treatment of malaria is two-fold, 1) prophylaxis or prevention of infection, and 2) treat symptoms of prior or new infection. Fortunately, we have several good studies showing that the transfer of most antimalarials into human milk is quite low. Because infants who travel or live in these endemic areas must be prophylaxed anyway, the amount in breastmilk, which is small, is seldom relevant. For a complete review of medications used for malaria by country, contact the Centers for Disease Control.

Treatment

* The strain of Plasmodium can usually be determined by the Geimsa stain, although 6% of malaria cases include multiple strains. The choice of medication is based on the strain, as well as the area where the patient likely contracted malaria, as resistance varies.

* WHO Treatment recommendations include:
    1. artemether-lumefantrine (six-dose regimen)
    2. Amodiaquine + artesunate
    3. Mefloquine + artesunate
    4. artesunate + sulfadoxine-pyrimethamine
    5. amodiaquine + sulfadoxine-pyrimethamine

* Most drugs used in treatment are active against the parasite forms in the blood (the form that causes disease) and include:
    1. Chloroquine
    2. Sulfadoxine-pyrimethamine (Fansidar®)
    3. Mefloquine (Lariam®)
    4. Atovaquone-proguanil (Malarone®)

5. Quinine
6. Doxycycline
7. Artemisin derivatives (not licensed for use in the United States, but often found overseas)

Medications

- ATOVAQUONE AND PROGUANIL   (*Malarone*)
  - ○ AAP = Not reviewed
  - ○ LRC = L3
  - ○ RID =
  - ○ Pregnancy = C
  - ○ Comment: Malarone is a fixed combination of atovaquone (250 mg) and proguanil (100 mg) (adult dose). The pediatric chewable tablet contains atovaquone (62.5) and proguanil (25 mg). Malarone is used both to prevent and treat malaria, particularly malaria resistant to certain other drugs. Both adult and pediatric formulations are available for treating pediatric patients down to 11 kg. There are no data available for transfer of these agents into human milk, although the pharmaceutical company suggests that atovaquone concentrations in rodent milk were 30% of the concurrent concentrations in the maternal plasma. It is this author's experience that rodent levels are much higher than the levels found in humans. Only trace quantities of proguanil were found in human milk. Further, while the pharmacokinetics of proguanil is similar in adults and pediatric patients, the elimination half-life of atovaquone is much shorter in pediatric patients (one to two days) than in adult patients (two to three days). Elimination half-life ranges from 32 to 84 hours for atovaquone and 12 to 21 hours for proguanil; the half-life of cycloguanil is approximately 14 hours.

- CHLOROQUINE   (*Aralen, Novo-Chloroquine*)
  - ○ AAP = Maternal Medication Usually Compatible with Breastfeeding
  - ○ LRC = L2
  - ○ RID = 0.6 - 1.1%
  - ○ Pregnancy = C
  - ○ Comment: Chloroquine is an antimalarial drug. In a group of six women who received 5 mg/kg IM during delivery, and then again at 17 days postpartum, milk levels averaged 0.227 mg/L and ranged from 0.192 to 0.319 mg/L. The milk/blood ratio ranged from 0.268 to 0.462. Based on these levels, the infant would consume approximately 34 µg/kg/day, an amount considered safe. If an infant consumed 500 mL/day of milk, it would receive an average of 113.5 µg of chloroquine per day. Other studies have shown absorption to vary from 2.2 to 4.2% of maternal dose. The breastmilk concentration of chloroquine in this study averaged 0.58 mg/L following a single dose of 600 mg.

    In a recent study of 16 women day three to 17-21 postpartum, the average concentration in milk (AUC) during the sampling time was 167 µg/L for chloroquine and 54 µg/L for desethylchloroquine, the possibly active metabolite.   Estimated absolute and relative infant doses were 34 µg/kg/day and 15 µg/kg/day, and 2.3% and 1.0% for chloroquine and desethylchloroquine, respectively. The authors suggested that chloroquine was compatible with breastfeeding.

    The current recommended pediatric dose for patients exposed to malaria is 8.3 mg/kg per week, which greatly exceeds that present in breastmilk.

- DOXYCYCLINE   (*Doxychel, Vibramycin, Periostat*)
  - ○ AAP = Not reviewed
  - ○ LRC = L3
  - ○ RID = 4.2-13.3%
  - ○ Pregnancy = D
  - ○ Comment: Doxycycline is a long half-life tetracycline antibiotic. In a study of 15 subjects, the average doxycycline level in milk was 0.77 mg/L following a 200 mg oral dose. One oral dose of 100 mg was administered 24 hours later, and the breastmilk levels were 0.380 mg/L.

    Following a dose of 100 mg daily in 10 mothers, doxycycline levels in milk on day two averaged 0.82 mg/L (range 0.37-1.24 mg/L) at three hours after the dose, and 0.46 mg/L (range 0.3-0.91 mg/L) 24 hours after the dose. The relative infant dose in an infant would be < 6% of the maternal weight-adjusted dosage. Following a single dose of 100 mg in three women or 200 mg in three women, peak milk levels occurred between two and four hours following the dose. The average "peak" milk levels were 0.96 mg/L (100 mg dose) or 1.8 mg/L (200 mg dose). After repeated dosing for five days, milk levels averaged 3.6 mg/L at doses of 100 mg twice daily. In a study of 13 women receiving 100-200 mg doses of doxycycline, peak levels in milk were 0.6 mg/L (n=3 @100 mg dose) and 1.1 mg/L (n=11 @ 200 mg dose).

    Tetracyclines administered orally to infants are known to bind in teeth, producing discoloration and inhibiting bone growth, although doxycycline and oxytetracycline stain teeth the least severe. Although most tetracyclines secreted into milk are generally bound to calcium, thus inhibiting their absorption, doxycycline is the least bound (20%) and may be better absorbed in a breastfeeding infant than the older tetracyclines. While the absolute absorption of older tetracyclines may be dramatically reduced by calcium salts, the newer doxycycline and minocycline analogs bind less and their overall absorption, while slowed, may be significantly higher than earlier versions. Prolonged use (months) could potentially alter GI flora and induce dental staining, although doxycycline produces the least dental staining. Short term use (three-four weeks) is not contraindicated. No harmful effects have yet been reported in breastfeeding infants, but prolonged use is not advised.

- HYDROXYCHLOROQUINE   (*Plaquenil*)
  - ○ AAP = Maternal Medication Usually Compatible with Breastfeeding
  - ○ LRC = L2
  - ○ RID = 2.9%
  - ○ Pregnancy = C
  - ○ Comment: HCQ is known to produce significant retinal damage and blindness if used over a prolonged period, and this could occur (theoretically but unlikely) in breastfed infants. Patients on this product should see an ophthalmologist routinely. It has a huge volume of distribution (Vd) which suggests milk levels will be quite low.

    In one study of a mother receiving 400 mg HCQ daily, the concentrations of HCQ in breastmilk were 1.46, 1.09, and 1.09 mg/L at 2.0, 9.5, and 14 hours after the dose. The average milk concentration was 1.1 mg/L. The milk/plasma ratio was approximately 5.5. On a body-weight basis, the infant's dose would be 2.9% of the maternal dose. In another study of one mother receiving 200 mg twice daily, milk levels were much lower than the previous study. Only a total of 3.2 micrograms of HCQ was detected in her milk over 48 hours.

Two breastfeeding mothers taking hydroxychloroquine were tested to determine the concentration in their breastmilk one week after delivery. The concentrations were 344 and 1424 ng/mL, which corresponded to an infant dose of 0.06 and 0.2 mg/kg/d, respectively. HCQ is mostly metabolized to chloroquine and has an incredibly long half-life. The pediatric dose for malaria prophylaxis is 5 mg/kg/week, far larger than the dose received via milk. See chloroquine.

- MEFLOQUINE (*Lariam*)
  - ○ AAP = Not reviewed
  - ○ LRC = L2
  - ○ RID = 0.1-0.2%
  - ○ Pregnancy = C
  - ○ Comment: Mefloquine is an antimalarial and a structural analog of quinine. It is concentrated in red cells and, therefore, has a long half-life. Following a single 250 mg dose in two women, the milk/plasma ratio was only 0.13 to 0.16 the first four days of therapy. The concentration of mefloquine in milk ranged from 32 to 53 µg/L. Unfortunately, these studies were not carried out after steady state conditions, which would probably increase to some degree the amount transferred to the infant. According to the manufacturer, mefloquine is secreted in small concentrations approximating 3% of the maternal dose. Assuming a milk level of 53 µg/L and a daily milk intake of 150 mL/kg/day, an infant would ingest approximately 8 µg/kg/day of mefloquine, which is not sufficient to protect the infant from malaria. The therapeutic dose for malaria prophylaxis is 62 mg in a 15-19 kg infant. Thus far, no untoward effects have been reported.

- QUINIDINE (*Quinaglute, Quinidex*)
  - ○ AAP = Maternal Medication Usually Compatible with Breastfeeding
  - ○ LRC = L2
  - ○ RID = 14.4%
  - ○ Pregnancy = C
  - ○ Comment: Quinidine is used to treat cardiac arrhythmias. Three hours following a dose of 600 mg, the level of quinidine in the maternal serum was 9.0 mg/L and the concentration in breastmilk was 6.4 mg/L. Subsequently, a level of 8.2 mg/L was noted in breastmilk. Quinidine is selectively stored in the liver. Long-term use could expose an infant to liver toxicity. Monitor liver enzymes.

- QUININE (*Quinamm*)
  - ○ AAP = Maternal Medication Usually Compatible with Breastfeeding
  - ○ LRC = L2
  - ○ RID = 0.7-1.3%
  - ○ Pregnancy = D
  - ○ Comment: Quinine is a cinchona alkaloid primarily used in malaria prophylaxis and treatment. Small to trace amounts are secreted into milk. No reported harmful effects have been reported, except in infants with G6PD deficiencies. In a study of six women receiving 600-1300 mg/day, the concentration of quinine in breastmilk ranged from 0.4 to 1.6 mg/L at 1.5 to 6 hours postdose. The authors suggest these levels are clinically insignificant. In another study, with maternal plasma concentrations of 0.5 to 8 mg/L, the milk/plasma ratio ranged from 0.11 to 0.53. The total daily consumption by a breastfed infant was estimated to be 1-3 mg/day.

- PRIMAQUINE PHOSPHATE
  - AAP = Not reviewed
  - LRC = L3
  - RID =
  - Pregnancy = C
  - Comment: Primaquine is a typical antimalarial medication that is primarily used as chemoprophylaxis after the patient has returned from the region of exposure, with the intention of preventing relapses of plasmodium vivax and or ovale. It is used in pediatric patients at a dose of 0.3 mg/kg/day for 14 days. No data are available on its transfer into human milk. Maternal plasma levels are rather low, only 53-107 nanogram/mL, suggesting that milk levels might be rather low as well.

Clinical Tips

Before any decision to treat or provide malaria prophylaxis is made, the clinician should closely review the excellent CDC website for current recommendations. In addition, the World Health Organization has issued a set of new guidelines on malaria treatment, and treatment with the artemisins has rapidly become one of the major recommendations due to high cure rates with uncomplicated malaria.

Artesunate is now recommended by the World Health Organization (WHO) in preference to quinidine for the treatment of severe malaria and has been used worldwide for many years. In the USA, Coartem (artemether 20 mg/lumefantrine 120 mg) has recently been approved for the treatment of malaria.

Resistance of *P. falciparum* to chloroquine is widespread, but in those areas where it is NOT resistant, once weekly doses of chloroquine are still effective. The clinical dose of chloroquine transferred via milk is quite low, only about 113 μg per day in mothers who received 5 mg/kg IM doses. This is minimal compared to the pediatric dose required for chemoprophylaxis (8.3 mg/kg/week). The amount of hydroxychloroquine transferred into milk is low as well, only about 1.1 mg per liter of milk. The average infant would, therefore, ingest about 0.6 mg per day. Studies with mefloquine indicate that milk levels are very low, less than 53 μg per liter of milk. This is minimal compared to the prophylaxis dose of 4.6 mg/kg/week. The CDC considers mefloquine the drug of choice for chemoprophylaxis in children. The CDC also recommends that mefloquine is preferred for breastfeeding mothers with infants less than 11 kg.

Doxycycline is a suitable choice for antimalarial prophylaxis in many parts of the world. While milk levels of doxycycline and oral bioavailability are low, long-term use (> three to four weeks) is probably not wise in breastfeeding mothers or children less than eight years of age. Quinine transfer into milk is extremely low and is unlikely to be clinically relevant. Estimated transfer of quinine varies with dose, but would likely be less than 1-3 mg daily. In places where quinine is not available, quinidine may be substituted. Quinidine transfer into milk is believed less than 6.4 mg/L of milk. This would be significantly less than pediatric therapeutic doses.

The treament of malaria is a multifaceted and rapidly emerging science. The authors recommend a thorough review of current protocols from the CDC or WHO.

Suggested Reading

CDC. Malaria. Accessed on Jan. 10, 2010 from http://wwwnc.cdc.gov/travel/

CDC. Travelers' Health. Accessed on Jan 10,2010 from http://wwwnc.cdc.gov/travel/

Freedman, D. O. (2008). Clinical practice. Malaria prevention in short-term travelers. *N Engl J Med, 359*(6), 603-612.

Orton, L. C., & Omari, A. A. (2008). Drugs for treating uncomplicated malaria in pregnant women. *Cochrane Database Syst Rev,* (4), CD004912.

Sayang, C., Gausseres, M., Vernazza-Licht, N., Malvy, D., Bley, D., & Millet, P. (2009). Treatment of malaria from monotherapy to artemisinin-based combination therapy by health professionals in urban health facilities in Yaounde, central province, Cameroon. *Malar J, 8*, 176.

Schlagenhauf, P., & Petersen, E. (2008). Malaria chemoprophylaxis: strategies for risk groups. *Clin Microbiol Rev, 21*(3), 466-472.

White, N. J., McGready, R. M., & Nosten, F. H. (2008). New medicines for tropical diseases in pregnancy: catch-22. *PLoS Med, 5*(6), e133.

Wiltz, S. A., Crawford, P., Nichols, W., & Hayes, M. (2008). Clinical inquiries. What is the most effective and safe malaria prophylaxis during pregnancy? *J Fam Pract, 57*(1), 51-53.

Mastitis / Breast Abscess

Principles of Therapy

Mastitis is a common and debilitating condition most often found in lactating women. It occurs most commonly in primigravida, rather than multipara women. Both inflammatory and infectious mastitis have been described, but it is often difficult to differentiate. Most cases are considered infectious and are treated with antibiotic therapy, with more often and complete emptying of the breast. The reported incidence varies, but approximately 20% of lactating women in the first six months postpartum will experience mastitis, with the highest incidence two to three weeks postpartum. Mastitis most likely occurs as a result of introduction of organisms from the infant's mouth and nostrils into an injured nipple. *Staphylococcus aureus* (occasionally penicillin resistant), streptococcus, and to a lesser degree *Escherichia coli* are the primary pathogens. Culture of breastmilk in routine circumstances is probably unwarranted, but certan circumstances may indicate otherwise, such as recurrent or persistent infections. Additionally, hospital acquired infections in areas of high methicillin resistant *Staphylococcus aureus* may provide reason to consider culture. Purported predisposing factors include stress, fatigue, anemia, prior breast surgery, improper fitting bras, poor emptying of the breast, missed feeding with engorgement, overabundant milk supply, too frequent or infrequent feeds, cracked or damaged nipples, and plugged ducts. A recent study of mastitis occurring in 946 breastfeeding women found an incidence of 9.5% in the first three months postpartum. In this particular study, factors associated with mastitis include a history of mastitis with a prior infant, cracks and sore nipple within the preceding week, using anti-fungal cream within the preceding three weeks, and using a manual breast pump. Discomfort for the mother can range from mild tenderness to severe breast pain with fever, chills, malaise, flu-like symptoms, and myalgias. Wedge-shaped areas of the breast will appear pink, hot, swollen, and extremely tender. Breast abscess occurs in 5-10% of cases of mastitis and may be associated with delayed or inadequate treatment of mastitis. Treatment of mastitis includes antibiotics, rest, frequent milk removal, and pain control, often with an anti-inflammatory medication, such as ibuprofen. Most authorities recommend antibiotic treatment for 10 to 14 days. There is no evidence that continued breastfeeding is harmful to the healthy full term nursing infant, and weaning during this time should be discouraged due to the potential increased risk for abscess formation. Mastitis in the setting of a preterm infant and exclusive breastpumping may benefit from identification of the organism and communication with the infant's healthcare provider regarding the safety of providing the pumped milk prior to control of the infection with antibiotics. An abscess should be suspected when a treated patient fails to defervesce within 24-48 hours after antibiotic therapy or when a mass is noted in the breast.

Treatment

- Treatment of mastitis includes antibiotics, rest, frequent milk removal, massage of the breast to remove plugs if present.

- Analgesics such as acetaminophen, ibuprofen, or perhaps hydrocodone can be used.

- As 85% of cases are due to *Staphylococcus aureus*, most authorities recommend antibiotic treatment for 10 to 14 days.

- Prior to the use of antibiotics, cultures of milk are suggested.

- Antibiotic selection should be based on safety in lactation and sensitivities determined from culture. Popular first choices include dicloxacillin, flucloxacillin, cloxacillin, floxacillin, amoxicillin + clavulanate, and perhaps cephalexin.

- Clindamycin, azithromycin, or clarithromycin should be used in cases of penicillin allergies.

- Methicillin Resistant *Staphylococcus aureus* should be treated with clindamycin initially, oral rifampin, or in more severe cases, intravenous vancomycin. Sulfonamides (including Co-Trimoxazole) can be used, but are slow and seldom recommended.

- There is no evidence that continued breastfeeding is harmful to the healthy term nursing infant.

- Weaning during this time should be discouraged due to the potential increased risk for abscess formation.

Medications

- AZITHROMYCIN   (*Zithromax*)
  - AAP = Not reviewed
  - LRC = L2
  - RID   = 5.9%
  - Pregnancy = B
  - Comment: Azithromycin belongs to the erythromycin family. It has an extremely long half-life, particularly in tissues. Azithromycin is concentrated for long periods in phagocytes, which are known to be present in human milk. In one study of a patient who received 1 gm initially followed by 500 mg doses each at 24 hour intervals, the concentration of azithromycin in breastmilk varied from 0.64 mg/L (initially) to 2.8 mg/L on day three. The predicted dose of azithromycin received by the infant would be approximately 0.4 mg/kg/day. This would suggest that the level of azithromycin ingested by a breastfeeding infant is not clinically relevant.

- CEFAZOLIN   (*Ancef, Kefzol*)
  - AAP = Maternal Medication Usually Compatible with Breastfeeding
  - LRC = L1
  - RID   = 0.8%
  - Pregnancy = B
  - Comment: Cefazolin is a typical first-generation cephalosporin antibiotic that has adult and pediatric indications. It is only used IM or IV, never orally. In 20 patients who received a 2 gm STAT dose over 10 minutes, the average concentration of cefazolin in milk two, three, and four hours after the dose was 1.25, 1.51, and 1.16 mg/L, respectively. A very small milk/plasma ratio (0.023) indicates insignificant transfer into milk. Cefazolin is poorly absorbed orally; therefore, the infant would absorb a minimal amount. Plasma levels in infants are reported to be too small to be detected.

- CEPHALEXIN   (*Keflex*)
  - AAP = Not reviewed
  - LRC = L1
  - RID = 0.5-1.5%
  - Pregnancy = B
  - Comment: Cephalexin is a typical first-generation cephalosporin antibiotic. Only minimal concentrations are secreted into human milk. Following a 1000 mg maternal oral dose, milk levels at one, two, three, four, and five hours ranged from 0.20, 0.28, 0.39, 0.50, and 0.47 mg/L, respectively. These levels are probably too low to be clinically relevant. In a group of two to three patients who received 500 mg orally, milk levels averaged 0.7 mg/L at four hours, although the average milk level was 0.36 mg/L over six hours. In another case report of a mother taking probenecid along with cephalexin to prolong the half-life of the cephalexin, the baby developed severe diarrhea. The average milk concentration of probenecid and cephalexin was 964 μg/L and 0.745 μg/L, respectively. This corresponds to a relative infant dose of 0.7% for probenecid and 0.5% for cephalexin.

- CO-TRIMOXAZOLE   (*TMP-SMZ, Bactrim, Cotrim, Septra*)
  - AAP = Maternal Medication Usually Compatible with Breastfeeding
  - LRC = L3
  - RID =
  - Pregnancy = C
  - Comment: Co-trimoxazole is the mixture of trimethoprim and sulfamethoxazole. See individual monographs for each of these products.

- CLARITHROMYCIN   (*Biaxin*)
  - AAP = Not reviewed
  - LRC = L1
  - RID = 2.1%
  - Pregnancy = C
  - Comment: Antibiotic that belongs to erythromycin family. In a study of 12 mothers receiving 250 mg twice daily, the Cmax occurred at 2.2 hours. The estimated average dose of clarithromycin via milk was reported to be 150 μg/kg/day, or 2% of the maternal dose. Clarithromycin is probably compatible with breastfeeding. Observe for diarrhea and thrush in the infant.

- CLINDAMYCIN   (*Cleocin, Cleocin T*)
  - AAP = Maternal Medication Usually Compatible with Breastfeeding
  - LRC = L2
  - RID = 1.7%
  - Pregnancy = B
  - Comment: Clindamycin is a broad-spectrum antibiotic frequently used for anaerobic infections. In one study of two nursing mothers and following doses of 600 mg IV every six hours, the concentration of clindamycin in breastmilk was 3.1 to 3.8 mg/L at 0.2 to 0.5 hours after dosing. Following oral doses of 300 mg every six hours, the breastmilk levels averaged 1.0 to 1.7 mg/L at

1.5 to 7 hours after dosing. In another study of two to three women who received a single oral dose of 150 mg, milk levels averaged 0.9 mg/L at four hours with a milk/plasma ratio of 0.47.

An alteration of GI flora is possible, even though the dose is low. One case of bloody stools (pseudomembranous colitis) has been associated with clindamycin and gentamicin therapy on day five postpartum, but this is considered rare. In this case, the mother of a newborn infant was given 600 mg IV every six hours. In rare cases, pseudomembranous colitis can appear several weeks later. In a study by Steen in five breastfeeding patients who received 150 mg three times daily for seven days, milk concentrations ranged from <0.5 to 3.1 mg/L, with the majority of levels <0.5 mg/L. In another study of 15 women who received 600 mg clindamycin intravenously, levels of clindamycin in milk averaged 1.03 mg/L at two hours following the dose.

With the rise of resistant staphlococcal infections, clindamycin use in infants has risen enormously. The amount in milk is unlikely to harm a breastfeeding infant.

- CLOXACILLIN   (*Tegopen, Cloxapen*)
  - AAP = Not reviewed
  - LRC = L2
  - RID = 0.4-0.8%
  - Pregnancy = B
  - Comment: Cloxacillin is an oral penicillinase-resistant penicillin frequently used for peripheral (non-CNS) Staphylococcus aureus and S. epidermidis infections, particularly mastitis. Following a single 500 mg oral dose of cloxacillin in lactating women, milk concentrations of the drug were zero to 0.2 mg/L one and two hours after the dose, respectively, and 0.2 to 0.4 mg/L after six hours. Usual dose for adults is 250-500 mg four times daily for at least 10-14 days. As with most penicillins, it is unlikely these levels would be clinically relevant.

- DAPTOMYCIN   (*Cubicin*)
  - AAP = Not reviewed
  - LRC = L3
  - RID = 0.1%
  - Pregnancy = B
  - Comment: Daptomycin is used intravenously for the treatment of complicated skin and skin structure infections caused by susceptible strains of Staphylococcus aureus (including methicillin-resistant or MRSA strains), Streptococcus pyogenes, S. agalactiae, S. dysgalactiae, Equisimilis, and Enterococcus faecalis. In a mother five months postpartum who received 500 mg IV daily (6.7 mg/kg/d), the highest concentration measured in milk was 44.7 ng/mL at eight hours following administration. Reported levels in milk were 33.5, 44.7, 40.8, 39.3, and 29.2 ng/mL at 4, 8, 12, 16, and 20 hours, respectively. The mother and infant received therapy for four weeks, and no adverse events were noted in mother or infant. In addition, the daptomycin present in milk is poorly absorbed orally.

- DICLOXACILLIN   (*Pathocil, Dycill, Dynapen*)
  - AAP = Not reviewed
  - LRC = L1
  - RID = 0.6-1.4%

- ○ Pregnancy = B
- ○ Comment: Dicloxacillin is an oral penicillinase-resistant penicillin frequently used for peripheral (non CNS) infections caused by *Staphylococcus aureus* and *Staphylococcus epidermidis* infections, particularly mastitis. Following oral administration of a 250 mg dose, milk concentrations of the drug were 0.1, and 0.3 mg/L at two and four hours after the dose, respectively. Levels were undetectable after one to six hours. It is compatible with breastfeeding.

- **FLOXACILLIN** (*Flucil*)
  - ○ AAP = Not reviewed
  - ○ LRC = L1
  - ○ RID =
  - ○ Pregnancy = B1
  - ○ Comment: Floxacillin, also called flucloxacillin, is a penicillinase-resistant penicillin frequently used for resistant staphylococcal infections. Only trace amounts are secreted into human milk. Its congener, cloxacillin, is commonly used to treat mastitis in breastfeeding mothers and has been used in thousands of breastfeeding patients without problem. Changes in gut flora are possible but unlikely.

- **LINEZOLID** (*Zyvox, Zyvoxam, Zyvoxid*)
  - ○ AAP = Not reviewed
  - ○ LRC = L3
  - ○ RID =
  - ○ Pregnancy = C
  - ○ Comment: Linezolid is a new oxazolidinone family of antibiotics primarily used for gram positive infections, but it has some spectrum for gram negative and anaerobic bacteria. It is active against many strains, including resistant *Staph aureus* (MRSA), *Streptococcus pneumonia*, *Streptococcus pyogenes*, and others. It is indicated for use in patients with vancomycin resistant *Enterococcus faecium* infections, *Staph aureus pneumonias*, resistant *Streptococcus pneumonia* infections, etc.

    Linezolid was found in the milk of lactating rats at concentrations similar to plasma levels, although the dose was not indicated (rat milk levels are always higher than humans). Using these data, with an average maternal plasma concentration of 11.5 µg/mL and a theoretical milk/plasma ratio of 1.0, an infant would ingest approximately 1.7 mg/kg/day following a maternal dose of 1200 mg/day. This amount is likely a high estimate, as doses given animals are extraordinarily high, and rodent milk levels are generally many times higher than human milk. A number of recent studies in children have found linezolid safe. The half-life is shorter in children, which requires dosing more often. Side effects in children are the same as adults and are significant. Observe for changes in gut flora and diarrhea.

- **NAFCILLIN** (*Unipen, Nafcil*)
  - ○ AAP = Not reviewed
  - ○ LRC = L1
  - ○ RID =
  - ○ Pregnancy = B

- Comment: Nafcillin is a penicillin antibiotic that is poorly and erratically absorbed orally. The only formulations are IV and IM. No data are available on concentration in milk, but it is likely small. Oral absorption in the infant would be minimal. See other penicillins.

- **RIFAMPIN**   (*Rifadin, Rimactane*)
  - AAP = Maternal Medication Usually Compatible with Breastfeeding
  - LRC = L2
  - RID = 11.4%
  - Pregnancy = C
  - Comment: Rifampin is a broad-spectrum antibiotic with particular activity against tuberculosis. It is secreted into breastmilk in very small levels. One report indicates that following a single 450 mg oral dose, maternal plasma levels averaged 21.3 mg/L and milk levels averaged 3.4 - 4.9 mg/L. Vorherr reported that after a 600 mg dose of rifampin, peak plasma levels were 50 mg/L, while milk levels were 10-30 mg/L.

- **VANCOMYCIN**   (*Vancocin*)
  - AAP = Not reviewed
  - LRC = L1
  - RID = 6.7%
  - Pregnancy = C
  - Comment: Vancomycin is an antimicrobial agent. Only low levels are secreted into human milk. Milk levels were 12.7 mg/L four hours after infusion in one woman receiving 1 gm every 12 hours for seven days. Its poor oral absorption from the infant's GI tract would limit its systemic absorption. Low levels in infant could provide alterations of GI flora.

Clinical Tips

Mastitis: Management of lactational mastitis includes the use of antibiotics when appropriate and effective draining of the breast always. Most protocols suggest that the mother should continue to breastfeed on both breasts. Complete emptying of each breast is important, so pumping may be required. Patients should be encouraged to reduce stress and use maternity bras (or none at all), rather than wear restrictive ill-fitting bras. The physician should insist on increased rest with frequent breastfeeding or emptying of the breast.

Even normal human breastmilk contains rather high colony counts of bacteria, including *Staphylococcus aureus, Staphylococcus epidermidis, streptococcus viridans,* group B streptococcus, *E. coli,* and various other species. The presence of rather high levels of bacteria, without symptoms, does not necessarily indicate infection, as most milk is rather heavily contaminated with staphylococcal species. The most important factor is the sensitivity of the species, not the absolute colony count.

Antibiotic therapy, particularly that which covers resistant *Staphylococcus aureus* (MSSA), is now required. The clinician is urged to review sensitivities of staphylococcal organisms for their individual regions. Orally, in most individuals, dicloxacillin, or flucloxacillin, and co-trimoxazole are still quite effective at doses of 500 mg four times daily for 10-14 days, and these products should be the first-line drugs of choice. Shorter courses are prone to relapse, though controlled studies have not been done evaluating optimal length of treatment. If treatment is effective, pain and flu symptoms regress rapidly, generally within 24 hours. If the bacteria are resistant, symptoms persist, indicating a change in antibiotic is required.

Amoxicillin with clavulanate (Augmentin) is an additional choice, but sensitivities may be useful prior to use. In individuals hypersensitive to penicillins and cephalosporins, clindamycin, azithromycin or clarithromycin can be used if the organism is sensitive. In those individuals with severe infections, nafcillin IV, cefazolin IV, clindamycin IV, rifampin (IV or oral), co-trimoxazole or vancomycin IV, have been efficacious. When using nafcillin IV, the addition of three to five days of gentamicin (2-5 mg/kg/day) greatly stimulates synergism and increases efficacy. In methicillin-resistant *Staphylococcus aureus* (MRSA) infections, clindamycin orally (in some cases), rifampin (oral), co-trimoxazole, or vancomycin IV are the drugs of choice. New data suggests that adding rifampin will greatly reduce emergence of resistance. MRSA should no longer be treated with fluoroquinolones or macrolides.

While erythromycin, other macrolide antibiotics, and sulfonamides have been useful in the past, the high degree of resistance to these agents may preclude their use today. Use of an anti-inflammatory medication, such as ibuprofen, is recommended for initial treatment of mastitis. This provides pain relief, and the anti-inflammatory properties may assist with resolution of the inflammation during the early therapy of this infection. In patients with severe abscess, surgical drainage is required, along with appropriate antibiotic therapy. Drainage may be accomplished by ultrasound guided needle aspiration. Repeated aspirations may be required while continuing antibiotic therapy, and abscesses larger than 3 cm may benefit from placement of a drainage catheter. Traditional open incision and drainage is typically reserved for failure of aspiration and antibiotics. Milk fistula is a rare (approximately 10%) complication of open drainage of breast abscesses. This is a self-limited condition, and reassurance and techniques to contain the milk drainage should be offered. Needle aspiration of breast abscesses may result in a more pleasing cosmetic result than incision.

In cases with two or three recurrences in the same location, underlying masses should be ruled out.

Suggested Reading

Academy of Breastfeeding Medicine Committee. (2008). ABM clinical protocol #4: mastitis. Revision, May 2008. *Breastfeed Med, 3*(3), 177-180.

Betzold, C. M. (2007). An update on the recognition and management of lactational breast inflammation. *J Midwifery Womens Health, 52*(6), 595-605.

Berth, W. L., Schauberger, C. W., Alvarado, M. A., & Mathiason, M. A. (2009). Telephone-based management of lactation mastitis. *J Reprod Med, 54*(5), 291-294.

Dener C, Inan A. (2003). Breast abscesses in lactating women. *World Journal of Surgery. 27*:130–133

Deshpande, W. (2007). Mastitis. *Community Pract, 80*(5), 44-45.

Foxman B., D'Arcy H., Gillespie B., Bobo J.K., Schwartz K. (2002). Lactation Mastitis: Occurrence and Medical Management among 946 Breastfeeding Women in the United States. *American Journal of Epidemiology 155*:103–114.

Kvist, L. J., Larsson, B. W., Hall-Lord, M. L., Steen, A., & Schalén, C. (2008). The role of bacteria in lactational mastitis and some considerations of the use of antibiotic treatment. *Int Breastfeed J, 3*, 6.

Kvist LJ, Rydhstroem H. (2005). Factors related to breast abscess after delivery: a population-based study. *BJOG 112*:1070–1074

Martin, J. G. (2009). Breast abscess in lactation. *J Midwifery Womens Health, 54*(2), 150-151.

Potter, B. (2005). Women's experiences of managing mastitis. *Community Pract, 78*(6), 209-212.

Spencer, J. P. (2008). Management of mastitis in breastfeeding women. *Am Fam Physician, 78*(6), 727-731.

Ulitzsch D, Nyman MKG, Carlson RA. (2004). Breast Abscess in Lactating Women: US-guided Treatment. *Radiology 232*:904–909.

Walker, M. (2008). Conquering common breast-feeding problems. *J Perinat Neonatal Nurs, 22*(4), 267-274.

Metabolic Bone Disease

Principles of Therapy

Metabolic bone disease denotes a number of conditions producing diffusely decreased bone density (osteopenia) and reduced bone strength. Histologically, it is characterized as: osteoporosis (reduced bone matrix and decreased mineral content) and osteomalacia (bone matrix intact and decreased mineral content). Osteoporosis is the most common bone disease in the USA and accounts for thousands of bone fractures annually. Interestingly, in osteoporosis the rate of bone production is normal, while the rate of bone resorption is significantly elevated. Osteomalacia is generally a result of poor mineralization of the bone, simply put, a result of poor calcium intake. In children, this is called rickets, while in adults it is called osteomalacia. Treatment of these two syndromes largely depends on the etiology. In postmenopausal women, estrogen replacement is generally recommended in suitable cases. While calcium and phosphate replacement help, they only slow bone loss, they do not necessarily replace lost bone density. The chronic use of high dose steroids also predisposes to osteoporosis. The use of the medications below first require accurate diagnosis of the etiology of the syndrome prior to use.

Treatment

- Weight bearing exercises to increase bone formation.

- Smoking cessation.

- Calcium and vitamin D supplements. Recommendations vary, but at least 1000 mg of Calcium and 800-2000 IU Vitamin D daily are currently the most widely recommended.

- Bisphosphonates, including alendronate, risedronate, and ibandronate.

- Raloxifene.

Medications

- ALENDRONATE SODIUM   (*Fosamax*)
    - AAP = Not reviewed
    - LRC = L3
    - RID =
    - Pregnancy = C
    - Comment: Alendronate is a specific inhibitor of osteoclast-mediated bone resorption, thus reducing bone loss and bone turnover. While incorporated in bone matrix, it is not pharmacologically active. Because concentrations in plasma are too low to be detected (<5 ng/mL), it is very unlikely that

it would be secreted into human milk in clinically relevant concentrations. Concentrations in human milk have not been reported. Because this product has exceedingly poor oral bioavailability, particularly when ingested with milk, it is very unlikely that alendronate would be orally absorbed by a breastfeeding infant. In one case of an unknown pregnancy, the mother was taking alendronate 0.12 mg/kg/day orally. Her baby was born with no physical abnormalities, and the baby's growth was normal. No data were collected on the concentrations of alendronate in the mother's milk.

- CALCITONIN   (*Calcimar, Salmonine, Osteocalcin, Miacalcin*)
  - AAP = Not reviewed
  - LRC = L3
  - RID =
  - Pregnancy = C
  - Comment: Calcitonin is a large polypeptide hormone (32 amino acids) secreted by the parafollicular cells of the thyroid that inhibits osteoclastic bone resorption, thus maintaining calcium homeostasis in mammals. It is used for control of postmenopausal osteoporosis and other calcium metabolic diseases. Calcitonins are destroyed by gastric acids, requiring parenteral (SC, IM) or intranasal dosing. Calcitonin is unlikely to penetrate human milk due to its large molecular weight. Further, its oral bioavailability is nil due to destruction in the GI tract. It has been reported to inhibit lactation in animals, although this has not been reported in humans.

- ESTROGEN-ESTRADIOL   (*Estratab, Premarin, Menext, Elestrin*)
  - AAP = Maternal Medication Usually Compatible with Breastfeeding
  - LRC = L3
  - RID =
  - Pregnancy = X
  - Comment: Although small amounts may pass into breastmilk, the effects of estrogens on the infant appear minimal. Early postpartum use of estrogens may reduce volume of milk produced and the protein content, but it is variable and depends on dose and the individual. Breastfeeding mothers should attempt to wait until lactation is firmly established (six to eight weeks) prior to use of estrogen-containing oral contraceptives. In one study of six lactating women who received 50 or 100 mg vaginal suppositories of estradiol, the plasma levels peaked at three hours. These doses are extremely large and are not used clinically. In another study of 11 women, the mean concentration of estradiol in breastmilk was found to be 113 picograms/mL. This is very close to that seen when the woman begins ovulating during lactation. If oral contraceptives are used during lactation, the transfer of estradiol to human milk will be low and will not exceed the transfer during physiologic conditions when the mother has resumed ovulation. However, suppression of lactation is still the major concern with the use of these products in breastfeeding mothers. If at all possible, do not use in breastfeeding mothers.

- ETIDRONATE   (*Didronel*)
  - AAP = Not reviewed
  - LRC = L3
  - RID =
  - Pregnancy = C

○ Comment: Etidronate is a bisphosphonate that slows the dissolution of hydroxyapatite crystals in the bone, thus reducing bone calcium loss in certain syndromes, such as Paget's syndrome. Etidronate also reduces the remineralization of bone and can result in osteomalacia over time. It is not known how the administration of this product during active lactation would affect the maternal bone porosity. It is possible that milk calcium levels could be reduced, although this has not been reported. Etidronate is poorly absorbed orally (1%) and must be administered in between meals on an empty stomach. Its penetration into milk is possible due to its small molecular weight, but it has not yet been reported. However, due to the presence of fat and calcium in milk, its oral bioavailability in infants would be exceedingly low. Whereas the plasma half-life is approximately six hours, the terminal elimination half-life (from bone) is >90 days.

- FLUORIDE   (*Pediaflor, Flura*)
  - ○ AAP = Reported as having no effect on breastfeeding
  - ○ LRC = L2
  - ○ RID =
  - ○ Pregnancy = C
  - ○ Comment: Fluoride is an essential element required for bone and teeth development. It is available as salts of sodium and stannic (tin). Excessive levels are known to stain teeth irreversibly. One study shows breastmilk levels of 0.024-0.172 ppm in milk (mean= 0.077 ppm) of a population exposed to fluoridated water (0.7ppm). In another study of breastfeeding women from areas low and rich in fluoride, milk fluoride levels were similar. The mean fluoride concentration was 0.36 μmol/L for colostrum and 0.37 μmol/L for mature milk in the region with 1 ppm fluoride enriched water. In the region with 0.2 ppm fluoride, the mean fluoride concentration of colostrum was 0.28 μmol/L. There was no statistical difference in any of these milk fluoride levels. Fluoride probably forms calcium fluoride salts in milk,which may limit the oral bioavailability of the fluoride provided by human milk. Maternal supplementation is unnecessary and not recommended in areas with high fluoride content (>0.7 ppm) in water. Allergy to fluoride has been reported in one infant.

- PAMIDRONATE   (*Aredia*)
  - ○ AAP = Not reviewed
  - ○ LRC = L2
  - ○ RID =
  - ○ Pregnancy = D
  - ○ Comment: Pamidronate is an inhibitor of bone-resorption. Although its mechanism of action is obscure, it possibly absorbs to the calcium phosphate crystal in bone and blocks dissolution (reabsorption) of this mineral component in bone, thus reducing turnover of bone calcium. A 39-year-old patient presented in the first month of pregnancy with reflex sympathetic dystrophy. Because she wished to continue breastfeeding, she was treated with monthly IV doses of pamidronate (30 mg) postpartum. Following the first dose, breastmilk was assayed for pamidronate content. After infusion, breastmilk was pumped and collected into two portions: 0-24 hours and 25-48 hours. None was detected (limit of detection, 0.4 micromol/L). The authors suggested that pamidronate could be considered safe for use in lactating women. Pamidronate is poorly absorbed (0.3% to 3% of a dose) after oral administration, and thus any present in milk would not likely be absorbed by the infant.

- RALOXIFENE HCL   (*Evista*)
  - AAP = Not reviewed
  - LRC = L3
  - RID =
  - Pregnancy = X
  - Comment: Raloxifene is a selective estrogen receptor modulator. It blocks such estrogen effects as those that lead to breast cancer and uterine cancer. In addition, it also prevents bone loss and improves lipid profiles. It is used to prevent osteoporosis in postmenopausal women. It is poorly absorbed orally (2%).

- TERIPARATIDE   (*Forteo*)
  - AAP = Not reviewed
  - LRC = L3
  - RID =
  - Pregnancy = C
  - Comment: Teriparatide is the identical peptide hormone secreted by the parathyroid gland in humans. This leads to an increase in skeletal mass, markers of bone formation and resorption, and bone strength. Teriparatide is used to treat osteoporosis. No studies are available on the levels in breastmilk; however, due to the high molecular weight and poor oral bioavailabliltiy, it is unlikely that teriparatide will cross into the milk or be absorbed by an infant.

- VITAMIN D   (*Calciferol, Delta-D, Vitamin D*)
  - AAP = Maternal Medication Usually Compatible with Breastfeeding
  - LRC = L2
  - RID =
  - Pregnancy = A
  - Comment: Vitamin D is secreted into milk in limited concentrations and is somewhat proportional to maternal serum levels. Excessive doses can produce elevated calcium levels in the infant; therefore, doses lower than 10,000 IU/day are suggested in undernourished mothers. There has been some concern that mothers deficient in vitamin D may not provide sufficient vitamin D to the infant, and hence impede bone mineralization in their infants. In a study by Greer, breastfed infants who received oral vitamin D supplementation had greater bone mineralization than those who were not supplemented. However, a more recent study of Korean women in winter who were not supplemented with vitamin D and whose infants were either fed with human milk or artificial cow's formula (with vitamin D added), suggested that even though the breastfed groups plasma 25-hydroxyvitamin D concentration was lower, bone mineralization was equivalent in both breastfed and formula-fed infants. The authors speculated that adequate bone mineralization occurs during the breastfeeding period from a predominantly vitamin D independent passive transport mechanism.

    Human milk is known to have rather minimal concentrations of vitamin D. On average, breastmilk contains approximately 26 IU/L (range= 5-136). Supplementing a mother with even moderate doses of vitamin D does not substantially increase milk levels.

    The newest recommendation from the Academy of Pediatrics is that all infants should be supplemented with 400 IU per day. Mothers who have limited vitamin D intake due to poor nutrition or whose bodies have limited exposure to sunlight, probably need supplementation as their milk is likely deficient in vitamin D. In addition, infants of these mothers (who have limited or no exposure to sunlight or inadequate intake) may need supplementation, as these infants (particularly dark skinned) are most at risk for developing rickets.

The most recent study to evaluate the use of higher maternal doses of vitamin D and its transmission into human milk suggests that relatively higher maternal doses may actually increase milk levels of vitamin D significantly. In two groups of exclusively lactating women (n= 18) who were consuming 1600 IU vitamin D2 and 400 IU vitamin D3 (prenatal vitamin) or 3600 IU vitamin D2 and 400 IU vitamin D3, supplementation at these higher levels increased circulating 25-hydroxyvitamin D [25(OH)D] concentrations for both groups. The vitamin D activity of milk from mothers receiving 2000 IU/d vitamin D increased by 34.2 IU/L, on average, whereas the activity in the 4000 IU/d group increased by 94.2 IU/L. Infants of mothers receiving 4000 IU/d exhibited increases in circulating 25(OH)D3 and 25(OH)D2 concentrations from 12.7 to 18.8 ng/mL and from 0.8 to 12.0 ng/mL, respectively. Total circulating 25(OH)D concentrations increased from 13.4 to 30.8 ng/mL.

This latter study clearly shows that increasing the maternal intake of vitamin D significantly increases milk vitamin D content, but only to a limited degree. Further, using the typical 400 IU dose (RDA) in adults is all but worthless in increasing maternal or the infant's plasma 25(OH)D concentrations. Maternal doses of 4000 IU/day may be required to facilitate increased transfer of 25(OH)D to the infant.

Clinical Tips

Calcitonin is a large molecular weight protein and is unlikely to penetrate milk to any degree. It is not orally bioavailable. Estrogen replacement therapy in postmenopausal, or hypogonadal, women is known to reduce bone loss, but does not increase bone density to any degree. Unfortunately, the use of estrogen in breastfeeding women carries a high risk of significantly suppressing breastmilk production, particularly during the first four to six months postpartum and somewhat less thereafter. Studies suggest that with higher calcium doses, estrogen doses can be reduced. Vitamin D is an oil soluble vitamin. Although we know that only limited quantities transfer into milk, milk levels are apparently in equilibrium with the maternal plasma. Thus extremely high maternal doses should be used with caution in breastfeeding mothers. At this time, it is advisable to supplement both the mother and the infant (400 IU/day). Mothers who are osteopenic should be supplemented with larger doses sufficient to elevate their serum levels. Normal plasma levels of serum 25-hydroxyvitamin D should be maintained > 32 ng/mL. Optimal ranges are 32 to 100 ng/mL. Levels of vitamin D > 100 ng/mL are potentially toxic.

The biphosphonates (e.g., pamidronate, alendronate, etidronate) inhibit osteoclast mediated bone resorption by depositing in bone for long periods and have the best evidence for efficacy in treating osteoporosis. Potential side effects of bisphosphonate therapy may include bone pain, gastritis, esophagitis, risk of atrial fibrillation, risk of incapacitating bone, joint, and muscle pain, potential osteonecrosis of the jaw, and possible bone marrow abnormalities. A recent concern raised regarding long term use of bisphosponates (> six years) is that of femur fracture. Due to their plasma kinetics and poor oral bioavailability, they are not likely to induce problems in breastfed infants, but we have no data showing safety. We have one study done with pamidronate in which milk levels were undetectable. Any present in milk would be largely unabsorbed orally in the infant. In many cases of breastfeeding mothers, it is unclear that deferring this therapy until after weaning would be detrimental to long term bone health.

Intranasal Calcitonin has been shown to reduce bone loss and decrease the risk of vertebral fracture. Its use in breastfeeding mothers is probably compatible as it would be virtually unabsorbed orally in an infant.

Raloxifene has been found to reduce the risk of vertebral fracture in postmenopausal women, although they also have a higher risk of thromboembolism. We do not have breastfeeding data on this drug, although its oral bioavailability is low and milk levels are likely quite low.

Teriparatide has been found more effective than bisphosphonates in preventing fractures, although it is extraordinarily expensive (> $7000/year). It would not likely enter milk or be orally bioavailable in an infant.

Fluoride decreases bone turnover and has often been used in osteoporotic patients, although it is presently quite controversial. While it appears efficacious in improving bone mineral density, there is concern that it may be ineffective in fracture prevention and may increase the risk of fractures. While its transfer in milk is modest to low, the use of large doses of fluoride in breastfeeding mothers is unwise. Side effects in adult patients on high doses of fluoride are significant, and interestingly, although the bone density increased, the bone strength did not. Lower doses (30-50 mg) are now in vogue. These doses are still far too high for breastfeeding mothers.

Suggested Reading

Cooper, A. (2009). A fractured service: the latest advice on osteoporosis. *Br J Gen Pract, 59*(561), 239-241.

Cooper, A. (2009). Osteoporosis guideline. *Br J Gen Pract, 59*(563), 451.

Godfrey, J. R., & Rosen, C. J. (2008). Toward optimal health: advances in diagnosis and preventive strategies to promote bone health in women. *J Womens Health (Larchmt), 17*(9), 1425-1430.

Khosla, S., & Melton, L. Jr. (2007). Clinical practice. Osteopenia. *N Engl J Med, 356*(22), 2293-2300.

Lim, L. S., Hoeksema, L. J., & Sherin, K. (2009). Screening for osteoporosis in the adult U.S. population: ACPM position statement on preventive practice. *Am J Prev Med, 36*(4), 366-375.

McClung, M. R. (2008). European guidance for osteoporosis: an American perspective. *Pol Arch Med Wewn, 118*(9), 462-463.

Poole, K. E., & Compston, J. E. (2006). Osteoporosis and its management. *BMJ, 333*(7581), 1251-1256.

Sweet, M. G., Sweet, J. M., Jeremiah, M. P., & Galazka, S. S. (2009). Diagnosis and treatment of osteoporosis. *Am Fam Physician, 79*(3), 193-200.

Multiple Sclerosis (MS)

Principles of Therapy

Multiple sclerosis (MS) is an autoimmune disease that affects the brain, spinal cord, and optic nerve in approximately 1 million individuals worldwide. It is a demyelinating disorder of the CNS. It most commonly affects women more than men and generally starts between the ages of 18 to 45, although it can be seen at any age. The demylinization of the neurons is due to inflammation. The risk of developing the disease may be partially due to genetic or perhaps infectious factors (human herpes virus 6). New data seems to suggest that low vitamin D levels may also trigger MS.

MS is characterized by continuous neurologic deterioration without treatment, although brief remittences can occur. Pregnancy may have a protective effect on the disease with fewer and less severe relapses reported, especially in the third trimester. The exacerbation rate is increased however in the initial three months postpartum. While some patients differ, most seem to have a relapsing, remitting course. Without treatment, most patients transition to a more progressive form of the disease, with a steady decline of neurologic function.

Treatment

- Short term high-dose steroids.

- Disease-modifying agents, such as glatiramer, interferons, natalizumab, IVIG, mitoxantrone.

- Cyclosporine, methotrexate, and azathioprine have occasionally been used.

- Plasma exchange.

Medications

- BACLOFEN   (*Lioresal, Atrofen*)
    - AAP = Maternal Medication Usually Compatible with Breastfeeding
    - LRC = L2
    - RID = 6.9%
    - Pregnancy = C
    - Comment: Baclofen inhibits spinal reflexes and is used to reverse spasticity associated with multiple sclerosis or spinal cord lesions. Animal studies indicate baclofen inhibits prolactin release and may inhibit lactation. Small amounts of baclofen are secreted into milk. In one mother given a 20 mg oral dose, total consumption by the infant over a 26 hour period is estimated to be 22 µg, about 0.1% of the maternal dose. Milk levels ranged from 0.6 µmol/L (Cmax) to 0.052 µmol/L at 26 hours. The maternal plasma and milk half-lives were 3.9 hours and 5.6 hours, respectively. It is quite unlikely that baclofen administered intrathecally would be secreted into milk in clinically relevant quantities.

- DIAZEPAM (*Valium*)
  - AAP = Drugs whose effect on nursing infants is unknown but may be of concern
  - LRC = L3
  - RID = 7.1%
  - Pregnancy = D
  - Comment: Diazepam is a powerful CNS depressant and anticonvulsant. Published data on milk and plasma levels are highly variable, and many are poor studies. In three mothers receiving 10 mg three times daily for up to six days, the maternal plasma levels of diazepam averaged 491 ng/mL (day four) and 601 ng/mL (day six). Corresponding milk levels were 51 ng/mL (day 4) and 78 ng/mL (day six). The milk/plasma ratio was approximately 0.1.

    In a case report of a patient taking 6-10 mg of diazepam daily, her milk levels varied from 7.5 to 87 μg/L. In a study of nine mothers receiving diazepam postpartum, milk levels varied from approximately 0.01 to 0.08 mg/L. Other reports suggest slightly higher values. Taken together, most results suggest that the dose of diazepam and its metabolite, desmethyldiazepam, to a suckling infant will be on average 0.78-9.1% of the weight-adjusted maternal dose The active metabolite, desmethyldiazepam, in general has a much longer half-life in adults and pediatric patients and may tend to accumulate on longer therapy. Some reports of lethargy, sedation, and poor suckling have been found. The acute use, such as in surgical procedures, is not likely to lead to significant accumulation. Long-term, sustained therapy may prove troublesome. The benzodiazepine family, as a rule, is not ideal for breastfeeding mothers due to relatively long half-lives and the development of dependence. However, it is apparent that the shorter-acting benzodiazepines (lorazepam, alprazolam) are safest during lactation provided their use is short-term or intermittent, low dose, and after the first week of life.

- GLATIRAMER (*Copaxone*)
  - AAP = Not reviewed
  - LRC = L3
  - RID =
  - Pregnancy = B
  - Comment: Glatiramer is a synthetic polypeptide indicated for the treatment of relapsing, remitting multiple sclerosis. It is primarily indicated for those who do not respond to interferons. Glatiramer is a mixture of random polymers of four amino acids: L-alanine, L-glutamic acid, L-lysine, and L-tyrosine. Its molecular weight ranges from 4,700 to 13,000 daltons, which would reduce its ability to enter milk. It is antigenically similar to myelin basic protein, a natural component of the myelin sheath of neurons. No data are available on its transfer into human milk, but it is very unlikely. If ingested orally, it would likely be depolymerized into individual amino acids, so toxicity is unlikely.

- INTERFERON BETA-1A (*Avonex, Rebif*)
  - AAP = Not reviewed
  - LRC = L2
  - RID =
  - Pregnancy = C
  - Comment: Interferon Beta-1A is a moderately large glycoprotein (166 amino acids) with antiviral, antiproliferative, and immunomodulator activity. It is presently used for reducing the severity

and frequency of exacerbations of relapsing-remitting multiple sclerosis. Interferons are large in molecular weight, generally containing 166 amino acids, which would limit their transfer into human milk. Their oral absorption is controversial, but is believed to be minimal. In addition, most researchers find that plasma levels of interferons following IM injection are detectable for only a few hours, generally less than 15 hours following the dose. Thus the transfer of interferons into the plasma compartment are minimal and last only briefly. Generally, they are low to undetectable.

In a group of six women receiving 30 μg IM weekly, milk levels ranged were 0.0026% of the maternal dose.

Thus the transfer of interferon beta-1A into human milk is extraordinarly low (essentially nil) and would be of no risk to a breastfeeding infant.

- INTERFERON BETA-1B   (*Betaseron*)

  - AAP = Not reviewed
  - LRC = L2
  - RID =
  - Pregnancy = C
  - Comment: Interferon Beta-1B is a glycoprotein with antiviral, antiproliferative, and immunomodulatory activity presently used for treatment of multiple sclerosis. Very little is known about the secretion of interferons in human milk, although some interferons are known to be secreted normally and may contribute to the antiviral properties of human milk. However, interferons are large in molecular weight, generally containing 165 amino acids, which would limit their transfer into human milk. Further, their oral absorption is believed to be minimal. However, interferons are relatively nontoxic unless extraordinarily large doses are administered parenterally. Interferons are sometimes used in infants and children to treat idiopathic thromboplastinemia (ITP) in huge doses. The transfer of interferon Beta-1a (Avonex, Rebif) is essentially nil, and it is likely the same for this product, interferon Beta-1b.

- METHYLPREDNISOLONE   (*Solu-Medrol, Depo-Medrol, Medrol*)

  - AAP = Maternal Medication Usually Compatible with Breastfeeding
  - LRC = L2
  - RID =
  - Pregnancy = C
  - Comment: Methylprednisolone (MP) is the methyl derivative of prednisolone. A measurement of 4 mg of methylprednisolone is roughly equivalent to 5 mg of prednisone. Multiple dosage forms exist and include the succinate salt, which is rapidly active, the methylprednisolone base, which is the tablet formulation for oral use, and the methylprednisolone acetate suspension (Depo-Medrol), which is slowly absorbed over many days to weeks. Depo-Medrol is generally used intrasynovially, IM, or epidurally and is slowly absorbed from these sites. They would be very unlikely to affect a breastfed infant, but this depends on dose and duration of exposure. For a complete description of corticosteroid use in breastfeeding mothers, see the prednisone monograph. In general, the amount of methylprednisolone and other steroids transferred into human milk is minimal as long as the dose does not exceed 80 mg per day. However, relating side effects of steroids administered via breastmilk and their maternal doses is rather difficult, and each situation should be evaluated individually. Extended use of high doses could predispose the infant to steroid side effects, including

decreased linear growth rate, but these require rather high doses. Low to moderate doses are believed to have minimal effect on breastfed infants. See prednisone.

High dose pulsed intravenous or oral administrations of methylprednisolone (MP) have become increasingly important as a treatment for acute relapses or progressively worsening of multiple sclerosis (MS). Even though prednisolone is approved by the American Academy of Pediatrics for use in breastfeeding women, when MP is used in such high doses in patients with MS, questions concerning when mothers can return to breastfeeding have arisen. While there are extensive kinetic data on the plasma levels, metabolism, and clearance of methylprednisolone from normal and MS patients, no data are available on the transfer of MP into human milk subsequent to using such high pulse IV doses in breastfeeding mothers. Simulation of MP elimination curves by the author shows a rapid and complete elimination from the maternal plasma compartment. From this simulation, it would appear pumping and discarding of milk for a period of 8-24 hours following the IV administration of MP (at doses up to 1 gm) would significantly reduce an infant's exposure to this corticosteroid. This simulation estimates the infant dose at 12 hours post-administration of MP to be approximately 1.24 µg/kg/day. These are only theoretical predictions as no one yet has published milk levels following IV administration of 1 gram doses.

- MITOXANTRONE   (*Novantrone*)
  - ○ AAP = Not reviewed
  - ○ LRC = L5
  - ○ RID =
  - ○ Pregnancy = D
  - ○ Comment: Mitoxantrone is an antineoplastic agent used in the treatment of relapsing multiple sclerosis. It is a DNA-reactive agent that intercalates into DNA via hydrogen bonding, causing crosslinks. It inhibits B cell, T cell, and macrophage proliferation. In a study of a patient who received three treatments of mitoxantrone (6 mg/meter^2) on days one to five, mitoxantrone levels in milk measured 120 ng/mL just after treatment (on the third day of treatment), and dropped to a stable level of 18 ng/mL for the next 28 days. This agent has an enormous volume of distribution and is sequestered in at least seven organs, including the liver and bone marrow. In another study, 15% of the dose remained 35 days after exposure. Assuming a mother was breastfeeding, these levels would provide about 18 µg/L of milk consumed after the first few days following exposure to the drug. In addition, it would be sequestered for long periods in the infant as well. As this is a DNA-reactive agent and it has a huge volume of distribution leading to prolonged tissue, plasma, and milk levels, mothers should be strongly advised to not breastfeed following its use.

- MODAFINIL   (*Provigil*)
  - ○ AAP = Not reviewed
  - ○ LRC = L4
  - ○ RID =
  - ○ Pregnancy = C
  - ○ Comment: Modafinil is a wakefulness-promoting agent used for the treatment of narcolepsy. Although its pharmacologic results are similar to amphetamines and methylphenidate (Ritalin), its method of action is unknown. No data are available on its transfer into human milk. Some caution is recommended, as it is small in molecular weight and very lipid soluble, both characteristics which may ultimately lead to higher milk levels. In addition, it apparently stimulates dopamine levels.

Compounds that stimulate dopamine levels in the brain often reduce prolactin secretion. Milk production may suffer, but this is only supposition.

- NATALIZUMAB (*Tysabri*)
  - AAP = Not reviewed
  - LRC = L3
  - RID =
  - Pregnancy = C
  - Comment: Natalizumab is a recombinant humanized IgG4k monoclonal antibody used to suppress immunity in patients with multiple sclerosis. Because it is a large molecular IgG, its transfer into milk is probably negligible, but as yet, we do not have data on its transfer to human milk. The transfer of native IgG into human milk is low. When small amounts of this product are added to vast quantities of IgG in the plasma, only a small percentage of natalizumab would ever be available for transport into milk. It is rather unlikely this product would be detrimental to a breastfeeding infant, but we do not know this for sure at this time.

- OXYBUTYNIN (*Ditropan*)
  - AAP = Not reviewed
  - LRC = L3
  - RID =
  - Pregnancy = B
  - Comment: Oxybutynin is an anticholinergic agent used to provide antispasmodic effects for conditions characterized by involuntary bladder spasms, reducing urinary urgency and frequency. It has been used in children down to five years of age at doses of 15 mg daily. No data on transfer of this product into human milk are available. But oxybutynin is a tertiary amine which is poorly absorbed orally (only 6%). Further, the maximum plasma levels (Cmax) generally attained are less than 31.7 ng/mL. If one were to assume a theoretical M/P ratio of 1.0 (which is probably unreasonably high) and a daily ingestion of 1 L of milk, then the theoretical dose to the infant would be <2 µg/day, a dose that would be clinically irrelevant to even a neonate.

- TOLTERODINE (*Detrol*)
  - AAP = Not reviewed
  - LRC = L3
  - RID =
  - Pregnancy = C
  - Comment: Tolterodine is a muscarinic anticholinergic agent similar in effect to atropine, but it is more selective for the urinary bladder. Tolterodine levels in milk have been reported in mice, where offspring exposed to extremely high levels had slightly reduced body weight gain, but no other untoward effects. While it is more selective for the urinary bladder, preclinical trials still showed adverse effects, including blurred vision, constipation, and dry mouth in adults. While we have no data on human milk, it is unlikely concentrations will be high enough to produce untoward effects in infants. However, the infant should be monitored for classic anticholinergic symptoms, including dry mouth, constipation, poor tearing, etc.

- TIZANIDINE   (*Zanaflex*)
  - ◦ AAP = Not reviewed
  - ◦ LRC = L4
  - ◦ RID =
  - ◦ Pregnancy = C
  - ◦ Comment: Tizanidine is a centrally acting muscle relaxant. It has demonstrated efficacy in the treatment of tension headache and spasticity associated with multiple sclerosis. It is not known if it is transferred into human milk, although the manufacturer states that due to its lipid solubility, it likely penetrates milk. This product has a long half-life, high lipid solubility, and significant CNS penetration, all factors that would increase milk penetration. While the half-life of the conventional formulation is only four to eight hours, the half-life of the sustained release formulation is 13-22 hours. Further, 48% of patients complain of sedation. Use caution if used in a breastfeeding mother.

Clinical Therapy

The use of high-dose methylprednisolone has been found to hasten acute recovery, but not the long-term course of the disease. The use of high intravenous dose methylprednisolone is generally considered first-line treatment for acute exacerbations. High-dose corticosteroids rapidly leave the plasma compartment and are sequestered in tissues. Following these doses (1-2 grams/day for five days), levels in milk are probably moderately high for a few hours (three to four) and then fall rapidly with plasma levels. Plasma levels are quite low in 12-24 hours, and breastfeeding could presumably be reinstated after this brief interruption until the next dose. Milk pumped during this interval should be discarded.

Interferon beta-1a and beta-1b are the primary medications for long-term therapy. Interferons are large molecular weight proteins that enter milk poorly. Their prolonged use is probably compatible with breastfeeding in patients undergoing therapy for relapsing multiple sclerosis. In an unpublished group of six women receiving 30 μg (30,000,000 pg) IM weekly, milk levels ranged from 33 pg to 80 pg/mL milk. Thus the transfer of interferon beta-1A into human milk is extraordinarily low (essentially nil) and would be of no risk to a breastfeeding infant.

Glatiramer (Copaxone) is an immunomodulating agent that is a random polymer (mean=6.4 kD) composed of four amino acids commonly found in myelin basic protein. It apparently diverts the immune system and suppresses the inflammatory response. Because of its large molecular weight and no oral bioavailability, it would not likely transfer into human milk.

Mitoxantrone is an antineoplastic agent used in the treatment of relapsing multiple sclerosis. It is a DNA-reactive agent that intercalates into DNA via hydrogen bonding, causing crosslinks. It inhibits B cell, T cell, and macrophage proliferation. While levels in milk are low, it is sequestered in numerous tissues and is retained for long periods of time (> 35 days). As this is a DNA-reactive agent and it has a huge volume of distribution leading to prolonged tissue, plasma, and milk levels, mothers should be strongly advised to not breastfeed following its use.

Another agent occasionally used in patients with MS is modafinal, which has a wake-promoting or stimulating CNS action. It is sometimes used to treat mild or moderate MS-related fatigue. Antispasmotic agents, such as diazepam, baclofen, and tizanidine, can be used to reduce muscle spasticity, but the infant should be monitored for sedation.

Natalizumab (Tysabri) is a very effective, but quite hazardous, recombinant humanized IgG4k monoclonal antibody used to suppress immunity in patients with multiple sclerosis. Controlled trials have demonstrated that natalizumab significantly reduces rate of relapses and even reduces MRI lesions. Unfortunately, it has been found to be associated with progressive multifocal leukoencephalopathy. Its use is highly restricted. Because it is a large molecular IgG, its transfer into milk is probably negligible, but as yet, we have no data on its transfer to human milk.

Suggested Reading

Cuddy, M. L. (2007). Multiple sclerosis. *J Pract Nurs, 57*(2), 5-6, 12; quiz 13-14.

de Seze, J., Debouverie, M., Waucquier, N., Steinmetz, G., Pittion, S., Zephir, H., et al. (2007). Primary progressive multiple sclerosis: a comparative study of the diagnostic criteria. *Mult Scler, 13*(5), 622-625.

Ferreira Vasconcelos, C. C., Miranda Santos, C. M., Papais Alvarenga, M., Camargo, S. M., & Papais Alvarenga, R. M. (2008). The reliability of specific primary progressive MS criteria in an ethnically diverse population. *J Neurol Sci, 270*(1-2), 159-164.

Fox, C. M., Bensa, S., Bray, I., & Zajicek, J. P. (2004). The epidemiology of multiple sclerosis in Devon: a comparison of the new and old classification criteria. *J Neurol Neurosurg Psychiatry, 75*(1), 56-60.

Hatzakis, M. J., Jr., Allen, C., Haselkorn, M., Anderson, S. M., Nichol, P., Lai, C., et al. (2006). Use of medical informatics for management of multiple sclerosis using a chronic-care model. *J Rehabil Res Dev, 43*(1), 1-16.

O'Brien, A. R., Chiaravalloti, N., Goverover, Y., & Deluca, J. (2008). Evidenced-based cognitive rehabilitation for persons with multiple sclerosis: a review of the literature. *Arch Phys Med Rehabil, 89*(4), 761-769.

Muscle Cramps-Spasticity

Principles of Therapy

Muscle cramps and tetany arise from any number of causes, including sports or occupational muscle injury, hypocalcemia, diabetes mellitus, Parkinson's disease, spinal cord injury, hemodialysis, chemotherapy, etc. Various drugs have been found to cause cramps, including cimetidine and cholestyramine. Electrolyte deficiencies, such as calcium and magnesium, are also well known to induce muscle cramping. While correction of the primary etiology is often the wisest course, pharmacotherapy is nevertheless sometimes used along with rest and physical therapy. The medications employed are few, and their mechanism of actions largely unresolved. Because many of these products are poorly efficacious, a risk versus benefit justification is required prior to their use in breastfeeding mothers.

Treatment

- Muscle relaxants, such as metaxalone, orphenadrine, carisoprodol, and cyclobenzaprine

- Stretching, exercise

- Verapamil, pregabalin, and gabapentin may be useful in severe cases.

Medications

- BACLOFEN   (*Lioresal, Atrofen*)
  - AAP = Maternal Medication Usually Compatible with Breastfeeding
  - LRC = L2
  - RID = 6.9%
  - Pregnancy = C
  - Comment: Baclofen inhibits spinal reflexes and is used to reverse spasticity associated with multiple sclerosis or spinal cord lesions. Animal studies indicate baclofen inhibits prolactin release and may inhibit lactation. Small amounts of baclofen are secreted into milk. In one mother given a 20 mg oral dose, total consumption by the infant over a 26 hour period is estimated to be 22 µg, about 0.1% of the maternal dose. Milk levels ranged from 0.6 µmol/L (Cmax) to 0.052 µmol/L at 26 hours. The maternal plasma and milk half-lives were 3.9 hours and 5.6 hours, respectively. It is quite unlikely that baclofen administered intrathecally would be secreted into milk in clinically relevant quantities.

- CARISOPRODOL   (*Soma Compound, Solol*)
  - AAP = Not reviewed
  - LRC = L3

- ○ RID = 0.5-6.3%
- ○ Pregnancy = C
- ○ Comment: Carisoprodol is a commonly used skeletal muscle relaxant that is a CNS depressant. It is metabolized to an active metabolite called meprobamate. As Soma Compound, it also contains 325 mg of aspirin. In a study of one breastfeeding mother receiving 2100 mg/d, the average milk concentration of carisoprodol and meprobamate was 0.9 mg/L and 11.6 mg/L, respectively. Based on these combined values, the relative infant dose for carisoprodol and meprobamate would be 4.1% of the weight-adjusted maternal dose. No adverse effects on the infant were noted.

- CYCLOBENZAPRINE   (*Flexeril, Cycoflex*)
  - ○ AAP = Not reviewed
  - ○ LRC = L3
  - ○ RID =
  - ○ Pregnancy = B
  - ○ Comment: Cyclobenzaprine is a centrally acting skeletal muscle relaxant that is structurally and pharmacologically similar to the tricyclic antidepressants. Cyclobenzaprine is used as an adjunct to rest and physical therapy for the relief of acute, painful musculoskeletal conditions. Studies have not conclusively shown whether the skeletal muscle relaxation properties are due to the sedation or placebo effects. At least one study has found it no more effective than a placebo. It is not known if cyclobenzaprine is secreted in milk, but one must assume that its secretion would be similar to the tricyclics (see amitriptyline, desipramine). There are no pediatric indications for this product.

- METAXALONE   (*Skelaxin*)
  - ○ AAP = Not reviewed
  - ○ LRC = L3
  - ○ RID =
  - ○ Pregnancy =
  - ○ Comment: Metaxalone is a centrally acting sedative used primarily as a muscle relaxant. Its ability to relax skeletal muscle is weak and is probably due to its sedative properties. Hypersensitivity reactions in adults (allergic) have occurred, as well as liver toxicity. No data are available on its transfer into breastmilk.

- ORPHENADRINE CITRATE   (*Norflex, Banflex, Norgesic, Flexon*)
  - ○ AAP = Not reviewed
  - ○ LRC = L3
  - ○ RID =
  - ○ Pregnancy = C
  - ○ Comment: Orphenadrine is an analog of Benadryl (diphenhydramine). It is primarily used as a muscle relaxant, although its primary effects are anticholinergic. No data are available on its secretion into breastmilk.

- QUININE   (*Quinamm*)
  - ○ AAP = Maternal Medication Usually Compatible with Breastfeeding

- ○ LRC = L2
- ○ RID = 0.7-1.3%
- ○ Pregnancy = D
- ○ Comment: Quinine is a cinchona alkaloid primarily used in malaria prophylaxis and treatment. Small to trace amounts are secreted into milk. No reported harmful effects have been reported except in infants with G6PD deficiencies. In a study of six women receiving 600-1300 mg/day, the concentration of quinine in breastmilk ranged from 0.4 to 1.6 mg/L at 1.5 to 6 hours postdose. The authors suggest these levels are clinically insignificant. In another study, with maternal plasma concentrations of 0.5 to 8 mg/L, the milk/plasma ratio ranged from 0.11 to 0.53. The total daily consumption by a breastfed infant was estimated to be 1-3 mg/day.

- • TIZANIDINE (*Zanaflex*)
  - ○ AAP = Not reviewed
  - ○ LRC = L4
  - ○ RID =
  - ○ Pregnancy = C
  - ○ Comment: Tizanidine is a centrally acting muscle relaxant. It has demonstrated efficacy in the treatment of tension headache and spasticity associated with multiple sclerosis. It is not known if it is transferred into human milk, although the manufacturer states that due to its lipid solubility, it likely penetrates milk. This product has a long half-life, high lipid solubility, and significant CNS penetration, all factors that would increase milk penetration. While the half-life of the conventional formulation is only four to eight hours, the half-life of the sustained release formulation is 13-22 hours. Further, 48% of patients complain of sedation. Use caution if used in a breastfeeding mother.

Clinical Tips

Quinine is apparently effective for frequent nocturnal leg cramps, although the FDA advises against its use due to the risk of complications. We have two studies that show quinine is quite safe for a breastfeeding mother, as the milk levels are very low. The newer product, metaxalone, is moderately effective and produces minimal or only occasional sedation. While we have no breastfeeding data on metaxalone, it or quinine is probably preferred. For the most part, these medications have not shown themselves to be much more effective than placebo and rest. Therefore, their use in breastfeeding mothers may not be justified. Baclofen is used in more severe cases of muscle spasm, including those associated with spinal reflexes. It is used to reverse spasticity associated with multiple sclerosis or spinal cord lesions.

Suggested Reading

Anonymous. (2004). Muscle cramps. Common and often manageable. *Mayo Clin Health Lett, 22*(2), 6.

Chandira, A. R. (2002). Muscle cramps. *J Indian Med Assoc, 100*(3), 203.

Dobkin, B. H., Landau, W. M., Sahrmann, S., Thomas Thach, W., Simpson, D. M., Gracies, J. M., et al. (2009). Assessment: botulinum neurotoxin for the treatment of spasticity (an evidence-based review). *Neurology, 73*(9), 736; author reply 737-738.

Francisco, G. E., Yablon, S. A., Schiess, M. C., Wiggs, L., Cavalier, S., & Grissom, S. (2006). Consensus panel guidelines for the use of intrathecal baclofen therapy in poststroke spastic hypertonia. *Top Stroke Rehabil, 13*(4), 74-85.

Hantoushzadeh, S., Jafarabadi, M., & Khazardoust, S. (2007). Serum magnesium levels, muscle cramps, and preterm labor. *Int J Gynaecol Obstet, 98*(2), 153-154.

Miller, T. M., & Layzer, R. B. (2005). Muscle cramps. *Muscle Nerve, 32*(4), 431-442.

Nephrolithiasis

Principles of Therapy

Nephrolithiasis is the presence of calculus or stones within the kidney. Nephrolithiasis presents with acute flank pain in approximately 90% of cases. The pain often radiates to the groin or lower abdomen and is typically severe. Hematuria is usually present (75%+), but is only grossly visible in about one-third of cases.

Initial management includes hydration and pain control. Pain from ureteral colic is frequently treated with either morphine, an oral narcotic such as codeine, or a NSAID. Associated nausea can be treated with anti-emetics if needed. Stones < 3mm frequently pass spontaneously.

Medical expulsive therapy (MET) can be considered in situations of small stones. It is most often successful for stones < 1cm. Medications which may be effective include those with ureteral relaxation, such as NSAID's, calcium channel blockers (nifedipine), alpha blockers (terazosin or tamsulosin), and corticosteroids.

Extracorporeal shockwave therapy (lithotripsy) may be useful in breaking up the stone to allow passage, though it is contraindicated during pregnancy.

Long term recommendations to avoid recurrence include hydration, avoidance of excessive salt and protein, and occasionally medication to increase intestinal calcium binding in appropriate situations. The chemical components of the stone may be of assistance for long term management. A 24 hour urine study evaluating pH, calcium, uric acid, oxalate, magnesium, etc. may be of assistance.

Treatment

- Initial management with pain control (codeine, NSAIDS orally, or Morphine) and vigorous hydration.

- Medical expulsive therapy: NSAIDS, calcium channel blockers, alpha blockers, corticosteroids.

- Lithotripsy.

Medications

- KETOROLAC (*Toradol, Acular*)
    - AAP = Maternal Medication Usually Compatible with Breastfeeding
    - LRC = L2
    - RID = 0.2%
    - Pregnancy = C in first and second trimesters
    - Comment: Ketorolac is a popular, nonsteroidal analgesic. In a study of 10 lactating women who received 10 mg orally four times daily, milk levels of ketorolac were not detectable in four of the subjects. The maximum daily dose an infant could absorb (maternal dose = 40 mg/day) would

range from 3.16 to 7.9 µg/day, assuming a milk volume of 400 mL or 1000 mL. An infant would, therefore, receive less than 0.2% of the daily maternal dose.

- MORPHINE   (*Duramorph, Infumorph*)
  - ○ AAP = Maternal Medication Usually Compatible with Breastfeeding
  - ○ LRC = L3
  - ○ RID = 9.1%
  - ○ Pregnancy = C
  - ○ Comment: Morphine is a potent narcotic analgesic and a number of studies on its use in breastfeeding mothers are available. When used in normal clinical doses, it does not apparently sedate breastfeeding infants. While the highest reported RID has been 10.7%, virtually none of this passes the liver to enter the plasma compartment of the infant. Hence, present studies suggest morphine is a preferred potent analgesic for breastfeeding mothers. In summary, morphine is a preferred opiate in breastfeeding mothers primarily due to its poor oral bioavailability. It is unfortunate that the clinical studies above do not necessarily suggest this. High doses over prolonged periods could lead to sedation and respiratory problems in newborn infants.

- NIFEDIPINE   (*Adalat, Procardia*)
  - ○ AAP = Maternal Medication Usually Compatible with Breastfeeding
  - ○ LRC = L2
  - ○ RID = 2.3-3.4%
  - ○ Pregnancy = C
  - ○ Comment: Nifedipine is an effective antihypertensive. It belongs to the calcium channel blocker family of drugs. Two studies indicate that nifedipine is transferred to breastmilk in varying but generally low levels. In one study in which the dose was varied from 10-30 mg three times daily, the highest concentration (53.35 µg/L) was measured at one hour after a 30 mg dose. Other levels reported were 16.35 µg/L 60 minutes after a 20 mg dose and 12.89 µg/L 30 minutes after a 10 mg dose. The milk levels fell linearly with the milk half-lives estimated to be 1.4 hours for the 10 mg dose, 3.1 hours for the 20 dose, and 2.4 hours for the 30 mg dose. The milk concentration measured eight hours following a 30 mg dose was 4.93 µg/L. In this study, using the highest concentration found and a daily intake of 150 mL/kg of human milk, the amount of nifedipine intake would only be 8 µg/kg/day (less than 1.8% of the therapeutic pediatric dose). The authors conclude that the amount ingested via breastmilk poses little risk to an infant.

    In another study, concentrations of nifedipine in human milk one to eight hours after 10 mg doses varied from <1 to 10.3 µg/L (median 3.5 µg/L) in six of 11 patients. In this study, milk levels three days after discontinuing medication ranged from <1 to 9.4 µg/L. The authors concluded the exposure to nifedipine through breastmilk is not significant. In a study by Penny and Lewis, following a maternal dose of 20 mg nifedipine daily for 10 days, peak breastmilk levels at one hour were 46 µg/L. The corresponding maternal serum level was 43 µg/L. From these data the authors suggest a daily intake for an infant would be approximately 6.45 µg/kg/day.

    Nifedipine has been found clinically useful for nipple vasospasm. Because of the similarity to Raynaud's Phenomenon, sustained release formulations providing 30-60 mg per day are suggested.

- TAMSULOSIN HYDROCHLORIDE   (*Flomax*)
  - ○ AAP = Not reviewed

- ○ LRC = L3
- ○ RID =
- ○ Pregnancy = B
- ○ Comment: Tamsulosin is not approved for use in women, but is used in men for benign prostatic hyperplasia. It is occasionally used in women to assist in the passage of a kidney stone or for bladder motility problems. It works by blocking the alpha1A adrenoreceptors, thus reducing ureter contractility. Due to its high protein binding and larger molecular weight, it is unlikely that tamsulosin would be excreted in human milk. But no breastfeeding data are presently available.

- • TERAZOSIN HCL   (*Hytrin*)
  - ○ AAP = Not reviewed
  - ○ LRC = L4
  - ○ RID =
  - ○ Pregnancy = C
  - ○ Comment: Terazosin is an antihypertensive that belongs to the alpha-1 blocking family. This family is generally very powerful and produces significant orthostatic hypotension and other side effects. Terazosin has rather powerful effects on the prostate and testes, producing testicular atrophy in some animal studies (particularly newborn), and is therefore not preferred in pregnant or in lactating women. No data are available on transfer into human milk.

Clinical Tips

Initial treatment of this painful syndrome is primarily to control pain. While NSAIDs are useful, a combination of morphine and ketorolac is reportedly much more effective than either alone. Both morphine and ketorolac are suitable analgesics for breastfeeding mothers. Meperidine should be avoided due to complications, such as excessive vomiting. Alpha-1 blockers, such as tamsulosin, and calcium channel blockers, such as nifedipine, are effective in increasing stone expulsion from the kidney. We presently have no data on the use of these potent alpha blockers in breastfeeding mothers. Short-term use of a day or so is probably not contraindicated, but mothers should avoid prolonged therapy as it would be risky for the breastfed infant. Nifedipine has been extensively studied and used in breastfeeding mothers without problems.

Extracorporeal shock wave lithotripsy is effective in fracturing some stones and increasing the rate of expulsion. Success is highest with small intrarental calculi < 2.5 cm in diameter. It should not be used in pregnant patients, those with blood dyscrasias, or those with severe obstruction or infections. Not contraindicated in breastfeeding mothers.

Prevention of kidney stones is less successful, but reducing soft drink consumption, particularly those with high phosphoric acid content (cokes, etc.) has been successful in reducing recurrence of renal stones. Reducing salt, calcium, and animal protein intake may also help reduce recurrence.

Suggested Reading

1: Semins M.J., Matlaga B.R. (2010). Management of stone disease in pregnancy. *Curr Opin Urol.* 20(2):174-7.

2: Lingeman J.E., McAteer J.A., Gnessin E., Evan A.P. (2009). Shock wave lithotripsy: advances in technology and technique. *Nat Rev Urol.* 6(12):660-70.

3: Hall P.M. (2009). Nephrolithiasis: treatment, causes, and prevention. *Cleve Clin J Med.* 76(10):583-91.

Nipple Dermatitis

Principles of Therapy

The painful nipple is one of the most common complaints of breastfeeding mothers early on and is a major reason for premature weaning. Most nipple irritation is initiated with improper latching of the infant to the nipple. Correction of improper latch and positioning will frequently reduce the pain. The assistance of an experienced lactation consultant to the management of latch difficulties can not be underestimated. Discomfort generally ensues between three to five days postpartum, followed by steady improvement in most cases. However, in some cases, the pain increases and becomes chronic. While the initial problem may be associated with improper latch, ultimately skin breakdown occurs, and is often associated with superinfections with *Staphylococcus aureus* or other bacteria. Initial treatment should be aimed toward providing for a better latch. If the latch is considered adequate, certain medications may be helpful. Skin protectants, such as highly purified lanolin ointments, have been used with significant success to prevent skin breakdown in some patients. In some instances, antimicrobials and topical corticosteroids are quite effective and can be used safely in breastfeeding mothers, particularly those with inflamed or infected lesions. Care should be used to limit exposure of the infant to large amounts of topical steroids, particularly high potency steroids.

Treatment

- Improving latch

- Antimicrobials

- Topical corticosteroids

- Highly purified lanolin ointments

Medications

- GENTIAN VIOLET   (*Crystal Violet, Methylrosaniline chloride, Gentian Violet*)
    - AAP = Not reviewed
    - LRC = L3
    - RID =
    - Pregnancy = C
    - Comment: Gentian violet is an older product that, when used topically and orally, is an exceptionally effective antifungal and antimicrobial. It is a strong purple dye that is difficult to remove. Gentian violet has been found to be equivalent to ketoconazole, and far superior to nystatin, in treating oral (not esophageal) candidiasis in patients with advanced AIDS. It is also useful in treating purulent infections of the ear infected with methicillin-resistant *Staphlococcus Aureus*. Gentian violet (GV)

solutions generally come as 1-2% Gentian violet dissolved in a 10% solution of alcohol. For use with infants, the solution should be diluted with distilled water to 0.25 to 0.5% Gentian violet. This reduces the irritant properties of GV and reduces the alcohol content as well. While the alcohol is irritating to the nipple, it is not detrimental to the infant. Higher concentrations of GV are known to be very irritating, leading to oral ulceration and necrotic skin reactions in children. If used, a small swab should be soaked in the solution, and then swabbed in the infant's gingivae. Apply it directly to the affected areas in the mouth no more than once or twice daily for no more than three to seven days. Direct application to the nipple has been reported.

- **HYDROCORTISONE TOPICAL** (*Westcort*)
  - AAP = Not reviewed
  - LRC = L2
  - RID =
  - Pregnancy = C
  - Comment: Hydrocortisone is a typical corticosteroid with glucocorticoid and mineralocorticoid activity. When applied topically, it suppresses inflammation and enhances healing. Initial onset of activity when applied topically is slow and may require several days for response. Absorption topically is dependent on placement; percutaneous absorption is 1% from the forearm, 2% from the rectum, 4% from the scalp, 7% from the forehead, and 36% from the scrotal area. The amount transferred into human milk has not been reported, but as with most steroids is believed minimal. Topical application to the nipple is generally approved by most authorities if amounts applied and duration of use are minimized. Only small amounts should be applied, and then only after feeding; larger quantities should be removed prior to breastfeeding. 0.5 to 1% ointments, rather than creams, are generally preferred.

- **MOMETASONE** (*Elocon, Nasonex*)
  - AAP = Not reviewed
  - LRC = L3
  - RID =
  - Pregnancy = C
  - Comment: Mometasone is a corticosteroid primarily intended for intranasal and topical use. It is considered a medium-potency steroid, similar to betamethasone and triamcinolone. Following topical application to the skin, less than 0.7% is systemically absorbed over an eight hour period. It is extremely unlikely mometasone would be excreted into human milk in clinically relevant levels following topical or intranasal administration.

- **MUPIROCIN OINTMENT** (*Bactroban*)
  - AAP = Not reviewed
  - LRC = L1
  - RID =
  - Pregnancy = B
  - Comment: Mupirocin is a topical antibiotic used for impetigo, Group A beta-hemolytic strep, and strep pyogenes. Mupirocin is only minimally absorbed following topical application. In one study, less than 0.3% of a topical dose was absorbed after 24 hours. Most remained adsorbed to the

corneum layer of the skin. The drug is absorbed orally, but it is so rapidly metabolized that systemic levels are not sustained. It is quite safe for breastfeeding mothers.

- TRIAMCINOLONE ACETONIDE   *(Nasacort, Azmacort, Tri-Nasal)*
  ○ AAP = Not reviewed
  ○ LRC = L3
  ○ RID =
  ○ Pregnancy = C
  ○ Comment: Triamcinolone is a typical corticosteroid (see prednisone) that is available for topical, intranasal, injection, inhalation, and oral use. When applied topically to the nose (Nasacort) or to the lungs (Azmacort), only minimal doses are used and plasma levels are exceedingly low to undetectable. Although no data are available on triamcinolone secretion into human milk, it is likely that the milk levels would be exceedingly low and not clinically relevant when administered via inhalation or intranasally. While the oral adult dose is 4-48 mg/day, the inhaled dose is 200 μg three times daily, and the intranasal dose is 220 μg/day. There is virtually no risk to the infant following use of the intranasal products in breastfeeding mothers.

Clinical Tips

Initial therapy for the sore nipple is to closely evaluate the positioning and latch of the infant. Clinically, the inflamed nipple is either due to trauma, inflammation, infection, or all of the above, and it may be difficult to discern the offending agent. Simple correction of the latch will provide comfort for the vast majority of patients.

For the nipple with severe trauma or cracking, topical anti-staphylococcal preparations, such as mupirocin (Bactroban), are ideal. Bactroban has limited oral bioavailability. Another anti-infective agent growing in popularity is gentian violet. Topical application of 0.5-1% strength aqueous solutions once daily for three to seven days (Do NOT Exceed Seven Days) is effective in treating superficial candida or bacterial infections of the nipple. Only use weak solutions, such as 0.5% to 1% solutions, or the infant may suffer from a severe mucocitis.

Patients with severe inflammation often respond to the topical application of moderate strength corticosteroids in combination with mupirocin (Bactroban). Hydrocortisone, triamcinolone, or mometasone ointments are ideal. The clinician should warn the mother to limit the amount to an absolute minimum, use them only after the infant has breastfed, and use them no more than four to six times daily. Hydrocortisone ointments, while inexpensive, are only moderately efficacious and slow in acting. Moderate to high potency topical steroids should be avoided. If high-potency steroids are overused on the nipple, an infant may show signs of "steroid" acne around the mouth. Finally, all of these treatments should be considered acute only, chronic use should be strictly avoided. For application to the nipple, ointments are always preferred. While the infant will ingest minor amounts of medication from the nipple, on an acute basis, this is seldom enough to produce clinical effects in the infant. Blotting off of any excess ointment prior to the next feeding may limit infant exposure, but attempting to remove all ointment with vigorous cleaning should be discouraged as it may propetuate the trauma to the nipple.

Suggested Reading

Akkuzu, G., & Taskin, L. (2000). Impacts of breast-care techniques on prevention of possible postpartum nipple problems. *Prof Care Mother Child, 10*(2), 38-41.

Amato, L., Berti, S., Chiarini, C., & Fabbri, P. (2005). Atopic dermatitis exclusively localized on nipples and areolas. *Pediatr Dermatol, 22*(1), 64-66.

Amir, L. H., & Lumley, J. (2001). The treatment of Staphylococcus aureus infected sore nipples: a randomized comparative study. *J Hum Lact, 17*(2), 115-117.

Anderson, J. E., Held, N., & Wright, K. (2004). Raynaud's phenomenon of the nipple: a treatable cause of painful breastfeeding. *Pediatrics, 113*(4), e360-364.

Barankin, B., & Gross, M. S. (2004). Nipple and areolar eczema in the breastfeeding woman. *J Cutan Med Surg, 8*(2), 126-130.

Blair, A., Cadwell, K., Turner-Maffei, C., & Brimdyr, K. (2003). The relationship between positioning, the breastfeeding dynamic, the latching process and pain in breastfeeding mothers with sore nipples. *Breastfeed Rev, 11*(2), 5-10.

Cady, B., Steele, G. D., Jr., Morrow, M., Gardner, B., Smith, B. L., Lee, N. C., et al. (1998). Evaluation of common breast problems: guidance for primary care providers. *CA Cancer J Clin, 48*(1), 49-63.

Centuori, S., Burmaz, T., Ronfani, L., Fragiacomo, M., Quintero, S., Pavan, C., et al. (1999). Nipple care, sore nipples, and breastfeeding: a randomized trial. *J Hum Lact, 15*(2), 125-130.

Dollberg, S., Botzer, E., Grunis, E., & Mimouni, F. B. (2006). Immediate nipple pain relief after frenotomy in breast-fed infants with ankyloglossia: a randomized, prospective study. *J Pediatr Surg, 41*(9), 1598-1600.

Fentiman, I. S., & Hamed, H. (2001). Assessment of breast problems. *Int J Clin Pract, 55*(7), 458-460.

Graves, S., Wright, W., Harman, R., & Bailey, S. (2003). Painful nipples in nursing mothers: fungal or staphylococcal? A preliminary study. *Aust Fam Physician, 32*(7), 570-571.

Hardwick, J. C., McMurtrie, F., & Melrose, E. B. (2002). Raynaud's syndrome of the nipple in pregnancy. *Eur J Obstet Gynecol Reprod Biol, 102*(2), 217-218.

Kapur, N., & Goldsmith, P. C. (2001). Nipple dermatitis -- not all what it 'seams'. *Contact Dermatitis, 45*(1), 44-45.

Livingstone, V., & Stringer, L. J. (1999). The treatment of Staphyloccocus aureus infected sore nipples: a randomized comparative study. *J Hum Lact, 15*(3), 241-246.

Lochner, J. E., Livingston, C. J., & Judkins, D. Z. (2009). Clinical inquiries: Which interventions are best for alleviating nipple pain in nursing mothers? *J Fam Pract, 58*(11), 612a-612c.

Mass, S. (2004). Breast pain: engorgement, nipple pain and mastitis. *Clin Obstet Gynecol, 47*(3), 676-682.

McClellan, H., Geddes, D., Kent, J., Garbin, C., Mitoulas, L., & Hartmann, P. (2008). Infants of mothers with persistent nipple pain exert strong sucking vacuums. *Acta Paediatr, 97*(9), 1205-1209.

Morland-Schultz, K., & Hill, P. D. (2005). Prevention of and therapies for nipple pain: a systematic review. *J Obstet Gynecol Neonatal Nurs, 34*(4), 428-437.

Tait, P. (2000). Nipple pain in breastfeeding women: causes, treatment, and prevention strategies. *J Midwifery Womens Health, 45*(3), 212-215.

Walker, M. (2008). Conquering common breast-feeding problems. *J Perinat Neonatal Nurs, 22*(4), 267-274.

Whitaker-Worth, D. L., Carlone, V., Susser, W. S., Phelan, N., & Grant-Kels, J. M. (2000). Dermatologic diseases of the breast and nipple. *J Am Acad Dermatol, 43*(5 Pt 1), 733-751; quiz 752-734.

Nipple Vasospasm

Principles of Therapy

Nipple vasospasm is believed to be a variant of Raynaud's Syndrome in which intense vasospasm of the vessels contiguous with the nipple undergo blanching and cause extreme pain. Classically, there is a triphasic color change of the nipple similar to digital ischemia in typical Raynaud's Syndrome. Initially, there is a pallor induced by exaggerated sympathetic adrenergic activity, followed by cyanosis and ischemia. Finally, rubor associated with a reflex vasodilation is probably due to release of local cytokines. Symptoms aside from color change include numbness, burning, tingling, and extreme pain. Treatment is largely palliative and is directed toward reducing the conditions that predispose to the symptoms, namely, reducing cold exposure or emotional situations. Preventive measures include warm clothing and avoidance of the following: tobacco in all forms, ergot alkaloids (ergotamine, bromocriptine), beta-blockers, oral contraceptives, and sympathomimetic medications (stimulants, pseudoephedrine, phenylephrine, phenylpropanolamine, etc.). Pharmacotherapy is not always effective, and often the side effects of the medications preclude continued therapy, particularly with breastfeeding infants.

Treatment

- Preventive measures include warm clothing.

- Avoidance of the following: tobacco in all forms, ergot alkaloids (ergotamine, bromocriptine), estrogens, beta-blockers, and sympathomimetic medications (stimulants, pseudoephedrine, phenylephrine, phenylpropanolamine, etc.)

- Pharmacotherapy is not always effective and often the side effects of the medications preclude continued therapy, particularly with breastfeeding infants.

- Calcium channel blockers such as Nifedipine

Medications

- FLUOXETINE   (*Prozac*)
  - AAP = Drugs whose effect on nursing infants is unknown but may be of concern
  - LRC = L2
  - RID = 1.6-14.6%
  - Pregnancy = C
  - Comment: Fluoxetine is a very popular serotonin reuptake inhibitor (SSRI) currently used for depression and a host of other syndromes. Fluoxetine absorption is rapid and complete, and the parent compound is rapidly metabolized to norfluoxetine, which is an active, long half-life metabolite

(360 hours). Both fluoxetine and norfluoxetine appear to permeate breastmilk to levels approximately 1/5 to 1/4 of maternal plasma. In one patient at steady-state (dose =20mg/day), plasma levels of fluoxetine were 100.5 μg/L and levels of norfluoxetine were 194.5 μg/L. Fluoxetine levels in milk were 28.8 μg/L and norfluoxetine levels were 41.6 μg/L. Milk/plasma ratios were 0.286 for fluoxetine, and 0.21 for norfluoxetine. For more data, consult *Medications and Mothers' Milk*.

- LOSARTAN   (*Cozaar, Hyzaar*)
  - AAP = Not reviewed
  - LRC = L3
  - RID =
  - Pregnancy = C in first trimester
  - Comment: Losartan is a new ACE-like antihypertensive. Rather than inhibiting the enzyme that makes angiotensin, such as the ACE inhibitor family, this medication selectively blocks the ACE receptor site, preventing attachment of angiotensin II. Although it penetrates the CNS significantly, its high protein binding would probably reduce its ability to enter milk. This product is only intended for those few individuals who cannot take ACE inhibitors. No data on transfer into human milk are available. The trade name Hyzaar contains losartan plus hydrochlorothiazide.

- METHYLDOPA   (*Aldomet*)
  - AAP = Maternal Medication Usually Compatible with Breastfeeding
  - LRC = L2
  - RID = 0.1-0.3%
  - Pregnancy = B
  - Comment: Alpha-methyldopa is a centrally acting antihypertensive. It is frequently used to treat hypertension during pregnancy. In a study of two lactating women who received a dose of 500 mg, the maximum breastmilk concentration of methyldopa ranged from 0.2 to 0.66 mg/L. In another patient who received 1000 mg dose, the maximum concentration in milk was 1.14 mg/L. The milk/plasma ratios varied from 0.19 to 0.34. The authors indicated that if the infant were to ingest 750 mL of milk daily (with a maternal dose = 1000 mg), the maximum daily ingestion would be less than 855 μg or approximately 0.02% of the maternal dose.

    In another study of seven women who received 0.750-2.0 gm/day of methyldopa, the free methyldopa concentrations in breastmilk ranged from zero to 0.2 mg/L, while the conjugated metabolite had concentrations of 0.1 to 0.9 mg/L. These studies generally indicate that the levels of methyldopa transferred to a breastfeeding infant would be too low to be clinically relevant.

    However, gynecomastia and galactorrhea have been reported in one full-term two week old female neonate following seven days of maternal therapy with methyldopa, 250 mg three times daily.

- NIFEDIPINE   (*Adalat, Procardia*)
  - AAP = Maternal Medication Usually Compatible with Breastfeeding
  - LRC = L2
  - RID = 2.3-3.4%
  - Pregnancy = C
  - Comment: Nifedipine is an effective antihypertensive. It belongs to the calcium channel blocker family of drugs. Two studies indicate that nifedipine is transferred to breastmilk in varying, but

generally low levels. In one study in which the dose was varied from 10-30 mg three times daily, the highest concentration (53.35 µg/L) was measured at one hour after a 30 mg dose. Other levels reported were 16.35 µg/L 60 minutes after a 20 mg dose and 12.89 µg/L 30 minutes after a 10 mg dose. The milk levels fell linearly with the milk half-lives estimated to be 1.4 hours for the 10 mg dose, 3.1 hours for the 20 dose, and 2.4 hours for the 30 mg dose. The milk concentration measured eight hours following a 30 mg dose was 4.93 µg/L. In this study, using the highest concentration found and a daily intake of 150 mL/kg of human milk, the amount of nifedipine intake would only be 8 µg/kg/day (less than 1.8% of the therapeutic pediatric dose). The authors conclude that the amount ingested via breastmilk poses little risk to an infant. In another study, concentrations of nifedipine in human milk one to eight hours after 10 mg doses varied from <1 to 10.3 µg/L (median 3.5 µg/L) in 6 of 11 patients. In this study, milk levels three days after discontinuing medication ranged from <1 to 9.4 µg/L. The authors concluded the exposure to nifedipine through breastmilk is not significant. In a study by Penny and Lewis, following a maternal dose of 20 mg nifedipine daily for 10 days, peak breastmilk levels at one hour were 46 µg/L. The corresponding maternal serum level was 43 µg/L. From these data, the authors suggest a daily intake for an infant would be approximately 6.45 µg/kg/day.

Nifedipine has been found clinically useful for nipple vasospasm. Because of the similarity to Raynaud's Phenomenon, sustained release formulations providing 30-60 mg per day are suggested.

- SILDENAFIL   (*Viagra*)
  - ◦ AAP = Not reviewed
  - ◦ LRC = L3
  - ◦ RID =
  - ◦ Pregnancy = B
  - ◦ Comment: Sildenafil is an inhibitor of nitrous oxide metabolism, that causes increased levels of nitrous oxide, smooth muscle relaxation, and an increased flow of blood in the corpus cavernosum of the penis. While not currently indicated for women, off label use for other conditions is increasing. No data are available on the transfer of sildenafil into human milk, but it is unlikely that significant transfer will occur due to its larger molecular weight and short half-life. However, caution is recommended in breastfeeding mothers. While not reported, persistent abnormal erections (priapism) could potentially occur in male infants.

- TERBUTALINE   (*Bricanyl, Brethine*)
  - ◦ AAP = Maternal Medication Usually Compatible with Breastfeeding
  - ◦ LRC = L2
  - ◦ RID = 0.2-0.3%
  - ◦ Pregnancy = B
  - ◦ Comment: Terbutaline is a popular beta-2 adrenergic used for bronchodilation in asthmatics. It is secreted into breastmilk, but in low quantities. Following doses of 7.5 to 15 mg/day of terbutaline, milk levels averaged 3.37 µg/L. Assuming a daily milk intake of 165 mL/kg, these levels would suggest a daily intake of less than 0.5 µg/kg/day, which corresponds to 0.2 to 0.7% of maternal dose.

    In another study of a patient receiving 5 mg three times daily, the mean milk concentrations ranged from 3.2 to 3.7 µg/L. The authors calculated the daily dose to infant at 0.4-0.5 µg/kg body weight.

Terbutaline was not detectable in the infant's serum. No untoward effects have been reported in breastfeeding infants.

Clinical Tips

Initially, preventive measures, such as evaluation of the infant's latch (poor positioning and attachment), and other breastfeeding factors must be explored. Patients should be advised to avoid stressful situations and cold environments when breastfeeding. Failing this, pharmacologic therapy is indicated in those individuals for whom preventive measures have been ineffective. While numerous medications are effective, all of the sympatholytics, alpha-adrenergic blockers, beta-receptor agonists, and calcium channel blockers may create intolerable side effects for the patient. At present, most agree that the newer slow-channel calcium channel blockers are greatly preferred due to efficacy and minimal side effects. These act by reducing vasospasm and vasoconstriction by reducing calcium influx into the vascular smooth muscle cell. Of these, nifedipine is greatly preferred because it has the most potent peripheral action and its concentration in human milk is minimal. The recommended starting dose is 10 mg orally three times daily, increasing the dose in a stepwise fashion as dictated by clinical response. Experience with long-acting dosage forms now suggests that they are preferred. Recent studies suggest that the SSRI fluoxetine may actually work better than calcium channel blockers, although these studies are few and small in size. While other agents have been used successfully, they are somewhat more risky in a breastfeeding mother. ACE inhibitors, such as captopril and losartan, have been used, but are only about 30% effective in Raynaud's syndrome. New data on sildenanfil (50 mg twice daily) suggests it is signficiantly effective at reducing symptoms of Raynaud's disease.

Methyldopa is about 50% effective and several studies show low milk levels. Although nicotinic acid is marginally effective (<40%), its use in high doses could be problematic for a breastfed infant (liver damage). Alpha-adrenergic blockers have not been studied in breastfeeding mothers, but due to their high potency, they are probably too toxic to risk (prazosin, phenoxybenzamine). There are numerous other medications that are poorly efficacious and have not been studied in breastfeeding mothers. These include griseofulvin, papaverine, nitrates, guanethidine, reserpine, prostaglandins (PGI2, PGE1), thyroid, dextran, and pentoxifylline. Topical nitroglycerine is not recommended as oral absorption by the infant could be significant.

Suggested Reading

Coates, M. M. (1992). Nipple pain related to vasospasm in the nipple? *J Hum Lact, 8*(3), 153.

Nicolas, J., & D., L. (2004). Rhytidectomy and Raynaud's phenomenon: about two cases]. *Ann Chir Plast Esthet, 49*(6), 564-568.

Page, S. M., & McKenna, D. S. (2006). Vasospasm of the nipple presenting as painful lactation. *Obstet Gynecol, 108*(3 Pt 2), 806-808.

Reilly, A., & Snyder, B. (2005). Raynaud phenomenon. *Am J Nurs, 105*(8), 56-65.

Thompson, A. E., & Pope, J. E. (2005). Calcium channel blockers for primary Raynaud's phenomenon: a meta-analysis. *Rheumatology, 44*, 145-150.

Obesity

Principles of Therapy

Obesity is a growing epidemic in the US. Discussion regarding appropriate pregnancy weight gain and goals for weight loss in the postpartum period should be standard obstetrical practice. BMI is defined as the weight in kilograms divided by height in meters squared. Overweight is defined as a BMI of 25 to 29.9 kg/m^2 and obesity is defined as a BMI of $\geq$30 kg/m^2. Most current obesity data suggests that the prevalence is over 30% of the adult population.

Mean pre-pregnancy BMI has increased in recent time. A study comparing pre-pregnancy BMI from the 1960's found a mean of 21.9 kg/m^2 compared to 23.7 kg/m^2 during the mid-1980's. Overweight women were also likely to gain more weight than recommended during pregnancy. Obese pregnant women are then at increased risk for various pregnancy complications, such as fetal macrosomia, diabetes, hypertension, and cesarean delivery, while their infants are more likely to require neonatal intensive care unit admission. A meta-analysis of 12 articles on postpartum weight retention found that two-thirds of women exceeded their pre-pregnancy weight at six weeks postpartum. Another study found that women who lost all weight by six months postpartum gained an average of 2.4 kg at follow-up 10 years later compared with an average of 8.3 kg for those who had not returned to pre-pregnancy weight by six months. Women who breastfed and those who participated in aerobic exercise also had lower weight gains.

Management of overweight and obesity should involve recommendations and support from healthcare providers for dietary changes and exercise as appropriate. However, these measures may not always be successful.

Drug therapies and, occasionally, surgical options may be pursued. In women with PCOS and evidence of insulin resistance, metformin may be useful in reversing disease characteristics and may promote weight loss. Additionally, certain medications aimed at reducing fat absorption may be employed. OTC products, such as Orlistat, are marketed for this use.

Bariatric surgical options are available. These procedures have different risk and benefit characteristics and detailed counseling should be pursued prior to proceeding. Gastric banding procedures (restrictive) can be performed and may be adjustable. Additionally, various gastric bypass procedures, such as Roux-en-Y(both restrictive and malabsorptive), are options. Procedures such as the Roux-en-Y bypass actually decrease the absorptive surface of the intestine. The procedures often result in signficiant weight loss over time, but have both surgical complications and associated nutritional deficiencies. Breastfeeding may not be the ideal time to proceed with these more drastic surgical options.

There is now a growing body of evidence for the management of subsequent pregnancy after bariatric surgery. It is best to defer pregnancy until 12-18 months after the surgical procedure so that weight loss has stabilized. Possible supplementation depends on the procedure performed and the patient's specific evaluation, but may include vitamin B12, folate, iron, vitamin D, and calcium. Women who have subsequent pregnancies may choose to breastfeed. There is little scientific evidence available about breastfeeding after bariatric surgery.

Treatment

- Cornerstones of initial therapy include behavioral therapy, dietary therapy and exercise.

- Drug therapy

- Surgical therapy

Medications

- ORLISTAT   (*Xenical, Alli*)
    - AAP = Not reviewed
    - LRC = L3
    - RID =
    - Pregnancy = B
    - Comment: Orlistat, now available over the counter as well as prescription, is used in the management of obesity. It is a reversible inhibitor of gastric and pancreatic lipases, thus it inhibits absorption of dietary fats by 30%. No studies have been performed on the transmission of orlistat into the breastmilk. With high protein binding, moderately high molecular weight, and poor oral absorption, it is unlikely that orlistat would enter breastmilk in clinically relevant amounts or affect a breastfeeding infant. However, due to orlistat's effect on the absorption of fat soluble vitamins and other fats, nutritional status of a breastfeeding mother should be closely monitored.

- METFORMIN   (*Glucophage, Glucovance*)
    - AAP = Not reviewed
    - LRC = L1
    - RID = 0.3-0.7%
    - Pregnancy = B
    - Comment: Metformin belongs to the biguanide family and is used to reduce glucose levels in non-insulin dependent diabetics. Oral bioavailability is only 50%. In a study of seven women taking metformin (median dose 1500 mg/d), the mean milk-to-plasma ratio (AUC) for metformin was 0.35. The mean average concentration in milk over the dose interval was 0.27 mg/L. The absolute infant dose averaged 0.04 mg/kg/d and the mean relative infant dose was 0.28%. Metformin was present in very low or undetectable concentrations in the plasma of four of the infants who were studied. No health problems were found in the six infants who were evaluated.

        In another study of five subjects the median milk/plasma ratio (AUC) for metformin was 0.47. The median calculated infant dose was 0.2% of the weight-adjusted maternal dose. None of the infants exposed to their mothers' milk had detectable levels of metformin in their plasma, nor were any side effects noted.

        In a recent study of five women consuming an average dose of 500 mg twice daily, the mean peak and trough metformin concentrations in breastmilk were 0.42 mg/L (range 0.38-0.46 mg/L) and

0.39 mg/L (range 0.31-0.52 mg/L), respectively. The average milk/serum ratio was 0.63 (range 0.36-1.00) and the estimated relative infant dose was 0.65% (range 0.43-1.08%). Blood glucose concentrations in three infants were normal, ranging from 47-77 mg/dL. The mothers reported no side effects were noted in the breastfed infants.

Metformin is also used to treat polycystic ovary syndrome. In one study of 61 nursing infants whose mothers were taking a median of 2.55 g/day throughout pregnancy and lactation, the growth, motor, and social development of the infants was recorded to be normal. The authors concluded that metformin was safe and effective during lactation in the first six months of an infant's life.

Clinical Tips

The cornerstone of weight therapy is still the reduction of caloric intake. The use of phentermine and sibutramine is associated with numerous clinical effects, and if ingested by an infant, complications could be serious. Neither of these products are worth the increased risk to the infant. Sibutamaine (Meridia) may be associated with increased cardiovascular risk (heart attack, stroke, etc.). Sibutramine is rather small in molecular weight, active in the CNS, extremely lipid soluble, and has two 'active' metabolites with long half-lives (14-16 hours). Although no data are available on its transfer into human milk, the pharmacokinetics of this drug theoretically suggest that it might have a rather high milk/plasma ratio and could enter milk in significant levels. Until we know more, a risk assessment may not support the use of this product in breastfeeding mothers.

Orlistat appears modestly effective in adults with only an average loss of 6.4 pounds in numerous studies. In severely obese patients and when taken for more than two years, orlistat may produce an average weight loss of 9.3 pounds. Patients must be advised to supplement with vitamins, particularly oil-soluble vitamins (vitamin D, E, A, K) as they are lost fecally. Orlistat is a reversible inhibitor of gastric and pancreatic lipases, thus it inhibits absorption of dietary fats by 30%. No studies have been performed on the transmission of orlistat into the breastmilk. It is very unlikely this product would ever be transferred into human milk as it is virtually unabsorbed by adults. However, due to orlistat's effect on the absorption of fat soluble vitamins and other fats, nutritional status of a breastfeeding mother should be closely monitored. Mothers should continue to take vitamins during lactation if using this product.

In patients with type 2 diabetes, metformin is a good choice and is weight negative, thus leading to significant weight loss in some patients. Levels in milk are low and it is compatible with breastfeeding. It may be particularly suitable for patients with polycystic ovarian syndrome. Another effect of metformin is to partially correct the endocrinopathy associated with polycystic ovarian syndrome.

Other medications, such as caffeine, ephedrine (Ma huang), should be avoided as they can be associated with numerous complications in breastfed infants.

An herbal product, Hoodia, has recently become quite popular for weight loss, although its efficacy in humans when taken orally is unresolved. A succulent plant from the Kalahari desert in Africa, the Hoodia species (very rare) suggested to suppress appetite is *Hoodia gordonii*. While the active extract believed to produce the anorexigenic effect, hoodigogenin A, which is the aglycone of the oxypregnane steroidal glycoside P57AS3 (P57), has been known since the early 1990s, little has been done to commercially develop this product. The one study done was flawed and its evidence of anorexia is questionable. Further, there are not enough Hoodia plants in the whole world to account for all the products available on today's market, so many products probably contain little or no Hoodia. We do not know if this product is safe for a breastfeeding mother. In these cases, numerous other adulterant drugs could be present and hazardous to the infant. Hoodia products should not be used by breastfeeding mothers until more is known.

Suggested Reading

Baumer, J. H. (2007). Obesity and overweight: its prevention, identification, assessment and management. *Arch Dis Child Educ Pract Ed, 92*(3), ep92-96.

Burguera, B., Agusti, A., Arner, P., Baltasar, A., Barbe, F., Barcelo, A., et al. (2007). Critical assessment of the current guidelines for the management and treatment of morbidly obese patients. *J Endocrinol Invest, 30*(10), 844-852.

Dick, J. J. (2004). Weight loss interventions for adult obesity: evidence for practice. *Worldviews Evid Based Nurs, 1*(4), 209-214.

Hendricks, E. J., Rothman, R. B., & Greenway, F. L. (2009). How physician obesity specialists use drugs to treat obesity. *Obesity (Silver Spring), 17*(9), 1730-1735.

King, D. E., Mainous, A. G., 3rd, Carnemolla, M., & Everett, C. J. (2009). Adherence to healthy lifestyle habits in US adults, 1988-2006. *Am J Med, 122*(6), 528-534.

Kinnunen T.I., Luoto R., Gissler M., Hemminki E. (2003). Pregnancy weight gain from 1960s to 2000 in Finland. *Int J Obes Relat Metab Disord. 27*(12), 1572-7

Lautz, D. B., Jiser, M. E., Kelly, J. J., Shikora, S. A., Partridge, S. K., Romanelli, J. R., et al. (2009). An update on best practice guidelines for specialized facilities and resources necessary for weight loss surgical programs. *Obesity (Silver Spring), 17*(5), 911-917.

Malik, V. S., & Hu, F. B. (2007). Popular weight-loss diets: from evidence to practice. *Nat Clin Pract Cardiovasc Med, 4*(1), 34-41.

McDonald, S. D. (2007). Management and prevention of obesity in adults and children. *CMAJ, 176*(8), 1109-1110.

Ockenden, J. (2007). Midwifery basics: diet matters (3). Obesity in pregnancy. *Pract Midwife, 10*(11), 39-40, 42-35.

Ockenden, J. (2008). Midwifery basics: diet matters (5). Obesity and complications of pregnancy and birth. *Pract Midwife, 11*(3), 36-39.

Rooney B.L., Schauberger C.W. (2002). Excess pregnancy weight and long-term obesity: one decade later. *Obstet Gynecol. 100*(2), 245-52.

Serci, I. (2007). Midwifery basics: diet matters (2). Maternal overweight in pregnancy. *Pract Midwife, 10*(10), 36-40, 42.

Walker L.O., Sterling B.S., Timmerman G.M. (2005). Retention of pregnancy-related weight in the early postpartum period: implications for women's health services. *J Obstet gynecol Neonatal Nurs. 34*(4), 418-27.

Wellesley, H., & Wharton, N. M. (2008). Maternal obesity and anaesthesia. *Int J Obstet Anesth, 17*(3), 279-280; author reply 280.

Wylie-Rosett, J., Albright, A. A., Apovian, C., Clark, N. G., Delahanty, L., Franz, M. J., et al. (2007). 2006-2007 American Diabetes Association Nutrition Recommendations: issues for practice translation. *J Am Diet Assoc, 107*(8), 1296-1304.

Pain

Principles of Therapy

Pain is the most common symptom causing patients to seek medical attention. Proper treatment depends largely on the careful diagnosis and source of the pain. As such, the medications used are largely determined by the source and cause of pain. The following medications are those generally used as analgesics for a variety of pain. More complete descriptions of pain by syndrome, such as 'Migraine Headaches' are provided under their specific categories.

Treatment

- NSAID drugs.

- Opiate drugs.

- Non-opiate drugs.

Medications

- ACETAMINOPHEN   (*Tempra, Tylenol, Paracetamol*)
    - AAP = Maternal Medication Usually Compatible with Breastfeeding
    - LRC = L1
    - RID = 8.8-24.2%
    - Pregnancy = B
    - Comment: Only small amounts are secreted into breastmilk and are considered too small to be hazardous. In a study of 11 mothers who received 650 mg of acetaminophen orally, the highest milk levels reported were from 10-15 mg/L. The milk/plasma ratio was 1.08. In another study of three patients who received a single 500 mg oral dose, the reported milk and plasma concentrations of acetaminophen was 4.2 mg/L and 5.6 mg/L, respectively. The milk/plasma ratio was 0.76. The maximum observed concentration in milk was 4.4 mg/L. In another study of women who ingested 1000 mg acetaminophen, milk levels averaged 6.1 mg/L and provided an average dose of 0.92 mg/kg/d according to the authors. There seems to be wide variation in the milk concentrations in these studies, but the relative infant dose is probably less than 6.4% of the maternal dose. This is significantly less than the pediatric therapeutic dose. Acetaminophen is compatible with breastfeeding.

- ASPIRIN   (*Anacin, Aspergum, Empirin, Genprin, Arthritis Foundation Pain Reliever, Ecotrin*)
    - AAP = Drugs associated with significant side effects and should be given with caution

- LRC = L3
- RID = 2.5 - 10.8%
- Pregnancy = C during first and second trimester
- Comment: Extremely small amounts are secreted into breastmilk. Few harmful effects have been reported. In one study, salicylic acid (active metabolite of Aspirin) penetrated poorly into milk (dose =454 mg ASA), with peak levels of only 1.12 to 1.60 µg/mL, whereas peak plasma levels were 33 to 43.4 µg/mL. In another study of a rheumatoid arthritis patient who received 4 gm/day aspirin, none was detectable in her milk (<5mg/100cc). Extremely high doses in the mother could potentially produce slight bleeding in the infant. Because aspirin is implicated in Reye syndrome, it is a poor choice of analgesic to use in breastfeeding mothers. However, in rheumatic fever patients, it is still one of the anti-inflammatory drugs of choice and a risk-vs-benefit assessment must be done in this case.

  While the direct use of aspirin in infants and children is definitely implicated in Reye syndrome, the use of the 82 mg/d dose in breastfeeding mothers is unlikely to increase the risk of this syndrome. Unfortunately, we do not at present know of any dose-response relationship between aspirin and Reye syndrome, other than in older children where even low plasma levels of aspirin were implicated in Reye syndrome during viral syndromes, such as flu or chickenpox. Therefore, the use of aspirin in breastfeeding mothers is questionable, but the risk is probably low. See ibuprofen or acetaminophen as better choices. Never use these products if the infant has a viral syndrome.

- **BUPRENORPHINE**   (*Buprenex, Subutex*)

  - AAP = Not reviewed
  - LRC = L2
  - RID = 1.9%
  - Pregnancy = C
  - Comment: Buprenorphine is a potent, long-acting narcotic agonist and antagonist and may be useful as a replacement for methadone treatment in addicts. It is also recently approved for the treatment of opiate dependence. Its elimination half-life varies from paper to paper, but new recent sublingual studies suggests it ranges from 23-30 hours.

    In one patient who received 4 mg/day to facilitate withdrawal from other opiates, the amount of buprenorphine transferred via milk was only 3.28 µg/day, an amount that was clinically insignificant. No symptoms were noted in this breastfed infant. In another study of continuous epidural bupivacaine and buprenorphine in post cesarean women for three days, it was suggested that buprenorphine may suppress the production of milk (and infant weight gain) although this was not absolutely clear.

    In another study of one patient on buprenorphine maintenance for seven months, and who received 8 mg daily sublingually over four days, milk levels of buprenorphine and norbuprenorphine ranged from 1.0 to 14.7 ng/mL and 0.6 to 6.3 ng/mL, respectively. Plasma concentrations of both analytes ranged from 0.2 to 20.1 ng/mL (buprenorphine) and 1.2 to 4.4 ng/mL (norbuprenorphine) over four days of study. Using peak levels only, the concentration of buprenorphine and norbuprenorphine were 1.47 and 0.63 µg/100 mL of breastmilk, respectively. Assuming an intake of 150 mL/kg/day, the authors estimated the daily dose would be less than 10 µg for a 4 kg infant, a dose that is probably far subclinical.

- BUTORPHANOL   (*Stadol*)
  - ◦ AAP = Maternal Medication Usually Compatible with Breastfeeding
  - ◦ LRC = L2
  - ◦ RID = 0.5%
  - ◦ Pregnancy = C during first and second trimester
  - ◦ Comment: Butorphanol is a potent narcotic analgesic. It is available as IV, IM, and a nasal spray. Butorphanol passes into breastmilk in low to moderate concentrations. The amount an infant would receive is probably clinically insignificant (estimated 4 µg/L of milk in a mother receiving 2 mg IM four times a day). Levels produced in infants are considered very low to insignificant. Butorphanol undergoes first-pass extraction by the liver, thus only 17% of the oral dose reaches the plasma. Butorphanol has been frequently used in labor and delivery in women who subsequently nursed their infants, although it has been noted to produce a sinusoidal fetal heart rate pattern and dysphoric or psychotomimetic responses in infants. Butorphanol use in breastfeeding mothers is, however, of minimum risk to the normal term infant.

- CODEINE   (*Empirin #3 # 4, Tylenol # 3 # 4*)
  - ◦ AAP = Maternal Medication Usually Compatible with Breastfeeding
  - ◦ LRC = L3
  - ◦ RID = 8.1%
  - ◦ Pregnancy = C
  - ◦ Comment: Codeine is considered a mild opiate analgesic whose action is probably due to its metabolism to small amounts (about 7%) of morphine. The amount of codeine secreted into milk is low and dose dependent. Infant response is higher during the neonatal period (first or second week). Four cases of neonatal apnea have been reported following administration of 60 mg codeine every four to six hours to breastfeeding mothers, although codeine was not detected in serum of the infants tested. Apnea resolved after discontinuation of maternal codeine. Tylenol # 3 tablets contain 30 mg and Tylenol #4 tablets contain 60 mg of codeine in the USA. In a study of seven mothers, codeine and morphine levels were studied in breastmilk of 17 samples, and neonatal plasma of 24 samples from 11 healthy, term neonates. Milk codeine levels ranged from 33.8 to 314 µg/L 20 to 240 minutes after administration of codeine; morphine levels ranged from 1.9 to 20.5 µg/L. Infant plasma samples one to four hours after feeding had codeine levels ranging from <0.8 to 4.5 µg/L; morphine ranged from <0.5 to 2.2 µg/L. The authors suggest that moderate codeine use during breastfeeding (< or = four 60 mg doses) is probably safe. In a recent report, an infant death was reported following the use of codeine (initially two tablets every 12 hours, reduced to half that dose from day two to two weeks because of maternal somnolence and constipation) in a mother. Codeine levels in milk were reported to be 87 µg/L, while the average reported milk levels in most mothers range from 1.9 to 20.5 µg/L at doses of 60 mg every six hours. Genotype analysis of this specific mother indicated that she was an ultra-rapid metabolizer of codeine. This genotype (which is very rare) leads to increased formation of morphine from codeine.

    Ultimately, each infant's response to exposure to codeine should be independently determined. In the vast majority of mothers, codeine taken in moderation should be safe for their breastfed infant. However, any report of overt somnolence, apnea, poor feeding, or grey skin should be reported to the physician and could be associated with exposure to codeine.

- FENTANYL (*Sublimaze*)
    - AAP = Maternal Medication Usually Compatible with Breastfeeding
    - LRC = L2
    - RID = 3-5%
    - Pregnancy = C
    - Comment: The transfer of fentanyl into human milk has been documented, but is low. In a group of 10 women receiving a total dose of 50 to 400 μg fentanyl IV during labor, the concentration of fentanyl in milk was exceedingly low, generally below the level of detection (<0.05 ng/mL). In a few samples, the levels were between 0.05 and 0.15 ng/mL. Using these data, an infant would ingest less than 3% of the weight-adjusted maternal dose per day. In another study of 13 women who received 2 μg/kg IV after delivery and cord clamping, fentanyl concentration in colostrum was extremely low. Colostrum levels dropped rapidly and were undetectable after ten hours. The authors conclude that with these small concentrations and fentanyl's low oral bioavailability, intravenous fentanyl analgesia may be used safely in breastfeeding women. It is apparent that fentanyl transfer to milk under most clinical conditions is poor and is probably clinically unimportant.

- FLURBIPROFEN (*Ansaid, Froben, Ocufen*)
    - AAP = Not reviewed
    - LRC = L2
    - RID = 0.7-1.4%
    - Pregnancy = B during first and second trimester
    - Comment: Flurbiprofen is a nonsteroidal analgesic similar in structure to ibuprofen, but used both as an ophthalmic preparation (in eyes) and orally. In one study of 12 women and following nine oral doses (50 mg/dose, three to five days postpartum), the concentration of flurbiprofen in two women ranged from 0.05 to 0.07 mg/L of milk, but was <0.05 mg/L in 10 of the 12 women. Concentrations in breastmilk and plasma of nursing mothers suggest that a nursing infant would receive less than 0.1 mg flurbiprofen per day, a level considered exceedingly low.

        In another study of 10 nursing mothers following a single 100 mg dose, the average peak concentration of flurbiprofen in breastmilk was 0.09 mg/L, or about 0.05% of the maternal dose. Both of these studies suggest that the amount of flurbiprofen transferred in human milk would be clinically insignificant to the infant.

- HYDROCODONE (*Lortab, Vicodin*)
    - AAP = Not reviewed
    - LRC = L3
    - RID = 3.1-3.7%
    - Pregnancy = B
    - Comment: Hydrocodone is a narcotic analgesic and antitussive structurally related to codeine although somewhat more potent. It is commonly used in breastfeeding mothers throughout the USA. In a study of two breastfeeding women taking hydrocodone for various periods, patient one received a total of 63,525 μg (998.8 μg/kg) over 86.5 hours. Patient two, received 9075 μg (123.5 μg/kg) over 36 hours.

        In patient one, the AUC of the drug concentration in milk was 4946.1 μg/L.hr and an average milk concentration of 57.2 μg/L. The authors estimate the relative infant dose at 3.1%. In patient two, the AUC of the drug concentration in milk was 735.6 μg/L.hr and an average milk concentration of 20.4 μg/L. The authors estimate the relative infant dose at 3.7%. This paper concluded that high doses of hydrocodone in mothers who are nursing newborn or premature infants can be concerning. Mothers should be advised to watch for sedation and appropriate weight gain in their infants.

- IBUPROFEN   (*Advil, Nuprin, Motrin, Pediaprofen*)
  - ○ AAP = Maternal Medication Usually Compatible with Breastfeeding
  - ○ LRC = L1
  - ○ RID = 0.1-0.7%
  - ○ Pregnancy = B in first and second trimester
  - ○ Comment: Ibuprofen is a nonsteroidal anti-inflammatory analgesic. It is frequently used for fever in infants. Ibuprofen enters milk only in very low levels (less than 0.6% of maternal dose). Even large doses produce very small milk levels. In one patient receiving 400 mg twice daily, milk levels were less than 0.5 mg/L.

    In another study of 12 women who received 400 mg doses every six hours for a total of five doses, all breastmilk levels of ibuprofen were less than 1.0 mg/L, the lower limit of the assay. Data in these studies document that no measurable concentrations of ibuprofen are detected in breastmilk following the above doses. Ibuprofen is presently popular for therapy of fever in infants. Current recommended dose in children is 5-10 mg/kg every six hours. Ibuprofen is an ideal analgesic for breastfeeding mothers.

- HYDROMORPHONE   (*Dilaudid*)
  - ○ AAP = Not reviewed
  - ○ LRC = L3
  - ○ RID = 0.7%
  - ○ Pregnancy = C
  - ○ Comment: Hydromorphone is a potent semisynthetic narcotic analgesic used to alleviate moderate to severe pain. It is approximately seven to ten times more potent that morphine, but is used in equivalently lower doses. In a group of eight women who received intranasal hydromorphone (2 mg), milk levels ranged from a high of about 6000 pg/mL at about one hour, to about 200 pg/mL at 24 hours, but averaged about 1.04 pg/mL. The observed milk/plasma ratio averaged 2.57. The half-life of hydromorphone in milk was estimated at 10.5 hours. The authors estimate a Relative Infant Dose of 0.67% of the maternal dose, although this author calculates it at 0.52%. Using these data an infant would consume (via milk) approximately 2.2 μg per day. This is significantly less than the clinical dose in infants and children of 15-30 μg/kg/dose every four to six hours.

- KETOROLAC   (*Toradol, Acular*)
  - ○ AAP = Maternal Medication Usually Compatible with Breastfeeding
  - ○ LRC = L2
  - ○ RID = 0.2%
  - ○ Pregnancy = C in first and second trimesters
  - ○ Comment: Ketorolac is a popular, nonsteroidal analgesic. Although previously used in labor and delivery, its use has subsequently been contraindicated because it is believed to adversely effect fetal circulation and inhibit uterine contractions, thus increasing the risk of hemorrhage. In a study of

10 lactating women who received 10 mg orally four times daily, milk levels of ketorolac were not detectable in four of the subjects. In the six remaining patients, the concentration of ketorolac in milk two hours after a dose ranged from 5.2 to 7.3 µg/L on day one and 5.9 to 7.9 µg/L on day two. In most patients, the breastmilk level was never above 5 µg/L. The maximum daily dose an infant could absorb (maternal dose = 40 mg/day) would range from 3.16 to 7.9 µg/day assuming a milk volume of 400 mL or 1000 mL. An infant would, therefore, receive less than 0.2% of the daily maternal dose. Please note, the original paper contained a misprint on the daily intake of ketorolac (mg instead of µg).

- MEPERIDINE   (*Demerol*)
  - ◦ AAP = Maternal Medication Usually Compatible with Breastfeeding
  - ◦ LRC = L2
  - ◦ RID = 1.4-13.9%
  - ◦ Pregnancy = C
  - ◦ Comment: Meperidine is a potent opiate analgesic. It is rapidly and completely metabolized by the adult and neonatal liver to an active form, normeperidine. Significant but small amounts of meperidine are secreted into breastmilk. In a study of nine nursing mothers two hours after a 50 mg IM injection, the average concentration of meperidine in milk was 82 µg/L and a milk/plasma ratio of 1.12. The highest concentration of meperidine in breastmilk at two hours after dose was 0.13 mg/L. In another study, the maximum concentration of meperidine in milk ranged from 134 to 244 µg/L in five patients at one to two hours after administration and 76 to 318 µg/L at two to four hours after administration of 25 mg intravenously (in three patients). According to these authors, the maximum dose to an infant would be approximately 9.5 µg/kg or 1.2% to 3.5% of the weight-adjusted maternal dose. In a study of two nursing mothers who received varying amounts of meperidine following delivery (up to 1275 mg within 72 hours), the concentration of meperidine ranged from 36.2 to 314 µg/L, with an average of 225 µg/L. Breastmilk levels of normeperidine ranged from zero to 333 µg/L, with an average of 142 µg/L. This study clearly shows a much longer half-life for the active metabolite, normeperidine. Normeperidine levels were detected after 56 hours post-administration in human milk (8.1 ng/mL), following a single 50 mg dose. The milk/plasma ratios varied from 0.82 to 1.59 depending on dose and timing of sampling.

    Published half-lives for meperidine in neonates (13 hours) and normeperidine (63 hours) are long and, with time, could concentrate in the plasma of a neonate. Wittels studies clearly indicate that infants from mothers treated with meperidine (PCA post-cesarean) were neurobehaviorally depressed after three days. Infants from similar groups treated with morphine were not affected.

- MORPHINE   (*Duramorph, Infumorph*)
  - ◦ AAP = Maternal Medication Usually Compatible with Breastfeeding
  - ◦ LRC = L3
  - ◦ RID = 9.1%
  - ◦ Pregnancy = C
  - ◦ Comment: Morphine is a potent narcotic analgesic. In a group of five lactating women, the highest morphine concentration in breastmilk following two epidural doses was only 82 µg/L at 30 minutes. The highest breastmilk level following 15 mg IV/IM was only 0.5 mg/L, although it dropped to almost 0.01 mg/L in four hours. In this study and following two 4 mg epidural doses, the peak milk level was 82 µg/L or a relative infant dose of 10.7%.

In another study of women receiving morphine via PCA pumps for 12-48 hours postpartum, the concentration of morphine in breastmilk ranged from 50-60 µg/L (estimated from graph). None of the infants in this study were neurobehaviorally delayed at three days. Because of the poor oral bioavailability of morphine (26%), it is unlikely these levels would be clinically relevant in a stable breastfeeding infant.

However, data from Robieux suggests the levels transferred to the infant are higher. In this study of a single patient, plasma levels in the breastfed infant were within therapeutic range (4 ng/mL), although the infant showed no untoward signs or symptoms. However, this case was somewhat unique in that the mother received daily morphine (50 mg PO every six hours) during the third trimester for severe back pain. One week postpartum, the morphine was discontinued and then five days later reinstated due to withdrawal effects in the mother. The reported concentration in foremilk and hindmilk was 100 ng/mL and 10 ng/mL, respectively, and the authors suggested that the dose to the infant would be 0.8 to 12% of the maternal oral dose (0.15 to 2.41 mg/day). Although this study suggests that the amount of morphine transferred in milk can be clinically relevant, the authors calculated the infant dose from the highest milk concentration and a milk intake of 150 mL/kg/day, thus the dose of morphine to the infant would have been substantially lower (53 µg/day). This study seems flawed because the plasma levels and the doses via milk just don't correlate. That this infant showed no untoward effects can be explained by the fact that it may have exhibited tolerance after long exposure, that the reported analgesic-therapeutic level required in neonates is actually slightly higher than in adults, or that the plasma levels assayed in this infant were in error.

Infants under one month of age have a prolonged elimination half-life and decreased clearance of morphine relative to older infants. The clearance of morphine and its elimination begins to approach adult values by two months of age. In summary, morphine is probably the preferred opiate in breastfeeding mothers primarily due to its poor oral bioavailability. It is unfortunate that the clinical studies above do not necessarily suggest this. However, high doses over prolonged periods could lead to sedation and respiratory problems in newborn infants.

- NALBUPHINE   (*Nubain*)
  - ○ AAP = Not reviewed
  - ○ LRC = L2
  - ○ RID = 0.6%
  - ○ Pregnancy = B
  - ○ Comment: Nalbuphine is a potent narcotic analgesic similar in potency to morphine. Nalbuphine is both an antagonist and agonist of opiate receptors and should not be mixed with other opiates due to interference with analgesia. In a group of 20 postpartum mothers who received a single 20 mg IM nalbuphine dose, the total amount of nalbuphine excreted into human milk during a 24 hour period averaged 2.3 micrograms, which is equivalent to 0.012% of the maternal dosage. The mean milk/plasma ratio using the AUC was 1.2. According to the authors, an oral intake of 2.3 µg nalbuphine per day by an infant would not show any measurable plasma concentrations in the neonate. In another study of 18 mothers who received 0.2 mg/kg every four hours over two to three days, the average concentration in breastmilk was 42 µg/L, with a maximum of 61 µg/L. The reported infant dose was an average of 7 µg/kg/day, with a maximum of 9 µg/kg/day. The authors estimate the RID = 0.59% of the weight-adjusted maternal daily dose and suggest breastfeeding is permissible.

- NAPROXEN   (*Anaprox, Naprosyn, Aleve*)
  - ○ AAP = Maternal Medication Usually Compatible with Breastfeeding

- LRC = L3
- RID = 3.3%
- Pregnancy = C
- Comment: Naproxen is a popular NSAID analgesic. In a study done at steady state in one mother consuming 375 mg twice daily, milk levels ranged from 1.76-2.37 mg/L at four hours. Total naproxen excretion in the infant's urine was only 0.26% of the maternal dose. Although the amount of naproxen transferred via milk is minimal, one should use with caution in nursing mothers because of its long half-life and its effects on infant cardiovascular system, kidneys, and GI tract. However, its short term use postpartum or infrequent or occasional use would not necessarily be incompatible with breastfeeding. One case of prolonged bleeding, hemorrhage, and acute anemia has been reported in a seven-day-old infant. The relative infant dose on a weight-adjusted maternal daily dose would probably be less than 3.3%.

- OXYCODONE   (*Tylox, Percodan, OxyContin, Roxicet, Endocet, Roxiprin, Percocet*)
  - AAP = Not reviewed
  - LRC = L3
  - RID = 3.5%
  - Pregnancy = B
  - Comment: Oxycodone is similar to hydrocodone and is a mild analgesic somewhat stronger than codeine. Small amounts are secreted in breastmilk. Following a dose of 5-10 mg every four to seven hours, maternal levels peaked at one to two hours, and analgesia persisted for up to four hours. Reported milk levels range from <5 to 226 µg/L. Maternal plasma levels were 14-35 µg/L. The authors suggest a milk/plasma ratio of approximately 3.4. Although active metabolites were not measured, the authors suggest that an exclusively breastfed infant would receive a maximum 8% of the maternal dosage of oxycodone. No reports of untoward effects in infants have been found, although sedation is a possibility in some infants.

    In another study, 50 post-cesarean women received 30 mg oxycodone rectally, and 10 mg orally up to every two hours as needed. The average maternal plasma levels at 0-24 hours and 24-48 hours were 18 (range 0-42) ng/mL and 12 (range 0-40) ng/mL, respectively. Average milk concentrations in samples taken during 0-24 hours and 24-48 hours were 58 (range 7-130) ng/mL and 49 (range 0-168) ng/mL, respectively. Milk/Plasma ratios were therefore calculated to be 3.2-3.4. Only one infant had a detectable level of oxycodone in their plasma, with a concentration of 6.6-7.4 ng/mL. These plasma and milk levels suggest that oxycodone concentrates in the milk compartment. However, the authors suggest that at doses less than 90 mg/day for up to three days, maternal use of oxycodone poses only a minimal threat to breastfeeding infants. This study did not measure plasma or milk concentrations at steady state or during peak plasma concentrations; therefore, levels may have been higher at times.

- TRAMADOL   (*Ultram, Ultracet*)
  - AAP = Not reviewed
  - LRC = L2
  - RID = 2.9%
  - Pregnancy = C
  - Comment: Tramadol is a new class analgesic that most closely resembles the opiates, although it is not a controlled substance and appears to have reduced addictive potential. It appears to be slightly

more potent than codeine. After oral use, its onset of analgesia is within one hour and reaches a peak in two to three hours. Following a single IV 100 mg dose of tramadol, the cumulative excretion in breastmilk within 16 hours was 100 µg of tramadol (0.1% of the maternal dose) and 27 µg of the M1 metabolite.

In a recent study of 75 mothers who received 100 mg every six hours after Cesarean section, milk samples were taken on days two to four postpartum in transitional milk. At steady state, the Milk/Plasma ratio averaged 2.4 for rac-tramadol and 2.8 for rac-O-desmethyltramadol. The estimated absolute and relative infant doses were 112 µg/kg/day and 30 µg/kg/day for rac-tramadol and its desmethyl metabolite. The relative infant dose was 2.24% and 0.64% for rac-tramadol and its desmethyl metabolite, respectively. No significant neurobehavioral adverse effects were noted between controls and exposed infants.

Clinical Tips

The control of pain largely depends on the source. For severe pain, the opioids are preferred and include morphine, codeine, hydrocodone, fentanyl, hydromorphone, and less preferred, meperidine. In several studies, morphine seems to be an ideal analgesic for breastfeeding mothers, as its bioavailability (via milk) is low and it seems to produce the least sedation in breastfed infants. Levels of fentanyl and hydromorphone are quite low, but prolonged use is cautioned.

Codeine should be used cautiously due to the reported complications with a mother who was an ultra-rapid metabolizer of codeine. This genotype (which is very rare) leads to increased formation of morphine from codeine. We would suggest hydrocodone as a suitable alternative to codeine, as it does not require metabolism to become active. Some caution is recommended with high doses of oxycodone. Its RID is relatively high, although in one large study, little was found in the plasma of breastfed infants.

Meperidine (pethidine) has a long half-life 'active' metabolite and is not a preferred analgesic pre- or postnatally, or in breastfeeding women. Its long half-life active metabolite, normeperidine, is present in milk days after the discontinuation of meperidine and has been found to sedate infants.

Morphine and the codeine derivatives, such as hydrocodone, have been used extensively in breastfeeding women with only occasional neonatal sedation reported. For rheumatic pain, the NSAID family is ideal. Of this family, ibuprofen is preferred, due to poor transfer into milk and its safety in infants. Longer half-life NSAIDS, such as naproxen, should only be used for short periods, thus eliminating accumulation in the infant's plasma. Ketorolac (Toradol) is somewhat controversial, as the manufacturer's information suggests it should not be used in breastfeeding women. However, an excellent study clearly shows that milk levels are far subclinical, and ketorolac should be an ideal NSAID for use in certain breastfeeding women. The transfer of flurbiprofen into milk is reported to be very low, and it should be used cautiously.

Suggested Reading

Freburger, J. K., Carey, T. S., Holmes, G. M., Wallace, A. S., Castel, L. D., Darter, J. D., et al. (2009). Exercise prescription for chronic back or neck pain: who prescribes it? who gets it? What is prescribed? *Arthritis Rheum, 61*(2), 192-200.

Halpern, S. (2009). SOGC Joint Policy Statement on Normal Childbirth. *J Obstet Gynaecol Can, 31*(7), 602; author reply 602-603.

Marucci, M. (2009). Women in labor and the quality obstetric care system: the role of evidence-based neuraxial analgesia. *Minerva Anestesiol, 75*(3), 99-101.

Samuels, J. G., & Fetzer, S. J. (2009). Evidence-based pain management: analyzing the practice environment and clinical expertise. *Clin Nurse Spec, 23*(5), 245-251.

Wilbeck, J., Schorn, M. N., & Daley, L. (2008). Pharmacologic management of acute pain in breastfeeding women. *J Emerg Nurs, 34*(4), 340-344.

PCOS (Polycystic Ovarian Syndrome)

Principles of Therapy

Polycystic ovarian syndrome is characterized by chronic anovulation (amenorrhea or oligomenorrhea), hyperandrogenism, and polycystic ovaries. There is no specific diagnostic test which is pathonomonic. Diagnosis requires more than one sign or symptom, and certain laboratory and ultrasound findings are suggestive of the diagnosis. Other diagnoses should be excluded (including congenital adrenal hyperplasia, androgen secreting tumors, or hyperprolactinemia). Insulin resistance is a frequent feature, and women with PCOS appear to be at risk for metabolic syndrome later in life.

In women with a confirmed diagnosis of PCOS, treatment will depend on the patient's current goal. Weight loss should be a therapy discussed with all obese women with PCOS. Often women with PCOS will present with anovulatory infertility, and in that situation fertility treatment will be their current goal. Please refer to the section on infertility for further discussion of treatment options. For PCOS women who are not interested in pursuing pregnancy, goals will often include avoidance of long term complications of disease, such as diabetes, hyperlipidemia, and cardiovascular disease. Appropriate laboratory evaluation should be pursued, including testing for diabetes with a hemoglobin A1C and a fasting lipid profile. Insulin sensitizing agents, such as biguanides or thiazolidinediones, may be used in some situations for management of insulin resistance or diabetes. The potential advantage of biguanides (such as metformin) is the tendency to decrease weight.

Women with PCOS are also at risk for endometrial pathyology, such as irregular menstruation and hyperplasia. These risks can be minimized by the use of oral contraceptive pills or other estrogen containing contraceptives for appropriate candidates. For those women with contraindications to estrogen, other options to provide endometrial protection include progesterone-only options, such as a progesterone-releasing IUD (Mirena), Depo-provera injections, progesterone-only pills, or cyclic progestin withdrawal (though this last option does not provide contraception). Unfortunately, progestins may also be associated with risk of weight gain and irregular bleeding patterns, despite their effectiveness in providing endometrial protection. Management of hirsuitism and acne often begins with oral contraceptives. Oral contraceptives increase sex hormone binding globulins, which then decrease free levels of circulating testosterone. Acne can be managed with usual dermatologic options.

Other options for hirsuitism are available including spironolactone, which binds to the androgen receptor as an antagonist, in addition to other actions.

Other anti-androgens are available, but are much less popular due to concerns related to teratogenicity, such as flutamide and finasteride. Eflornithine is available and is effective for treating female facial hirsuitism with 605 women noting improvement after six months. Other options include mechanical hair removal (shaving, plucking, electrolysis, waxing, depilatory creams, laser vaporization, etc.). Hirsuitism requires extended time of therapy to appreciate change; therefore, mechanical options are often included in the initial management. Sleep apnea may also be more common in women with PCOS. Evaluation and therapy may be indicated for patients with excessive daytime somulence.

Treatment

- Lifestyle modifications, maintainance of healthy BMI, diet, and exercise.

- Appropriate fertility treatment if conception desired (clomiphene citrate first line therapy).

- Avoidance and early detection of long term disease complications: diabetes, hyperlipidemia, cardiovascular disease.

- Insulin sensitization agents for insulin resistance.

- Treatment of menstrual irregularities and endometrial protection: Oral contraceptives, NuvaRing, or progestin therapies (Mirena IUD, Depo-provera, Progestine-only pills, Progestin withdrawal).

- Statins may play a role, though this is presently unclear.

- Acne: oral contraceptives and usual dermatologic options (see acne).

- Hirsuitism: oral contraceptives, spironolactone, mechanical methods

Medications

- CLOMIPHENE   (*Clomid, Serophene, Milophene*)
  - AAP = Not reviewed
  - LRC = L3 in late stage lactation
  - RID =
  - Pregnancy = X
  - Comment: Clomiphene appears to stimulate the release of the pituitary gonadotropins, follicle-stimulating hormone (FSH), and luteinizing hormone (LH), which result in development and maturation of the ovarian follicle, ovulation, and subsequent development and function of the corpus luteum. It has both estrogenic and anti-estrogenic effects. LH and FSH peak at five to nine days after completing clomiphene therapy. In a study of 60 postpartum women (one to four days postpartum), clomiphene was effective in totally inhibiting lactation early postnatally and in suppressing established lactation (day four). Only seven of 40 women receiving clomiphene to inhibit lactation had signs of congestion or discomfort. In the 20 women who received clomiphene to suppress established lactation (on day four), a rapid amelioration of breast engorgement and discomfort was produced. After five days of treatment, no signs of lactation were present. In another study of 177 postpartum women, clomiphene was very effective at inhibiting lactation.

    Clomiphene appears to be very effective in suppressing lactation when used up to four days postpartum. However, its efficacy in reducing milk production in women months after lactation is established is unknown, but believed to be minimal.

- METFORMIN   (*Glucophage, Glucovance*)
  - AAP = Not reviewed
  - LRC = L1
  - RID = 0.3-0.7%

- Pregnancy = B
- Comment: Metformin belongs to the biguanide family and is used to reduce glucose levels in non-insulin dependent diabetics. Oral bioavailability is only 50%. In a study of seven women taking metformin (median dose 1500 mg/d), the mean milk-to-plasma ratio (AUC) for metformin was 0.35. The mean average concentration in milk over the dose interval was 0.27 mg/L. The absolute infant dose averaged 0.04 mg/kg/d, and the mean relative infant dose was 0.28%. Metformin was present in very low or undetectable concentrations in the plasma of four of the infants who were studied. No health problems were found in the six infants who were evaluated. In a recent study of five women consuming an average dose of 500 mg twice daily, the mean peak and trough metformin concentrations in breastmilk were 0.42 mg/L (range 0.38-0.46 mg/L) and 0.39 mg/L (range 0.31-0.52 mg/L), respectively. The average milk/serum ratio was 0.63 (range 0.36-1.00) and the estimated relative infant dose was 0.65% (range 0.43-1.08%). Blood glucose concentrations in three infants were normal, ranging from 47-77 mg/dL. The mothers reported no side effects were noted in the breastfed infants. Metformin is also used to treat polycystic ovary syndrome. In one study of 61 nursing infants whose mothers were taking a median of 2.55 g/day throughout pregnancy and lactation, the growth, motor, and social development of the infants was recorded to be normal. The authors concluded that metformin was safe and effective during lactation in the first six months of an infant's life.

- **ORLISTAT** (*Xenical, Alli*)
  - AAP = Not reviewed
  - LRC = L3
  - RID =
  - Pregnancy = B
  - Comment: Orlistat, now available over the counter as well as prescription, is used in the management of obesity. It is a reversible inhibitor of gastric and pancreatic lipases, thus it inhibits absorption of dietary fats by 30%. No studies have been performed on the transmission of orlistat into the breastmilk. With high protein binding, moderately high molecular weight, and poor oral absorption, it is unlikely that orlistat would enter breastmilk in clinically relevant amounts or affect a breastfeeding infant. However, due to orlistat's effect on the absorption of fat soluble vitamins and other fats, nutritional status of a breastfeeding mother should be closely monitored.

- **SPIRONOLACTONE** (*Aldactone*)
  - AAP = Maternal Medication Usually Compatible with Breastfeeding
  - LRC = L2
  - RID = 4.3%
  - Pregnancy = D
  - Comment: Spironolactone is metabolized to canrenone, which is known to be secreted into breastmilk. In one mother receiving 25 mg of spironolactone, at two hours postdose, the maternal serum and milk concentrations of canrenone were 144 and 104 µg/L, respectively. At 14.5 hours, the corresponding values for serum and milk were 92 and 47 µg/L, respectively. Milk/plasma ratios varied from 0.51 at 14.5 hours to 0.72 at two hours.

Clinical Tips

Polycystic ovary syndrome (PCOS) is one of the most common endocrine disorders in women of fertile age. Associated with suboptimal fertility (and complete infertility), miscarriage, gestational diabetes, and pre-eclampsia, PCOS has been reported to impede many women's ability to breastfeed. While it is not known what the etiology of poor breastmilk production may be, it is possibly due to the enhanced levels of testosterone. While metformin has been used in many of these patients to treat the endocrinopathy, we do not know for sure that it enhances milk production, although it is believed to do so.

Clomiphene, while not a treament for PCOS itself, is known to dramatically increase the fertility rates following its use, particularly in PCOS patients. Its use in breastfeeding mothers is only problematic when used early postpartum, where it known to suppress lactation. Used months later, it is unlikely to suppress lactation.

Medications known to reduce testosterone levels in women with PCOS, such as flutamide and finasteride, are horribly teratogenic and should not be used in women in childbearing years, particularly breastfeeding women. Finasteride may cause abnormalities of the external genitalia of a male fetus of a pregnant woman who receives it. The transfer of this drug into human milk could have devastating effects on male infant development. While their use prior to or during the first few days of pregnancy may be possible, the risks for the infant are high.

Eflornithine is available and is effective for treating female facial hirsuitism with 605 women noting improvement after six months. Used topically, less than 1% is absorbed transcutaneously.

Suggested Reading

Alexander, C. J., Tangchitnob, E. P., & Lepor, N. E. (2009). Polycystic ovary syndrome: a major unrecognized cardiovascular risk factor in women. *Rev Cardiovasc Med, 10*(2), 83-90.

Azziz, R., Carmina, E., Dewailly, D., Diamanti-Kandarakis, E., Escobar-Morreale, H. F., Futterweit, W., et al. (2006). Positions statement: criteria for defining polycystic ovary syndrome as a predominantly hyperandrogenic syndrome: an Androgen Excess Society guideline. *J Clin Endocrinol Metab, 91*(11), 4237-4245.

Bhattacharya, S. M. (2008). Metabolic syndrome in females with polycystic ovary syndrome and International Diabetes Federation criteria. *J Obstet Gynaecol Res, 34*(1), 62-66.

Carmina, E. (2006). Polycystic ovary syndrome: an update on diagnostic evaluation. *J Indian Med Assoc, 104*(8), 439-440, 442, 444.

Dunaif, A., & Lobo, R. A. (2002). Toward optimal health: the experts discuss polycystic ovary syndrome. *J Womens Health Gend Based Med, 11*(7), 579-584.

Meurer, L. N., Kroll, A. P., Jamieson, B., & Yousefi, P. (2006). Clinical inquiries. What is the best way to diagnose polycystic ovarian syndrome? *J Fam Pract, 55*(4), 351-352, 354.

Rosenfield, R. L. (2005). Clinical practice. Hirsutism. *N Engl J Med, 353*(24), 2578-2588.

Stadtmauer, L., & Oehninger, S. (2005). Management of infertility in women with polycystic ovary syndrome : a practical guide. *Treat Endocrinol, 4*(5), 279-292.

Stankiewicz, M., & Norman, R. (2006). Diagnosis and management of polycystic ovary syndrome: a practical guide. *Drugs, 66*(7), 903-912.

Pediculosis

Principles of Therapy

Pediculosis (lice) is caused by various species of lice. On the head, they are called Pediculus humanus capitis and on the body Pediculosis humanus humanus (sometimes called corporis). Lice are most commonly found behind the ears or on the back of the head, as the skin is warmer, but may also be found in eyelashes and eyebrows. Close examination reveals egg cases (nits) and active lice. Lice are transmitted by body contact, clothing, shared sports equipment, combs, and hats, and occur without regard to social status. Treatment of lice is primarily by the use of external insecticides. Patients with eczematous inflammation or signs of infections should be treated with appropriate antibiotics.

Treatment

- Permethrin on affected areas.

- Ivermectin is reserved for cases resistant to permethrin.

- Lindane is the last choice with higher side effects (neurotoxicity) and should not be used in infants or children.

- Cephalexin for secondary bacterial infections.

- Topical diphenhydramine or hydrocortisone for pruritis.

- All clothing, bedding, and stuffed animals must be washed in hot water.

Medications

- IVERMECTIN   (*Mectizan*)
    - AAP = Maternal Medication Usually Compatible with Breastfeeding
    - LRC = L3
    - RID = 1.3%
    - Pregnancy = C
    - Comment: Ivermectin is now widely used to treat human onchocerciasis, lymphatic filariasis, and other worms and parasites, such as head lice. In a study of four women given 150 µg/kg orally, the maximum breastmilk concentration averaged 14.13 µg/L. Milk/plasma ratios ranged from 0.39 to 0.57, with a mean of 0.51. Highest breastmilk concentration was at four to six hours. Average daily ingestion of ivermectin was calculated at 2.1 µg/kg, which is ten fold less than the adult dose. No adverse effects were reported.

- PERMETHRIN   (*Nix, Elimite, A-200, Pyrinex, Pyrinyl, Acticin*)
  - AAP = Not reviewed
  - LRC = L2
  - RID =
  - Pregnancy = B
  - Comment: Permethrin is a synthetic pyrethroid structure of the natural ester pyrethrum, a natural insecticide, and is used to treat lice, mites, and fleas. Permethrin absorption through the skin following application of a 5% cream is reported to be less than 2%. Permethrin is rapidly metabolized by serum and tissue enzymes to inactive metabolites and rapidly excreted in the urine. Overt toxicity is very low. It is not known if permethrin is secreted in human milk, although it has been found in animal milk after injection of significant quantities intravenously. In spite of its rapid metabolism, some residuals are sequestered in fat tissue.

    To use, recommend that the hair be washed with detergent and then saturated with permethrin liquid for 10 minutes before rinsing with water. One treatment is all that is required. At 14 days, a second treatment may be required if viable lice are seen. Elimite cream is generally recommended for scabies infestations and should be applied head to toe for 8-12 hours in infants, and body (not head) only in adults. Reapplication may be needed in seven days if live mites appear.

- MALATHION SOLUTION (*Ovide, A-Lices, Prioderm, Quellada, Suleo-M*)
  - AAP = Not reviewed
  - LRC = L3
  - RID =
  - Pregnancy = B
  - Comment: Malathion is a common pediculicide. It is used in lotions (0.5%) for the treatment of resistant lice and scabies. It should be applied to dry hair and scalp in high enough quantities to thoroughly wet the hair and scalp. The hair should be allowed to dry naturally and shampooed 8-12 hours later. A second application at seven to nine days is required if lice are still present. It should not be used in neonates, although one case report of its use in a seven-month-old infant suggests it is relatively safe. Less than 10% of malathion is absorbed transcutaneously and is rapidly metabolized and excreted. While it belongs to the organophosphate family of insecticides, it is so rapidly metabolized and eliminated by humans (10 times) that it is relatively nontoxic under normal conditions.

Clinical Tips

Permethrin is a synthetic pyrethroid structure derived from the ester pyrethrum, a natural insecticide in plants. Permethrin is very effective against body and head lice and scabies, although some species are becoming resistant. Permethrin is ideal for breastfeeding mothers because its transcutaneous absorption is minimal and it is very unlikely to ever enter milk. Further, it is very nontoxic. To use for body and head lice, recommend that the hair be washed with detergent and then saturated with permethrin liquid for 10 minutes before rinsing with water. After 14 days, another treatment is often recommended.

In some countries, malathion, an organophosphate insecticide, has been safely used, as it is not overtly toxic to humans. It is probably most useful for resistant cases of lice.

For resistant scabies, oral ivermectin (200 μg/kg PO, one dose) is the most recent recommendation. It is extremely effective and has virtually no side effects. For treament of head lice (and probably scabies), Ivermectin in an 0.8% topical solution is under development.

Due to significant transcutaneous absorption and the possibility of seizures, lindane solutions are no longer recommended for breastfeeding mothers. Never use lindane in pregnant women, infants, or children. Permethrin can be be safely used in pregnant women and in infants two months or older.

The most common reasons for treatment failure are: 1) other patient contacts have not been treated, 2) bedding and living areas have not been treated and cleaned, 3) areas under the toenail and fingernails have not been treated effectively, 4) eggs are not removed from the hair.

Numerous non-pharmacologic treatments are available, but none are as effective as the above measures.

Suggested Reading

Anonymous. (2009). Getting the bugs out: FDA approves new treatment for head lice. (2009). *Child Health Alert, 27*, 2.

Anonymous. (2009). Head lice--new options for treatment. *Child Health Alert, 27*, 3.

Burkhart, C. G., & Burkhart, C. N. (2006). Safety and efficacy of pediculicides for head lice. *Expert Opin Drug Saf, 5*(1), 169-179.

CDC, Workowski, K. A., & Berman, S. M. (2006). Sexually transmitted diseases treatment guidelines, 2006. *MMWR Recomm Rep, 55*(RR-11), 1-94 Section on Pediculosis.

Idriss S, L. J. (2009). Malathion for head lice and scabies: treatment and safety considerations. *J Drugs Dermatol, 8*(8), 715-720.

Lebwohl, M., Clark, L., & Levitt, J. (2007). Therapy for head lice based on life cycle, resistance, and safety considerations. *Pediatrics, 119*(5), 965-974.

Mumcuoglu, K. Y. (2006). Effective treatment of head louse with pediculicides. *J Drugs Dermatol, 5*(5), 451-452.

Takano-Lee, M., Edman, J. D., Mullens, B. A., & Clark, J. M. (2004). Home remedies to control head lice: assessment of home remedies to control the human head louse, Pediculus humanus capitis (Anoplura: Pediculidae). *J Pediatr Nurs, 19*(6), 393-398.

Weisberg, L. (2009). The goal of evidence-based pediculosis guidelines. *Nasnewsletter, 24*(4), 165-166.

Pelvic Inflammatory Disease

Principles of Therapy

Pelvic Inflammatory Disease (PID) is used to describe a spectrum of inflammatory diseases of the upper female genital tract, including non-puerperal endometritis, mucopurulent cervicitis, peritonitis, salpingitis, and tubo-ovarian abscess. Most affected are females from 15-24 years of age, those with increased number of sexual partners, and those who seldom use barrier contraceptives. Sexually transmitted organisms, such as *Neisseria gonorrhoeae* and *Chlamydia trachomatis*, may instigate the infection, though once established, this is a polymicrobial infection often involving organisms from vaginal flora. *Escherichia coli* and bacteroides are other commonly involved organisms. Clinical diagnosis of PID is imperfect as symptoms are frequently mild. The classic clinical symptoms of acute PID, including lower abdominal pain, fever, adnexal tenderness or mass, purulent discharge from the cervix, elevated white cell count and sedimentation rate, are rarely found. Laparoscopy can provide a more accurate diagnosis, but remains an invasive surgical procedure that is usually reserved for cases unresponsive to antibiotic therapy or with unclear diagnosis. Risk factors for development of PID include multiple sexual partners, a new partner, unprotected intercourse, and a history of an untreated sexually transmitted disease. Diagnostic criteria are imperfect. Minimal criteria for diagnosis include lower abdominal pain, adnexal tenderness, and cervical motion tenderness, with no other apparent cause for these symptoms. Additional criteria to support this diagnosis include fever, abnormal vaginal discharge, and documentation of cervical infection with chlamydia or gonorrhea. Pelvic ultrasound may also be useful in cases of suspected tubo-ovarian abscess. Treatment of PID is largely based on the use of multiple antibiotic regimens to ensure broad spectrum coverage, but must also cover Gonorrhea and Chlamydia. Therapy can be given either in an inpatient or outpatient setting. Criteria for hospitalization include inability to tolerate oral medications due to nausea and vomiting, uncertain diagnosis, evidence of peritonitis or pelvic abscess, suspected non-compliance, immunodeficiency, and failed outpatient therapy. Women who have not responded by 72 hours after initial therapy should return for reevaluation, and inpatient therapy should be pursued if the diagnosis is confirmed. PID has many late sequelae, including infertility, ectopic pregnancy, and chronic pelvic pain.

In addition to hospitalization, women with tubo-ovarian abscess may require broader antibiotic coverage. Hospitalization is continued until at least 48 hours after defervescing and resolution of pain. Follow-up of the pelvic abscess may be indicated depending on the extent of disease.

Treatment

- Treatment regimens are highly varied and depend on the pathogen.

- Intravenous regimen: cefoxitin 2 g IV every six hours or cefotetan 2 gm IV every 12 hours, plus doxycycline 100 mg orally every 12 hours.

- Another regimen includes: clindamycin 900 mg IV every eight hours, plus gentamicin 1.5 mg/kg every eight hours after loading dose.

- Oral regimen: ceftriaxone 250 mg IM once, plus doxycycline 100 mg orally twice daily for 14 days. Metronidazole may be included (50 mg twice daily X 14 days).

- Sexual partners need to be evaluated; men are often asymptomatic carriers and will re-infect their treated partners, as well as spread infection to other partners.

Medications

- AZITHROMYCIN   (*Zithromax*)
  - ○   AAP = Not reviewed
  - ○   LRC = L2
  - ○   RID = 5.9%
  - ○   Pregnancy = B
  - ○   Comment: Azithromycin belongs to the erythromycin family. It has an extremely long half-life, particularly in tissues. Azithromycin is concentrated for long periods in phagocytes, which are known to be present in human milk. In one study of a patient who received 1 gm initially followed by 500 mg doses each at 24 hour intervals, the concentration of azithromycin in breastmilk varied from 0.64 mg/L (initially) to 2.8 mg/L on day three. The predicted dose of azithromycin received by the infant would be approximately 0.4 mg/kg/day. This would suggest that the level of azithromycin ingested by a breastfeeding infant is not clinically relevant. New pediatric formulations of azithromycin have been recently introduced. Pediatric dosing is 10 mg/kg STAT followed by 5 mg/kg per day for up to five days.

- CEFOTETAN   (*Cefotan*)
  - ○   AAP = Not reviewed
  - ○   LRC = L2
  - ○   RID = 0.2-0.3%
  - ○   Pregnancy = B
  - ○   Comment: Cefotetan is a third generation cephalosporin that is poorly absorbed orally and is only available via IM and IV injection. The drug is distributed into human milk in low concentrations. Following a maternal dose of 1000mg IM every 12 hours in five patients, breastmilk concentrations ranged from 0.29 to 0.59 mg/L. Plasma concentrations were almost 100 times higher. In a group of two to three women who received 1000 mg IV, the maximum average milk level reported was 0.2 mg/L at four hours with a milk/plasma ratio of 0.02.

- CEFTRIAXONE   (*Rocephin*)
  - ○   AAP = Maternal Medication Usually Compatible with Breastfeeding
  - ○   LRC = L2
  - ○   RID = 4.1-4.2%
  - ○   Pregnancy = B
  - ○   Comment: Ceftriaxone is a very popular third-generation broad-spectrum cephalosporin antibiotic. Small amounts are transferred into milk (3-4% of maternal serum level). Following a 1 gm IM dose, breastmilk levels were approximately 0.5-0.7 mg/L at between four to eight hours. The estimated

mean milk levels at steady state were 3-4 mg/L. Another source indicates that following a 2 g/d dose, and at steady state, approximately 4.4% of dose penetrates into milk. In this study, the maximum breastmilk concentration was 7.89 mg/L after prolonged therapy (seven days). Poor oral absorption of ceftriaxone would further limit systemic absorption by the infant. The half-life of ceftriaxone in human milk varies from 12.8 to 17.3 hours (longer than maternal serum). Even at this high dose, no adverse effects were noted in the infant. Ceftriaxone levels in breastmilk are probably too low to be clinically relevant, except for changes in GI flora. Ceftriaxone is commonly used in neonates.

- CEFOXITIN (*Mefoxin*)
  - ○ AAP = Maternal Medication Usually Compatible with Breastfeeding
  - ○ LRC = L1
  - ○ RID = 0.1-0.3%
  - ○ Pregnancy = B
  - ○ Comment: Cefoxitin is a cephalosporin antibiotic with a spectrum similar to the second generation family. It is transferred into human milk in very low levels. In a study of 18 women receiving 2000-4000 mg doses, only one breastmilk sample contained cefoxitin (0.9 mg/L), all the rest were too low to be detected. In another study of two to three women who received 1000 mg IV, only trace amounts were reported in milk over six hours. In a group of five women who received an IM injection of 2000 mg, the highest milk levels were reported at four hours after dose. The maternal plasma levels varied from 22.5 at two hours to 77.6 µg/mL at four hours. Maternal milk levels ranged from <0.25 to 0.65 mg/L. Observe for changes in gut flora.

- CLINDAMYCIN (*Cleocin, Cleocin T*)
  - ○ AAP = Maternal Medication Usually Compatible with Breastfeeding
  - ○ LRC = L2
  - ○ RID = 1.66%
  - ○ Pregnancy = B
  - ○ Comment: Clindamycin is a broad-spectrum antibiotic frequently used for anaerobic infections. In one study of two nursing mothers and following doses of 600 mg IV every six hours, the concentration of clindamycin in breastmilk was 3.1 to 3.8 mg/L at 0.2 to 0.5 hours after dosing. Following oral doses of 300 mg every six hours, the breastmilk levels averaged 1.0 to 1.7 mg/L at 1.5 to 7 hours after dosing. In another study of two to three women who received a single oral dose of 150 mg, milk levels averaged 0.9 mg/L at four hours, with a milk/plasma ratio of 0.47. An alteration of GI flora is possible, even though the dose is low. One case of bloody stools (pseudomembranous colitis) has been associated with clindamycin and gentamicin therapy on day five postpartum, but this is considered rare. In this case, the mother of a newborn infant was given 600 mg IV every six hours. In rare cases, pseudomembranous colitis can appear several weeks later.

    In a study of 15 women who received 600 mg clindamycin intravenously, levels of clindamycin in milk averaged 1.03 mg/L at two hours following the dose. With the rise of resistant Staphlococcal infections, clindamycin use in infants has risen enormously. The amount in milk is unlikely to harm a breastfeeding infant.

- DOXYCYCLINE (*Doxychel, Vibramycin, Periostat*)
  - ○ AAP = Not reviewed
  - ○ LRC = L3

- RID = 4.2-13.3%
- Pregnancy = D
- Comment: Doxycycline is a long half-life tetracycline antibiotic. In a study of 15 subjects, the average doxycycline level in milk was 0.77 mg/L following a 200 mg oral dose. One oral dose of 100 mg was administered 24 hours later, and the breastmilk levels were 0.380 mg/L. Following a dose of 100 mg daily in 10 mothers, doxycycline levels in milk on day two averaged 0.82 mg/L (range 0.37-1.24 mg/L) at three hours after the dose, and 0.46 mg/L (range 0.3-0.91 mg/L) 24 hours after the dose. The relative infant dose in an infant would be < 6% of the maternal weight-adjusted dosage. Tetracyclines administered orally to infants are known to bind in teeth, producing discoloration and inhibiting bone growth, although doxycycline and oxytetracycline stain teeth the least severe. Although most tetracyclines secreted into milk are generally bound to calcium, thus inhibiting their absorption, doxycycline is the least bound (20%) and may be better absorbed in a breastfeeding infant than the older tetracyclines. While the absolute absorption of older tetracyclines may be dramatically reduced by calcium salts, the newer doxycycline and minocycline analogs bind less, and their overall absorption while slowed, may be significantly higher than earlier versions. Prolonged use (months) could potentially alter GI flora and induce dental staining, although doxycycline produces the least dental staining. Short term use (three-four weeks) is not contraindicated. No harmful effects have yet been reported in breastfeeding infants, but prolonged use is not advised. For prolonged administration, such as for exposure to anthrax, check the CDC web site as they have published specific dosing guidelines.

- GENTAMICIN   (*Garamycin*)
  - AAP = Maternal Medication Usually Compatible with Breastfeeding
  - LRC = L2
  - RID = 2.1%
  - Pregnancy = C
  - Comment: Gentamicin is a narrow spectrum antibiotic generally used for gram negative infections. The oral absorption of gentamicin (<1%) is generally nil, with the exception of premature neonates, where small amounts may be absorbed. In one study of 10 women given 80 mg three times daily IM for five days postpartum, milk levels were measured on day four. Gentamicin levels in milk were 0.42, 0.48, 0.49, and 0.41 mg/L at one, three, five, and seven hours, respectively. The milk/plasma ratios were 0.11 at one hour and 0.44 at seven hours. Plasma gentamicin levels in neonates were small, found in only five of the ten neonates, and averaged 0.41 µg/mL. The authors estimate that daily ingestion via breastmilk would be 307 µg for a 3.6 Kg neonate (normal neonatal dose = 2.5 mg/kg every 12 hours). These amounts would be clinically irrelevant in most infants.

- METRONIDAZOLE   (*Flagyl, Metizol, Trikacide, Protostat, Noritate*)
  - AAP = Drugs whose effect on nursing infants is unknown but may be of concern
  - LRC = L2
  - RID = 12.6-13.5%
  - Pregnancy = B
  - Comment: Metronidazole is indicated in the treatment of vaginitis, due to Trichomonas Vaginalis and various anaerobic bacterial infections, including Giardiasis, H. Pylori, B. Fragilis, and Gardnerella vaginalis. Metronidazole has become the treatment of choice for pediatric giardiasis

(AAP). Metronidazole absorption is time and dose dependent and also depends on the route of administration (oral vs. vaginal). Following a 2 gm oral dose, milk levels were reported to peak at 50-57 mg/L at two hours. Milk levels after 12 hours were approximately 19 mg/L and at 24 hours were approximately 10 mg/L. The average drug concentration reported in milk at 2, 8, 12, and 12-24 hours was 45.8, 27.9, 19.1, and 12.6 mg/L, respectively. If breastfeeding were to continue uninterrupted, an infant would consume 21.8 mg via breastmilk. With a 12 hour discontinuation, an infant would consume only 9.8 mg.

It is true that the relative infant dose via milk is moderately high depending on the dose and timing. Infants whose mothers ingest 1.2 gm/d will receive approximately 13.5% or less of the maternal dose or approximately 2.3 mg/kg/day. Bennett has calculated the relative infant dose from 11.7% to as high as 24% of the maternal dose. Heisterberg found metronidazole levels in infant plasma to be 16% and 19% of the maternal plasma levels following doses of 600 mg/d and 1200 mg/d. While these levels seem significant, it is still pertinent to remember that metronidazole is a commonly used drug in premature neonates, infants, and children, and 2.3 mg/kg/d is still much less than the therapeutic dose used in infants/children (7.5-30 mg/kg/d). Thus far, virtually no adverse effects have been reported. Numerous other studies have been carried out. See *Medications and Mothers' Milk* for complete listing.

Clinical Tips

Treatment regimens vary enormously depending on the suitability of oral verses intravenous therapy. Typical intravenous therapy involves cefotetan or cefoxitin combined with doxycycline. Alternatively, clindamycin and gentamycin can be used. There is no advantage to intravenous doxycycline if oral medication can be tolerated, as infusion is associated with significant pain. Cefoxitin 2 gm every six hours or cefotetan 2 gm IV every 12 hours plus doxycycline 100 mg IV/PO every 12 hours is suitable. Azithromycin can be substituted for doxycycline regimens in hypersensitive individuals. In fact, some studies suggest that azithromycin regimens are more effective than doxycycline. In addition, some studies now suggest that all regimens should be supplemented with metronidazole in non-pregnant females. In pregnant patients, the CDC recommends the use of clindamycin plus gentamicin. Male partners should be treated as well.

The CDC no longer recommends the use of fluoroquinolones in treating gonococcal infections, such as pelvic inflammatory disease.

Suggested Reading

CDC. (2007). Updated recommended treatment regimens for gonococcal infections and associated conditions - United States, April 2007. Retrieved Jan 12, 2010, from http://www.cdc.gov/std/treatment/2006/updated-regimens.htm.

Crossman, S. H. (2006). The challenge of pelvic inflammatory disease. *Am Fam Physician, 73*(5), 859-864.

Kropp, R. Y., Latham-Carmanico, C., Steben, M., Wong, T., & Duarte-Franco, E. (2007). What's new in management of sexually transmitted infections? Canadian Guidelines on Sexually Transmitted Infections, 2006 Edition. *Can Fam Physician, 53*(10), 1739-1741.

Sweet, R. L. (2009). Treatment strategies for pelvic inflammatory disease. *Expert Opin Pharmacother, 10*(5), 823-837.

Trigg, B. G., Kerndt, P. R., & Aynalem, G. (2008). Sexually transmitted infections and pelvic inflammatory disease in women. *Med Clin North Am, 92*(5), 1083-1113.

Walker, C. K., & Wiesenfeld, H. C. (2007). Antibiotic therapy for acute pelvic inflammatory disease: the 2006 Centers for Disease Control and Prevention sexually transmitted diseases treatment guidelines. *Clin Infect Dis, 44 Suppl 3*, S111-122.

Peptic Ulcer Disease

Principles of Therapy

The normal gastric and duodenal mucosa are remarkably capable of defending against injury from the acid of peptic activity in gastric fluids. Peptic ulcers are an erosion that penetrates the muscularis mucosa and ultimately heals with granulation tissue. It is now clear that the two most important insults predisposing to peptic ulceration (PUD) are infection with *Helicobacter pylori* (HP) and the use of nonsteroidal anti-inflammatory drugs (NSAIDS). Although other forms of ulceration exist, such as with Crohn's disease, extreme acid hypersecretion, etc., these are rare. The medications used for PUD consist of acid suppressors, such as the H_2 blockers (famotidine, ranitidine, etc.) or the proton-pump inhibitors (omeprazole, lansoprazole), coating agents (e.g., sucralfate), antacids, and antibiotics for treating HP infections.

Treatment

- Discontinue NSAIDs; avoid caffeine, bisphosphonates, and alcohol.

- Proton pump inhibitors, including omeprazole, lansoprazole, dexlansoprazole, esomeprazole and pantoprazole

- Treatment to eradicate *H. pylori*, which usually includes a proton pump inhibitor, clarithromycin, and either metronidazole or amoxicillin.

Medications

- AMOXICILLIN   (*Larotid, Amoxil*)
  - AAP = Maternal Medication Usually Compatible with Breastfeeding
  - LRC = L1
  - RID   = 1%
  - Pregnancy = B
  - Comment: Amoxicillin is a popular oral penicillin used for otitis media and many other pediatric/ adult infections. In one group of six mothers who received 1 gm oral doses, the concentration of amoxicillin in breastmilk ranged from 0.68 to 1.3 mg/L of milk (average= 0.9 mg/L). Peak levels occurred at four to five hours. Milk/plasma ratios at one, two, and three hours were 0.014, 0.013, and 0.043. Less than 0.95% of the maternal dose is secreted into milk. No harmful effects have been reported.

- BISMUTH SUBSALICYLATE   (*Pepto-Bismol*)
  - AAP = Drugs whose effect on nursing infants is unknown but may be of concern
  - LRC = L3
  - RID =
  - Pregnancy = C during first trimester
  - Comment: Bismuth subsalicylate is present in many diarrhea mixtures. Although bismuth salts are poorly absorbed from the maternal GI tract, significant levels of salicylate could be absorbed from these products. As such, these drugs should not be routinely used due to the association of salicylates in Reye's syndrome in children. Some forms (Parepectolin, Infantol Pink) may contain a tincture of opium (morphine).

- CLARITHROMYCIN   (*Biaxin*)
  - AAP = Not reviewed
  - LRC = L1
  - RID = 2.1%
  - Pregnancy = C
  - Comment: Antibiotic that belongs to erythromycin family. In a study of 12 mothers receiving 250 mg twice daily, the Cmax occurred at 2.2 hours. The estimated average dose of clarithromycin via milk was reported to be 150 µg/kg/day, or 2% of the maternal dose. Clarithromycin is probably compatible with breastfeeding. Observe for diarrhea and thrush in the infant.

- ESOMEPRAZOLE   (*Nexium*)
  - AAP = Not reviewed
  - LRC = L2
  - RID =
  - Pregnancy = C
  - Comment: Esomeprazole is just the L isomer of omeprazole (Prilosec) and is essentially identical to Prilosec. See omeprazole for breastfeeding recommendations.

- FAMOTIDINE   (*Pepcid, Axid-AR, Pepcid-AC*)
  - AAP = Not reviewed
  - LRC = L1
  - RID = 1.9%
  - Pregnancy = B
  - Comment: Famotidine is a typical Histamine-2 antagonist that reduces stomach acid secretion. In one study of eight lactating women receiving a 40 mg/day dose, the peak concentration in breastmilk was 72 µg/L and occurred at six hours postdose. The milk/plasma ratios were 0.41, 1.78, and 1.33 at 2, 6, and 24 hours, respectively. These levels are apparently much lower than other histamine H-2 antagonists (ranitidine, cimetidine) and make it a preferred choice.

- LANSOPRAZOLE   (*Prevacid, Prevpac, Prevacid NapraPak*)
  - AAP = Not reviewed

- ○ LRC = L3
- ○ RID =
- ○ Pregnancy = B
- ○ Comment: Lansoprazole is a new proton pump inhibitor that suppresses the release of acid protons from the parietal cells in the stomach, effectively raising the pH of the stomach. Structurally similar to omeprazole, it is very unstable in stomach acid and to a large degree is denatured by acidity of the infant's stomach. A new study shows milk levels of omeprazole are minimal (see omeprazole), and it is likely milk levels of lansoprazole are small as well. Although there are no studies of lansoprazole in breastfeeding mothers, transfer to milk and its oral absorption (via milk) is likely to be minimal in a breastfed infant. Lansoprazole is secreted in animal milk, although no data are available on the amount secreted in human milk. The only likely untoward effects would be reduced stomach acidity. This product has no current pediatric indications, although it is occasionally used in severe cases of erosive gastritis.

  Prevpac contains Lansoprazole, Amoxicillin, and Clarithromycin. It is primarily indicated for treatment of H. Pylori infections which cause stomach ulcers.

  Prevacid NapraPAC contains 15 mg lansoprazole and 500 mg naproxen. It is used in reducing the risk of NSAID-associated gastric ulcers in patients with a history of documented gastric ulcer that require the use of an NSAID.

- **METRONIDAZOLE** (*Flagyl, Metizol, Trikacide, Protostat, Noritate*)
  - ○ AAP = Drugs whose effect on nursing infants is unknown but may be of concern
  - ○ LRC = L2
  - ○ RID = 12.6-13.5%
  - ○ Pregnancy = B
  - ○ Comment: Metronidazole is indicated in the treatment of vaginitis due to Trichomonas Vaginalis and various anaerobic bacterial infections, including Giardiasis, H. Pylori, B. Fragilis, and Gardnerella vaginalis. Metronidazole has become the treatment of choice for pediatric giardiasis (AAP). Metronidazole absorption is time and dose dependent and also depends on the route of administration (oral vs. vaginal). Following a 2 gm oral dose, milk levels were reported to peak at 50-57 mg/L at two hours. Milk levels after 12 hours were approximately 19 mg/L and at 24 hours were approximately 10 mg/L. The average drug concentration reported in milk at 2, 8, 12, and 12-24 hours was 45.8, 27.9, 19.1, and 12.6 mg/L, respectively. If breastfeeding were to continue uninterrupted, an infant would consume 21.8 mg via breastmilk. With a 12 hour discontinuation, an infant would consume only 9.8 mg.

    It is true that the relative infant dose via milk is moderately high depending on the dose and timing. Infants whose mothers ingest 1.2 gm/d will receive approximately 13.5% or less of the maternal dose or approximately 2.3 mg/kg/day. Bennett has calculated the relative infant dose from 11.7% to as high as 24% of the maternal dose. Heisterberg found metronidazole levels in infant plasma to be 16% and 19% of the maternal plasma levels following doses of 600 mg/d and 1200 mg/d. While these levels seem significant, it is still pertinent to remember that metronidazole is a commonly used drug in premature neonates, infants, and children, and 2.3 mg/kg/d is still much less than the therapeutic dose used in infants/children (7.5-30 mg/kg/d). Thus far, virtually no adverse effects have been reported. Numerous other studies have been carried out. See *Medications and Mothers' Milk* for complete listing.

- NIZATIDINE (*Axid*)
  - AAP = Not reviewed
  - LRC = L2
  - RID = 0.5%
  - Pregnancy = B
  - Comment: Nizatidine is an antisecretory, histamine-2 antagonist that reduces stomach acid secretion. In one study of five lactating women using a dose of 150 mg, milk levels of nizatidine were directly proportional to circulating maternal serum levels, yet were very low. Over a 12 hour period, 96 μg (less than 0.1% of dose) was secreted into the milk. No effects on infant have been reported.

- OMEPRAZOLE (*Prilosec, Zegerid*)
  - AAP = Not reviewed
  - LRC = L2
  - RID = 1.1%
  - Pregnancy = C
  - Comment: Omeprazole is a potent inhibitor of gastric acid secretion. In a study of one patient receiving 20 mg omeprazole daily, the maternal serum concentration was negligible until 90 minutes after ingestion, and then reached 950 nM at 240 minutes. The breastmilk concentration of omeprazole began to rise minimally at 90 minutes after ingestion and peaked after 180 minutes at only 58 nM, or less than 7% of the highest serum level. This would indicate a maximum dose of 3 μg/kg/day in a breastfed infant. Omeprazole milk levels were essentially flat over four hours of observation. Omeprazole is extremely acid labile with a half-life of 10 minutes at pH values below four. Virtually all omeprazole ingested via milk would probably be destroyed in the stomach of the infant prior to absorption.

- RANITIDINE (*Zantac*)
  - AAP = Not reviewed
  - LRC = L2
  - RID = 1.3-4.6%
  - Pregnancy = B
  - Comment: Ranitidine is a prototypic histamine-2 blocker used to reduce acid secretion in the stomach. It has been widely used in pediatrics without significant side effects primarily for gastroesophageal reflux (GER). Following a dose of 150 mg for four doses, concentrations in breastmilk were 0.72, 2.6, and 1.5 mg/L at 1.5, 5.5 and 12 hours, respectively. The milk/serum ratios varied from 6.81, 8.44 to 23.77 at 1.5, 5.5 and 12 hours, respectively. Although the milk/plasma ratios are quite high, using these data, an infant would ingest at most 0.4 mg/kg/d. This amount is quite small considering the pediatric dose currently recommended is 2-4 mg/kg/24 hours. See nizatidine or famotidine for alternatives.

- SUCRALFATE (*Carafate*)
  - AAP = Not reviewed
  - LRC = L2
  - RID =

- ○ Pregnancy = B
- ○ Comment: Sucralfate is a sucrose aluminum complex used for stomach ulcers. When administered orally, sucralfate forms a complex that physically covers stomach ulcers. Less than 5% is absorbed orally. At these plasma levels, it is very unlikely to penetrate into breastmilk.

- **TETRACYCLINE** (*Achromycin, Sumycin, Terramycin*)
  - ○ AAP = Maternal Medication Usually Compatible with Breastfeeding
  - ○ LRC = L2
  - ○ RID = 0.6%
  - ○ Pregnancy = D
  - ○ Comment: Tetracycline is a broad-spectrum antibiotic with significant side effects in pediatric patients, including dental staining and reduced bone growth. It is secreted into breastmilk in extremely small levels. Because tetracyclines bind to milk calcium, they would have reduced oral absorption in the infant. Posner reports that in a patient receiving 500 mg four times daily, the average concentration of tetracycline in milk was 1.14 mg/L. The maternal plasma level was 1.92 mg/L and the milk/plasma ratio was 0.59. The absolute dose to the infant ranged from 0.17 to 0.39 mg/kg/day. None was detected in the plasma compartment of the infant (limit of detection 0.05 mg/L).

    In a mother receiving 275 mg/d, milk levels averaged 1.25 mg/L, with a maximum of 2.51 mg/L. None was detected in the infant's plasma. In another study of two to three patients receiving a single 150 mg/d dose, milk levels ranged from 0.3 to 1.2 mg/L at four hours (Cmax). The maximum reported milk level was 1.2 mg/L. A milk/plasma ratio of 0.58 was reported. From the above studies, the relative infant dose is 0.6%, 4.77%, and 8.44%. Thus a high degree of variability exists in these studies. Invariably mixture of tetracyclines in milk would greatly limit their oral bioavailability. The short-term (<3 weeks) exposure of infants to tetracyclines (via milk) is not contraindicated. However, the long-term exposure of breastfeeding infants to tetracyclines, such as when used daily for acne, could cause problems. The absorption of even small amounts over a prolonged period could result in dental staining.

Clinical Tips

Therapy of gastric ulceration largely depends on etiology. NSAID ulcers should be treated by withdrawal of the offending agent and adding an H2 blocker, such as famotidine. Peptic ulceration of *H. pylori* etiology requires up to two weeks of therapy with omeprazole and one of numerous antibiotic regimens. Antibiotic regimens include clarithromycin, tetracycline, metronidazole, amoxicillin, bismuth and others. Due to the emergence of resistance, monotherapy is not considered a treatment of choice for eradicating *H. pylori*. For this reason, the above antibiotics/proton pump inhibitors are used in combination, such as omeprazole + clarithromycin + amoxicillin or metronidazole. Alternative therapy includes: bismuth subsalicylate + metronidazole + tetracycline + proton pump inhibitor. Although most of the above antibiotics transfer poorly into human milk, some changes in the infant's GI flora may result in diarrhea (rarely). Although not FDA approved, amoxicillin has been substituted for tetracycline for patients for whom tetracycline is not recommended. Treatment regimens and dosage change routinely. Check the CDC and other references for current regimen.

Suggested Reading

Anonymous. (2007). Choice of antibacterial drugs. *Treat Guidel Med Lett, 5*(57), 33-50.

Anonymous. (2008). Treatment of peptic ulcers and GERD. *Treat Guidel Med Lett, 6*(72), 55-60.

Chan, F. K. (2008). Proton-pump inhibitors in peptic ulcer disease. *Lancet, 372*(9645), 1198-1200.

de Sousa Falcão, H., Leite, J. A., Barbosa-Filho, J. M., de Athayde-Filho, P. F., de Oliveira Chaves, M. C., Moura, M. D., et al. (2008). Gastric and duodenal antiulcer activity of alkaloids: a review. *Molecules, 13*(12), 3198-3223.

McColl, K. E. (2009). How I manage H. pylori-negative, NSAID/aspirin-negative peptic ulcers. *Am J Gastroenterol, 104*(1), 190-193.

Thukral, C., & Wolf, J. L. (2006). Therapy insight: drugs for gastrointestinal disorders in pregnant women. *Nat Clin Pract Gastroenterol Hepatol, 3*(5), 256-266.

Postpartum Depression

Principles of Therapy

During the early postpartum period, up to 85% of women suffer some type of mood disorder. In most women, the symptoms are transitory and relatively mild (postpartum blues). However, up to 20% of postpartum women may suffer from a more severe and persistent disorder, postpartum depression. The cardinal symptoms of major depressive disorder, and postpartum depression are poor mood, decreased or increased sleep, poor appetite, feelings of worthlessness or guilt, decreased energy, and anhedonia or lack of interest in most things ordinarily found to be interesting by the patient. Postpartum depression is diagnosed when an episode of major depression occurs within four to six weeks postpartum. Often women report similar symptoms were present during pregnancy. Depression within a year after birth is commonly refered to as postpartum depression as well. The use of a postpartum screening tool may be useful to assist with diagnosis. PPD can also include anxiety and symptoms of obsessive-compulsive disorder. Although breastfeeding women may have lower rates of postpartum depression as compared to formula-feeding women, it is still prevalent in breastfeeding mothers. Approximately 10% to 20% of mothers in the year following childbirth suffer depression. In some vulnerable groups, the incidence of depression may be as high as 50%. Severe postpartum depression may be accompanied by suicidal thoughts. Postpartum psychosis is more rare and occurs in approximately 1 out of 1000 births. Psychosis can include delusions and hallucinations, and may include thoughts of infanticide.

Treatment

- Cognitive-behavioral or interpersonal psychotherapy

- Psychotherapy with additional medical therapy indicated for more severe symptoms

- Antidepressant medications, including SSRIs or SNRIs, as first-line medical treatment

- Tricyclic antidepressants (TCA) are less frequently used, but may be appropriate in some circumstances.

- Frequent follow-up is needed.

Medications

- AMITRIPTYLINE   (*Elavil, Endep*)
    - AAP = Drugs whose effect on nursing infants is unknown but may be of concern
    - LRC = L2
    - RID = 1.9-2.8%
    - Pregnancy = C

○ Comment: Amitriptyline and its active metabolite, nortriptyline, are secreted into breastmilk in small amounts. In one report of a mother taking 100 mg/day of amitriptyline, milk levels of amitriptyline and nortriptyline (active metabolite) averaged 143 µg/L and 55.5 µg/L, respectively; maternal serum levels averaged 112 µg/L and 72.5 µg/L, respectively. No drug was detected in the infant's serum. From these data, an infant would consume approximately 21.5 µg/kg/day, a dose that is unlikely to be clinically relevant.

In another study following a maternal dose of 25 mg/day, the amitriptyline and nortriptyline (active metabolite) levels in milk were 30 µg/L and <30 µg/L, respectively. In the same study when the dosage was 75 mg/day, milk levels of amitriptyline and nortriptyline averaged 88 µg/L and 69 µg/L, respectively. Both drugs were essentially undetectable in the infant's serum. Therefore, the authors estimated that a nursing infant would receive less than 0.1 mg/day.

In another mother taking 175 mg/day, amitriptyline levels in the mother's milk were the same as in her serum on day one (24-27 µg/mL), but milk levels decreased to 54% of the serum concentration on days 2 to 26. Milk concentrations of nortriptyline were 74% of that in the mother's serum (87 ng/mL). Thus the authors reported the absolute infant dose as 35 µg/kg, 80 times lower than the mother's dose. Neither compound could be detected in the infant's serum on day 26, nor were there any signs of sedation or other adverse effects.

- AMOXAPINE (*Asendin*)
  - ○ AAP = Drugs whose effect on nursing infants is unknown but may be of concern
  - ○ LRC = L2
  - ○ RID = 0.6%
  - ○ Pregnancy = C
  - ○ Comment: Amoxapine and its metabolite are both secreted into breastmilk at relatively low levels. Following a dose of 250 mg/day, milk levels of amoxapine were less than 20 µg/L and 113 µg/L of the active metabolite. Milk levels of the active metabolite varied from 113 to 168 µg/L in two other milk samples. Maternal serum levels of amoxapine and metabolite at steady state were 97 µg/L and 375 µg/L, respectively.

- BUPROPION (*Wellbutrin, Zyban*)
  - ○ AAP = Drugs whose effect on nursing infants is unknown but may be of concern
  - ○ LRC = L3
  - ○ RID = 0.2-2%
  - ○ Pregnancy = C
  - ○ Comment: Bupropion is an older antidepressant with a structure unrelated to tricyclics. One report in the literature indicates that bupropion probably accumulates in human milk, although the absolute dose transferred appears minimal. In three infants studied, no bupropion was detected in the plasma compartment.

    Following one 100 mg dose in a mother, the milk/plasma ratio ranged from 2.51 to 8.58, clearly suggesting a concentrating mechanism for this drug in human milk. However, plasma levels of bupropion (or its metabolites) in the infant were undetectable, indicating that the dose transferred to the infant was low, and accumulation in infant plasma apparently did not occur under these conditions (infant was fed 7.5 to 9.5 hours after dosing). The peak milk bupropion level (0.189 mg/L) occurred two hours after a 100 mg dose. This milk level would provide 0.66% of the maternal dose, a dose that is likely to be clinically insignificant to a breastfed infant.

In a recent study of two breastfeeding patients consuming 75 mg twice daily and 150 mg (sustained release) daily, respectively, no bupropion or metabolite were detected in either breastfed infant. In the first patient at 17 weeks postpartum, plasma levels were drawn at two hours postdose, and bupropion or hydroxybupropion levels were undetectable. In the second patient at 29 weeks postpartum, bupropion and hydroxybupropion were undetectable as well. The limit of detection for bupropion was 5-10 ng/mL and for hydroxybupropion was 100-200 ng/mL.

In a study of 10 breastfeeding patients who received 150 mg bupropion SR daily for two days and then 300 mg bupropion SR daily thereafter for five more days, milk concentrations of bupropion averaged 45 µg/L. The average infant dose via milk was 6.75 µg/kg/day. The reported relative infant dose was 0.14% of the weight-normalized maternal dose. When the active metabolites present in milk were added, the RID would be 2% of the maternal dose. No side effects were noted in any of the infants.

Seizures in a six-month-old breastfed infant were recently reported four days following administration of 150 mg/day bupropion in the mother. The mother discontinued bupropion and continued breastfeeding. No further seizures were reported.

- CITALOPRAM   (*Celexa*)
  - ◦   AAP = Not reviewed
  - ◦   LRC = L2
  - ◦   RID = 3.6%
  - ◦   Pregnancy = C
  - ◦   Comment: Citalopram is an SSRI antidepressant. In one study of a 21-year-old patient receiving 20 mg citalopram per day, citalopram levels in milk peaked at three to nine hours following administration. Peak milk levels varied during the day, but the mean daily concentration was 298 nM (range 270-311). The milk/serum ratio was approximately three. The metabolite, desmethylcitalopram, was present in milk in low levels (23-28 nM). The concentration of metabolite in milk varied little during the day. Assuming a milk intake of 150 mL/kg in the infant, approximately 272 nM (88 µg or 16 ng/kg) of citalopram was passed to the baby each day. This amounts to only 0.4% of the dose administered to the mother. At three weeks, maternal serum levels of citalopram were 185 nM, compared to the infant's plasma level of just 7 nM. No untoward effects were noted in this breastfed infant. In another study, a milk/serum ratio of 1.16 to 1.88 was reported. This study suggests the infant would ingest 4.3 µg/kg/day and a relative dose of 0.7 to 5.9% of the weight-adjusted maternal dose.

    In another study of seven women receiving an average of 0.41 mg/kg/d citalopram, the average peak level (Cmax) of citalopram was 154 µg/L and 50 µg/L for desmethylcitalopram (metabolite is eight times less potent than citalopram). However, average milk concentrations (AUC) were lower and averaged 97 µg/L for citalopram and 36 µg/L for desmethylcitalopram during the dosing interval. The mean peak milk/plasma AUC ratio was 1.8 for citalopram. Low concentrations of citalopram (around 2-2.3 µg/L) were detected in only three of the seven infant plasmas. No adverse effects were found in any of the infants. The authors estimate the daily intake to be approximately 3.7% of the maternal dose.

    In a study of a single patient receiving 40 mg/day of citalopram, the concentration in milk and serum were 205 µg/L and 98.9 ng/mL, respectively. Infant serum levels were 12.7 ng/mL. This infant was noted to have 'uneasy' sleep patterns, which were reduced upon lowering the maternal dose.

In a recent study of women (n=31) who were consuming citalopram while breastfeeding, no significant difference was noted in infant side effect profiles, as compared to depressed and non-depressed control patients who were not consuming citalopram. In one infant, colic, decreased feeding, and irritability/restlessness was reported. In another infant, irritability and restlessness was reported. The authors recommend continued breastfeeding while consuming citalopram.

Eleven mothers taking citalopram and their babies were monitored during pregnancy and lactation. Plasma and milk samples were taken that suggested citalopram and its metabolite concentrations in milk were two to three times higher than in maternal plasma, but infant plasma levels were very low or undetectable.

One case reported an infant experiencing neonatal withdrawal syndrome after in utero exposure. The mother was taking 20-30 mg/day. The symptoms started upon delivery, and the child was discharged at day seven with no medical treatment needed.

- CLOMIPRAMINE   (*Anafranil*)
  - AAP = Drugs whose effect on nursing infants is unknown but may be of concern
  - LRC = L2
  - RID = 2.8%
  - Pregnancy = C
  - Comment: Clomipramine is a tricyclic antidepressant frequently used for obsessive-compulsive disorder. In one patient taking 125 mg/day, on the fourth and sixth day postpartum, milk levels were 342.7 and 215.8 µg/L, respectively. Maternal plasma levels were 211 and 208.4 µg/L at day four and six, respectively. Milk/plasma ratio varied from 1.62 to 1.04 on day four to six, respectively. Neonatal plasma levels continued to drop from a high of 266.6 ng/mL at birth to 127.6 ng/mL at day four, to 94.8 ng/mL at day six, to 9.8 ng/mL at 35 days. In a study of four breastfeeding women who received doses of 75 to 125 mg/day, plasma levels of clomipramine in the breastfed infants were below the limit of detection, suggesting minimal transfer to the infant via milk. No untoward effects were noted in any of the infants.

- DESIPRAMINE   (*Pertofrane, Norpramin*)
  - AAP = Drugs whose effect on nursing infants is unknown but may be of concern
  - LRC = L2
  - RID = 0.3-0.9%
  - Pregnancy = C
  - Comment: Desipramine is a prototypic tricyclic antidepressant. In one case report, a mother taking 200 mg of desipramine at bedtime had milk/plasma ratios of 0.4 to 0.9, with milk levels ranging between 17-35 µg/L. Desipramine was not found in the infant's blood, although these levels are probably too low to measure. In another study of a mother consuming 300 mg of desipramine daily, the milk levels were 30% higher than the maternal serum. The milk concentrations of desipramine were reported to be 316 to 328 µg/L, with peak concentrations occurring at four hours postdose. Assuming an average milk concentration of 280 µg/L, an infant would receive approximately 42 µg/kg/day. No untoward effects have been reported.

- DOTHIEPIN   (*Prothiaden*)
  - AAP = Drugs whose effect on nursing infants is unknown but may be of concern

- ○ LRC = L2
- ○ RID = 0.8-2.2%
- ○ Pregnancy = D
- ○ Comment: This is a new analog of the older tricyclic antidepressant amitriptyline. Dothiepin appears in breastmilk in a concentration of 11 µg/L following a dose of 75 mg/day, while the maternal plasma level was 33 µg/L. If the infant ingests 150 mL/kg/day of milk, the total daily dose of dothiepin ingested by the infant in this case would be approximately 1.7 µg/kg/day, approximately 1/650th of the adult dose. In an outcome study of 15 mother/infant pairs three to five years postpartum, no overall cognitive differences were noted in dothiepin treated mothers/infants, suggesting that this medication did not alter cognitive abilities in breastfed infants.

  In a study by Ilett, dothiepin concentrations in the milk of eight mothers was determined (dose ranged from 25-225 mg/day). The mean post-feeding milk/plasma ratio was 1.59, and the mean post-feeding dothiepin concentration in milk ranged from 20-475 µg/L (median=52 µg/L). Mean daily infant doses on a weight basis (in dothiepin equivalents) was 4.4% for dothiepin and its metabolites. Blood levels in all five infants were low (>10 µg/L). No untoward effects were noted in any of the eight infants following chronic maternal use.

- DULOXETINE   (*Cymbalta*)
  - ○ AAP = Not reviewed
  - ○ LRC = L3
  - ○ RID = 0.14%
  - ○ Pregnancy = C
  - ○ Comment: Duloxetine is a selective serotonin and norepinephrine reuptake inhibitor (SNRI) that is indicated for depression and for patients with neuropathic pain. The primary role of SNRIs is as an alternative in patients with major depressive disorder who have responded poorly to other agents (e.g., tricyclics or SSRIs). The transfer of duloxetine into breastmilk was studied in six women who were at least 12 weeks postpartum and taking 40 mg twice daily for 3.5 days. Paired blood and breastmilk samples were taken at 0, 1, 2, 3, 6, 9, and 12 hours postdose. The milk/plasma ratio was reported to be about 0.267. The daily dose of duloxetine was estimated to be 7 µg/day (range=4-15 µg/day). According to the manufacturer, the weight-adjusted infant dose would be approximately 0.141% of the maternal dose. Further, even this is unlikely absorbed, as duloxetine is unstable under acid conditions of the infant's stomach.

- ESCITALOPRAM   (*Lexapro*)
  - ○ AAP = Not reviewed
  - ○ LRC = L2
  - ○ RID = 5.2-8%
  - ○ Pregnancy = C
  - ○ Comment: Escitalopram is a selective serotonin reuptake inhibitor (SSRI) used in the treatment of depression. It is the active S(+)-enantiomer of citalopram (Celexa). While this agent is very specific for the serotonin receptor site, it does apparently have a number of other side effects which may be related to activities at other receptors. Antagonism of muscarinic, histaminergic, and adrenergic receptors has been hypothesized to be associated with various anticholinergic, sedative, and cardiovascular side effects.

In a case report of a 32-year-old mother taking escitalopram (5 mg/day) while breastfeeding her newborn, the reported milk level was 24.9 ng/mL at one week postpartum. The infant's daily dose was estimated to be 3.74 µg/kg. At 7.5 weeks of age, the mother was taking 10 mg/day, and the milk concentration level was 76.1 ng/mL. The infant daily dose was 11.4 µg/kg. There were no adverse events reported in the infant.

In a recent study of eight breastfeeding women taking an average of 10 mg/day, the total relative infant dose of escitalopram and its metabolite was reported to be 5.3% of the mother's dose. The mean M/P ratio (AUC) was 2.2 for escitalopram and 2.2 for demethylescitalopram. Absolute infant doses were 7.6 µg/kg/day for escitalopram and 3.0 µg/kg/day for demethylescitalopram. The drug and its metabolite were undetectable in most of the infants tested. No adverse events in the infants were reported. Because the absolute infant dose of escitalopram is less than an equivalent antidepressant dose of racemic citalopram (Celexa), its use is preferred over citalopram in treating depression in lactating women.

- FLUOXETINE   (*Prozac*)
  - ○ AAP = Drugs whose effect on nursing infants is unknown but may be of concern
  - ○ LRC = L2
  - ○ RID = 1.6-14.6%
  - ○ Pregnancy = C
  - ○ Comment: Fluoxetine is a very popular serotonin reuptake inhibitor (SSRI) currently used for depression and a host of other syndromes. Fluoxetine absorption is rapid and complete, and the parent compound is rapidly metabolized to norfluoxetine, which is an active, long half-life metabolite (360 hours). Both fluoxetine and norfluoxetine appear to permeate breastmilk to levels approximately 1/5 to 1/4 of maternal plasma. In one patient at steady-state (dose =20mg/day), plasma levels of fluoxetine were 100.5 µg/L and levels of norfluoxetine were 194.5 µg/L. Fluoxetine levels in milk were 28.8 µg/L and norfluoxetine levels were 41.6 µg/L. Milk/plasma ratios were 0.286 for fluoxetine, and 0.21 for norfluoxetine.

    In another patient receiving 20 mg daily at bedtime, the milk concentration of fluoxetine was 67 µg/L and norfluoxetine was 52 µg/L at four hours. At eight hours postdose, the concentration of fluoxetine was 17 µg/L and norfluoxetine was 13 µg/L. Using these data, the authors estimated that the total daily dose was only 15-20 µg/kg per day, which represents a low exposure.

    In another study of ten breastfeeding women receiving 0.39 mg/kg/day of fluoxetine, the average breastmilk levels for fluoxetine and norfluoxetine ranged from 24.4-181.1 µg/L and 37.4-199.1 µg/L, respectively. Peak milk concentrations occurred within six hours. The milk/plasma ratios for fluoxetine and norfluoxetine were 0.88 and 0.72, respectively. Fluoxetine plasma levels in one infant were undetectable (<1 ng/mL). Using these data, an infant consuming 150 mL/kg/day would consume approximately 9.3-57 µg/kg/day total fluoxetine (and metabolite), which represents 5-9% of the maternal dose. No adverse effects were noted in the infants in this study.

    Severe colic, fussiness, and crying have been reported in one case report. The mother was receiving a dose of 20 mg fluoxetine per day. Concentrations of fluoxetine and norfluoxetine in breastmilk were 69 µg/L and 90 µg/L, respectively. The plasma levels in the infant for fluoxetine and norfluoxetine were 340 ng/mL and 208 ng/mL, respectively, which is almost twice that of normal maternal ranges. The author does not report the maternal plasma levels, but suggests they were similar to Isenberg's adult levels (100.5 ng/mL and 194.5 ng/mL for fluoxetine and norfluoxetine). In this infant, the plasma levels would approach those of a mother receiving twice the above 20 mg dose per day (40 mg/day). The symptoms resolved upon discontinuation of fluoxetine by the mother.

In a study by Brent, an infant exposed in utero and postpartum via milk had moderate plasma fluoxetine levels that increased in the three weeks postpartum due to breastmilk ingestion. The infant's plasma levels of fluoxetine went from none detectable at day 13 to 61 ng/mL at day 21. The mean adult therapeutic range is 145 ng/mL. The infant in this study exhibited slight seizure activity at three weeks, four months, and five months.

Ilett reports that in a group of 14 women receiving 0.51 mg/kg/day fluoxetine, the mean M/P ratio was 0.67 (range 0.35 to 0.13) and 0.56 for norfluoxetine. Mean total infant dose in fluoxetine equivalents was 6.81% of the weight-adjusted maternal dose. The reported infant's fluoxetine and norfluoxetine plasma levels ranged from 20-252 µg/L and 17-187 µg/L, respectively.

Neonatal withdrawl syndrome was reported in one infant exposed in utero. The mother was taking 20 mg/day, and delivered at 27 weeks. The baby was treated with nasal CPAP and phenobarbital at a dose of 5 mg/kg/day because the symptoms were interpreted as convulsions. The clinical picture was interpreted as neonatal withdrawl syndrome.

It is not known if these reported side effects (seizures, colic, fussiness, crying) are common, although this author has received numerous other personal communications similar to this. Indeed in one case, the infant became comatose at 11 days postpartum, with high plasma levels of norfluoxetine. At present, fluoxetine is the only antidepressant cleared for use in pregnancy. This may pose an added problem in breastfed infants. Infants born of mothers receiving fluoxetine are born with full steady state plasma levels of the medication, and each time they are breastfed, the level in the infant may rise further.

While we do not know the real risk of side effects, they are apparently low for the population. If the patient cannot tolerate switching to another antidepressant, then fluoxetine should be continued.

Age at initiation of therapy is of importance. Use in older infants (four to six months or older) is virtually without complications because they can metabolize and excrete the medication more rapidly. Data published in 1999 also suggest that weight gain in infants breastfed from mothers who were taking fluoxetine demonstrated a growth curve significantly below that of infants who were breastfed by mothers who did not take the drug. The average deficit in measurements taken between two and six months of age was 392 grams body weight. None of these infants were noted to have unusual behavior. Another report suggests that fluoxetine may induce a state of anesthesia of the vagina and nipples, although the relevance of this to breastfeeding mothers is unknown. The author has had another report of a paroxetine-induced reduction of milk ejection reflex. Whether or not a loss of MER is related to an anesthesia of the nipples is purely speculative.

One case reported toxicity in a preterm infant whose mother was taking 40 mg/day. At four hours of age, the infant was tachypneic, with a respiratory rate of 100. The infant had an erythematous rash on both cheeks; petechiae on the abdomen, chest, and extremeties; and scleral icterus. Plasma levels of fluoxetine and norfluoxetine at 96 hours of age were 92 and 34 ng/mL, respectively, which is within the adult therapeutic range. This infant at four months of age had normal neurodevelopment. This study suggests that seizure-like activity and toxicity can be expected in preterm infants.

Current data on Sertraline and escitalopram suggest these medications have difficulty entering milk, and more importantly, the infant. Therefore, they are preferred agents over fluoxetine for therapy of depression in breastfeeding mothers. However, it is important to remember that the risks of not breastfeeding far outweigh the risk of using fluoxetine, and women who can only take fluoxetine should be advised to continue breastfeeding and observe the infant for side effects. Finally, fluoxetine therapy during breastfeeding is by no means contraindicated and has been used in many thousands of women.

The new product Symbyax contains both fluoxetine and olanzapine for treatment of Bipolar Depression.

- FLUVOXAMINE (*Luvox*)

  ○ AAP = Drugs whose effect on nursing infants is unknown but may be of concern

  ○ LRC = L2

  ○ RID = 0.3-1.4%

  ○ Pregnancy = C

  ○ Comment: Although structurally dissimilar to the other serotonin reuptake inhibitors, fluvoxamine provides increased synaptic serotonin levels in the brain. It has several hepatic metabolites which are not active. Its primary indications are for the treatment of obsessive-compulsive disorders (OCD), although it also functions as an antidepressant. There are a number of significant drug-drug interactions with this product.

    In a case report of one 23-year-old mother and following a dose of 100 mg twice daily for two weeks, the maternal plasma level of fluvoxamine base was 0.31 mg/L and the milk concentration was 0.09 mg/L. The authors reported a theoretical dose to infant of 0.0104 mg/kg/day of fluvoxamine, which is only 0.5% of the maternal dose. According to the authors, the infant suffered no unwanted effects as a result of this intake and that this dose poses little risk to a nursing infant.

    In a study of one patient receiving 100 mg twice daily, the AUC milk/serum ratio averaged 1.32. The absolute daily dose of fluvoxamine ingested by the newborn was calculated to be 48 μg/kg/d and the relative dose was calculated to be 1.58% of the weight-adjusted maternal dose.

    In another study of two breastfeeding women, the AUC average concentration of fluvoxamine in milk was 36 and 256 μg/L, respectively. The absolute infant dose was estimated at 5.4 and 38.4 μg/kg/d, with a relative infant dose (% of maternal dose) of 0.8% and 1.38%. A Denver assessment on one infant indicated normal development. Fluvoxamine was not detected in the plasma of either infant (limit of detection = 2 μg/L).

    In a case report of a single mother receiving 25 mg three times daily, the highest milk concentration was 40 μg/L. Using these data, an infant would ingest approximately 6 μg/kg/day, which is 0.62% of the maternal weight-adjusted dose. Interestingly, the maternal serum concentration at 10 hours was 20 ng/mL, while the infant plasma level was 9 ng/mL. Considering the clinical dose to the infant is low, this plasma level in the infant appears high. The authors suggest this may be an atypical case or that this infant's clearance of fluvoxamine is poor. The infant showed no symptoms of adverse effects.

    Yoshida reported a case of a mother receiving 100 mg/day in an infant 15 weeks postpartum. The concentration of fluvoxamine in maternal serum and milk was 170 μg/L and 50 μg/L, respectively, with a milk/plasma ratio of 0.29. The authors estimated the dose to the infant at 7.5 μg/kg/day. Developmental assessments of the infant at four months and 21 months suggested normal development. In a report of two breastfeeding women receiving 300 mg/d, Piontek was unable to detect any fluvoxamine in the plasma of two breastfed infants.

In summary, the data from these eight cases suggests that only minuscule amounts of fluvoxamine are transferred to infants, that plasma levels in infants are too low to be detected, and no adverse effects have been noted.

- IMIPRAMINE   (*Tofranil, Janimine*)
    - AAP = Drugs whose effect on nursing infants is unknown but may be of concern
    - LRC = L2
    - RID   = 0.1-4.4%
    - Pregnancy = D
    - Comment: Imipramine is a classic tricyclic antidepressant. Imipramine is metabolized to desipramine, the active metabolite. Milk levels approximate those of maternal serum. In a patient receiving 200 mg daily at bedtime, the milk levels at 1, 9, 10, and 23 hours were 29, 24, 12, and 18 µg/L, respectively. However, in this previous study, the mother was not in a therapeutic range. In a mother with full therapeutic levels, it is suggested that an infant would ingest approximately 0.2 mg/L of milk. This represents a dose of only 30 µg/kg/day, far less than the 1.5 mg/kg dose recommended for older children. The long half-life of this medication in infants could, under certain conditions, lead to high plasma levels, although they have not been reported. Although no untoward effects have been reported, the infant should be monitored closely. Therapeutic plasma levels in children 6-12 years are 200-225 ng/mL. Two good reviews of psychotropic drugs in breastfeeding patients are available.

- NORTRIPTYLINE   (*Aventyl, Pamelor*)
    - AAP = Drugs whose effect on nursing infants is unknown but may be of concern
    - LRC = L2
    - RID   = 1.7-3.1%
    - Pregnancy = D
    - Comment: Nortriptyline (NT) is a tricyclic antidepressant and is the active metabolite of amitriptyline (Elavil). In one patient receiving 125 mg of nortriptyline at bedtime, milk concentrations of NT averaged 180 µg/L after six to seven days of administration. Based on these concentrations, the authors estimate the average daily infant exposure would be 27 µg/kg/d. The relative dose in milk would be 1.5% of the maternal dose. Several other authors have been unable to detect NT in maternal milk nor in the serum of infants after prolonged exposure. So far, no untoward effects have been noted.

    A pooled analysis of 35 studies with an average dose of 78 mg/day reported a detectable level of nortriptyline in breastmilk in only one patient, with a concentration of 230 ng/mL. The authors suggest that breastfeeding infants exposed to nortriptyline are unlikely to develop detectable concentrations in plasma; therefore, breastfeeding during nortriptyline therapy is not contraindicated.

- PAROXETINE   (*Paxil*)
    - AAP = Drugs whose effect on nursing infants is unknown but may be of concern
    - LRC = L2
    - RID   = 1.2-2.8%
    - Pregnancy = D
    - Comment: Paroxetine is a typical serotonin reuptake inhibitor. Although it undergoes hepatic metabolism, the metabolites are not active. Paroxetine is exceedingly lipophilic and distributes

throughout the body with only 1% remaining in plasma. In one case report of a mother receiving 20 mg/day paroxetine at steady state, the breastmilk level at peak (four hours) was 7.6 µg/L. While the maternal paroxetine dose was 333 µg/kg, the maximum daily dose to the infant was estimated at 1.14 µg/kg, or 0.34% of the maternal dose.

In two studies of six and four nursing mothers, respectively, the mean dose of paroxetine received by the infants in the first study was 1.13% (range 0.5-1.7) of the weight adjusted maternal dose. The mean M/P (AUC) was 0.39 (range 0.32-0.51), while the predicted M/P was 0.22.

In the second study, the mean dose of paroxetine received by the infants was 1.25% (range 0.38-2.24%) of the weight adjusted maternal dose, with a mean M/P of 0.96 (range 0.31-3.33). The drug was not detected in the plasma of seven of the eight infants studied and was detected (<4 mg/L) in only one infant. No adverse effects were observed in any of the infants.

In a recent study of 16 mothers by Stowe, paroxetine levels in milk were low and varied according to maternal dose. Milk/plasma ratios varied from 0.056 to 1.3. Milk levels ranged from approximately 17 µg/L, 45 µg/L, 70 µg/L, 92 µg/L, and 101 µg/L in mothers receiving a dose of 10, 20, 30, 40, and 50 mg/day, respectively. Levels of paroxetine were below the limit of detection (<2 ng/mL) in all 16 infants.

In a study of six women receiving 20-40 mg/day, the milk/plasma ratio ranged from 0.39 to 1.11, but averaged 0.69. The average estimated dose to the infants ranged from 0.7 to 2.9% of the weight-adjusted maternal dose. In a seventh patient, and based on area-under-the-curve data, the milk/plasma ratio was 0.69 at a dose of 20 mg and 0.72 at a dose of 40 mg/day. The estimated dose to the infant was 1.0% and 2.0% of the weight-adjusted maternal dose at 20 and 40 mg, respectively. Paroxetine levels in milk averaged 44.3 and 78.5 µg/L over six hours following 20 and 40 mg doses, respectively. No adverse reactions or unusual behaviors were noted in any of the infants.

In another study of 24 breastfeeding mothers who received an average dose of 17.6 mg/d (range 10-40 mg/d), the average level of paroxetine in maternal serum and milk was 45.2 ng/mL and 19.2 ng/mL, respectively. The average milk/plasma ratio was 0.53. The authors estimated the average infant dose to be 2.88 µg/kg/d or 2.88% of the weight-adjusted maternal dose. All infant serum levels were below the limit of detection. Yet another study of 16 mothers taking an average of 18.75 mg/day showed that paroxetine was undetectable in any of the breastfeeding infants exposed to paroxetine. A pooled analysis of 68 breastfeeding mothers taking between 10-50 mg/day reported breastmilk levels between 0-153 µg/mL, with an average of 28 µg/mL. No untoward effects were noted in any of these infants exposed to paroxetine through breastmilk. One infant did experience lethargy and poor weight gain, but this infant had prenatal exposure.

These studies generally conclude that paroxetine can be considered relatively 'safe' for breastfeeding infants, as the absolute dose transferred is quite low. Plasma levels in the infant were generally undetectable. Recent data suggests that a neonatal withdrawal syndrome may occur in newborns exposed in utero to paroxetine, although there is significant difficulty in differentiating between withdrawal and toxicity. Symptoms include jitteriness, vomiting, irritability, hypoglycemia, and necrotizing enterocolitis. Suicide ideation and withdrawal sympmtoms seem worse with this product, and it should not be used in adolescent patients due to the risk of suicide. In addition, the Swedish birth registries have found that pregnant women who consumed Paroxetine were 1.5-2.0 times more likley to give birth to a baby with severe heart defects. Paroxetine is no longer recommended for use in pregnancy. While all of these complications may arise in pregnancy and in adolescents, paroxetine is still a suitable SSRI for breastfeeding women simply because the clinical dose consumed by the infant via breastmilk is exceedingly low. This said, it is still probably smart to use sertraline or another SSRI at this time.

- SERTRALINE (*Zoloft*)
  - AAP = Drugs whose effect on nursing infants is unknown but may be of concern
  - LRC = L2
  - RID = 0.4-2.2%
  - Pregnancy = C
  - Comment: Sertraline is a typical serotonin reuptake inhibitor similar to Prozac and Paxil, but unlike Prozac, the longer half-life metabolite of sertraline is only marginally active. In one study of a single patient taking 100 mg of sertraline daily for three weeks postpartum, the concentration of sertraline in milk was 24, 43, 40, and 19 µg/L of milk at 1, 5, 9, and 23 hours, respectively, following the dose. The maternal plasma levels of sertraline after 12 hours was 48 ng/mL. Sertraline plasma levels in the infant at three weeks were below the limit of detection (<0.5 ng/mL) at 12 hours postdose. Routine pediatric evaluation after three months revealed a neonate of normal weight who had achieved the appropriate developmental milestones.

    In another study of three breastfeeding patients who received 50-100 mg sertraline daily, the maternal plasma levels ranged from 18.4 to 95.8 ng/mL, whereas the plasma levels of sertraline and its metabolite, desmethylsertraline, in the three breastfed infants was below the limit of detection (<2 ng/mL). Milk levels were not measured. Desmethylsertraline is poorly active, less than 10% of the parent sertraline.

    Another recent publication reviewed the changes in platelet serotonin levels in breastfeeding mothers and their infants who received up to 100 mg of sertraline daily. Mothers treated with sertraline had significant decreases in their platelet serotonin levels, which is expected. However, there was no change in platelet serotonin levels in breastfed infants of mothers consuming sertraline, suggesting that only minimal amounts of sertraline are actually transferred to the infant. This confirms other studies.

    Studies by Stowe of 11 mother/infant pairs (maternal dose = 25-150 mg/day) further suggest minimal transfer of sertraline into human milk. From this superb study, the concentration of sertraline peaked in the milk at seven to eight hours and the metabolite (desmethylsertraline) at 5-11 hours. The reported concentrations of sertraline and desmethylsertraline in breastmilk were 17-173 µg/L and 22-294 µg/L, respectively. The reported dose of sertraline to the infant via milk varied from undetectable (5 of 11) to 0.124 mg/day in one infant. The infant's serum concentration of sertraline varied from undetectable to 3.0 ng/mL, but was undetectable in 7 of 11 patients. No developmental abnormalities were noted in any of the infants studied.

    In a study of eight women taking sertraline (1.05 mg/kg/d), the mean milk/plasma ratio was 1.93 and 1.64 for sertraline and N-desmethylsertraline. Infant exposure estimated from actual milk produced was 0.2% and 0.3% of the weight-adjusted maternal dose for sertraline and N-desmethylsertraline (sertraline equivalents), respectively. Assuming a 150 mL/kg/d intake, infant exposure was significantly greater at 0.90% and 1.32% for sertraline and N-desmethylsertraline, respectively. Neither sertraline nor its N-desmethyl metabolite could be detected in plasma samples from the four infants tested. No adverse effects were observed in any of the eight infants, and all had achieved normal developmental milestones.

    Sertraline is a potent inhibitor of 5-HT transporter function, both in the CNS and platelets. One recent study assessed the effect of sertraline on platelet 5-HT transporter function in 14 breastfeeding mothers (dose = 25-200 mg/d) and their infants to determine if even low levels of sertraline exposure could perhaps lead to changes in the infant's blood platelet 5-HT levels and, therefore, CNS serotonin levels. While a significant reduction in platelet levels of 5-HT were noted in the mothers, no changes in 5-HT levels were noted in the 14 infants. Thus it appears that at typical clinical doses, maternal sertraline has a minimal effect on platelet 5-HT transport in breastfeeding infants.

These studies generally confirm that the transfer of sertraline and its metabolite to the infant is minimal, and that attaining clinically relevant plasma levels in infants is remote at maternal doses less than 150 mg/day. Thorough reviews of antidepressant use in breastfeeding mothers are available.

- TRAZODONE (*Desyrel*)
  - ○ AAP = Drugs whose effect on nursing infants is unknown but may be of concern
  - ○ LRC = L2
  - ○ RID = 2.8%
  - ○ Pregnancy = C
  - ○ Comment: Trazodone is an antidepressant whose structure is dissimilar to the tricyclics and to the other antidepressants. In six mothers who received a single 50 mg dose, the milk/plasma ratio averaged 0.14. Peak milk concentrations occurred at two hours and were approximately 110 µg/L (taken from graph), and declined rapidly thereafter. On a weight basis, an adult would receive 0.77 mg/kg, whereas a breastfeeding infant, using these data, would consume only 0.005 mg/kg. The authors estimate that about 0.6% of the maternal dose was ingested by the infant over 24 hours.

- VENLAFAXINE (*Effexor*)
  - ○ AAP = Not reviewed
  - ○ LRC = L3
  - ○ RID = 6.8-8.1%
  - ○ Pregnancy = C
  - ○ Comment: Venlafaxine is a new serotonin reuptake inhibitor antidepressant. It inhibits both serotonin reuptake and norepinephrine reuptake. It is somewhat similar in mechanism to other antidepressants, such as Prozac, but has fewer anticholinergic side-effects.

    In an excellent study of three mothers (mean age = 34.5 years, 84.5 kg) receiving venlafaxine (225-300 mg/d), the mean milk/plasma ratios for venlafaxine (V) and O-desmethylvenlafaxine (ODV) were 2.5 and 2.7, respectively. The mean maximum concentrations of V and ODV in milk were 1.16 mg/L and 0.796 mg/L. The Cmax for milk was 2.25 hours. The mean infant exposure was 3.2% for V and 3.2% for ODV of the weight-adjusted maternal dose. Venlafaxine was detected in the plasma of one of seven infants, while ODV was detected in four of the seven infants. The infants were healthy and showed no acute adverse effects.

    However, recent data (MedWatch, FDA) has suggested that infants exposed in utero to various SNRIs, such as venlafaxine, may have profound adverse effects immediately upon delivery. These include respiratory distress, cyanosis, apnea, seizures, temperature instability, etc. It is not known if these adverse events are due to a direct toxic effect of venlafaxine on the fetus or to a discontinuation (withdrawal) syndrome. Studies have shown that these adverse effects may be partially relieved with venlafaxine received through breastmilk.

    The new product Pristiq (desvenlafaxine) consists of the active component from venlafaxine (ODV).

Clinical Tips

Current studies now suggest that infants of depressed mothers may be neurobehaviorally delayed at one year. In essence, the clinician must weigh the risk of untreated maternal depression (major) with the risk-benefit of exposure to these medications (relatively minor) and the risk-benefit of breastfeeding for the mother and infant dyad.

Thus it is now considered the standard of care to treat both pregnant and breastfeeding mothers for depression or psychosis in order to prevent more severe complications in pregnancy and during breastfeeding. Treatment largely depends on symptom severity and a risk-benefit assessment. Mild to moderate depression may respond to non-pharmacological therapy. In patients with more severe symptoms, or those that do not initially respond, they may benefit from the addition of other medications. While some medications have been well studied, inevitably the choice of a specific antidepressent should be based on clinical factors, including prior use of various medications. In the naive user, sertraline and perhaps paroxetine should be the agents of first choice, as their levels in milk are extraordinarily low. The initial dose of the antidepressant should be low and slowly increased over time to observe for complications in the infant.

Three major new studies now suggest that there are no major differences in tolerability or efficacy in the major SSRI family. Further, there are no major predictors of outcome either. The selection of an SSRI is largely up to the clinician. In general, the selection of the SSRI is largely dependent on the characteristics of the patient, tolerability, and cost of treatment. However, in one study, reboxetine is the only SSRI found to produce significantly lower response rate as compared to others in this family.

While it is not clear, most data suggest that a minimum of four to six weeks of therapy were required to produce an antidepressant effect. Newer data now suggests that in some patients, an onset of activity may occur within one to two weeks. Early response also predicts a higher rate of remission. Indeed, new meta analysis suggests that patients who show minimal or no improvement after two weeks of therapy should have a change in therapy, such as an increase in dose or perhaps even a change to another antidepressant. But the standard of care is still at present to wait four to six weeks before making major changes in therapy.

In recent years, there has been considerable concern about the risk of emergent suicidality associated with treatment with the SSRI family. A number of recent randomized controlled trials have thrown into question the correlation with SSRIs and emergent suicidality. In only one group of 18-24 year-old individuals a slight trend was noted. In older groups, no association was found with SSRI treatment and suicidality. Thus while the situation with children and young adults is still in question, in older adults, there seems no documented relationship with antidepressants and emergent suicidality.

Side effects reported with the use of SSRIs primarily include GI tract complications, including bleeding, nausea, vomiting, diarrhea, and sedation. Treatment-emergent nausea is most severe the first two weeks of therapy and tends to wane thereafter. Administering the medication once daily at bedtime is recommended. In cases of severe symptoms, a change in SSRI or treatment with gastric anti-motility drugs may be useful. CNS side effects include headache, insomnia, tremor, sedation, and nervousness. Other unique side effects include seizures (with bupropion), osteoporosis, elevated liver profiles, sexual side effects, etc.

While treatment choice is best determined by the patient's prior history, of the newer SSRIs, sertraline appears safest, with more than 60 mother-infants pairs studied to date and no untoward effects noted in these studies. At present, approximately 48% of mothers consuming antidepressants during breastfeeding use sertraline. Less than half this number use fluoxetine. Other SSRIs, such as paroxetine and venlafaxine, have been studied and found to produce exceedingly low milk levels and few untoward effects on the infant.

While fluoxetine has probably been used in more than a million breastfeeding mothers, levels produced in breastmilk are slightly higher than with paroxetine or sertraline. Nevertheless, in patients who are presently using fluoxetine either during pregnancy or early postpartum, it is certainly advisable to continue the use of this antidepressant while breastfeeding.

Mothers ingesting citalopram have occasionally complained of sedation in the infant. This too was suggested from a pooled analysis, although newer data suggests that levels in the breastfed infant are virtually undetectable. New data with its metabolite, escitalopram, suggests that milk levels are quite low, and in one small study, no complications were reported in the infants.

Many studies show minimal to no effect of the tricyclics on infants or their neurobehavioral development. Bupropion levels in milk are quite low, but two cases of seizures have been reported in breastfed infants. Patients or their infants should have no history of seizures before recommending this medication.

Numerous cases of neonatal withdrawal syndrome (early postpartum) have been reported in infants of mothers who ingested (during gestation) the shorter half-life SSRIs, such as paroxetine, sertraline (while pregnant), and even one case of fluoxetine. Current estimates are that approximately 30% of newborns (exposed to gestation SSRIs) may have some symptoms of discontinuation. These symptoms generally arise early postpartum (24-72 hours). Neonatal withdrawal symptoms include irritability, constant crying, shivering, increased tonus, eating and sleeping difficulties, and convulsions. Withdrawal symptoms seen early postpartum generally resolve without treatment within a few days. Breastfeeding should continue in these cases.

Suggested Reading

Barnett, B., & Austin, M. P. (2009). Reflections on perinatal depression treatment. *J Clin Psychiatry, 70*(9), 1315-1316.

Dossett, E. C. (2008). Perinatal depression. *Obstet Gynecol Clin North Am, 35*(3), 419-434, viii.

Field, T. (2008). Breastfeeding and antidepressants. *Infant Behav Dev, 31*(3), 481-487.

Freeman, M. P. (2007). Antenatal depression: navigating the treatment dilemmas. *Am J Psychiatry, 164*(8), 1162-1165.

Freeman, M. P. (2009). Breastfeeding and antidepressants: clinical dilemmas and expert perspectives. *J Clin Psychiatry, 70*(2), 291-292.

Gjerdingen, D. K., & Yawn, B. P. (2007). Postpartum depression screening: importance, methods, barriers, and recommendations for practice. *J Am Board Fam Med, 20*(3), 280-288.

Kendall-Tackett, K., & Hale, T. W. (2009). Use of Antidepressants in Pregnant and Breastfeeding Women: A Review of Recent Studies. *J Hum Lact 26*, 2, 187-195

Kennedy, S. H., Lam, R. W., Parikh, S. V., Patten, S. B., & Ravindran, A. V. (2009). Canadian Network for Mood and Anxiety Treatments (CANMAT) clinical guidelines for the management of major depressive disorder in adults. Introduction. *J Affect Disord, 117 Suppl 1*, S1-2.

Lam, R. W., Kennedy, S. H., Grigoriadis, S., McIntyre, R. S., Milev, R., Ramasubbu, R., et al. (2009). Canadian Network for Mood and Anxiety Treatments (CANMAT) clinical guidelines for the management of major depressive disorder in adults. III. Pharmacotherapy. *J Affect Disord, 117 Suppl 1*, S26-43.

Lanza di Scalea, T., & Wisner, K. L. (2009). Antidepressant medication use during breastfeeding. *Clin Obstet Gynecol, 52*(3), 483-497.

Leung, B. M., & Kaplan, B. J. (2009). Perinatal depression: prevalence, risks, and the nutrition link--a review of the literature. *J Am Diet Assoc, 109*(9), 1566-1575.

Logsdon, M. C., Wisner, K., & Shanahan, B. (2007). Evidence on postpartum depression: 10 publications to guide nursing practice. *Issues Ment Health Nurs, 28*(5), 445-451.

McQueen, K., & Dennis, C. L. (2007). Development of a postpartum depression best practice guideline: a review of the systematic process. *J Nurs Care Qual, 22*(3), 199-204.

McQueen, K., Montgomery, P., Lappan-Gracon, S., Evans, M., & Hunter, J. (2008). Evidence-based recommendations for depressive symptoms in postpartum women. *J Obstet Gynecol Neonatal Nurs, 37*(2), 127-136.

Muzik, M., Marcus, S. M., & Flynn, H. A. (2009). Psychotherapeutic treatment options for perinatal depression: emphasis on maternal-infant dyadic outcomes. *J Clin Psychiatry, 70*(9), 1318-1319.

Sharma, V. (2008). Treatment of postpartum psychosis: challenges and opportunities. *Curr Drug Saf, 3*(1), 76-81.

Sit, D. K., Flint, C., Svidergol, D., White, J., Wimer, M., Bish, B., et al. (2009). Best practices: An emerging best practice model for perinatal depression care. *Psychiatr Serv, 60*(11), 1429-1431.

Sit, D. K., Perel, J. M., Helsel, J. C., & Wisner, K. L. (2008). Changes in antidepressant metabolism and dosing across pregnancy and early postpartum. *J Clin Psychiatry, 69*(4), 652-658.

Postpartum Psychosis

Principles of Therapy

Postpartum psychosis is a mood disorder accompanied by loss of contact with reality and other psychotic symptoms. While considered one of the worst, it is also the rarest of the mood disorders. It occurs following delivery of an infant, with an incidence of one to two per 1000 deliveries. Symptoms include: hallucinations, delusions, illogic thought, insomnia, anorexia, anxiety, agitation, delirium, mania, and suicidal and infanticidal thoughts. Some patients have symptoms of mania, such as euphoria, overactivity, decreased sleep, disinhibition, irritability, and delusions of religious content. Others may have symptoms of severe depression with hallucinations, stupor, and hypomania. Women with a history of bipolar disorder, schizophrenia, or psychosis are at highest risk, but it can occur in naïve individuals without a prior psychiatric history. The etiology is unknown, but various theories include: fluctuating hormone levels, low self esteem about appearance early postpartum, feelings of inadequacy as a mother, etc.

Treatment of postpartum psychosis should be considered an emergency. Severe mania or depression requires rapid treatment starting with atypical antipsychotic agents. The atypical antipsychotics, such as olanzapine, risperidone, quetiapine, ziprasidone, and aripiprazole, are the most effective acute treatment for this condition. Most of these atypical antipsychotics have been studied in breastfeeding mothers and are considered compatible with breastfeeding.

Mood stabilizing drugs, such as lithium, valproic acid, carbamazepine, lamotrigine and others, may be useful, but less so with patients in acute crisis. Electroconvulsive therapy may be useful in situations when other therapy has failed.

Treatment

- Atypical antipsychotics: quetiapine, olanzapine, ziprasidone, aripiprazole, risperidone. These agents generally cause weight gain, but cause fewer central nervous system side effects.

- Typical antipsychotics: haloperidol, chlorpromazine, fluphenazine. These agents are effective and inexpensive, but carry a higher side effect profile than the atypical antipsychotics.

- Mood stabilizing agents, such as lithium, valproic acid, carbamazepine and lamotrigine, may be used, but are not as effective as the atypical antipsychotics.

- Psychosis during pregnancy and/or in the postpartum period is associated with adverse pregnancy and infant outcome and careful monitoring to assure infant safety is indicated.

Medications

- ARIPIPRAZOLE (*Abilify, Abilitat*)
    - AAP = Not reviewed
    - LRC = L3
    - RID = 1%
    - Pregnancy = C
    - Comment: Aripiprazole is a second-generation antipsychotic, now first-line treatment for schizophrenia. In a small study of a single patient receiving 10 mg/day initially, and then 15 mg subsequently, levels of aripiprazole in milk were reported to be 13 and 14 µg/L on two consecutive days (15 and 16 after initiation of therapy). Maternal plasma levels at the same time were 71 and 71 µg/L. Levels were drawn in the morning before aripiprazole administration. Thus it appears from this brief report that they were drawn approximately 24 hours postdose

      Several reports (personal communication) of somnolence have been reported to this author. The infant should be monitored for somnolence.

- CLOZAPINE (*Clozaril*)
    - AAP = Drugs whose effect on nursing infants is unknown but may be of concern
    - LRC = L3
    - RID = 1.4%
    - Pregnancy = B
    - Comment: Clozapine is an atypical antipsychotic, sedative drug somewhat similar to the phenothiazine family. In a study of one patient receiving 50 mg/d clozapine at delivery, the maternal and fetal plasma were reported to be 14.1 ng/mL and 27 ng/mL, respectively. After 24 hours postpartum, the maternal plasma level was 14.7 ng/mL and maternal milk levels were 63.5 ng/mL. On day seven postpartum and receiving a dose of 100 mg/d clozapine, the maternal plasma and milk levels were 41.1 ng/mL and 115.6 µg/L, respectively. From these data, it is apparent that clozapine concentrates in milk, with a milk/plasma ratio of 4.3 at a dose of 50 mg/d and 2.8 at a dose of 100 mg/d. The change from day one to seven suggests that clozapine entry into mature milk is less. From these data, the weight-adjusted relative infant dose would be 1.2% of the maternal dose.

- HALOPERIDOL (*Haldol*)
    - AAP = Drugs whose effect on nursing infants is unknown but may be of concern
    - LRC = L2
    - RID = 2.1-12%
    - Pregnancy = C
    - Comment: Haloperidol is a potent antipsychotic agent that is reported to increase prolactin levels in some patients. In one study of a woman treated for puerperal hypomania and receiving 5 mg twice daily, the concentration of haloperidol in milk was 0.0, 23.5, 18.0, and 3.25 µg/L on day 1, 6, 7, and 21, respectively. The corresponding maternal plasma levels were 0, 40, 26, and 4 µg/L at day 1, 6, 7, and 21, respectively. The milk/plasma ratios were 0.58, 0.69, and 0.81 on days 6, 7, and 21, respectively. After four weeks of therapy, the infant showed no symptoms of sedation and was feeding well.

In another study, after a mean daily dose of 29.2 mg, the concentration of haloperidol in breastmilk was 5 μg/L at 11 hours postdose. In a study of three women on chronic haloperidol therapy receiving 3, 4, and 6 mg daily, milk levels were reported to be 32, 17, and 4.7 ng/mL. The latter levels (4.7) were taken from a patient believed to be noncompliant.

Bennett calculates the relative infant dose to be 0.2-2.1% to 9.6% of the weight-adjusted maternal daily dose.

- OLANZAPINE   (*Zyprexa, Symbyax*)
  - AAP = Not reviewed
  - LRC = L2
  - RID = 1.2%
  - Pregnancy = C
  - Comment: Olanzapine is a typical antipsychotic agent, structurally similar to clozapine, and may be used for treating schizophrenia. It is rather unusual in that it blocks serotonin receptors rather than dopamine receptors.

    In a recent and excellent study of seven mother-infant nursing pairs receiving a median dose of olanzapine of 7.5 mg/day (range = 5-20 mg/day), the median infant dose ingested via milk was approximately 1.02% of the maternal dose. The median milk/plasma AUC ratio was 0.38. Olanzapine was undetected in the plasma of six infants tested. All infants were healthy and experienced no observable side effects. The maximum relative infant dose was approximately 1.2%.

    In a case report of a mother taking 20 mg/day, the milk/plasma ratio was 0.35, giving a relative infant dose of about 4% at steady state. This milk was not fed to the infant, so infant plasma levels were not performed.

    A study of five mothers receiving olanzapine at a dose of 2.5-20 mg/day reported milk/plasma ratios of 0.2 to 0.84, with an average relative infant dose of 1.6%. The authors reported no untoward effects on the infants attributable to olanzapine.

    The new product Symbyax contains both fluoxetine and olanzapine for treatment of Bipolar Depression.

- QUETIAPINE FUMARATE   (*Seroquel*)
  - AAP = Not reviewed
  - LRC = L2
  - RID = 0.07-0.1%
  - Pregnancy = C
  - Comment: Quetiapine (Seroquel) is indicated for the treatment of psychotic disorders. It has some affinity for histamine receptors, which may account for its sedative properties. It has been shown to increase the incidence of seizures, prolactin levels, and to lower thyroid levels in adults.

    In a patient (92 kg) receiving 200 mg/day of quetiapine throughout pregnancy, samples were expressed just before dosing, and at one, two, four and six hours postdose. The average milk concentration (AUC) of quetiapine over the six hours was 13 μg/L, with a maximum concentration of 62 μg/L at one hour. Levels of quetiapine rapidly fell to almost predose levels by two hours. The authors report that an exclusively breastfed infant would ingest only 0.09% of the weight-adjusted maternal dose. At maximum, the infant would ingest 0.43% of the weight-adjusted maternal dose. Although only one patient was studied, the data suggests levels in milk are minimal at this maternal dose.

One study of six mothers taking a combination of quetiapine, paroxetine, clonazepam, trazodone, and/or venlafaxine showed that no medication was detectable in three of the mothers' milk. In two of the other cases, quetiapine levels were below 0.01 mg/kg/day infant dose, while the final mother expressed an infant dose of less than 0.10 mg/kg/day. The mothers' doses of quetiapine ranged from 25-400 mg. The authors reported that no correlation was noted between drug exposure and developmental outcomes.

In another study of one mother receiving 400 mg quetiapine per day three months postpartum, expressed milk contained with an average drug concentration of 41 µg/L and a milk-to-plasma ratio of 0.29. The relative infant dose reported was 0.09% of the mother's dose. The infant's plasma concentration was 1.4 µg/L, or 6% of the mother's plasma concentration. No adverse effects were reported in the infant, but the authors suggest monitoring the infant's progress and quetiapine serum concentration.

- RISPERIDONE   (*Risperdal, Invega*)
    - AAP = Not reviewed
    - LRC = L3
    - RID = 2.8-9.1%
    - Pregnancy = C
    - Comment: Risperidone is a potent antipsychotic agent, belonging to a new chemical class, and is a dopamine and serotonin antagonist. Risperidone is metabolized to an active metabolite, 9-hydroxyrisperidone. In a study of one patient receiving 6 mg/day of risperidone at steady state, the peak plasma level of approximately 130 µg/L occurred four hours after an oral dose. Peak milk levels of risperidone and 9-hydroxyrisperidone were approximately 12 µg/L and 40 µg/L, respectively. The estimated daily dose of risperidone and metabolite (risperidone equivalents) was 4.3% of the weight-adjusted maternal dose. The milk/plasma ratios calculated from areas under the curve over 24 hours were 0.42 and 0.24, respectively, for risperidone and 6-hydroxyrisperidone.

      In another study, the transfer of risperidone and 9-hydroxyrisperidone into milk was studied in two breastfeeding women and one woman with risperidone-induced galactorrhea. In case two (risperidone dose = 42.1 µg/kg/d), the average concentration of risperidone and 9-hydroxyrisperidone in milk (Cav) was 2.1 and 6 µg/L, respectively. The relative infant dose was 2.8% of the maternal dose. In case three (risperidone dose = 23.1µg/kg/d), the average concentration of risperidone and 9-hydroxyrisperidone in milk (Cav) was 0.39 and 7.06 µg/L, respectively. The milk/plasma ratio determined in two women was <0.5 for both risperidone compounds. The relative infant doses were 2.3%, 2.8%, and 4.7% (as risperidone equivalents) of the maternal weight-adjusted doses in these three cases. Risperidone and 9-hydroxyrisperidone were not detected in the plasma of the two breastfed infants studied, and no adverse effects were noted.

      Paliperidone (Invega), the active metabolite of risperidone, is available in extended release tablets. This formulation has a volume of distribution of 6.95 L/kg, 74% protein binding, and a bioavailability of 28%.

- ZIPRASIDONE   (*Geodon*)
    - AAP = Not reviewed
    - LRC = L4
    - RID = 0.1-1.2%
    - Pregnancy = C

○ Comment: Ziprasidone is an atypical antipsychotic agent, chemically unrelated to phenothiazines or butyrophenones. No data are available on its transfer into human milk. Until data are available, risperidone or olanzapine should be suggested.

Clinical Tips

The mainstay of treatment for acute postpartum psychosis is the atypical antipsychotic agents. The onset of postpartum psychosis is as early as several days to a week after delivery, but can range up to four weeks. Acute pharmacotherapy with antipsychotics is essential. Olanzapine, risperidone, quetiapine, and ziprasidone have indications for acute psychosis, schizophrenia, and bipolar disorders. With exception of ziprasidone, all have data published in breastfeeding mothers. All together, the data suggest the levels in milk are generally low and side effects in the infants are reportedly low to nil.

Antiepileptic drugs, such as valproic acid and carbamazepine, have indications for mania, and all have data in breastfeeding mothers. Lamotrigine produces the highest levels in milk, and infants generally develop levels in the low to mid therapeutic range. Some caution is recommended with newborns and lamotrigine. Older infants (> 2 months) can probably metabolize and clear lamotrigine more efficiently.

As for haloperidol, levels in milk appear quite low, and this drug would be an optimal choice as a rapid neuroleptic agent. The older clozapine, despite its rather high incidence of agranulocytosis (1-2%), is still commonly used in treatment-refractory patients. Its use in breastfeeding mothers should be viewed very cautiously, and monitoring of the infant for agranulcytosis is probably mandatory.

Suggested Reading

ACOG Practice Bulletin: Clinical management guidelines for obstetrician-gynecologists number 92, April 2008 (replaces practice bulletin number 87, November 2007). Use of psychiatric medications during pregnancy and lactation. (2008). *Obstet Gynecol, 111*(4), 1001-1020.

Brockington, I. F. (2007). The present importance of the organic psychoses of pregnancy, parturition and the puerperium. *Arch Womens Ment Health, 10*(6), 305-306.

Chaudron, L. H., & Pies, R. W. (2003). The relationship between postpartum psychosis and bipolar disorder: a review. *J Clin Psychiatry, 64*(11), 1284-1292.

Epperson, C. N. (1999). Postpartum major depression: detection and treatment. *Am Fam Physician, 59*(8), 2247-2254, 2259-2260.

Ernst, C. L., & Goldberg, J. F. (2002). The reproductive safety profile of mood stabilizers, atypical antipsychotics, and broad-spectrum psychotropics. *J Clin Psychiatry, 63 Suppl 4*, 42-55.

Gentile, S. (2004). Clinical utilization of atypical antipsychotics in pregnancy and lactation. *Ann Pharmacother, 38*(7-8), 1265-1271.

Hay, P. J. (2009). Post-partum psychosis: which women are at highest risk? *PLoS Med, 6*(2), e27.

Iqbal, M. M., Kunwar, A., Lee, K., Khan, S., Megna, J., Iqbal, M. D., et al. (2005). Effects of commonly used antipsychotics (typical and atypical) in pregnancy and lactation. *J La State Med Soc, 157*(2), 94-97.

Jain, A. E., & Lacy, T. (2005). Psychotropic drugs in pregnancy and lactation. *J Psychiatr Pract, 11*(3), 177-191.

Seeman, M. V. (2004). Gender differences in the prescribing of antipsychotic drugs. *Am J Psychiatry, 161*(8), 1324-1333.

Sit, D., Rothschild, A. J., & Wisner, K. L. (2006). A review of postpartum psychosis. *J Womens Health (Larchmt), 15*(4), 352-368.

Posttraumatic Stress Disorder (PTSD)

Principles of Therapy

Posttraumatic stress disorder is a complex of somatic, cognitive, and other disorders. Patients with PTSD typically present with various nonspecific complaints, such as chronic pain, nausea, tremors, and mood swings. Sleep-related problems are common and include insomnia, rapid leg movements, confusional arousals, and even sleep walking. Gastric complaints, such as irritable bowel syndrome and chronic pelvic pain, are often associated with PTSD. PTSD also accompanies major mood disorders, including depression and generalized anxiety disorders. Patients with PTSD have a higher incidence of other disorders, such as asthma, hypertension, gastro-erosive disease, fibromyalgia, and chronic fatigue syndrome. PTSD is now best managed with a combination of SSRIs and cognitive behavioral therapy. New data seems to suggest that while the SSRIs are effective, they are self-limited, and the patient may regress after discontinuing the medication. On the other hand, cognitive behavioral therapy seems to be lasting, even after therapy is discontinued.

Treatment

- SSRI/SNRIs.

- Cognitive behavioral therapy.

- Exposure or trauma-focused therapy.

- Peer support.

- Eye Movement Desensitization and Reprocessing (EMDR).

- Noradrenergic agents.

- Atypical antipsychotics.

Medications

- CITALOPRAM   (*Celexa*)
    - AAP = Not reviewed
    - LRC = L2
    - RID = 3.6%
    - Pregnancy = C
    - Comment: Citalopram is an SSRI antidepressant. In one study of a 21-year-old patient receiving 20 mg citalopram per day, citalopram levels in milk peaked at three to nine hours following administration.

Peak milk levels varied during the day, but the mean daily concentration was 298 nM (range 270-311). The milk/serum ratio was approximately three. The metabolite, desmethylcitalopram, was present in milk in low levels (23-28 nM). The concentration of metabolite in milk varied little during the day. Assuming a milk intake of 150 mL/kg in the infant, approximately 272 nM (88 μg or 16 ng/kg) of citalopram was passed to the baby each day. This amounts to only 0.4% of the dose administered to the mother. At three weeks, maternal serum levels of citalopram were 185 nM, compared to the infant's plasma level of just 7 nM. No untoward effects were noted in this breastfed infant. In another study, a milk/serum ratio of 1.16 to 1.88 was reported. This study suggests the infant would ingest 4.3 μg/kg/day and would have a relative dose of 0.7 to 5.9% of the weight-adjusted maternal dose.

In another study of seven women receiving an average of 0.41 mg/kg/d citalopram, the average peak level (Cmax) of citalopram was 154 μg/L and 50 μg/L for desmethylcitalopram (metabolite is eight times less potent than citalopram). However, average milk concentrations (AUC) were lower and averaged 97 μg/L for citalopram and 36 μg/L for desmethylcitalopram during the dosing interval. The mean peak milk/plasma AUC ratio was 1.8 for citalopram. Low concentrations of citalopram (around 2-2.3 μg/L) were detected in only three of the seven infant plasmas. No adverse effects were found in any of the infants. The authors estimate the daily intake to be approximately 3.7% of the maternal dose.

In a study of a single patient receiving 40 mg/day of citalopram, the concentration in milk and serum were 205 μg/L and 98.9 ng/mL, respectively. Infant serum levels were 12.7 ng/mL. This infant was noted to have 'uneasy' sleep patterns, which were reduced upon lowering the maternal dose.

In a recent study of women (n=31) who were consuming citalopram while breastfeeding, no significant difference was noted in infant side effect profiles, as compared to depressed and non-depressed control patients who were not consuming citalopram. In one infant, colic, decreased feeding, and irritability/restlessness was reported. In another infant, irritability and restlessness was reported. The authors recommend continued breastfeeding while consuming citalopram.

Eleven mothers taking citalopram and their babies were monitored during pregnancy and lactation. Plasma and milk samples were taken that suggested citalopram and its metabolite concentrations in milk were two to three times higher than in maternal plasma, but infant plasma levels were very low or undetectable.

One case reported an infant experiencing neonatal withdrawal syndrome after in utero exposure. The mother was taking 20-30 mg/day. The symptoms started upon delivery, and the child was discharged at day seven with no medical treatment needed.

- CLONIDINE   (*Catapres*)
    - AAP = Not reviewed
    - LRC = L3
    - RID = 0.9-7.1%
    - Pregnancy = C
    - Comment: Clonidine is an antihypertensive that reduces sympathetic nerve activity from the brain. Clonidine is excreted in human milk. In a study of nine nursing women receiving between 241.7 and 391.7 μg/day of clonidine, milk levels varied from approximately 1.8 μg/L to as high as 2.8 μg/L on postpartum day 10-14. In another report following a maternal dose of 37.5 μg twice daily, maternal plasma was determined to be 0.33 ng/mL and milk level was 0.60 μg/L. Clinical symptoms of

neonatal toxicity are unreported and are unlikely in normal full term infants. Clonidine may reduce prolactin secretion and could conceivably reduce milk production early postpartum. Transdermal patches produce maternal plasma levels of 0.39, 0.84, and 1.12 ng/mL, using the 3.5, 7, and 10.5 cm square patches, respectively. The 3.7 square cm patch would produce maternal plasma levels equivalent to the 37.5 µg oral dose and would likely produce milk levels equivalent to the above study.

- ESCITALOPRAM   (*Lexapro*)
  - ◦ AAP = Not reviewed
  - ◦ LRC = L2
  - ◦ RID = 5.2-8%
  - ◦ Pregnancy = C
  - ◦ Comment: Escitalopram is a selective serotonin reuptake inhibitor (SSRI) used in the treatment of depression. It is the active S(+)-enantiomer of citalopram (Celexa). While this agent is very specific for the serotonin receptor site, it does apparently have a number of other side effects which may be related to activities at other receptors. Antagonism of muscarinic, histaminergic, and adrenergic receptors has been hypothesized to be associated with various anticholinergic, sedative, and cardiovascular side effects.

    In a case report of a 32-year-old mother taking escitalopram (5 mg/day) while breastfeeding her newborn, the reported milk level was 24.9 ng/mL at one week postpartum. The infant's daily dose was estimated to be 3.74 µg/kg. At 7.5 weeks of age, the mother was taking 10 mg/day, and the milk concentration level was 76.1 ng/mL. The infant daily dose was 11.4 µg/kg. There were no adverse effects reported in the infant.

    In a recent study of eight breastfeeding women taking an average of 10 mg/day, the total relative infant dose of escitalopram and its metabolite was reported to be 5.3% of the mother's dose. The mean M/P ratio (AUC) was 2.2 for escitalopram and 2.2 for demethylescitalopram. Absolute infant doses were 7.6 µg/kg/day for escitalopram and 3.0 µg/kg/day for demethylescitalopram. The drug and its metabolite were undetectable in most of the infants tested. No adverse effects in the infants were reported. Because the absolute infant dose of escitalopram is less than an equivalent antidepressant dose of racemic citalopram (Celexa), its use is preferred over citalopram in treating depression in lactating women.

- FLUOXETINE   (*Prozac*)
  - ◦ AAP = Drugs whose effect on nursing infants is unknown but may be of concern
  - ◦ LRC = L2
  - ◦ RID = 1.6-14.6%
  - ◦ Pregnancy = C
  - ◦ Comment: Fluoxetine is a very popular serotonin reuptake inhibitor (SSRI) currently used for depression and a host of other syndromes. Fluoxetine absorption is rapid and complete, and the parent compound is rapidly metabolized to norfluoxetine, which is an active, long half-life metabolite (360 hours). Both fluoxetine and norfluoxetine appear to permeate breastmilk to levels approximately 1/5 to 1/4 of maternal plasma. In one patient at steady-state (dose =20mg/day), plasma levels of fluoxetine were 100.5 µg/L and levels of norfluoxetine were 194.5 µg/L. Fluoxetine levels in milk were 28.8 µg/L and norfluoxetine levels were 41.6 µg/L. Milk/plasma ratios were 0.286 for fluoxetine and 0.21 for norfluoxetine.

In another patient receiving 20 mg daily at bedtime, the milk concentration of fluoxetine was 67 µg/L and norfluoxetine was 52 µg/L at four hours. At eight hours postdose, the concentration of fluoxetine was 17 µg/L and norfluoxetine was 13 µg/L. Using these data, the authors estimated that the total daily dose was only 15-20 µg/kg per day, which represents a low exposure.

In another study of 10 breastfeeding women receiving 0.39 mg/kg/day of fluoxetine, the average breastmilk levels for fluoxetine and norfluoxetine ranged from 24.4-181.1 µg/L and 37.4-199.1 µg/L, respectively. Peak milk concentrations occurred within six hours. The milk/plasma ratios for fluoxetine and norfluoxetine were 0.88 and 0.72, respectively. Fluoxetine plasma levels in one infant were undetectable (<1 ng/mL). Using these data, an infant consuming 150 mL/kg/day would consume approximately 9.3-57 µg/kg/day total fluoxetine (and metabolite), which represents 5-9% of the maternal dose. No adverse effects were noted in the infants in this study.

Severe colic, fussiness, and crying have been reported in one case report. The mother was receiving a dose of 20 mg fluoxetine per day. Concentrations of fluoxetine and norfluoxetine in breastmilk were 69 µg/L and 90 µg/L, respectively. The plasma levels in the infant for fluoxetine and norfluoxetine were 340 ng/mL and 208 ng/mL, respectively, which is almost twice that of normal maternal ranges. The author does not report the maternal plasma levels, but suggests they were similar to Isenberg's adult levels (100.5 ng/mL and 194.5 ng/mL for fluoxetine and norfluoxetine). In this infant, the plasma levels would approach those of a mother receiving twice the above 20 mg dose per day (40 mg/day). The symptoms resolved upon discontinuation of fluoxetine by the mother.

In a study by Brent, an infant exposed in utero and postpartum via milk had moderate plasma fluoxetine levels that increased in the three weeks postpartum due to breastmilk ingestion. The infant's plasma levels of fluoxetine went from none detectable at day 13 to 61 ng/mL at day 21. The mean adult therapeutic range is 145 ng/mL. The infant in this study exhibited slight seizure activity at three weeks, four months, and five months.

Ilett reports that in a group of 14 women receiving 0.51 mg/kg/day fluoxetine, the mean M/P ratio was 0.67 (range 0.35 to 0.13) and 0.56 for norfluoxetine. Mean total infant dose in fluoxetine equivalents was 6.81% of the weight-adjusted maternal dose. The reported infant fluoxetine and norfluoxetine plasma levels ranged from 20-252 µg/L and 17-187 µg/L, respectively.

Neonatal withdrawl syndrome was reported in one infant exposed in utero. The mother was taking 20 mg/day and delivered at 27 weeks. The baby was treated with nasal CPAP and phenobarbital at a dose of 5 mg/kg/day because the symptoms were interpreted as convulsions. The clinical picture was interpreted as neonatal withdrawl syndrome..

It is not known if these reported side effects (seizures, colic, fussiness, crying) are common, although this author has received numerous other personal communications similar to this. Indeed in one case, the infant became comatose at 11 days postpartum, with high plasma levels of norfluoxetine. At present, fluoxetine is the only antidepressant cleared for use in pregnancy. This may pose an added problem in breastfed infants. Infants born of mothers receiving fluoxetine are born with full steady state plasma levels of the medication, and each time they are breastfed the level in the infant may rise further.

While we do not know the real risk of side effects, they are apparently low for the population. If the patient cannot tolerate switching to another antidepressant, then fluoxetine should be continued.

Age at initiation of therapy is of importance. Use in older infants (four to six months or older) is virtually without complications because they can metabolize and excrete the medication more rapidly. Data published in 1999 also suggest that weight gain in infants breastfed from mothers who were taking fluoxetine demonstrated a growth curve significantly below that of infants who were breastfed by mothers who did not take the drug. The average deficit in measurements taken between two and six months of age was 392 grams body weight. None of these infants were noted to have unusual behavior. Another report suggests that fluoxetine may induce a state of anesthesia of the vagina and nipples, although the relevance of this to breastfeeding mothers is unknown. The author has had another report of a paroxetine-induced reduction of milk ejection reflex. Whether or not a loss of MER is related to an anesthesia of the nipples is purely speculative.

One case reported toxicity in a preterm infant whose mother was taking 40 mg/day. At four hours of age, the infant was tachypneic, with a respiratory rate of 100. The infant had an erythematous rash on both cheeks; petechiae on the abdomen, chest, and extremeties; and scleral icterus. Plasma levels of fluoxetine and norfluoxetine at 96 hours of age were 92 and 34 ng/mL, respectively, which is within the adult therapeutic range. This infant at four months of age had normal neurodevelopment. This study suggests that seizure-like activity and toxicity can be expected in preterm infants.

Current data on Sertraline and escitalopram suggest these medications have difficulty entering milk, and more importantly, the infant. Therefore, they are preferred agents over fluoxetine for therapy of depression in breastfeeding mothers. However, it is important to remember that the risks of not breastfeeding far outweigh the risk of using fluoxetine, and women who can only take fluoxetine should be advised to continue breastfeeding and observe the infant for side effects. Finally, fluoxetine therapy during breastfeeding is by no means contraindicated and has been used in many thousands of women.

The new product Symbyax contains both fluoxetine and olanzapine for treatment of Bipolar Depression.

- OLANZAPINE   (*Zyprexa, Symbyax*)
  - AAP = Not reviewed
  - LRC = L2
  - RID = 1.2%
  - Pregnancy = C
  - Comment: Olanzapine is a typical antipsychotic agent, structurally similar to clozapine, and may be used for treating schizophrenia. It is rather unusual in that it blocks serotonin receptors rather than dopamine receptors.

    In a recent and excellent study of seven mother-infant nursing pairs receiving a median dose of olanzapine of 7.5 mg/day (range = 5-20 mg/day), the median infant dose ingested via milk was approximately 1.02% of the maternal dose. The median milk/plasma AUC ratio was 0.38. Olanzapine was undetected in the plasma of six infants tested. All infants were healthy and experienced no observable side effects. The maximum relative infant dose was approximately 1.2%.

    In a case report of a mother taking 20 mg/day, the milk/plasma ratio was 0.35, giving a relative infant dose of about 4% at steady state. This milk was not fed to the infant, so infant plasma levels were not performed.

    A study of five mothers receiving olanzapine at a dose of 2.5-20 mg/day reported milk/plasma ratios of 0.2 to 0.84, with an average relative infant dose of 1.6%. The authors reported no untoward effects on the infants attributable to olanzapine.

    The new product Symbyax contains both fluoxetine and olanzapine for treatment of Bipolar Depression.

- MIRTAZAPINE   (*Remeron*)
  - AAP = Not reviewed

- ○ LRC = L3
- ○ RID = 1.6-6.3%
- ○ Pregnancy = C
- ○ Comment: Mirtazapine is a unique antidepressant structurally dissimilar to the SSRIs, tricyclics, or the monoamine oxidase inhibitors. Mirtazapine has little or no serotonergic-like side effects, fewer anticholinergic side effects than amitriptyline, produces less sexual dysfunction, and has not demonstrated cardiotoxic or seizure potential in a limited number of overdose cases.

  In a study of three women who received 45, 60, and 45 mg/day mirtazapine, the average concentration (AUC) in milk was 77, 75, and 47 µg/L, respectively. The absolute infant dose was 10, 11.3, and 7.1 µg/kg/d, respectively. The relative infant dose was 1.9%, 1.1%, and 1.5% of the weight-normalized maternal dose, respectively. Mirtazapine was below the limit of quantitation in two of the infants and only 1.5 ng/mL in the third infant. The infants were meeting all developmental milestones and were without side effects.

  Another study of eight women taking an average of 38 mg/day showed average milk concentrations of 53 µg/L and 13 µg/L of mirtazapine and its metabolite, respectively. The average absolute infant dose was 495 µg/kg/day, indicating a relative infant dose of 1.9%. The authors of this study suggest that breastfeeding is safe during mirtazapine therapy.

  In another mother who took 22.5 mg/day, milk levels were 130 µg/L four hours after dosing and 61 µg/L 10 hours after the dose (foremilk). This suggests the relative infant dose was 3.9-4.4% and 1.8-2.7%, respectively, of the weight-adjusted maternal dose at these two times. At 12.5 hours postdose, infant plasma levels were undetectable.

- PAROXETINE (*Paxil*)
  - ○ AAP = Drugs whose effect on nursing infants is unknown but may be of concern
  - ○ LRC = L2
  - ○ RID = 1.2-2.8%
  - ○ Pregnancy = D
  - ○ Comment: Paroxetine is a typical serotonin reuptake inhibitor. Although it undergoes hepatic metabolism, the metabolites are not active. Paroxetine is exceedingly lipophilic and distributes throughout the body, with only 1% remaining in plasma. In one case report of a mother receiving 20 mg/day paroxetine at steady state, the breastmilk level at peak (four hours) was 7.6 µg/L. While the maternal paroxetine dose was 333 µg/kg, the maximum daily dose to the infant was estimated at 1.14 µg/kg or 0.34% of the maternal dose.

    In two studies of six and four nursing mothers, respectively, the mean dose of paroxetine received by the infants in the first study was 1.13% (range 0.5-1.7) of the weight adjusted maternal dose. The mean M/P (AUC) was 0.39 (range 0.32-0.51), while the predicted M/P was 0.22.

    In the second study, the mean dose of paroxetine received by the infants was 1.25% (range 0.38-2.24%) of the weight adjusted maternal dose, with a mean M/P of 0.96 (range 0.31-3.33). The drug was not detected in the plasma of seven of the eight infants studied and was detected (<4 mg/L) in only one infant. No adverse effects were observed in any of the infants.

    In a recent study of 16 mothers by Stowe, paroxetine levels in milk were low and varied according to maternal dose. Milk/plasma ratios varied from 0.056 to 1.3. Milk levels ranged from approximately 17 µg/L, 45 µg/L, 70 µg/L, 92 µg/L, and 101 µg/L in mothers receiving a dose of 10, 20, 30, 40, and 50 mg/day, respectively. Levels of paroxetine were below the limit of detection (<2 ng/mL) in all 16 infants.

In a study of six women receiving 20-40 mg/day, the milk/plasma ratio ranged from 0.39 to 1.11, but averaged 0.69. The average estimated dose to the infants ranged from 0.7 to 2.9% of the weight-adjusted maternal dose. In a seventh patient, and based on area-under-the-curve data, the milk/plasma ratio was 0.69 at a dose of 20 mg and 0.72 at a dose of 40 mg/day. The estimated dose to the infant was 1.0% and 2.0% of the weight-adjusted maternal dose at 20 and 40 mg, respectively. Paroxetine levels in milk averaged 44.3 and 78.5 μg/L over six hours following 20 and 40 mg doses, respectively. No adverse reactions or unusual behaviors were noted in any of the infants.

In another study of 24 breastfeeding mothers who received an average dose of 17.6 mg/d (range 10-40 mg/d), the average level of paroxetine in maternal serum and milk was 45.2 ng/mL and 19.2 ng/mL, respectively. The average milk/plasma ratio was 0.53. The authors estimated the average infant dose to be 2.88 μg/kg/d or 2.88% of the weight-adjusted maternal dose. All infant serum levels were below the limit of detection.

Yet another study of 16 mothers taking an average of 18.75 mg/day showed that paroxetine was undetectable in any of the breastfeeding infants exposed to paroxetine.

A pooled analysis of 68 breastfeeding mothers taking between 10-50 mg/day reported breastmilk levels between 0-153 μg/mL, with an average of 28 μg/mL. No untoward effects were noted in any of these infants exposed to paroxetine through breastmilk. One infant did experience lethargy and poor weight gain, but this infant had prenatal exposure.

These studies generally conclude that paroxetine can be considered relatively 'safe' for breastfeeding infants, as the absolute dose transferred is quite low. Plasma levels in the infant were generally undetectable. Recent data suggests that a neonatal withdrawal syndrome may occur in newborns exposed in utero to paroxetine, although there is significant difficulty in differentiating between withdrawal and toxicity. Symptoms include jitteriness, vomiting, irritability, hypoglycemia, and necrotizing enterocolitis. Suicide ideation and withdrawal symptoms seem worse with this product, and it should not be used in adolescent patients due to the risk of suicide. In addition, the Swedish birth registries have found that pregnant women who consumed Paroxetine were 1.5-2.0 times more likely to give birth to a baby with severe heart defects. Paroxetine is no longer recommended for use in pregnancy. While all of these complications may arise in pregnancy and in adolescents, paroxetine is still a suitable SSRI for breastfeeding women simply because the clinical dose consumed by the infant via breastmilk is exceedingly low. This said, it is still probably smart to use sertraline or another SSRI at this time.

- PRAZOSIN (*Minipress*)
    - AAP = Not reviewed
    - LRC = L4
    - RID =
    - Pregnancy = C
    - Comment: Prazosin is a selective alpha-1-adrenergic antagonist used to control hypertension. It is structurally similar to doxazosin and terazosin. Antihypertensives may reduce breastmilk production and prazosin may do likewise. Others in this family (doxazosin) are known to concentrate in milk. Exercise extreme caution when administering to nursing mothers.

- PROPRANOLOL   (*Inderal*)
  - ◦ AAP = Maternal Medication Usually Compatible with Breastfeeding
  - ◦ LRC = L2
  - ◦ RID = 0.3-0.5%
  - ◦ Pregnancy = C
  - ◦ Comment: Propranolol is a popular beta blocker used in treating hypertension, cardiac arrhythmia, migraine headache, and numerous other syndromes. In general, the maternal plasma levels are exceedingly low; hence, the milk levels are low as well. Milk/plasma ratios are generally less than one. In one study of three patients, the average milk concentration was only 35.4 μg/L after multiple dosing intervals. The milk/plasma ratio varied from 0.33 to 1.65. Using these data, the authors suggest that an infant would receive only 70 μg/L of milk per day, which is <0.1% of the maternal dose.

    In another study of a patient receiving 20 mg twice daily, milk levels varied from 4 to 20 μg/L, with an estimated average dose to infant of 3 μg/day. In another patient receiving 40 mg four times daily, the peak concentration occurred at three hours after dosing. Milk levels varied from zero to 9 μg/L.

    After a 30 day regimen of 240 mg/day propranolol, the predose and postdose concentration in breastmilk was 26 and 64 μg/L, respectively. No symptoms or signs of beta blockade were noted in this infant. The above amounts in milk would likely be clinically insignificant. Long term exposure has not been studied, and caution is urged. Of the beta blocker family, propranolol is probably preferred in lactating women. Use with great caution, if at all, in mothers or infants with asthma.

- QUETIAPINE FUMARATE   (*Seroquel*)
  - ◦ AAP = Not reviewed
  - ◦ LRC = L2
  - ◦ RID = 0.07-0.1%
  - ◦ Pregnancy = C
  - ◦ Comment: Quetiapine (Seroquel) is indicated for the treatment of psychotic disorders. It has some affinity for histamine receptors, which may account for its sedative properties. It has been shown to increase the incidence of seizures and prolactin levels and to lower thyroid levels in adults.

    In a patient (92 kg) receiving 200 mg/day of quetiapine throughout pregnancy, samples were expressed just before dosing, and at one, two, four and six hours postdose. The average milk concentration (AUC) of quetiapine over the six hours was 13 μg/L, with a maximum concentration of 62 μg/L at one hour. Levels of quetiapine rapidly fell to almost predose levels by two hours. The authors report that an exclusively breastfed infant would ingest only 0.09% of the weight-adjusted maternal dose. At maximum, the infant would ingest 0.43% of the weight-adjusted maternal dose. Although only one patient was studied, the data suggest levels in milk are minimal at this maternal dose.

    One study of six mothers taking a combination of quetiapine, paroxetine, clonazepam, trazodone, and/or venlafaxine showed that no medication was detectable in three of the mothers' milk. In two of the other cases, quetiapine levels were below 0.01 mg/kg/day infant dose, while the final mother expressed an infant dose of less than 0.10 mg/kg/day. The mothers' doses of quetiapine ranged from 25-400 mg. The authors reported that no correlation was noted between drug exposure and developmental outcomes.

In another study of one mother receiving 400 mg quetiapine per day three months postpartum, expressed milk contained an average drug concentration of 41 µg/L, and a milk-to-plasma ratio of 0.29. The relative infant dose reported was 0.09% of the mother's dose. The infant's plasma concentration was 1.4 µg/L, or 6% of the mother's plasma concentration. No adverse effects were reported in the infant, but the authors suggest monitoring the infant's progress and quetiapine serum concentration.

- **RISPERIDONE**   (*Risperdal, Invega*)
  - ◦   AAP = Not reviewed
  - ◦   LRC = L3
  - ◦   RID   = 2.8-9.1%
  - ◦   Pregnancy = C
  - ◦   Comment: Risperidone is a potent antipsychotic agent, belonging to a new chemical class, and is a dopamine and serotonin antagonist. Risperidone is metabolized to an active metabolite, 9-hydroxyrisperidone. In a study of one patient receiving 6 mg/day of risperidone at steady state, the peak plasma level of approximately 130 µg/L occurred four hours after an oral dose. Peak milk levels of risperidone and 9-hydroxyrisperidone were approximately 12 µg/L and 40 µg/L, respectively. The estimated daily dose of risperidone and metabolite (risperidone equivalents) was 4.3% of the weight-adjusted maternal dose. The milk/plasma ratios calculated from areas under the curve over 24 hours were 0.42 and 0.24, respectively, for risperidone and 6-hydroxyrisperidone.

    In another study, the transfer of risperidone and 9-hydroxyrisperidone into milk was studied in two breastfeeding women and one woman with risperidone-induced galactorrhea. In case two (risperidone dose = 42.1 µg/kg/d), the average concentration of risperidone and 9-hydroxyrisperidone in milk (Cav) was 2.1 and 6 µg/L, respectively. The relative infant dose was 2.8% of the maternal dose. In case three (risperidone dose = 23.1µg/kg/d), the average concentration of risperidone and 9-hydroxyrisperidone in milk (Cav) was 0.39 and 7.06 µg/L, respectively. The milk/plasma ratio determined in two women was <0.5 for both risperidone compounds. The relative infant doses were 2.3%, 2.8%, and 4.7% (as risperidone equivalents) of the maternal weight-adjusted doses in these three cases. Risperidone and 9-hydroxyrisperidone were undetected in the plasma of the two breastfed infants studied, and no adverse effects were noted.

    Paliperidone (Invega), the active metabolite of risperidone, is available in extended release tablets. This formulation has a volume of distribution of 6.95 L/kg, 74% protein binding, and a bioavailability of 28%.

- **SERTRALINE**   (*Zoloft*)
  - ◦   AAP = Drugs whose effect on nursing infants is unknown but may be of concern
  - ◦   LRC = L2
  - ◦   RID   = 0.4-2.2%
  - ◦   Pregnancy = C
  - ◦   Comment: Sertraline is a typical serotonin reuptake inhibitor similar to Prozac and Paxil, but unlike Prozac, the longer half-life metabolite of sertraline is only marginally active. In one study of a single patient taking 100 mg of sertraline daily for three weeks postpartum, the concentration of sertraline in milk was 24, 43, 40, and 19 µg/L of milk at 1, 5, 9, and 23 hours, respectively, following the dose. The maternal plasma levels of sertraline after 12 hours was 48 ng/mL. Sertraline plasma levels in the infant at three weeks were below the limit of detection (<0.5 ng/mL) at 12 hours postdose. Routine

pediatric evaluation after three months revealed a neonate of normal weight who had achieved the appropriate developmental milestones.

In another study of three breastfeeding patients who received 50-100 mg sertraline daily, the maternal plasma levels ranged from 18.4 to 95.8 ng/mL, whereas the plasma levels of sertraline and its metabolite, desmethylsertraline, in the three breastfed infants was below the limit of detection (<2 ng/mL). Milk levels were not measured. Desmethylsertraline is poorly active, less than 10% of the parent sertraline.

Another recent publication reviewed the changes in platelet serotonin levels in breastfeeding mothers and their infants who received up to 100 mg of sertraline daily. Mothers treated with sertraline had significant decreases in their platelet serotonin levels, which is expected. However, there was no change in platelet serotonin levels in breastfed infants of mothers consuming sertraline, suggesting that only minimal amounts of sertraline are actually transferred to the infant. This confirms other studies.

Studies by Stowe of 11 mother/infant pairs (maternal dose = 25-150 mg/day) further suggest minimal transfer of sertraline into human milk. From this superb study, the concentration of sertraline peaked in the milk at seven to eight hours and the metabolite (desmethylsertraline) at 5-11 hours. The reported concentrations of sertraline and desmethylsertraline in breastmilk were 17-173 µg/L and 22-294 µg/L, respectively. The reported dose of sertraline to the infant via milk varied from undetectable (5 of 11) to 0.124 mg/day in one infant. The infant's serum concentration of sertraline varied from undetectable to 3.0 ng/mL, but was undetectable in 7 of 11 patients. No developmental abnormalities were noted in any of the infants studied.

In a study of eight women taking sertraline (1.05 mg/kg/d), the mean milk/plasma ratio was 1.93 and 1.64 for sertraline and N-desmethylsertraline. Infant exposure estimated from actual milk produced was 0.2% and 0.3% of the weight-adjusted maternal dose for sertraline and N-desmethylsertraline (sertraline equivalents), respectively. Assuming a 150 mL/kg/d intake, infant exposure was significantly greater at 0.90% and 1.32% for sertraline and N-desmethylsertraline, respectively. Neither sertraline nor its N-desmethyl metabolite could be detected in plasma samples from the four infants tested. No adverse effects were observed in any of the eight infants, and all had achieved normal developmental milestones.

Sertraline is a potent inhibitor of 5-HT transporter function, both in the CNS and platelets. One recent study assessed the effect of sertraline on platelet 5-HT transporter function in 14 breastfeeding mothers (dose = 25-200 mg/d) and their infants to determine if even low levels of sertraline exposure could perhaps lead to changes in the infant's blood platelet 5-HT levels and, therefore, CNS serotonin levels. While a significant reduction in platelet levels of 5-HT were noted in the mothers, no changes in 5-HT levels were noted in the 14 infants. Thus it appears that at typical clinical doses, maternal sertraline has a minimal effect on platelet 5-HT transport in breastfeeding infants.

These studies generally confirm that the transfer of sertraline and its metabolite to the infant is minimal, and that attaining clinically relevant plasma levels in infants is remote at maternal doses less than 150 mg/day. Thorough reviews of antidepressant use in breastfeeding mothers are available.

- TRAZODONE (*Desyrel*)
  - ∘ AAP = Drugs whose effect on nursing infants is unknown but may be of concern
  - ∘ LRC = L2
  - ∘ RID = 2.8%

- Pregnancy = C
- Comment: Trazodone is an antidepressant whose structure is dissimilar to the tricyclics and to the other antidepressants. In six mothers who received a single 50 mg dose, the milk/plasma ratio averaged 0.14. Peak milk concentrations occurred at two hours and were approximately 110 μg/L (taken from graph) and declined rapidly thereafter. On a weight basis, an adult would receive 0.77 mg/kg, whereas a breastfeeding infant, using these data, would consume only 0.005 mg/kg. The authors estimate that about 0.6% of the maternal dose was ingested by the infant over 24 hours.

Clinical Tips

A wide range of treatments now exist for PTSD; however, treatment with SSRIs and cognitive behavior therapy are now the mainstays of treatment. The objectives are to reduce the core symptoms of the disorder and improve the patient's ability to cope with daily stresses.

The psychological treatment presently considered most effective is trauma-focused cognitive behavioral therapy. This therapy includes a combination of exposure therapy, trauma-focused cognitive therapy, and eye movement desensitization (Eye Movement Desensitization and Reprocessing). Exposure therapy involves the patient reviewing the traumatic event in great detail, taping this interview, and listening to it repeatedly. In trauma-focused cognitive therapy, the therapist challenges the distorted beliefs and misinterpretations concerning the traumatic event. Current evidence suggests that patients who do well following cognitive behavioral therapy retain this benefit, even following discontinuation of therapy.

The use of medications is somewhat controversial and open to debate. Recommended SSRIs include sertraline, fluoxetine, citalopram, paroxetine, and probably others. Most all were considerably better than placebo in numerous studies. The addition of an antipsychotic (olanzapine) to an antidepressant seems effective in patients who do not respond fully to antidepressant drugs alone.

Other medications, such as prazosin, propranolol, and topliramate, may reduce nightmares and flashbacks. Medications not recommended as first-line treatment include nefazodone, buspirone, venlafaxine, bupropion, mirtazapine, etc.

Suggested Reading

Campbell, D. G., Felker, B. L., Liu, C. F., Yano, E. M., Kirchner, J. E., Chan, D., et al. (2007). Prevalence of depression-PTSD comorbidity: implications for clinical practice guidelines and primary care-based interventions. *J Gen Intern Med, 22*(6), 711-718.

Copeland-Linder, N. (2008). Posttraumatic stress disorder. *Pediatr Rev, 29*(3), 103-104; discussion 104.

Katzman, M. A., Struzik, L., Vivian, L. L., Vermani, M., & McBride, J. C. (2005). Pharmacotherapy of post-traumatic stress disorder: a family practitioners guide to management of the disease. *Expert Rev Neurother, 5*(1), 129-139.

Kozaric-Kovacic, D. (2009). Pharmacotherapy treatment of PTSD and comorbid disorders. *Psychiatr Danub, 21*(3), 411-414.

Seng, J. S., Low, L. K., Sperlich, M., Ronis, D. L., & Liberzon, I. (2009). Prevalence, trauma history, and risk for posttraumatic stress disorder among nulliparous women in maternity care. *Obstet Gynecol, 114*(4), 839-847.

Stein, D. J., Ipser, J. C., & Seedat, S. (2006). Pharmacotherapy for post traumatic stress disorder (PTSD). *Cochrane Database Syst Rev*(1), CD002795.

Stein, M. B., Kerridge, C., Dimsdale, J. E., & Hoyt, D. B. (2007). Pharmacotherapy to prevent PTSD: Results from a randomized controlled proof-of-concept trial in physically injured patients. *J Trauma Stress, 20*(6), 923-932.

Psoriasis

Principles of Therapy

Psoriasis is a chronic inflammatory papulosquamous dermatosis characterized by excessive keratinocytes, resulting in the formation of thick, scaly plaques that are puritic and inflammatory. It affects between 1 to 3% of the population and has a peak onset of 60 years of age. The main goal of psoriasis treatment is to rapidly gain control of the disease and prevent spread across the body. Treatment involves both topical and systemic therapy. Long term complications include psoriatic arthritis, which occurs in approximately 10-205 of patients. Topical therapy includes the use of topical corticosteroids, calcipotriene, anthralin, keratolytics, and tazarotene. Oral therapy includes the use of methotrexate, acitretin, biologic agents, and cyclosporine.

Treatment

- Avoid medications that trigger psoriatic outbreaks: NSAIDs, lithium, ACE inhibitors, antimalarials, beta blockers, salicylates, withdrawal of steroids.

- Discontinue smoking and the use of alcohol.

- Topical corticosteroids, calcipotriene, anthralin, keratolytics, and tazarotene.

- Treatment with immunomodulators, such as methotrexate, cyclosporine, adalimumab (Humira), alefacept (Amevive), etanercept (Enbrel), and infliximab (Remicade).

- Acitretin.

Medications

- ADALIMUMAB   (*Humira*)
    - AAP = Not reviewed
    - LRC = L3
    - RID =
    - Pregnancy = B
    - Comment: Adalimumab is a recombinant human IgG1 monoclonal antibody specific for human tumor necrosis factor (TNF). TNF is implicated in the pain and destructive component of arthritis and other autoimmune syndromes. This product would be similar to others, such as etanercept (Enbrel) and infliximab (Remicade). IgG transfer into human milk is significant the first four days postpartum, then is minimal afterwards. The primary immunoglobulin in mature human milk is IgA. Immunoglobulins are transferred into human milk by a very specific carrier protein which inhibits the transfer of IgG-like products. It is not known if these unusual immunoglobulins are transferred

into milk, but it is unlikely. Specific data from my laboratories suggests that no infliximab transfers into human milk in mothers receiving IV doses. It is not likely that Adalimumab would transfer in clinically relevant amounts after the first week postpartum, but no data are available at this time.

- ANTHRALIN   (*Anthra-Derm, Drithocreme, Dritho-Scalp, Micanol*)
  - ○ AAP = Not reviewed
  - ○ LRC = L3
  - ○ RID =
  - ○ Pregnancy = C
  - ○ Comment: Anthralin is a synthetic tar derivative used topically for suppression of psoriasis. Anthralin, when applied topically, induces burning and inflammation of the skin, but is one of the most effective treatments for psoriasis. Purple-brown staining of skin and permanent staining of clothing and porcelain bathroom fixtures is frequent. Anthralin, when applied topically, is absorbed into the surface layers of the skin, and only minimal amounts enter the systemic circulation. That absorbed is rapidly excreted via the kidneys almost instantly; plasma levels are very low to undetectable. No data are available on its transfer into human milk. Most anthralin is eliminated by washing off and desquamation of dead surface cells. For this reason, when placed directly on lesions on the areola or nipple, breastfeeding should be discouraged. Another similar anthraquinone is Senna (laxative), which even in high doses does not enter milk. While undergoing initial intense treatment, it would perhaps be advisable to interrupt breastfeeding temporarily, but this may be overly conservative. Observe the infant for diarrhea. It has been used in children over two years of age for psoriasis.

- CYCLOSPORINE   (*Sandimmune, Neoral, Restasis*)
  - ○ AAP = Cytotoxic drug that may interfere with cellular metabolism of the nursing infant
  - ○ LRC = L3
  - ○ RID = 0.4-3%
  - ○ Pregnancy = C
  - ○ Comment: Cyclosporine is an immunosuppressant used to reduce organ rejection following transplant, and in autoimmune syndromes, such as arthritis, etc. In a recent report of seven breastfeeding mothers treated with cyclosporine, the levels of cyclosporine in breastmilk ranged from 50 to 227 μg/L. Corresponding plasma levels in the breastfed infants were undetectable (<30 ng/mL) in all infants. In this study, the infants received less than 300 μg per day via breastmilk. In another, following a dose of 320 mg/d, the milk level at 22 hours postdose was 16 μg/L and the milk/plasma ratio was 0.28. In another report of a mother receiving 250 mg twice daily, the maternal plasma level of cyclosporine was measured at 187 μg/L and the breastmilk level was 167 μg/L. None was detected in the plasma of the infant. In a study of a breastfeeding transplant patient who received 300 mg twice daily, maternal serum levels were 193, 273, and 123 ng/mL at 23 days, 6.5 and 9.7 weeks postpartum. Corresponding milk cyclosporine levels were 160, 286, and 79 μg/L, respectively. Using the higher milk level, an infant would receive less than 0.4% of the weight-adjusted maternal dose.

    In another mother receiving cyclosporine (3 mg/kg/d), the concentration of cyclosporine in milk averaged 596 μg/L, or a dose of about <0.1 mg/kg to the infant. The infant's trough blood level was always <3 μg/L, while the mother's was 260 μg/L. No untoward effects were noted in the infant.

    In a more recent study of five patients receiving 5.3, 4.0, 5, 4.11, and 5 mg/kg/day cyclosporine, respectively, the average concentration of cyclosporine in the mothers was 403 μg/L, 465 μg/L,

97.6 µg/L, 117.7 µg/L, and 84-144 µg/L (range), respectively. Hind milk levels were much higher in one case, probably due to the high lipid content. In mother one, the cyclosporine blood levels in the infant were 131 µg/L and 117 µg/L on two occasions, which were near a therapeutic trough. In none of the other infants were blood levels of cyclosporine determinable (<25 µg/L). This study clearly suggests that some infants could potentially attain near-therapeutic levels from ingesting breastmilk. From these data, the relative infant dose would be approximately 0.78% of the weight-normalized maternal dose.

These studies together suggest cyclosporine transfer to milk is generally low, but the latter study suggests that some infants may receive more than has been expected from the prior studies. Therefore, cyclosporine use in breastfeeding mothers should be followed by close observation of the infant to probably include monitoring of the infant's plasma levels.

- ETANERCEPT   (*Enbrel*)
    - ◦ AAP = Not reviewed
    - ◦ LRC = L3
    - ◦ RID =
    - ◦ Pregnancy = B
    - ◦ Comment: Etanercept is a dimeric fusion protein consisting of the extracellular ligand-binding portion of tumor necrosis factor bound to human IgG1. Etanercept binds specifically to tumor necrosis factor (TNF) and blocks its inflammatory and immune activity in rheumatoid arthritis patients. Elevated levels of TNF are found in the synovial fluid of arthritis patients. In a recent study of a non-breastfeeding mother who received 25 mg twice weekly, etanercept was measured in the milk retained in the breast. This mother was not breastfeeding, but retained some milk in the breast after 30 days. The author reported milk levels of 75 ng/mL on the day after injection. While there data are interesting, measuring drug transfer in residual breastmilk following involution of alveolar tissues is simply not clinically relevant. After involution, the alveolar system would be totally open to drug transfer due to the breakdown of the tight intercellular junctions between lactocytes.

        Due to its enormous molecular weight (150,000 daltons), it is extremely unlikely that clinically relevant amounts would transfer into milk in actively breastfeeding mothers. In addition, due to its protein structure, it would not be orally bioavailable in an infant. Infliximab is somewhat similar and is apparently not secreted into human milk (see infliximab).

- FLUTICASONE   (*Cutivate*)
    - ◦ AAP = Not reviewed
    - ◦ LRC = L3
    - ◦ RID =
    - ◦ Pregnancy = C
    - ◦ Comment: Fluticasone is a moderate to high potency steroid used intranasally for allergic rhinitis, topically for psoriasis, and intrapulmonary for asthma. Oral absorption following inhaled fluticasone is approximately 30%, although almost instant first-pass absorption virtually eliminates plasma levels of fluticasone. Topically, absorption depends on the amount applied and most importantly the surface area treated. Adrenocortical suppression following oral or even systemic absorption at normal doses is extremely rare due to limited plasma levels. Plasma levels are not detectable when using suggested doses. Although fluticasone is secreted into milk of rodents, the dose used was many times higher than found under normal conditions. With the above limited oral and systemic

bioavailability and rapid first-pass uptake by the liver, it is not likely that milk levels will be clinically relevant, even with rather high doses.

- HYDROCORTISONE TOPICAL   (*Westcort*)
  - AAP = Not reviewed
  - LRC = L2
  - RID =
  - Pregnancy = C
  - Comment: Hydrocortisone is a typical corticosteroid with glucocorticoid and mineralocorticoid activity. When applied topically, it suppresses inflammation and enhances healing. Initial onset of activity when applied topically is slow and may require several days for response. Absorption topically is dependent on placement; percutaneous absorption is 1% from the forearm, 2% from the rectum, 4% from the scalp, 7% from the forehead, and 36% from the scrotal area. The amount transferred into human milk has not been reported, but as with most steroids, is believed minimal. Topical application to the nipple is generally approved by most authorities if amounts applied and duration of use are minimized. Only small amounts should be applied, and then only after feeding; larger quantities should be removed prior to breastfeeding. 0.5 to 1% ointments, rather than creams, are generally preferred.

- INFLIXIMAB   (*Remicade*)
  - AAP = Not reviewed
  - LRC = L2
  - RID =
  - Pregnancy = B
  - Comment: Infliximab is a monoclonal antibody to tumor necrosis factor-alpha (TNF-alpha) used to treat Crohn's disease and rheumatoid arthritis. Infliximab is a very large molecular weight antibody and is largely retained in the vascular system. In a study of one breastfeeding patient who received 5 mg/kg IV, infliximab levels were determined in milk at 0, 2, 4, 8, 24, 48, and 72 hours and four, five and seven days. None was detected in milk at any time (detection limit <0.1 µg/mL). In another study, a breastfeeding mother receiving five infusions of 10 mg/kg during pregnancy did not have a detectable amount of infliximab in her milk at any point. The baby's serum level after delivery was 39.5 µg/mL, likely due to placental transfer. The half-life of the drug appeared to be prolonged in the newborn. Another breastfeeding mother's milk was tested 24 hours and one week following her first infusion of a 5 mg/kg dose, with milk levels below the limit of quantification in both cases. Infliximab is probably too large to enter milk in clinically measurable amounts. It would not be orally bioavailable.

- PIMECROLIMUS   (*Elidel*)
  - AAP = Not reviewed
  - LRC = L2
  - RID =
  - Pregnancy = C
  - Comment: Pimecrolimus is a topical agent used as a cytokine inhibitor for atopic dermatitis. While its mechanism of action is unknown, it inhibits the release of various inflammatory cytokines for T

cells and many others. Systemic absorption following topical application is minimal, with reported blood concentrations consistently below 0.5 ng/mL following twice-daily application of the 1% cream. Oral absorption is unreported, but probably low to moderate, as plasma levels of 54 ng/mL have been reported following twice daily oral doses of 30 mg. Pimecrolimus is cleared for use in pediatric patients two years and older.

No data are available on its transfer to human milk, but because the maternal plasma levels are so low, it is extremely remote that this agent would penetrate milk in clinically relevant amounts. However, its use on or around the nipples should be avoided, as the clinical dose absorbed orally in the infant could be significant.

- TACROLIMUS   *(Protopic)*
  - ○ AAP = Not reviewed
  - ○ LRC = L3
  - ○ RID = 0.1-0.5%
  - ○ Pregnancy = C
  - ○ Comment: Tacrolimus is an immunosuppressant formerly known as SK506. It is used to reduce rejection of transplanted organs, including liver and kidney.

    Recently, the FDA has approved a topical form of tacrolimus (Protopic) for use in moderate to severe eczema, in those for whom standard eczema therapies are deemed inadvisable because of potential risks, or who are not adequately treated by, or who are intolerant of standard eczema therapies. Absorption via skin is minimal to nil. In a study of 46 adult patients after multiple doses, plasma levels ranged from undetectable to 20 ng/mL, with 45 of the patients having peak blood concentrations less than 5 ng/mL. In another study, the peak blood levels averaged 1.6 ng/mL, which is significantly less than the therapeutic range in kidney transplantation (7-20 ng/mL). While the absolute transcutaneous bioavailability is unknown, it is apparently very low. Combined with the poor oral bioavailability of this product, it is not likely a breastfed infant will receive enough following topical use (maternal) to produce adverse effects.

- TAZAROTENE   *(Tazorac)*
  - ○ AAP = Not reviewed
  - ○ LRC = L3
  - ○ RID =
  - ○ Pregnancy = X
  - ○ Comment: Tazarotene is a specialized retinoid for topical use and is used for the topical treatment of stable plaque psoriasis and acne. Following topical application, tazarotene is converted to an active metabolite; transcutaneous absorption is minimal (<1%). Applied daily, it is indicated for treatment of stable plaque psoriasis of up to 20% of the body surface area. Only 2-3% of the topically applied drug is absorbed transcutaneously. Tazarotene is metabolized to the active ingredient, tazarotenic acid. Little compound could be detected in the plasma. At steady state, plasma levels were only 0.09 ng/mL, although this value is largely a function of surface area treated. When applied to large surface areas, systemic absorption is increased. Data on transmission to breastmilk are not available. The manufacturer reports some is transferred to rodent milk, but it has not been tested in humans.

- TRIAMCINOLONE ACETONIDE
  - ○ AAP = Not reviewed

- ○ LRC = L3
- ○ RID =
- ○ Pregnancy = C
- ○ Comment: Triamcinolone is a typical corticosteroid (see prednisone) that is available for topical, intranasal, injection, inhalation, and oral use. When applied topically to the nose (Nasacort) or to the lungs (Azmacort), only minimal doses are used and plasma levels are exceedingly low to undetectable. Although no data are available on triamcinolone secretion into human milk, it is likely that the milk levels would be exceedingly low and not clinically relevant when administered via inhalation or intranasally. While the oral adult dose is 4-48 mg/day, the inhaled dose is 200 µg three times daily, and the intranasal dose is 220 µg/day. There is virtually no risk to the infant following use of the intranasal products in breastfeeding mothers.

Clinical Tips

The therapy of psoriasis normally starts with the use of topical steroids, although it may be inadvisable. Two factors are of major concern in the choice of treatment: one is the severity of the lesions and secondly, the surface area of the body affected. Topical steroids rarely return the skin to a normal state, and when discontinued, the psoriatic lesion rapidly recurs. In moderate to limited conditions, topical steroids are probably suitable. However, after continued treatment, a steroid-resistant state ensues with permanent atrophy of the skin and a more aggressive psoriatic lesion. Treatment of large surface areas with steroids can induce adrenal suppression. General consensus is that systemic steroids have no place in the treatment of psoriasis because rebound spreading of the disease is a major result. However, steroids can be used initially if 'pulse therapy' is employed. One technique is to use high potency steroids, but only on two days of the week such as Saturday and Sunday. This prevents the rapid tachyphylaxis to steroids and can help many patients. Newer therapies (newer formulations) using anthralin have increased in popularity because it can clear psoriasis and produce remissions for many months without continued treatment. Anthralin is poorly absorbed through the skin. Studies show plasma levels are brief and hardly detectable. Milk levels of anthralin have not been determined, but are probably very low.

Tar is an effective treatment, but it is messy to use, and it may be carcinogenic in humans over time. Unfortunately, the safer, refined tar preparations are poorly effective. Phototherapy with lubrication is an effective treatment of psoriasis. Almost 95% of patients will benefit from ultraviolet B irradiation when applied under medical supervision in correct doses. Lubrication is applied to each lesion prior to irradiation, as it facilitates penetration.

Systemic therapy with methotrexate is highly effective, but has two major problems. One is that it is highly teratogenic; it suppresses bone marrow and may be sequestered in the GI cells of infants for long periods. And two, it appears to alter the nature of psoriasis, ultimately making it a more severe and aggressive disease with each rebound. Hence, the type and severity of the disease can be negatively affected after treatment with methotrexate. Treatment of breastfeeding mothers with methotrexate is not recommended. The retinoids, particularly etretinate (Tegison), have been found to be effective, but they have so many untoward effects that they are seldom used. Side effects include lipid abnormalities, calcification of tendons, teratogenicity, and a half-life of more than 120 days. The use of etretinate during breastfeeding should be discouraged. Tazarotene is an effective retinoid for psoriasis and, fortunately, does not penetrate skin effectively; hence, milk levels would likely be minimal. Transcutaneous absorption is less than 1%. Virtually none is detected in the plasma. While it is teratogenic in pregnant women, it is not likely to cause untoward effects in a breastfed infant, but caution is recommended.

Pimecrolimus and tacrolimus are topical agents used as a cytokine inhibitor for atopic dermatitis. While their mechanism of action is unknown, they inhibit the release of various inflammatory cytokines for T cells and many others. Systemic absorption following topical application is minimal, with reported blood concentrations consistently quite low. Both would probably be suitable products to use in breastfeeding mothers.

The use of biological response modifiers, such as infliximab, etanercept and adalimumab, has risen, and studies suggest they are highly effective treatments, although expensive and probably of limited duration. Many patients develop systemic reactions to these biologics over-time, as they are protein immunoglobulins.

Suggested Reading

Belazarian, L. (2008). New insights and therapies for teenage psoriasis. *Curr Opin Pediatr, 20*(4), 419-424.

Bissonnette, R., Ho, V., & Langley, R. G. (2009). Safety of conventional systemic agents and biologic agents in the treatment of psoriasis. *J Cutan Med Surg, 13 Suppl 2*, S67-76.

Boehncke, W. H., Prinz, J., & Gottlieb, A. B. (2006). Biologic therapies for psoriasis. A systematic review. *J Rheumatol, 33*(7), 1447-1451.

de Felice, C., Ardigo, M., & Berardesca, E. (2009). Biologic therapies for psoriasis. *J Rheumatol Suppl, 83*, 62-64.

Gisondi, P., & Girolomoni, G. (2007). Biologic therapies in psoriasis: a new therapeutic approach. *Autoimmun Rev, 6*(8), 515-519.

Griffiths, C. E., Taylor, H., Collins, S. I., Hobson, J. E., Collier, P. A., Chalmers, R. J., et al. (2006). The impact of psoriasis guidelines on appropriateness of referral from primary to secondary care: a randomized controlled trial. *Br J Dermatol, 155*(2), 393-400.

Guibal, F., Iversen, L., Puig, L., Strohal, R., & Williams, P. (2009). Identifying the biologic closest to the ideal to treat chronic plaque psoriasis in different clinical scenarios: using a pilot multi-attribute decision model as a decision-support aid. *Curr Med Res Opin, 25*(12), 2835-2843.

Mason, A. R., Mason, J., Cork, M., Dooley, G., & Edwards, G. (2009). Topical treatments for chronic plaque psoriasis. *Cochrane Database Syst Rev*(2), CD005028.

Menter, A. (2009). The status of biologic therapies in the treatment of moderate to severe psoriasis. *Cutis, 84*(4 Suppl), 14-24.

Naldi, L., & Rzany, B. (2009). Psoriasis (chronic plaque). *Clin Evid (Online), 2009*.

Nast, A., Erdmann, R., Hofelich, V., Reytan, N., Orawa, H., Sterry, W., et al. (2009). Do guidelines change the way we treat? Studying prescription behaviour among private practitioners before and after the publication of the German Psoriasis Guidelines. *Arch Dermatol Res, 301*(8), 553-559.

Roelofzen, J. H., Aben, K. K., Khawar, A. J., Van de Kerkhof, P. C., Kiemeney, L. A., & Van Der Valk, P. G. (2007). Treatment policy for psoriasis and eczema: a survey among dermatologists in the Netherlands and Belgian Flanders. *Eur J Dermatol, 17*(5), 416-421.

Strober, B. E., Siu, K., & Menon, K. (2006). Conventional systemic agents for psoriasis. A systematic review. *J Rheumatol, 33*(7), 1442-1446.

van de Kerkhof, P. C. (2006). Update on retinoid therapy of psoriasis in: an update on the use of retinoids in dermatology. *Dermatol Ther, 19*(5), 252-263.

Wakkee, M., Lugtenberg, M., Spuls, P. I., de Jong, E. M., Thio, H. B., Westert, G. P., et al. (2008). Knowledge, attitudes and use of the guidelines for the treatment of moderate to severe plaque psoriasis among Dutch dermatologists. *Br J Dermatol, 159*(2), 426-432.

Pulmonary Hypertension

Principles of Therapy

Symptoms of pulmonary hypertension may be difficult to recognize during the early stages of disease. Dyspnea is often present, but other symptoms, such as fatigue and syncope, are vague. Evaluation should be performed to distinguish primary from secondary pulmonary hypertension. Work up includes evaluation for autoimmune and connective tissue disease including; scleroderma with CREST, systemic lupus erythematosus, and mixed connective tissue disease (CREST: calcinosis cutis, Raynaud phenomenon, esophageal motility disorder, sclerodactyly, and telangiectasia). Thyroid disease and sleep apnea should also be excluded. Definitive diagnosis is made by cardiac catheterization.

Medications used for therapy include: vasodilators (either parenteral or inhaled), phosphodiesterase enzyme inhibitors, or other agents used for pulmonary hypertension. Calcium channel blockers may be useful for those responsive to inhaled nitric oxide and who do not have evidence of right-sided heart failure. Anticoagulation is typically indicated. Digoxin may be useful in patients with right heart failure. Pulmonary hypertension is not reversible.

Treatment

- Evaluate for primary verses secondary disease.

- Cardiac catheterization is confirmatory.

- Medications: vasodilators (inhaled or parenteral), phosphodiesterase enzyme inhibitors, bosentan.

- Calcium channel blockers for those responsive to inhaled nitric oxide and lacking right-sided heart failure.

- Anticoagulation with warfarin.

- Oxygen supplementation may be helpful in patients with resting or exercise induced hypoxemia.

Medications

- BOSENTAN   (Tracleer)
    - AAP = Not reviewed.
    - LRC = L4
    - RID =
    - Pregnancy = X

- ○ Comment: Bosentan is used in the treatment of pulmonary artery hypertension. It blocks endothelin receptors on vascular endothelium and smooth muscle, thus blocking vasoconstriction. No data are available on the transfer into human milk, but bosentan is a highly protein bound (98%), large molecular weight product; therefore, only small amounts are likely to be found unbound in the plasma. As a result, the amount in the milk compartment would probably be very low. However, this product is highly teratogenic, is 50% bioavailable orally, and has a high incidence of liver toxicity in patients. Great caution is recommended with this product in breastfeeding mothers until we have published milk levels.

- DIGOXIN   (*Lanoxin, Lanoxicaps*)
  - ○ AAP =   Maternal Medication Usually Compatible with Breastfeeding
  - ○ LRC = L2
  - ○ RID = 2.7-2.8%
  - ○ Pregnancy = C
  - ○ Comment: Digoxin is a cardiac stimulant used primarily to strengthen the contractile process. In one mother receiving 0.25 mg digoxin daily, the amount found in breastmilk ranged from 0.96 to 0.61 μg/L at four and six hours post-dose, respectively. Mean peak breastmilk levels varied from 0.78 μg/L in one patient to 0.41 μg/L in another. Plasma levels in the infants were undetectable.

    In another study of five women receiving digoxin therapy, the average breastmilk concentration was 0.64 μg/L. From these studies, it is apparent that a breastfeeding infant would receive less than 1 μg/day of digoxin, too low to be clinically relevant. The small amounts secreted into breastmilk have not produced problems in nursing infants. Poor and erratic GI absorption could theoretically reduce absorption in nursing infant.

    Digibind, or digoxin immune fab (ovine), is composed of antigen binding fragments made from antidigoxin antibodies. It is used for life-threatening digoxin toxicity or overdose. The dosage needed can be calculated using the ratio that one vial of Digibind (38 mg) will bind 0.5 mg of digoxin. The molecular weight of these fragments are approximately 46.000 daltons, and thus would not be able to transfer into the milk compartment.

- DILTIAZEM HCL   (*Cardizem SR, Dilacor-XR, Cardizem CD, Cartia XT*)
  - ○ AAP =   Maternal Medication Usually Compatible with Breastfeeding
  - ○ LRC = L3
  - ○ RID = 0.9%
  - ○ Pregnancy = C
  - ○ Comment: Diltiazem is an typical calcium channel blocker antihypertensive. In a report of a single patient receiving 240 mg/d on day 14 postpartum, levels in milk were parallel those of serum (milk/plasma ratio was approximately 1.0). Peak level in milk (and plasma) was slightly higher than 200 μg/L and occurred at eight hours. While nifedipine is probably a preferred choice calcium channel blocker, because of our experience with it, the relative infant dose with this agent is quite small, and it is not likely to be problematic.

- EPOPROSTENOL   (*Flolan*)
  - ○ AAP =   Not reviewed
  - ○ LRC = L3

- ○ RID =
- ○ Pregnancy = B
- ○ Comment: Epoprostenol (Prostacyclin; PGX; PGI-2) is a naturally occurring prostaglandin that is a potent inhibitor of platelet aggregation and a vasodilator. It is commonly used to treat primary pulmonary hypertension. It is rapidly metabolized in plasma to 6-keto-prostaglandin F1-alpha, which is biologically inactive, and has a half-life of only three to five minutes. Prostaglandins are known to be transferred into human milk, but they are believed derived from mammary tissue and synthesis by the cellular components of breastmilk. With the extraordinarily short half-life of this product, it is unlikely any would penetrate into milk, be retained for very long, or be stable in the infant's gut. Oral absorption by the infant is unlikely.

- **ILOPROST** *(Ventavis)*
  - ○ AAP = Maternal Medication Usually Compatible with Breastfeeding
  - ○ LRC = L3
  - ○ RID =
  - ○ Pregnancy = C
  - ○ Comment: Iloprost is a synthetic analogue of prostacyclin PGI2. It dilates systemic and pulmonary arterial vascular beds. It also affects platelet aggregation. It is indicated for the treatment of pulmonary arterial hypertension (WHO Group I) in patients with NYHA Class III or IV symptoms. No data are available on its transfer into human milk, but levels are probably low, and the oral bioavailability would be low as well.

- **NIFEDIPINE** *(Adalat, Procardia)*
  - ○ AAP = Maternal Medication Usually Compatible with Breastfeeding
  - ○ LRC = L2
  - ○ RID = 2.3-3.4%
  - ○ Pregnancy = C
  - ○ Comment: Nifedipine is an effective antihypertensive. It belongs to the calcium channel blocker family of drugs. Two studies indicate that nifedipine is transferred to breastmilk in varying, but generally low levels. In one study in which the dose was varied from 10-30 mg three times daily, the highest concentration (53.35 µg/L) was measured at one hour after a 30 mg dose. Other levels reported were 16.35 µg/L 60 minutes after a 20 mg dose and 12.89 µg/L 30 minutes after a 10 mg dose. The milk levels fell linearly, with the milk half-lives estimated to be 1.4 hours for the 10 mg dose, 3.1 hours for the 20 dose, and 2.4 hours for the 30 mg dose. The milk concentration measured eight hours following a 30 mg dose was 4.93 µg/L. In this study, using the highest concentration found and a daily intake of 150 mL/kg of human milk, the amount of nifedipine intake would only be 8 µg/kg/day (less than 1.8% of the therapeutic pediatric dose). The authors conclude that the amount ingested via breastmilk poses little risk to an infant.

    In another study, concentrations of nifedipine in human milk one to eight hours after 10 mg doses varied from <1 to 10.3 µg/L (median 3.5 µg/L) in six of 11 patients. In this study, milk levels three days after discontinuing medication ranged from <1 to 9.4 µg/L. The authors concluded the exposure to nifedipine through breastmilk is not significant. In a study by Penny and Lewis, following a maternal dose of 20 mg nifedipine daily for 10 days, peak breastmilk levels at one hour were 46 µg/L. The corresponding maternal serum level was 43 µg/L. From these data the authors suggest a daily intake for an infant would be approximately 6.45 µg/kg/day.

Nifedipine has been found clinically useful for nipple vasospasm. Because of the similarity to Raynaud's Phenomenon, sustained release formulations providing 30-60 mg per day are suggested.

- SILDENAFIL   (*Viagra*)
  - ○ AAP = Not reviewed
  - ○ LRC = L3
  - ○ RID =
  - ○ Pregnancy = B
  - ○ Comment: Sildenafil is an inhibitor of nitrous oxide metabolism, thus increasing levels of nitrous oxide, smooth muscle relaxation, and an increased flow of blood in the corpus cavernosum of the penis. While not currently indicated for women, illicit use is increasing. No data are available on the transfer of sildenafil into human milk, but it is unlikely that significant transfer will occur due to its larger molecular weight and short half-life. However, caution is recommended in breastfeeding mothers. While not reported, persistent abnormal erections (priapism) could potentially occur in male infants.

- TADALAFIL   (*Cialis, Adcirca*)
  - ○ AAP = Not reviewed
  - ○ LRC = L3
  - ○ RID =
  - ○ Pregnancy = B
  - ○ Comment: Tadalafil is a selective inhibitor of cyclic guanosine monophosphate (cGMP)-specific phosphodiesterase type 5 (PDE5). It is commonly used for erectile dysfuntion, but is also indicated for the treatment of pulmonary arterial hypertension (WHO Group I) to improve exercise ability. It is not apparently teratogenic. No data are available on its use in breastfeeding mothers, but its prolonged half-life (15 hours), high volume of distribution, and high protein binding suggest that milk levels when determined will probably be low.

- TREPROSTINIL (Tyvaso)
  - ○ AAP = Maternal Medication Usually Compatible with Breastfeeding
  - ○ LRC = L3
  - ○ RID =
  - ○ Pregnancy = C
  - ○ Comment: Treprostinil is a prostacyclin analogue that produces direct vasodilation of pulmonary and systemic arterial vascular bed. It is used for treatment of pulmonary hypertension. Mean estimates of bioavailability after inhalation were 64-72%. The mean Cmax was $0.91 - 1.32$ ng/mL. It is 91% protein bound with a half-life of four hours. Cough, headache, and throat irriation were the major reported side effects. No data are available on the use of this product in breastfeeding mothers. However, plasma levels are exceedingly low and oral bioavailability, although unreported, is likely low.

- WARFARIN   (*Coumadin, Panwarfin*)
  - ○ AAP = Maternal Medication Usually Compatible with Breastfeeding
  - ○ LRC = L2

- ◦ RID =
- ◦ Pregnancy = X
- ◦ Comment: Warfarin is a potent anticoagulant. Warfarin is highly protein bound in the maternal circulation; therefore, very little is secreted into human milk. Very small and insignificant amounts are secreted into milk, but it depends to some degree on the dose administered. In one study of two patients who were anticoagulated with warfarin, no warfarin was detected in the infant's serum, nor were changes in coagulation detectable. In another study of 13 mothers, less than 0.08 μmol per liter (25 ng/mL) was detected in milk, and no warfarin was detected in the infants' plasma.

  According to these authors, maternal warfarin apparently poses little risk to a nursing infant, and thus far has not produced bleeding anomalies in breastfed infants. Other anticoagulants, such as phenindione, should be avoided. Observe infant for bleeding, such as excessive bruising or reddish petechia (spots). While the risks in breastfeeding premature infants (which are more susceptible to intracranial bleeding) is still low, oral supplementation with vitamin K1 will preclude any chance of hemorrhage. Even modest doses of Vitamin K1 counteract high doses of warfarin.

Clinical Tips

Due to the idiopathic nature of pulmonary hypertension, many of the therapies found effective are not really supported by extensive randomized clinical trials. This includes: oxygen, calcium channel blockers, sildenafil, and other products. Limited but some data now exists for the prostacyclin and endothelin antagonists; however, these last two treatments are extremely expensive. Oxygen therapy should be tailored to maintain blood oxygen saturation greater than 90% continuously.

The treatment of pulmonary hypertension (PH) in a breastfeeding patient is extraordinarily difficult in that virtually none of the medications approved for this conditions have been studied in breastfeeding mothers. First-line therapy is generally the calcium channel blockers, pariticularly diltiazem or nifedipine. Calcium channel blockers improve pulmonary hemodynamic parameters and increase exercise tolerance in some individuals. Nifedipine and diltiazem would be useful for these individuals.

Intravenous epoprostenol dilates pulmonary vasculature and is recommended for patients with PH in classes III and IV who do not respond to CCBs. Another prostacyclin analog, treprostinil, increases exercise tolerance but is plagued with side effects.

Bosentan is an endothelin receptor antagonist. It competitively inhibits endothelin receptors type ETA and ETB, which results in vasodilation of endothelium and vascular smooth muscle, thus reducing vasoconstriction. Unfortunately, it is horribly teratogenic and should rarely be used in women at risk for pregnancy.

Sildenafil, an inhibitor of nitrous oxide metabolism, thus increasing levels of nitrous oxide, smooth muscle relaxation, and an increased flow of blood in the corpus cavernosum of the penis., and it increases exercise tolerance in PH patients. Numerous studies show significant efficacy in PH, particularly in class II and II PH.

Anticoagulant therapy with warfarin is used to minimize small vessel thrombosis, particularly those with idiopathic pulmonary arterial hypertension (IPAH). Warfarin poses no risk to a breastfed infant.

Suggested Reading

Rubin L.J. (2004). Diagnosis and management of pulmonary arterial hypertension: ACCP evidence-based clinical practice guidelines. *Chest* *126*:7S-10S

Archer S.L., Michelakis E.D. (2009). Phosphodiesterase type 5 inhibitors for pulmonary arterial hypertension. *N Engl J Med. 361*(19):1864-71. Review.

McLaughlin V.V., Archer S.L., Badesch D.B., Barst R.J., Farber H.W., Lindner J.R., Mathier M.A., McGoon M.D., Park M.H., Rosenson R.S., Rubin L.J., Tapson V.F., Varga J; American College of Cardiology Foundation Task Force on Expert Consensus Documents; American Heart Association; American College of Chest Physicians; American Thoracic Society, Inc; Pulmonary Hypertension Association. (2009). ACCF/AHA 2009 expert consensus document on pulmonary hypertension a report of the American College of Cardiology Foundation Task Force on Expert Consensus Documents and the American Heart Association developed in collaboration with the American College of Chest Physicians; American Thoracic Society, Inc.; and the Pulmonary Hypertension Association. *J Am Coll Cardiol. 53*(17):1573-619.

Beghetti M. (2009). Bosentan in pediatric patients with pulmonary arterial hypertension. *Curr Vasc Pharmacol. 7*(2):225-33. Review.

Radioactive Procedures

Principles of Therapy

The use of radioactive isotopes in diagnostic procedures in breastfeeding mothers is common. While it can be quite hazardous in some cases, it need not be in all cases. With proper timing, most all isotopes can be safely used. But you should always use caution and review the documentation on these products before recommending breastfeeding.

In general, the radioactive substances used in medicine are comprised of nuclides that decay and produce gamma rays, beta particle emissions, alpha particle emissions, and several other less common radioactive emissions. Radioactive nuclides are, in general, incorporated into chemical mixtures, so that they have affinity for various tissue sites. As such, they are chosen for their specific affinity. For instance, Iodine-131 has a high affinity for thyroid, so it is chosen for its biology in the thyroid gland. Technetium-99 nuclides, when incorporated into various salt forms, have affinity for bony tissue, tissues that are inflamed, and numerous other sites. Thallium-201 salts have a high affinity for myocardial tissues and can be used to diagnose certain myocardial diseases. While most all radioactive nuclides will pass into milk to some degree, many have very brief half-lives and are of minimal risk to the infant if a brief interruption of breastfeeding is used. Others, such as radioactive iodine, are highly risky and must be carefully used, if at all. A comprehensive table of guidelines for radioisotope use in breastfeeding mothers is provided in the Appendix.

Treatment

- Different radioactive isotopes have different cautions, please refer to appendix for specific information.

- Many isotopes are compatible with breastfeeding after a varying amount of time for clearance.

- I-131 is incompatible with lactation.

Medications

- I-^{125} I-^{131} I-^{123} (*Radioactive Iodine, Iodine-^{125}, Iodine-^{131}, Iodine-^{123}, Iodotope, I-^{125}, I-^{131}, I-^{123}*)
    - ○ AAP = Radioactive compound that requires temporary cessation of breastfeeding
    - ○ LRC = L4
    - ○ RID =
    - ○ Pregnancy =
    - ○ Comment: Radioactive iodine concentrates in the thyroid gland, as well as in breastmilk. If ingested by an infant, it may suppress its thyroid function or increase the risk of future thyroid carcinomas, and it may also produce thyroid destruction in the infant. Radioactive iodine is clinically used to

ablate or destroy the thyroid (dose = 355 MBq), or in much smaller doses (7.4 MBq), to scan the thyroid for malignancies. Following ingestion, radioactive iodine concentrates in the thyroid and lactating tissues, and it is estimated 27.9% of total radioactivity is secreted via breastmilk.

Two potential half-lives exist for radioactive iodine: one is the radioactive half-life, which is solely dependent on radioactive decay of the molecule; and two, the biological half-life, which is often briefer and is the half-life of the iodine molecule itself in the human being. The latter half-life is influenced most by elimination via the kidneys and other routes.

Previously published data have suggested that I-125 is present in milk for at least 12 days, and I-131 is present for 2-14 days, but these studies may be in error as they ignored the second component of the biexponential breastmilk disappearance curve. The radioactive half-life of I-131 is 8.1 days. The half-life of I-125 is 60.2 days, and the half-life of I-123 is 13.2 hours. The biological or effective half-life may be shorter due to excretion in urine, feces, and milk.

A well done study by Dydek reviewed the transfer of both tracer and ablation doses of I-131 into human milk. If the tracer doses are kept minimal (0.1 µCi or 3.7 kBq), breastfeeding could resume as early as the eighth day. However, if larger tracer doses (8.6 µCi or 0.317 MBq) are used, nursing could not resume until 46 days following therapy. Doses used for ablation of the maternal thyroid (111 MBq) would require an interruption of breastfeeding for a minimum of 106 days or more. However, an acceptable dose to an infant, as a result of ingestion of radioiodine, is a matter for debate, although an effective dose of <1 mSv has been suggested.

In another study of I-131 use in a mother, breastmilk levels were followed for 32 days. These authors recommend discontinuing breastfeeding for up to 50-52 days to ensure safety of the infant thyroid. Thyroid scans use either radioactive iodine or technetium-[99m] pertechnetate. Technetium has a very short half-life and should be preferred in breastfeeding mothers for thyroid scanning.

Due to the fact that significant concentrations of I-131 are concentrated in breastmilk, women should discontinue breastfeeding prior to treatment, as the cumulative exposure to breast tissues could be excessively high. It is sometimes recommended that women discontinue breastfeeding several days to weeks before undergoing therapy or that they pump and discard milk for several weeks after exposure to iodine to reduce the overall radioactive exposure to breast tissues. The estimated dose of radioactivity to the breasts would give a "theoretical" probability of induction of breast cancer of 0.32%. In addition, holding the infant close to the breast or thyroid gland for long periods may expose the infant to gamma irradiation and is not recommended. Patients should consult with the radiologist concerning exposure of the infant.

One case of significant exposure was reported in a breastfed infant. The mother received a 3.02 millicurie dose of I-131 and continued to breastfeed for the next seven days before the mother admitted breastfeeding. During this seven day period, the infant's thyroid contained 2.7 microcuries of I-131, which is an effective dose equivalent of 5.5 rads. Had the mother continued to breastfeed, the dose would have been much larger and potentially dangerous.

In another case report of a patient who received 14 microcuries of oral I-131, and then 5 millicuries of [99]Technetium, the mothers' milk was withdrawn and screened for radiation with a gamma counter. On day eight the measured radioactivity was 94 counts per minute (cpm). On day 13, the measured radioactivity was 30 cpm, and by day 20, the radioactivity was measured at background levels (20 cpm). These data suggests that if the I-131 levels administered are equal to or less than 14 microcuries, then the mother could potentially return to breastfeeding after 20 days.

Another alternative is I-123, a newer isotope that is increasing in popularity. I-123 has a short half-life of only 13.2 hours and is radiologically ideal for thyroid and other scans. If radioactive iodine compounds are mandatory for various "scanning" procedures, I-123 should be preferred, followed by pumping and dumping for 12-24 hours, depending on the dose. However, the return to breastfeeding following I-123 therapy is dependent on the purity of this product. During manufacture of I-123, I-124 and I-125 are created. If using I-123, breastfeeding should be temporarily interrupted (see Appendix). I-123 is not used for ablation of the thyroid.

In a study by Morita of the transfer of I-123 into breastmilk, I-123 was excreted exponentially with an effective half-life of 5.5 hours. A total of 2.5% of the total radioactivity administered was excreted in the breastmilk over the 93 hours, 95% of which was excreted within the first 24 hours, and 98.2% within 36 hours. The first milk sample collected at seven hours after administration contained 48.5% of the total radioactivity excreted. The authors estimated the potential absorption of radioactivity to an infant's thyroid in uninterrupted breastfeeding to be 30.3 mGy. With a 24-hour interruption, the absorbed radioactivity would be 1.25 mGy; with a 36-hour interruption, it would be 0.24 mGy. They recommend that breastfeeding should be curtailed for 36 hours to reduce the infant's exposure to I-123 radioactivity.

The Nuclear Regulatory Commission has released a table of instructions to mothers concerning the use of radioisotopes (see Appendix). These instructions conclude that patients should not breastfeed following the use of I-131. In a study by Hammami, radioactive I-131 was found to transfer into breasts for weeks following cessation of lactation. They suggest the breast is a "radioiodine reservoir".

Ultimately, the amount of radioiodine transferred into human milk depends on the clinical dose administered to the mother. Low scanning doses may present an opportunity to return to breastfeeding if the counts in milk are closely monitored in the coming weeks. Using extraordinarily high ablative doses may continue to be present in milk for many weeks. If one is able to measure the milk for radiation, then a return to baseline would allow a patient to reinitiate breastfeeding. See Appendix for more recommendations and other radiopharmaceuticals.

- TECHNETIUM-^{99m} (*Technetium-^{99m}*)

   ○ AAP = Radioactive compound that requires temporary cessation of breastfeeding

   ○ LRC = L4

   ○ RID =

   ○ Pregnancy = C

   ○ Comment: Radioactive technetium-^{99m} (Tc-^{99m}) is present in milk for at least 15 hours to three days, and significant quantities have been reported in the thyroid and gastric mucosa of infants ingesting milk from treated mothers. Technetium is one of the halide elements and is handled, biologically, much like iodine. Like iodine, it concentrates in thyroid tissues, the stomach, and breastmilk of nursing mothers. It has a radioactive half-life of 6.02 hours. Following a dose of 15 mCi of Tc-^{99m} for a brain scan, the concentration of Tc-^{99m} in breastmilk at 4, 8.5, 20, and 60 hours was 0.5 µCi, 0.1 µCi, 0.02 µCi, and 0.006 µCi, respectively. In another study, following a dose of 10 mCi of NaTcO4, breastmilk levels were 5.7, 1.5, 0.015 µCi/mL at 3.25, 7.5, and 24 hours, respectively. The estimated dose to infant was 1,036, 284, and 2.7 µCi/180 mL milk. These authors recommended pumping and discarding of milk for 48 hours. Technetium-^{99m} is used in many salt and chemical forms, but the radioactivity and decay are the same, although the concentration in milk may be influenced by the salt form.

   In another study using Technetium MAG3 in two mothers receiving 150 MBq of radioactivity, the total percent of ingested radioactivity ranged from 0.7 to 1.6% of the total. These authors suggested that the DTPA salt of technetium would produce the least breastmilk levels and would be preferred in breastfeeding mothers. The NRC table in the Appendix A suggests duration of interruption of breastfeeding of 12 to 24 hours for 12 and 30 mCi, respectively, but this depends on the salt form used.

- THALLIUM-201   (*Thallium-201*)
  - ◦ AAP = Not reviewed
  - ◦ LRC = L3 with interruption
  - ◦ RID =
  - ◦ Pregnancy =
  - ◦ Comment: Thallium-201 in the form of thallous chloride is used extensively for myocardial perfusion imaging to delineate ischemic myocardium. Following infusion, almost 85% of the administered dose is extracted into the heart on the first pass. Less than 5% of the dose remains free in the plasma in as little as five minutes after administration. Whereas Thallium-201 has a radioactive half-life of only 73 hours, the terminal elimination half-life of the Thallium ion from the body is about 10 days. Most all radiation will be decayed in five to six half-lives (15 days). In a study of one breastfeeding patient who received 111MBq (3 mCi) for a brain scan, the amount of Thallium-201 in breastmilk at four hours was 326 Bq/mL and subsequently dropped to 87 Bq/mL after 72 hours. Even without interrupting breastfeeding, the infant would have received less than the NCRP radiation safety guideline dose for infrequent exposure for a one-year-old infant. However, a brief interruption of breastfeeding was nevertheless recommended. The length of interrupted breastfeeding is dependent on age of infant and dose of Thallium. With an interruption time varying from 2, 24, 48, to 96 hours, the respective Thallium dose to the infant would be 0.442, 0.283, 0.197, and 0.101 MBq compared to the maternal dose of 111 MBq.

    In another study of a breastfeeding mother who received 111 MBq (3 mCi), the calculated dose an infant (without any interruption of breastfeeding and assuming the consumption of 1000 mL of milk daily) would receive is approximately 0.81 MBq, which is presently less than the maximal allowed radiation dose (NCRP) for an infant. The authors, therefore, recommend that breastfeeding be discontinued for at least 24-48 hours following the administration of 111 MBq of Thallium-201. The amount of infant exposure from close contact with the mother was also measured and found to be very small in comparison to the orally ingested dose via milk.

    Thus the interruption of breastfeeding largely depends on the dose and the volume of milk consumed by the infant. Most authors recommend interruption for 24 up to 96 hours, although the NRC commission (see Appendix) recommends interruption for two weeks. See Appendix for more recommendations.

Clinical Tips

As with any medication, exposure of the infant to risk is largely dependent on the dose. It is the same with radiation exposure from radionuclides. However, with radioisotopes, it is the radiation hazard rather than the chemical hazard that is important. With the shorter half-live isotopes, simply waiting a few hours or days eliminates all risk, and mothers can continue to breastfeed after the product is gone (eliminated or decayed). Two considerations are of utmost importance when counseling patients concerning the use of radioisotopes while breastfeeding. One is the type of radioisotope and its affinity for the milk compartment. Radioactive iodine is particularly hazardous because of its ability to enter milk. Approximately 27% of the dose of radioactive iodine is sequestered in the thyroid, and approximately 28% enters the milk compartment. If a mother were to breastfeed, this could dramatically increase the risk of thyroid cancer in her infant. Thus radioactive iodine must be avoided at all times.

The next most important component is the radioactive half-life of the isotope. Remember, after five to seven half-lives, virtually all of the radioactivity is decayed away and is completely nonhazardous. Thus after exposure to technetium products (radioactive half-life = 6 hours), virtually all of the product is cleared renally or decayed away in 24 hours, regardless of the dose. With exception of radioactive I-131 or I-125, most mothers can continue to breastfeed their infant following a brief interruption with pumping and discarding of the milk.

Both radioisotopes of iodine (I-131 and I-125) pose significant and long-term hazards, which include possible ablation of the infant's thyroid, a future increased risk of thyroid carcinoma in the infant, and an elevated theoretical risk of breast cancer (0.32%) in the mother due to the high dose of I-131 reposited in lactating breast tissues. Because of these issues, it is the recommendation of the NRC that breastfeeding mothers should discontinue breastfeeding if I-131 is required. It is a recommendation of these authors that breastfeeding should be discontinued for several weeks 'prior' to therapy to allow involution of the breasts and reduce exposure of the breast tissues to radioactive iodine (I-131 and I-125). The NRC table provided in the Appendix provides excellent guidelines on the use of radioisotopes and temporary interruption of breastfeeding as a function of dose.

Suggested Reading

Bakheet, S. M., & Hammami, M. M. (1994). Patterns of radioiodine uptake by the lactating breast. *Eur J Nucl Med, 21*(7), 604-608.

Chow, S. M., Yau, S., Lee, S. H., Leung, W. M., & Law, S. C. (2004). Pregnancy outcome after diagnosis of differentiated thyroid carcinoma: no deleterious effect after radioactive iodine treatment. *Int J Radiat Oncol Biol Phys, 59*(4), 992-1000.

Hicks, R. J., Binns, D., & Stabin, M. G. (2001). Pattern of uptake and excretion of (18)F-FDG in the lactating breast. *J Nucl Med, 42*(8), 1238-1242.

Lin, J. D., Wang, H. S., Weng, H. F., & Kao, P. F. (1998). Outcome of pregnancy after radioactive iodine treatment for well differentiated thyroid carcinomas. *J Endocrinol Invest, 21*(10), 662-667.

McCauley, E., & Mackie, A. (2002). Breastmilk activity during early lactation following maternal 99Tcm macroaggregated albumin lung perfusion scan. *Br J Radiol, 75*(893), 464-466.

Miller, R. W., & Zanzonico, P. B. (2005). Radioiodine fallout and breast-feeding. *Radiat Res, 164*(3), 339-340.

Pomeroy, K. M., Sawyer, L. J., & Evans, M. J. (2005). Estimated radiation dose to breast feeding infant following maternal administration of 57Co labelled to vitamin B12. *Nucl Med Commun, 26*(9), 839-841.

Sawka, A. M., Lakra, D. C., Lea, J., Alshehri, B., Tsang, R. W., Brierley, J. D., et al. (2008). A systematic review examining the effects of therapeutic radioactive iodine on ovarian function and future pregnancy in female thyroid cancer survivors. *Clin Endocrinol (Oxf), 69*(3), 479-490.

Radiopaque/Radiocontrast Agents

Principles of Therapy

Radiopaque or radiocontrast agents (except barium) are iodinated or gadolinium-containing compounds used to visualize various organs during X-ray, MRI scans, CT scans, and other radiological procedures. These compounds are of two chemical structures: 1) highly iodinated benzoic acid structures, or 2) gadoliniuim-containing structures. Iodinated compounds are universally used for CT scans. Gadoliniuim products are only used for MRI scans. Although under usual circumstances, iodine-containing products are moderately contraindicated in nursing mothers (due to active transport in milk), these products are unique in that the iodine is covalently bonded to the benzene ring and, as such, are not metabolized, nor free for transport into milk or the thyroid. While exceedingly small amounts may be released from some agents, thyroid function is only briefly altered. According to several manufacturers, less than 0.005% of the iodine is free for transfer into tissues. Further, the oral bioavailability of most of these compounds is poor to nil; hence, they can be used orally as radiopaque agents to visualize the gut. While dozens of these compounds are available, most have not been specifically studied in breastfeeding mothers. Those that have been studied do not appear to penetrate milk effectively.

Medications

- RADIOPAQUE AGENTS (*Omnipaque, Conray, Cholebrine, Telepaque, Oragrafin, Bilivist, Hypaque, Optiray*)

  ◦ AAP = Some approved by the American Academy of Pediatrics for use in breastfeeding mothers

  ◦ LRC = L2

  ◦ RID =

  ◦ Pregnancy =

  ◦ Comment: Radiocontrast or radiopaque agents are opaque to X-rays and are used to visualize blood vessels in various tissues. Barium sulfate was one of the original agents used, while organic iodinated compounds are used primarily in CAT scans and for various X-ray procedures. While iodinated products, in general, are contraindicated in breastfeeding mothers due to the high milk transfer of iodine, in these products, the iodine is covalently bound to the organic molecule, is metabolically stable, and essentially not bioavailable. For the most part, these organic radiocontrast agents are rapidly excreted without significant metabolism, and the amount of elemental iodine released is minimal. Virtually all of these agents have very short plasma half-lives (<1 h), and for those studied, milk concentrations are extremely low (see table below). Of the minimal amount in milk, virtually none is bioavailable to the infant, as these agents are largely unabsorbed orally. According to several manufacturers, less than 0.005% of the iodine is free. These contrast agents are in essence pharmacologically inert, not metabolized, unabsorbed, and are rapidly excreted by the kidney (80-90% with 24 hours). See Appendix for other information on these agents.

Clinical Tips

While there are perhaps a hundred or more of these radiopaque agents available, most differ only in iodine content and chemical structure. It is well documented that the iodine is largely not bioavailable, but rather is eliminated with the parent compound renally. These agents as a whole exhibit poor oral bioavailability; hence, they would not likely even be absorbed by a breastfeeding infant. Studies of two of the more prominent agents above used for CAT and MRI scans show milk levels are extremely low and the bioavailability low as well. While most manufacturer's suggest a 24-hour waiting period to reinitiate breastfeeding, there is no clear reason for such a prolonged interruption of breastfeeding. A brief interruption of several hours would be more than sufficient, although there are no good data to suggest that even this is required.

Radiocontrast Agents and Their Reported Milk Concentrations*

Drug	Milk (C_{max})	Clinical Significance	Bioavailability
Gadopentetate	3.09 umol/L	Only 0.023% of maternal dose; total dose = 0.013 umol/24h	0.8%
Iohexol	35 mg/L	Mean milk level was only 11.4 mg/L; virtually unabsorbed	<0.1%
Iopanoic Acid	20.8 mg/19-29 h	Only 0.08% of maternal dose; virtually unabsorbed	Nil
Metrizamide	32.9 mg/L	Only 0.02% maternal dose recovered over 44.3 hour; poor oral absorption	0.4%
Metrizoate	14 mg/L	Mean milk level 11.4 mg/24 hour; only 0.3% of maternal dose	Nil

Adapted from Hale TW, Ilett KF. (2002). Drug Therapy and Breastfeeding: From Theory to Clinical Practice, First Edition ed. London: Parthenon Publishing.

Suggested Reading

American College of Radiology Committee on Drug & Contrast Media. (2009). Administration of contrast medium to nursing mothers. Accessed on January 18, 2010, from http://www.infantrisk.org/sites/default/files/files/Radiocontrast%20Breastfeeding.pdf

Raynaud's Phenomenon

Principles of Therapy

Raynaud's phenomenon (RP) is characterized by episodic digital arteriospasm resulting in reduced digital blood flow (toes, fingers, tip of nose, ears, and nipple). Most patients are women between the ages of 20-45 years, with cold-induced or emotion-induced finger pallor that occurs in cold exposure. Upon rewarming, finger color returns to cyanosis and, subsequently, to intense redness (reactive hyperemia). Although the fingers are the most commonly involved, the toes, cheeks, nipples, and ears may also be affected. Episodes are most common in northern climates during the winter months. The exact etiology is unknown, but supra physiologic vasoconstrictor responses due to hyperreactive alpha-adrenergic receptor activity may predispose to the syndrome. In some cases, Raynaud's phenomenon is associated with a connective tissue disorder, such as scleroderma, systemic lupus ertyematosus, or rheumatoid arthritis. Raynaud's phenomenon affects young women more than any other demographic group. Treatment is largely palliative and is directed toward reducing the conditions that predispose to the symptoms, namely, reducing cold exposure or emotional situations. Preventive measures include warm clothing and gloves and avoidance of the following: tobacco in all forms, ergot alkaloids (ergotamine, bromocriptine), beta-blockers, oral contraceptives, and sympathomimetic medications (stimulants, pseudoephedrine, phenylephrine, phenylpropanolamine, etc.). Patients should also avoid vibrating machinery, particularly since 40-90% of loggers and 50% of miners who use vibrating equipment experience RP. Pharmacotherapy is not always effective and often the side effects of the medications preclude continued therapy. Raynaud's syndrome may be the first symptom noted in patients with scleroderma.

Treatment

- Avoidance of cold environments.

- Nifedipine.

- Topical nitroglycerin.

- Sildenafil.

Medications

- CAPTOPRIL (*Capoten*)
    - ○ AAP = Maternal Medication Usually Compatible with Breastfeeding
    - ○ LRC = L2
    - ○ RID = 0.02%
    - ○ Pregnancy = C in first trimester

- Comment: Captopril is a typical angiotensin converting enzyme inhibitor (ACE) used to reduce hypertension. Small amounts are secreted (4.7 μg/L) in milk. In one report of 12 women treated with 100 mg three times daily, maternal serum levels averaged 713 μg/L, while breastmilk levels averaged 4.7 μg/L at 3.8 hours after administration. Data from this study suggest that an infant would ingest approximately 0.002% of the free captopril consumed by its mother (300mg) on a daily basis. No adverse effects have been reported in this study. Use with care in mothers with premature infants.

- LOSARTAN   (*Cozaar*, *Hyzaar*)
  - AAP = Not reviewed
  - LRC = L3
  - RID =
  - Pregnancy = C in first trimester
  - Comment: Losartan is a new ACE-like antihypertensive. Rather than inhibiting the enzyme that makes angiotensin, such as the ACE inhibitor family, this medication selectively blocks the ACE receptor site preventing attachment of angiotensin II. No data are available on its transfer to human milk. Although it penetrates the CNS significantly, its high protein binding would probably reduce its ability to enter milk. This product is only intended for those few individuals who cannot take ACE inhibitors. No data on transfer into human milk are available. The trade name Hyzaar contains losartan plus hydrochlorothiazide.

- METHYLDOPA   (*Aldomet*)
  - AAP = Maternal Medication Usually Compatible with Breastfeeding
  - LRC = L2
  - RID = 0.1-0.3%
  - Pregnancy = B
  - Comment: Alpha-methyldopa is a centrally acting antihypertensive. It is frequently used to treat hypertension during pregnancy. In a study of two lactating women who received a dose of 500 mg, the maximum breastmilk concentration of methyldopa ranged from 0.2 to 0.66 mg/L. In another patient who received 1000 mg dose, the maximum concentration in milk was 1.14 mg/L. The milk/plasma ratios varied from 0.19 to 0.34. The authors indicated that if the infant were to ingest 750 mL of milk daily (with a maternal dose = 1000mg), the maximum daily ingestion would be less than 855 μg or approximately 0.02% of the maternal dose.

    In another study of seven women who received 0.750-2.0 gm/day of methyldopa, the free methyldopa concentrations in breastmilk ranged from zero to 0.2 mg/L, while the conjugated metabolite had concentrations of 0.1 to 0.9 mg/L. These studies generally indicate that the levels of methyldopa transferred to a breastfeeding infant would be too low to be clinically relevant.

    However, gynecomastia and galactorrhea have been reported in one full-term two-week-old female neonate following seven days of maternal therapy with methyldopa, 250 mg three times daily.

- NIFEDIPINE   (*Adalat, Procardia*)
  - AAP = Maternal Medication Usually Compatible with Breastfeeding
  - LRC = L2
  - RID = 2.3-3.4%

- ○ Pregnancy = C
- ○ Comment: Nifedipine is an effective antihypertensive. It belongs to the calcium channel blocker family of drugs. Two studies indicate that nifedipine is transferred to breastmilk in varying, but generally low levels. In one study in which the dose was varied from 10-30 mg three times daily, the highest concentration (53.35 µg/L) was measured at one hour after a 30 mg dose. Other levels reported were 16.35 µg/L 60 minutes after a 20 mg dose and 12.89 µg/L 30 minutes after a 10 mg dose. The milk levels fell linearly, with the milk half-lives estimated to be 1.4 hours for the 10 mg dose, 3.1 hours for the 20 dose, and 2.4 hours for the 30 mg dose. The milk concentration measured eight hours following a 30 mg dose was 4.93 µg/L. In this study, using the highest concentration found and a daily intake of 150 mL/kg of human milk, the amount of nifedipine intake would only be 8 µg/kg/day (less than 1.8% of the therapeutic pediatric dose). The authors conclude that the amount ingested via breastmilk poses little risk to an infant.

  In another study, concentrations of nifedipine in human milk one to eight hours after 10 mg doses varied from <1 to 10.3 µg/L (median 3.5 µg/L) in six of 11 patients. In this study, milk levels three days after discontinuing medication ranged from <1 to 9.4 µg/L. The authors concluded the exposure to nifedipine through breastmilk is not significant. In a study by Penny and Lewis, following a maternal dose of 20 mg nifedipine daily for 10 days, peak breastmilk levels at one hour were 46 µg/L. The corresponding maternal serum level was 43 µg/L. From these data, the authors suggest a daily intake for an infant would be approximately 6.45 µg/kg/day.

  Nifedipine has been found clinically useful for nipple vasospasm. Because of the similarity to Raynaud's Phenomenon, sustained release formulations providing 30-60 mg per day are suggested.

- • TERBUTALINE (*Bricanyl, Brethine*)
  - ○ AAP = Maternal Medication Usually Compatible with Breastfeeding
  - ○ LRC = L2
  - ○ RID = 0.2-0.3%
  - ○ Pregnancy = B
  - ○ Comment: Terbutaline is a popular Beta-2 adrenergic used for bronchodilation in asthmatics. It is secreted into breastmilk, but in low quantities. Following doses of 7.5 to 15 mg/day of terbutaline, milk levels averaged 3.37 µg/L. Assuming a daily milk intake of 165 mL/kg, these levels would suggest a daily intake of less than 0.5 µg/kg/day, which corresponds to 0.2 to 0.7% of maternal dose.

    In another study of a patient receiving 5 mg three times daily, the mean milk concentrations ranged from 3.2 to 3.7 µg/L. The authors calculated the daily dose to infant at 0.4-0.5 µg/kg body weight. Terbutaline was not detectable in the infant's serum. No untoward effects have been reported in breastfeeding infants.

Clinical Tips

At present, the calcium channel blockers appear most effective and include nifedipine, nicardipine, and diltiazem. Nifedipine, having the most potent peripheral action, is considered the agent of choice. There are no data available on nicardipine in breastfeeding mothers, but it is probably reasonably safe. Diltiazem may not be suitable for breastfeeding mothers due to higher milk levels. Recent data suggests that Losartan (an ACE inhibitor, 50 mg/day) may be as effective as the calcium channel blockers. Fluoxetine in a low dose (20 mg/day) has been found to be reasonably effective as well. New data on Sildenafil (Viagra) (50 mg twice daily) or vardenafil (10 mg twice daily) suggest they may be effective in reducing Raynaud attacks as well (avoid in migraine patients).

Methyldopa is about 50% effective in Raynaud's and several studies show low milk levels. Although nicotinic acid is marginally effective (< 40%), its use in high doses could be problematic for a breastfed infant (liver damage). Alpha-adrenergic blockers have not been studied in breastfeeding mothers, but due to incredible potency, they are probably too toxic to risk (prazosin, phenoxybenzamine). The ACE inhibitor captopril is marginally effective (30%). There are numerous other medications that are poorly efficacious and have not been studied in breastfeeding mothers. These include griseofulvin, papaverine, nitrates, guanethidine, reserpine, prostaglandins (PGI2, PGE1), thyroid, dextran, and pentoxifylline.

Suggested Reading

Anderson, J. E., Held, N., & Wright, K. (2004). Raynaud's phenomenon of the nipple: a treatable cause of painful breastfeeding. *Pediatrics, 113*(4), e360-364.

Bakst, R., Merola, J. F., Franks, A. G., Jr., & Sanchez, M. (2008). Raynaud's phenomenon: pathogenesis and management. *J Am Acad Dermatol, 59*(4), 633-653.

Flavahan, N. A. (2008). Regulation of vascular reactivity in scleroderma: new insights into Raynaud's phenomenon. *Rheum Dis Clin North Am, 34*(1), 81-87; vii.

Gayraud, M. (2007). Raynaud's phenomenon. *Joint Bone Spine, 74*(1), e1-8.

Lawlor-Smith, L., & Lawlor-Smith, C. (1997). Vasospasm of the nipple--a manifestation of Raynaud's phenomenon: case reports. *BMJ, 314*(7081), 644-645.

Lawlor-Smith, L. S., & Lawlor-Smith, C. L. (1997). Raynaud's phenomenon of the nipple: a preventable cause of breastfeeding failure? *Med J Aust, 166*(8), 448.

Morino, C., & Winn, S. M. (2007). Raynaud's phenomenon of the nipples: an elusive diagnosis. *J Hum Lact, 23*(2), 191-193.

Page, S. M., & McKenna, D. S. (2006). Vasospasm of the nipple presenting as painful lactation. *Obstet Gynecol, 108*(3 Pt 2), 806-808.

Tagliarino, H., Purdon, M., Jamieson, B., & Hoekzema, G. (2005). Clinical inquiries. What is the evaluation and treatment strategy for Raynaud's phenomenon? *J Fam Pract, 54*(6), 553-555.

Vinjar, B., & Stewart, M. (2008). Oral vasodilators for primary Raynaud's phenomenon. *Cochrane Database Syst Rev*(2), CD006687.

Rheumatoid Arthritis

Principles of Therapy

Rheumatoid arthritis (RA) is a chronic, insidious, autoimmune inflammatory disease of unknown etiology which is primarily characterized by symmetric polyarthritis. It primarily affects the small joints in the hands (PIP and MCP joints), the MTP joints in the feet, wrists, elbows, knees, shoulder, hips, and cervical spine. Spontaneous partial remissions occur in over 75% of patients, with about 10% progressing on to rapid degenerative arthritis. Treatment is highly varied and depends on the source and site of pain, age, and condition of patient (pregnant, breastfeeding), and length and severity of condition. While the salicylates have for ages been the primary tool for treating RA, their high side effect profile has relegated them to lesser status. Treatment of minor rheumatic pain generally begins with the use of acetaminophen, light doses of aspirin, or more likely, the NSAIDs. With increasing severity, intra-articular injections of steroids may be used. But none of these agents produce remissions in this syndrome. The disease modifying antirheumatic drugs (DMARD) (e.g., methotrexate, gold salts, azathioprine, etc.) can in some cases reduce or retard destruction of the joint, and with many rheumatologists, are being used far earlier than in the past. Timing is critical. Treatment guidelines emphasize that the initiation of DMARD therapy should not be delayed past three months for any patient with an established diagnosis who has ongoing joint pain, morning stiffness, active synovitis, and an elevated ESR (SED rate). However, the use of DMARD drugs in breastfeeding mothers is problematic at best, as many of these drugs are not well studied in breastfeeding mothers and are highly toxic. Their use in breastfeeding mothers is not generally advised.

Treatment

- NSAIDs.

- Corticosteroids.

- DMARDs, including methotrexate, hydroxychloroquine, and azathrioprine.

- Tumor Necrosis Factor Antagonists, including etanercept, abatacept, rituximab, and infliximab.

Medications

- ACETAMINOPHEN   (*Tempra, Tylenol, Paracetamol*)
    - AAP = Maternal Medication Usually Compatible with Breastfeeding
    - LRC = L1
    - RID   = 8.8-24.2%
    - Pregnancy = B

◦ Comment: Only small amounts are secreted into breastmilk and are considered too small to be hazardous. In a study of 11 mothers who received 650 mg of acetaminophen orally, the highest milk levels reported were from 10-15 mg/L. The milk/plasma ratio was 1.08. In another study of three patients who received a single 500 mg oral dose, the reported milk and plasma concentrations of acetaminophen was 4.2 mg/L and 5.6 mg/L, respectively. The milk/plasma ratio was 0.76. The maximum observed concentration in milk was 4.4 mg/L. In another study of women who ingested 1000 mg acetaminophen, milk levels averaged 6.1 mg/L and provided an average dose of 0.92 mg/kg/d according to the authors. There seems to be wide variation in the milk concentrations in these studies, but the relative infant dose is probably less than 6.4% of the maternal dose. This is significantly less than the pediatric therapeutic dose. Acetaminophen is compatible with breastfeeding.

- ADALIMUMAB   (*Humira*)
  ◦ AAP = Not reviewed
  ◦ LRC = L3
  ◦ RID =
  ◦ Pregnancy = B
  ◦ Comment: Adalimumab is a recombinant human IgG1 monoclonal antibody specific for human tumor necrosis factor (TNF). TNF is implicated in the pain and destructive component of arthritis and other autoimmune syndromes. This product would be similar to others, such as etanercept (Enbrel) and infliximab (Remicade). IgG transfer into human milk is significant the first four days postpartum, then is minimal afterwards. The primary immunoglobulin in mature human milk is IgA. Immunoglobulins are transferred into human milk by a very specific carrier protein which inhibits the transfer of IgG-like products. It is not known if these unusual immunoglobulins are transferred into milk, but it is unlikely. Specific data from our laboratories suggests that no infliximab transfers into human milk in mothers receiving IV doses. It is not likely that Adalimumab would transfer in clinically relevant amounts after the first week postpartum, but no data are available at this time.

- DICLOFENAC   (*Cataflam, Voltaren*)
  ◦ AAP = Not reviewed
  ◦ LRC = L2
  ◦ RID = 1.05%
  ◦ Pregnancy = B topical/ C oral
  ◦ Comment: Diclofenac is a typical nonsteroidal analgesic (NSAID). Voltaren is a sustained release product, whereas Cataflam is an immediate release product. In one study of six postpartum mothers receiving three 50 mg doses on day one, followed by two 50 mg doses on day two, the levels of diclofenac in breastmilk were approximately 5 ng/mL of milk, although the limit of detection was reported as <19 ng/mL.

  In another patient on long-term treatment with diclofenac, milk levels of 0.1 μg/mL milk were reported which would amount to 0.015 mg/kg/d ingested. These amounts are probably far too low to affect an infant.

- ETANERCEPT   (*Enbrel*)
  ◦ AAP = Not reviewed
  ◦ LRC = L3

- ○ RID =
- ○ Pregnancy = B
- ○ Comment: Etanercept is a dimeric fusion protein consisting of the extracellular ligand-binding portion of tumor necrosis factor bound to human IgG1. Etanercept binds specifically to tumor necrosis factor (TNF) and blocks its inflammatory and immune activity in rheumatoid arthritis patients. Elevated levels of TNF are found in the synovial fluid of arthritis patients.

  In a recent study of a non-breastfeeding mother who received 25 mg twice weekly, etanercept was measured in the milk retained in the breast. This mother was not breastfeeding, but retained some milk in the breast after 30 days. The author reported milk levels of 75 ng/mL on the day after injection. While these data are interesting, measuring drug transfer in residual breastmilk following involution of alveolar tissues is simply not clinically relevant. After involution, the alveolar system would be totally open to drug transfer due to the breakdown of the tight intercellular junctions between lactocytes.

  Due to its enormous molecular weight (150,000 daltons), I still believe it is extremely unlikely that clinically relevant amounts would transfer into milk in actively breastfeeding mothers. In addition, due to its protein structure, it would not be orally bioavailable in an infant. Infliximab is somewhat similar and is apparently not secreted into human milk (see infliximab).

- **FLURBIPROFEN** (*Ansaid, Froben, Ocufen*)
  - ○ AAP = Not reviewed
  - ○ LRC = L2
  - ○ RID = 0.7-1.4%
  - ○ Pregnancy = B during first and second trimester
  - ○ Comment: Flurbiprofen is a nonsteroidal analgesic similar in structure to ibuprofen, but used both as an ophthalmic preparation (in eyes) and orally. In one study of 12 women and following nine oral doses (50 mg/dose, three to five days postpartum), the concentration of flurbiprofen in two women ranged from 0.05 to 0.07 mg/L of milk, but was <0.05 mg/L in 10 of the 12 women. Concentrations in breastmilk and plasma of nursing mothers suggest that a nursing infant would receive less than 0.1 mg flurbiprofen per day, a level considered exceedingly low.

    In another study of 10 nursing mothers following a single 100 mg dose, the average peak concentration of flurbiprofen in breastmilk was 0.09 mg/L, or about 0.05% of the maternal dose. Both of these studies suggest that the amount of flurbiprofen transferred in human milk would be clinically insignificant to the infant.

- **HYDROXYCHLOROQUINE** (*Plaquenil*)
  - ○ AAP = Maternal Medication Usually Compatible with Breastfeeding
  - ○ LRC = L2
  - ○ RID = 2.9%
  - ○ Pregnancy = C
  - ○ Comment: Hydroxychloroquine (HCQ) is effective in the treatment of malaria, but is also used in immune syndromes, such as rheumatoid arthritis and Lupus erythematosus. HCQ is known to produce significant retinal damage and blindness if used over a prolonged period, and this could occur (theoretically but unlikely) in breastfed infants. Patients on this product should see an

ophthalmologist routinely. It has a huge volume of distribution (Vd) which suggests milk levels will be quite low.

In one study of a mother receiving 400 mg HCQ daily, the concentrations of HCQ in breastmilk were 1.46, 1.09, and 1.09 mg/L at 2.0, 9.5, and 14 hours after the dose. The average milk concentration was 1.1 mg/L. The milk/plasma ratio was approximately 5.5. On a body-weight basis, the infant's dose would be 2.9% of the maternal dose.

In another study of one mother receiving 200 mg twice daily, milk levels were much lower than the previous study. Only a total of 3.2 µg HCQ was detected in her milk over 48 hours.

Two breastfeeding mothers taking hydroxychloroquine were tested to determine the concentration in their breastmilk one week after delivery. The concentrations were 344 and 1424 ng/mL, which corresponded to an infant dose of 0.06 and 0.2 mg/kg/d, respectively. HCQ is mostly metabolized to chloroquine and has an incredibly long half-life. The pediatric dose for malaria prophylaxis is 5 mg/kg/week, far larger than the dose received via milk. See chloroquine.

- INFLIXIMAB   (*Remicade*)
    - ○ AAP = Not reviewed
    - ○ LRC = L2
    - ○ RID =
    - ○ Pregnancy = B
    - ○ Comment: Infliximab is a monoclonal antibody to tumor necrosis factor-alpha (TNF-alpha) used to treat Crohn's disease and rheumatoid arthritis. Infliximab is a very large molecular weight antibody and is largely retained in the vascular system. In a study of one breastfeeding patient who received 5 mg/kg IV, infliximab levels were determined in milk at 0, 2, 4, 8, 24, 48, 72 hours, and four, five and seven days. None was detected in milk at any time (detection limit <0.1 µg/mL).

    In another study, a breastfeeding mother receiving five infusions of 10 mg/kg during pregnancy did not have a detectable amount of infliximab in her milk at any point. The baby's serum level after delivery was 39.5 µg/mL, likely due to placental transfer. The half-life of the drug appeared to be prolonged in the newborn.

    Another breastfeeding mother's milk was tested 24 hours and one week following her first infusion of a 5 mg/kg dose, with milk levels below the limit of quantification in both cases.

    Infliximab is probably too large to enter milk in clinically measurable amounts. It would not be orally bioavailable.

- IBUPROFEN   (*Advil, Nuprin, Motrin, Pediaprofen*)
    - ○ AAP = Maternal Medication Usually Compatible with Breastfeeding
    - ○ LRC = L1
    - ○ RID = 0.1-0.7%
    - ○ Pregnancy = B in first and second trimester
    - ○ Comment: Ibuprofen is a nonsteroidal anti-inflammatory analgesic. It is frequently used for fever in infants. Ibuprofen enters milk only in very low levels (less than 0.6% of maternal dose). Even large doses produce very small milk levels. In one patient receiving 400 mg twice daily, milk levels were less than 0.5 mg/L.

    In another study of twelve women who received 400 mg doses every six hours for a total of five doses, all breastmilk levels of ibuprofen were less than 1.0 mg/L, the lower limit of the assay. Data in these studies document that no measurable concentrations of ibuprofen are detected in breastmilk following the above doses. Ibuprofen is presently popular for therapy of fever in infants. Current recommended dose in children is 5-10 mg/kg every six hours. Ibuprofen is an ideal analgesic for breastfeeding mothers.

- **KETOROLAC**   (*Toradol, Acular*)
  - ◦ AAP = Maternal Medication Usually Compatible with Breastfeeding
  - ◦ LRC = L2
  - ◦ RID = 0.2%
  - ◦ Pregnancy = C in first and second trimesters
  - ◦ Comment: Ketorolac is a popular, nonsteroidal analgesic. Although previously used in labor and delivery, its use has subsequently been contraindicated because it is believed to adversely effect fetal circulation and inhibit uterine contractions, thus increasing the risk of hemorrhage.

    In a study of 10 lactating women who received 10 mg orally four times daily, milk levels of ketorolac were not detectable in four of the subjects. In the six remaining patients, the concentration of ketorolac in milk two hours after a dose ranged from 5.2 to 7.3 µg/L on day one and 5.9 to 7.9 µg/L on day two. In most patients, the breastmilk level was never above 5 µg/L. The maximum daily dose an infant could absorb (maternal dose = 40 mg/day) would range from 3.16 to 7.9 µg/day, assuming a milk volume of 400 mL or 1000 mL. An infant would, therefore, receive less than 0.2% of the daily maternal dose. Please note, the original paper contained a misprint on the daily intake of ketorolac (mg instead of µg).

- **PIROXICAM**   (*Feldene*)
  - ◦ AAP = Maternal Medication Usually Compatible with Breastfeeding
  - ◦ LRC = L2
  - ◦ RID = 3.4-5.8%
  - ◦ Pregnancy = C
  - ◦ Comment: Piroxicam is a typical nonsteroidal anti inflammatory commonly used in arthritics. In one patient taking 40 mg/day, breastmilk levels were 0.22 mg/L at 2.5 hours after dose. In another study of long-term therapy in four lactating women receiving 20 mg/day, the mean piroxicam concentration in breastmilk was 78 µg/L, which is approximately 1-3% of the maternal plasma concentration. The daily dose ingested by the infant was calculated to average 3.5% of the weight-adjusted maternal dose of piroxicam. Even though piroxicam has a very long half-life, this report suggests its use to be safe in breastfeeding mothers.

- **PREDNISONE-PREDNISOLONE**   (*Prednisone, Prednisolone*)
  - ◦ AAP = Maternal Medication Usually Compatible with Breastfeeding
  - ◦ LRC = L2
  - ◦ RID = 1.8-5.3%
  - ◦ Pregnancy = C
  - ◦ Comment: Small amounts of most corticosteroids are secreted into breastmilk. Following a 10 mg oral dose of prednisone, peak milk levels of prednisolone and prednisone were 1.6 µg/L and 2.67 µg/L, respectively. In a group of 10 women who received 10-80 mg/d prednisolone, the milk levels were only 5-25% of the maternal serum levels.

In one patient who received 80 mg/day prednisolone, the Cmax at one hour was 317 µg/L. The AUC average milk concentration in this mother was 156 µg/L over six hours. This is significantly less than 2% of the weight-normalized maternal dose. Because this last estimate was only determined over 6 hours and this dose was administered once each 24 hours, the total daily estimate would be much less than the 2% estimate.

In another study of a single patient who received 120 mg prednisone/day, the total combined steroid levels (prednisone + prednisolone) peaked at two hours. The peak level of combined steroid was 627 µg/L. Assuming the infant received 120 mL of milk every four hours, the total possible ingestion would only be 47 µg/day.

In a group of seven women who received radioactive labeled prednisolone 5 mg, the total recovery per liter of milk during the 48 hours after the dose was 0.14%.

In small doses, most steroids are certainly not contraindicated in nursing mothers. Whenever possible use low-dose alternatives, such as aerosols or inhalers. Following administration, wait at least four hours if possible prior to feeding infant to reduce exposure. With high doses (>40 mg/day), particularly for long periods, steroids could potentially produce problems in infant growth and development, although we have absolutely no data in this area or know which doses would pose problems. Brief applications of high dose steroids are probably not contraindicated as the overall exposure is low. With prolonged high dose therapy, the infant should be closely monitored for growth and development.

- RITUXIMAB   (*Rituxan*)
  - ◦ AAP = Not reviewed
  - ◦ LRC = L3
  - ◦ RID =
  - ◦ Pregnancy = C
  - ◦ Comment: Rituximab, an IgG antibody, binds to the CD20 antigen found on the surface of B lymphocytes. It is used in the treatment of non-Hodgkin's lymphoma, rheumatoid arthritis, and lymphoid leukemia. There are no reported levels in human milk. Levels of IgG antibodies in human milk are generally low. In addition, oral bioavailability of this protein is likely to be nil.

Clinical Tips

Initial treatment of RA has always included the use of salicylates. However, with the high incidence of side effects, they are seldom used today. Acetaminophen, although not anti-inflammatory, may be useful in some patients and could be used safely in breastfeeding mothers. Of the NSAID family, very few have been studied in breastfeeding mothers, and of these, none are popular with RA patients. All patients respond differently to the various NSAIDs. Most patients try several brands prior to finding one that works best for their specific condition. Ibuprofen, while safe for breastfeeding mothers, requires up to four doses daily and has a rather higher incidence of renal and GI side effects when used chronically. Diclofenac is reportedly better for the GI tract, but has been reported to induce elevated liver enzymes in some patients. However, diclofenac levels in milk are reportedly small to undetectable. Naproxen is transferred into milk at low to moderate levels. However, several reports of GI symptoms in breastfed infants suggest that it should be used only briefly and cautiously. Flurbiprofen and ketorolac have been studied in breastfeeding mothers, and their transmission to milk is very low. Unfortunately, we do not have data on many of the newer, more popular NSAIDS. This does not necessarily preclude their use as long as the infant is closely observed for GI symptoms, cramping, and diarrhea.

Therapy of a chronic syndrome with daily prednisone is risky, and the incidence of osteoporosis is high. Low to moderate oral doses of prednisone (10 mg/day) (short-term) are useful in some patients and are not a contraindication to breastfeeding. Intra-articular injections of triamcinolone are very effective and seldom lead to systemic steroid side effects if they are used less than three or four injections per joint per year. Due to the minimal plasma levels attained, the amount of triamcinolone transferred into milk is likely small and would not preclude breastfeeding, just be observant of the infant's growth and development. Of the DMARD drugs, hydroxychloroquine (HCQ) and methotrexate are the only medications that have been studied. HCQ may be used in breastfeeding mothers with close observation of the infant as the dose transferred to the infant is less than one-third of the pediatric dose used in malaria regions. While the studies of methotrexate show milk levels are quite low, the reports of methotrexate storage in mucosal cells in the GI tract of infants is concerning, and we hesitate to recommend the use of methotrexate in breastfeeding mothers. The reported concentration of myochrysine(Gold) in milk is low, but due to its incredibly long half-life (up to 26 days), it may not be advisable to expose an infant for long periods to this potentially toxic compound.

Suggested Reading

Adams Waldorf, K. M., & Nelson, J. L. (2008). Autoimmune disease during pregnancy and the microchimerism legacy of pregnancy. *Immunol Invest, 37*(5), 631-644.

Berthelot, J. M., De Bandt, M., Goupille, P., Solau-Gervais, E., Liote, F., Goeb, V., et al. (2009). Exposition to anti-TNF drugs during pregnancy: outcome of 15 cases and review of the literature. *Joint Bone Spine, 76*(1), 28-34.

de Man, Y. A., Dolhain, R. J., van de Geijn, F. E., Willemsen, S. P., & Hazes, J. M. (2008). Disease activity of rheumatoid arthritis during pregnancy: results from a nationwide prospective study. *Arthritis Rheum, 59*(9), 1241-1248.

de Man, Y. A., Hazes, J. M., van der Heide, H., Willemsen, S. P., de Groot, C. J., Steegers, E. A., et al. (2009). Association of higher rheumatoid arthritis disease activity during pregnancy with lower birth weight: results of a national prospective study. *Arthritis Rheum, 60*(11), 3196-3206.

Gerosa, M., De Angelis, V., Riboldi, P., & Meroni, P. L. (2008). Rheumatoid arthritis: a female challenge. *Womens Health (Lond Engl), 4*(2), 195-201.

Karlson, E. W., Mandl, L. A., Hankinson, S. E., & Grodstein, F. (2004). Do breast-feeding and other reproductive factors influence future risk of rheumatoid arthritis? Results from the Nurses' Health Study. *Arthritis Rheum, 50*(11), 3458-3467.

Keeling, S. O., & Oswald, A. E. (2009). Pregnancy and rheumatic disease: "by the book" or "by the doc". *Clin Rheumatol, 28*(1), 1-9.

Keuken, D. G., Haafkens, J. A., Moerman, C. J., Klazinga, N. S., & ter Riet, G. (2007). Attention to sex-related factors in the development of clinical practice guidelines. *J Womens Health (Larchmt), 16*(1), 82-92.

Pikwer, M., Bergstrom, U., Nilsson, J. A., Jacobsson, L., Berglund, G., & Turesson, C. (2009). Breast feeding, but not use of oral contraceptives, is associated with a reduced risk of rheumatoid arthritis. *Ann Rheum Dis, 68*(4), 526-530.

Vroom, F., van de Laar, M. A., van Roon, E. N., Brouwers, J. R., & de Jong-van den Berg, L. T. (2008). Treatment of pregnant and non-pregnant rheumatic patients: a survey among Dutch rheumatologists. *J Clin Pharm Ther, 33*(1), 39-44.

Rosacea

Principles of Therapy

Rosacea is a chronic facial inflammatory skin disease. It is more common in women, but more severe in males. This disorder is common in older individuals (30-50 years), and characterized by exaggerated blushing or rosy hue of the cheeks, nose, and chin. Although sometimes called adult acne, it is not related. Rosacea often comes in periods of exacerbation, followed by quiescent periods; flare-ups are often triggered by sun, warmth, and alcohol. Follicular obstruction and comedones are not present in this disorder. It is instead an inflammatory disorder, characterized by telangiectasis, erythema, inflammatory papules, and pustules appearing in the central areas of the face. Tissue hypertrophy, particularly of the nose (rhinophyma), may result. The cause is unknown, but is most common in people with fair complexions. Facial skin is unusually sensitive to skin sensitizers, such as harsh soaps, abrasive cleaners, or those containing astringents. While this condition cannot be cured, effective treatments are available. Treatment generally consists of topical metronidazole gel or oral antibiotics, particularly tetracycline. There are strong indications that depression may play a significant role in the incidence of rosacea. Many dermatologists are now using antidepressants as an adjunctive treatment.

Treatment

- Sunscreen.

- Avoid alcohol.

- Topical metronidazole.

- Azelaic acid.

- Tetracycline or doxycycline.

- Benzoyl peroxide.

Medications

- AZELAIC ACID   (*Azelex, Finevin*)
    - AAP = Not reviewed
    - LRC = L3
    - RID =
    - Pregnancy = B
    - Comment: Azelaic is a dicarboxylic acid derivative normally found in whole grains and animal products. Azelaic acid, when applied as a cream, produces a significant reduction of P. acnes and has an antikeratinizing effect as well. Small amounts of azelaic acid are normally present in human milk.

Azelaic acid is only modestly absorbed via skin (<4%), and it is rapidly metabolized. The amount absorbed does not change the levels normally found in plasma nor milk. Due to its poor penetration into plasma and rapid half-life (45 minutes), it is not likely to penetrate milk or produce untoward effects in a breastfed infant.

- **CLARITHROMYCIN**   (*Biaxin*)
  - AAP = Not reviewed
  - LRC = L1
  - RID = 2.1%
  - Pregnancy = C
  - Comment: Antibiotic that belongs to erythromycin family. In a study of 12 mothers receiving 250 mg twice daily, the Cmax occurred at 2.2 hours. The estimated average dose of clarithromycin via milk was reported to be 150 µg/kg/day, or 2% of the maternal dose. Clarithromycin is probably compatible with breastfeeding. Observe for diarrhea and thrush in the infant.

- **CLINDAMYCIN LOTION/GEL** (*Cleocin T*)
  - AAP = Not reviewed
  - LRC =
  - RID = 1% - 7.3% (oral)
  - Pregnancy = B
  - Comment: Clindamycin gels are poorly absorbed (less than 0.2%). Clindamycin is a broad-spectrum antibiotic frequently used for anaerobic infections. In one study of two nursing mothers and following doses of 600 mg IV every six hours, the concentration of clindamycin in breastmilk was 3.1 to 3.8 mg/L at 0.2 to 0.5 hours after dosing. Following oral doses of 300 mg every six hours, the breastmilk levels averaged 1.0 to 1.7 mg/L at 1.5 to 7 hours after dosing. In another study of two to three women who received a single oral dose of 150 mg, milk levels averaged 0.9 mg/L at four hours with a milk/plasma ratio of 0.47.

    An alteration of GI flora is possible even though the dose is low. One case of bloody stools (pseudomembranous colitis) has been associated with clindamycin and gentamicin therapy on day five postpartum, but this is considered rare. In this case, the mother of a newborn infant was given 600 mg IV every six hours. In rare cases, pseudomembranous colitis can appear several weeks later.

    In a study by Steen, in five breastfeeding patients who received 150 mg three times daily for seven days, milk concentrations ranged from <0.5 to 3.1 mg/L, with the majority of levels <0.5 mg/L. There are a number of pediatric clinical uses of clindamycin (anaerobic infections, bacterial endocarditis, pelvic inflammatory disease, and bacterial vaginosis). The current pediatric dosage recommendation is 10-40 mg/kg/day divided every six to eight hours.

    In a study of 15 women who received 600 mg clindamycin intravenously, levels of clindamycin in milk averaged 1.03 mg/L at two hours following the dose.

    Cleocin T topical solution or lotion contain clindamycin phosphate equivalent to 10 mg/mL. Transcutaneous absorption is minimal (<1-4%) and reported plasma levels are low to nil. Some does appear in urine of treated patients. Due to low maternal plasma levels, virtually none should be expected in breastmilk.

    With the rise of resistant Staphlococcal infections, clindamycin use in infants has risen enormously. The amount in milk is unlikely to harm a breastfeeding infant.

- ERYTHROMYCIN   (*E-Mycin, Ery-Tab, Eryc, Ilosone*)
  - AAP = Maternal Medication Usually Compatible with Breastfeeding
  - LRC = L2
  - RID = 1.4-1.7%
  - Pregnancy = B
  - Comment: Erythromycin is an older, narrow-spectrum antibiotic. In one study of patients receiving 400 mg three times daily, milk levels varied from 0.4 to 1.6 mg/L. Doses as high as 2 gm per day produced milk levels of 1.6 to 3.2 mg/L. One case of hypertrophic pyloric stenosis apparently linked to erythromycin administration has been reported. In a study of two to three patients who received a single 500 oral dose, milk levels at four hours ranged from 0.9 to 1.4 mg/L, with a milk/plasma ratio of 0.92. Newer macrolide-like antibiotics (azithromycin) may preclude the use of erythromycin. A recent and large study now suggests a strong positive correlation between the use of erythromycin in breastfeeding mothers and infantile hypertrophic pyloric stenosis in newborns.

- METRONIDAZOLE TOPICAL GEL   (*MetroGel Topical*)
  - AAP = Not reviewed
  - LRC = L3
  - RID =
  - Pregnancy = B
  - Comment: Metronidazole topical gel is primarily indicated for acne and is a gel formulation containing 0.75% metronidazole. For metronidazole kinetics and entry into human milk, see metronidazole. Following topical application of 1 gm of metronidazole gel to the face (equivalent to 7.5 mg metronidazole base), the maximum serum concentration was only 66 ng/mL in only one of 10 patients. (In three of the ten patients, levels were undetectible). This concentration is 100 times less than the serum concentration achieved following the oral ingestion of just one 250 mg tablet. Therefore, the topical application of metronidazole gel provides only exceedingly low plasma levels in the mother and minimal to no levels in milk.

- TETRACYCLINE   (*Achromycin, Sumycin, Terramycin*)
  - AAP = Maternal Medication Usually Compatible with Breastfeeding
  - LRC = L2
  - RID = 0.6%
  - Pregnancy = D
  - Comment: Tetracycline is a broad-spectrum antibiotic with significant side effects in pediatric patients, including dental staining and reduced bone growth. It is secreted into breastmilk in extremely small levels. Because tetracyclines bind to milk calcium, they would have reduced oral absorption in the infant.

    Posner reports that in a patient receiving 500 mg four times daily, the average concentration of tetracycline in milk was 1.14 mg/L. The maternal plasma level was 1.92 mg/L and the milk/plasma ratio was 0.59. The absolute dose to the infant ranged from 0.17 to 0.39 mg/kg/day. None was detected in the plasma compartment of the infant (limit of detection 0.05 mg/L).

    In a mother receiving 275 mg/d, milk levels averaged 1.25 mg/L, with a maximum of 2.51 mg/L. None was detected in the infant's plasma. In another study of two to three patients receiving a single 150 mg/d dose, milk levels ranged from 0.3 to 1.2 mg/L at four hours (Cmax). The maximum reported milk level was 1.2 mg/L. A milk/plasma ratio of 0.58 was reported.

From the above studies, the relative infant dose is 0.6%, 4.77%, and 8.44%. Thus a high degree of variability exists in these studies. Invariably, mixture of tetracyclines in milk would greatly limit their oral bioavailability.

The short-term exposure of infants to tetracyclines (via milk) is not contraindicated (<3 weeks). However, the long-term exposure of breastfeeding infants to tetracyclines, such as when used daily for acne, could cause problems. The absorption of even small amounts over a prolonged period could result in dental staining.

Clinical Tips

First-line therapy is avoidance of factors that provoke flushing, such as heat, sunlight, and ingestion of hot beverages, spicy foods, and alcohol. The topical use of azelaic acid is ideal for a breastfeeding mother if it is effective. Interestingly, small amounts of azelaic are normally found in human milk. Applied topically, it is only modestly absorbed via the skin (< 4%) and it is rapidly metabolized and cleared.

Topical metronidazole gel 0.75% (MetroGel) or Clindamycin lotion 1% (Cleocin T) are the preferred therapies for rosacea and would be ideal for breastfeeding mothers. Systemic absorption of topical metronidazole or clindamycin is very low to nil. After control, the dose of topical metronidazole or clindamycin can be gently tapered until the next severe recurrence. In one study, topical clindamycin was equally efficacious with oral tetracycline. More severe cases may require oral erythromycin, clarithromycin, or tetracycline. The dose of oral erythromycin varies from 250-500 mg twice daily. Several more recent studies have suggested that oral clarithromycin (250 mg twice daily for one month, followed by 250 mg daily for one month) is more efficacious than doxycycline. This would be ideal oral therapy for a breastfeeding mother.

While the use of tetracycline is not ideal, the initial dose of oral tetracycline is 250 mg QID and may be decreased later to once daily and continued for up to one month. However, the 'chronic' use of oral tetracyclines (> 6 weeks) may be problematic in breastfeeding patients, and we do not recommend it. It is true that oral tetracycline, when ingested via milk, is poorly bioavailable (< 30-40%). While the absolute level of tetracycline in milk is low (< 2.58 mg/L) and bioavailability of this would be only 30-40%, taken over a long period of time (months), the amount of tetracycline reaching the infant could be significant. The newer tetracyclines are even more problematic. The bioavailability of the newer tetracyclines (minocycline, doxycycline) is much higher (80%), even in the presence of calcium salts, so that the chronic use of these tetracyclines should be discouraged in breastfeeding mothers. Further, due to chronic hypersensitivity syndrome, minocycline-induced scleral pigmentation, and acute eosinophilic pneumonia now associated with minocycline use, most dermatologists are using doxycycline for chronic acne or rosacea. If needed, the older tetracyclines should probably be used and in the lowest doses possible.

Resistant cases may respond to isotretinoin (Accutane), but we do not believe this drug is safe for breastfeeding mothers and infants, although there are no data to suggest this. Remember, topical, particularly fluorinated, steroids aggravate rosacea and are contraindicated. One of the most common reasons for the occurrence of rosacea is steroid-induced rosacea. Recently, there is increasing data to suggest that clinical depression may play a major role in the occurrence of rosacea. Many dermatologists have now begun using antidepressants (SSRIs) in these patients with good results.

Suggested Reading

Ceilley, R. I. (2004). Advances in the topical treatment of acne and rosacea. *J Drugs Dermatol, 3*(5 Suppl), S12-22.

Del Rosso, J. Q. (2007). Recently approved systemic therapies for acne vulgaris and rosacea. *Cutis, 80*(2), 113-120.

Del Rosso, J. Q., Baldwin, H., & Webster, G. (2008). American Acne & Rosacea Society rosacea medical management guidelines. *J Drugs Dermatol, 7*(6), 531-533.

Del Rosso, J. Q., Leyden, J. J., Thiboutot, D., & Webster, G. F. (2008). Antibiotic use in acne vulgaris and rosacea: clinical considerations and resistance issues of significance to dermatologists. *Cutis, 82*(2 Suppl 2), 5-12.

Schauber, J., & Gallo, R. L. (2009). Antimicrobial peptides and the skin immune defense system. *J Allergy Clin Immunol, 124*(3 Suppl 2), R13-18.

Schittek, B., Paulmann, M., Senyurek, I., & Steffen, H. (2008). The role of antimicrobial peptides in human skin and in skin infectious diseases. *Infect Disord Drug Targets, 8*(3), 135-143.

Salmonella Ileocolitis

Principles of Therapy

Salmonellosis includes infection by any of 2500 serotypes of salmonellae. It is the most common cause of gastroenteritis, following food-borne transmission, particularly from poultry/eggs. Human infections are generally caused by one of three major subtypes, S. *typhi, typhimurium,* and *choleraesuis.* Three clinical patterns of infections are most common and include enteric fever (typhoid fever caused by S. typhi), acute enterocolitis (S. *typhimurium*), and bacterial septicemia (S. *choleraesuis*). All such infections are due to the ingestion of contaminated food or drink. Treatment depends on the subtype of infection. Most, however, are self-limiting in healthy patients and may not require treatment. Indeed, antibiotics are generally more harmful than beneficial.

Treatment

- Antibiotics are not usually required unless the patient is very old or very young, extremely ill, or immunocompromised.

- Relapses are more common in those receiving antibiotics, particularly after three weeks.

- When antibiotics are needed, common choices include ciprofloxacin, azithromycin, amoxicillin, and trimethoprim/sulfamethoxazole.

Medications

- AMPICILLIN   (*Polycillin, Omnipen*)
  - AAP = Not reviewed
  - LRC = L1
  - RID   = 0.2-0.5%
  - Pregnancy = B
  - Comment: Low milk/plasma ratios of 0.2 have been reported. In a study by Matsuda of two to three breastfeeding patients who received 500 mg of ampicillin orally, levels in milk peaked at six hours and averaged only 0.14 mg/L of milk. The milk/plasma ratio was reported to be 0.03 at two hours. In a group of nine breastfeeding women sampled at various times and who received doses of 350 mg TID orally, milk concentrations ranged from 0.06 to 0.17 mg/L, with peak milk levels at three to four hours after the dose. Milk/plasma ratios varied between 0.01 and 0.58. The highest reported milk level (1.02 mg/L) was in a patient receiving 700 mg TID. Ampicillin was not detected in the plasma of any infant.

- CEFIXIME   (*Suprax*)
  - AAP = Not reviewed
  - LRC = L2

- $\circ$ RID =
- $\circ$ Pregnancy = B
- $\circ$ Comment: Cefixime is an oral, third-generation cephalosporin used in treating infections. It is poorly absorbed (30-50%) by the oral route. It is secreted to a limited degree in the milk, although in one study of a mother receiving 100 mg, it was undetected in the milk from one to six hours after the dose.

- CEFTRIAXONE (*Rocephin*)
  - $\circ$ AAP = Maternal Medication Usually Compatible with Breastfeeding
  - $\circ$ LRC = L2
  - $\circ$ RID = 4.1-4.2%
  - $\circ$ Pregnancy = B
  - $\circ$ Comment: Ceftriaxone is a very popular third-generation broad-spectrum cephalosporin antibiotic. Small amounts are transferred into milk (3-4% of maternal serum level). Following a 1 gm IM dose, breastmilk levels were approximately 0.5-0.7 mg/L at between four to eight hours. The estimated mean milk levels at steady state were 3-4 mg/L. Another source indicates that following a 2 g/d dose and at steady state, approximately 4.4% of dose penetrates into milk. In this study, the maximum breastmilk concentration was 7.89 mg/L after prolonged therapy (seven days). Poor oral absorption of ceftriaxone would further limit systemic absorption by the infant. The half-life of ceftriaxone in human milk varies from 12.8 to 17.3 hours (longer than maternal serum). Even at this high dose, no adverse effects were noted in the infant. Ceftriaxone levels in breastmilk are probably too low to be clinically relevant, except for changes in GI flora. Ceftriaxone is commonly used in neonates.

- CHLORAMPHENICOL (*Chloromycetin*)
  - $\circ$ AAP = Drugs whose effect on nursing infants is unknown but may be of concern
  - $\circ$ LRC = L4
  - $\circ$ RID = 3.2%
  - $\circ$ Pregnancy = C
  - $\circ$ Comment: Chloramphenicol is a broad-spectrum antibiotic. In one study of five women receiving 250 mg PO four times daily, the concentration of chloramphenicol in milk ranged from 0.54 to 2.84 mg/L. In the same study, but in another group receiving 500 mg four times daily, the concentration of chloramphenicol in milk ranged from 1.75 to 6.10 mg/L. In a group of patients being treated for typhus, milk levels were lower than maternal plasma levels. With maternal plasma levels of 49 and 26 mg/L in two patients, the milk levels were 26 and 16 mg/L, respectively.

    In a study of two to three patients who received a single 500 mg oral dose, the average milk concentration at four hours was 4.1 mg/L. The milk/plasma ratio at four hours was 0.84. Safety in infants is highly controversial. Milk levels are too low to produce overt toxicity in infants, but could produce allergic sensitization to subsequent exposures. Generally, chloramphenicol is considered contraindicated in nursing mothers, although it is occasionally used in infants. This antibiotic can be extremely toxic, particularly in newborns, and should not be used for trivial infections. Blood levels should be constantly monitored and kept below 20 μg/mL.

- CIPROFLOXACIN (*Cipro, Ciloxan*)
  - $\circ$ AAP = Maternal Medication Usually Compatible with Breastfeeding
  - $\circ$ LRC = L3

- ◦ RID = 2.1-6.3%
- ◦ Pregnancy = C
- ◦ Comment: Ciprofloxacin is a fluoroquinolone antibiotic primarily used for gram negative coverage and is presently the drug of choice for anthrax treatment and prophylaxis. Because it has been implicated in arthropathy in newborn animals, it is not normally used in pediatric patients. Levels secreted into breastmilk (2.26 to 3.79 mg/L) are somewhat conflicting. They vary from the low to moderate range to levels that are higher than maternal serum up to 12 hours after a dose. In one study of ten women who received 750 mg every 12 hours, milk levels of ciprofloxacin ranged from 3.79 mg/L at two hours postdose to 0.02 mg/L at 24 hours. In another study of a single patient receiving one 500 mg tablet daily at bedtime, the concentrations in maternal serum and breastmilk were 0.21 µg/mL and 0.98 µg/mL, respectively. Plasma levels were undetectable (<0.03 µg/mL) in the infant. The dose to the four-month-old infant was estimated to be 0.92 mg/day or 0.15 mg/kg/day. No adverse effects were noted in this infant. There has been one reported case of severe pseudomembranous colitis in an infant of a mother who self-medicated with ciprofloxacin for six days. In a patient 17 days postpartum, who received 500 mg orally, ciprofloxacin levels in milk were 3.02, 3.02, 3.02, and 1.98 mg/L at 4, 8, 12, and 16 hours postdose, respectively.

  If used in lactating mothers, observe the infant closely for GI symptoms, such as diarrhea. Current studies seem to suggest that the amount of ciprofloxacin present in milk is quite low. Ciprofloxacin was recently approved by the American Academy of Pediatrics for use in breastfeeding women, and it is becoming increasingly popular for use in pediatric patients.

- **CO-TRIMOXAZOLE** (*TMP-SMZ, Bactrim, Cotrim, Septra*)
  - ◦ AAP = Maternal Medication Usually Compatible with Breastfeeding
  - ◦ LRC = L3
  - ◦ RID =
  - ◦ Pregnancy = C
  - ◦ Comment: Co-trimoxazole is the mixture of trimethoprim and sulfamethoxazole. See individual monographs for each of these products.

- **FURAZOLIDONE** (*Furoxone*)
  - ◦ AAP = Not reviewed
  - ◦ LRC = L2
  - ◦ RID =
  - ◦ Pregnancy = C
  - ◦ Comment: Furazolidone belongs to the nitrofurantoin family of antibiotics (see nitrofurantoin). It has a broad-spectrum of activity against gram-positive and gram-negative enteric organisms, including cholera, but is generally used for giardiasis.

    Following an oral dose, furazolidone is poorly absorbed (<5%) and is largely inactivated in the gut. Concentrations transferred to milk are unreported, but the total amounts would be exceedingly low due to the low maternal plasma levels attained by this product. Due to poor oral absorption, systemic absorption in a breastfeeding infant would likely be minimal. Caution should be observed in early postpartum newborns.

- **OFLOXACIN** (*Floxin*)
  - ◦ AAP = Maternal Medication Usually Compatible with Breastfeeding

- LRC = L2
- RID = 3.1%
- Pregnancy = C
- Comment: Ofloxacin is a typical fluoroquinolone antimicrobial. Breastmilk concentrations are reported equal to maternal plasma levels. In one study in lactating women who received 400 mg oral doses twice daily, drug concentrations in breastmilk averaged 0.05-2.41 mg/L in milk (24 hours and two hours postdose, respectively). The drug was still detectable in milk 24 hours after a dose. The fluoroquinolones are becoming more popular in pediatrics due to recent studies and reviews showing their safe use. It is very unlikely that arthropathy would ensue following the dose received via milk. The only probable risk is a change in gut flora, diarrhea, and a remote risk of overgrowth of C. difficile. Ofloxacin levels in breastmilk are consistently lower (37%) than ciprofloxacin. If a fluoroquinolone is required, ofloxacin, levofloxacin, or norfloxacin are probably the better choices for breastfeeding mothers.

Clinical Tips

Antibiotic treatment of otherwise healthy individuals has not demonstrated a change in the length of non-thyphoid disease. Decision for antibiotic therapy should be individualized. For those requiring treatment, cefotaxime, ceftriaxone, or a fluoroquinolone (norfloxacin, ciprofloxacin) are preferred. Currently, due to the emergence of high resistance, ampicillin and chloramphenicol are seldom recommended. Trimethoprim-sulfamethoxazole (TMP/SMX) is also suitable. Of the cephalosporins, ceftriaxone (2 gm daily) for three to seven days is quite effective. Other effective cephalosporins include cefixime, cefotaxime, and cefoperazone. The fluoroquinolones, although not ideal in breastfeeding mothers, can be used with caution, particularly ofloxacin. Duration of therapy is five to seven days. Due to lower milk levels, ofloxacin and trovafloxacin are preferred.

Acute enterocolitis is the most common salmonella infection. Fluid and electrolyte therapy remains the best initial treatment as most cases are self-limited. Antimotility drugs, such as loperamide or diphenoxylate, should be discouraged, as they may increase complications and lead to bacteremia. Antibiotics are generally not needed for the uncomplicated salmonella enterocolitis in normal patients. However, in patients with co-morbid conditions, such as immunodeficiency states (HIV), then TMP/SMX or the fluoroquinolones as above are preferred. Treatment of salmonellosis with antibiotics, if possible, should be avoided, as it frequently leads to a permanent carrier state.

Suggested Reading

Crum-Cianflone, N. F. (2008). Salmonellosis and the gastrointestinal tract: more than just peanut butter. *Curr Gastroenterol Rep, 10*(4), 424-431.

Darby, J., & Sheorey, H. (2008). Searching for Salmonella. *Aust Fam Physician, 37*(10), 806-810.

Hendriksen, R. S., Seyfarth, A. M., Jensen, A. B., Whichard, J., Karlsmose, S., Joyce, K., et al. (2009). Results of use of WHO Global Salm-Surv external quality assurance system for antimicrobial susceptibility testing of Salmonella isolates from 2000 to 2007. *J Clin Microbiol, 47*(1), 79-85.

Hohmann, E. L. (2001). Nontyphoidal salmonellosis. *Clin Infect Dis, 32*(2), 263-269.

Parry, C. M., & Threlfall, E. J. (2008). Antimicrobial resistance in typhoidal and nontyphoidal salmonellae. *Curr Opin Infect Dis, 21*(5), 531-538.

Wegener, H. C. (2006). Risk management for the limitation of antibiotic resistance--experience of Denmark. *Int J Med Microbiol, 296 Suppl 41*, 11-13.

Scabies

Principles of Therapy

Scabies is a transmissible ectoparasite infection characterized by superficial burrows, secondary infection, and intense itching (especially at night). Scabies is caused by the itch mite Sarcoptes scabiei. The female parasite burrows into the stratum corneum and deposits eggs and feces along the burrow. They are transmitted by skin-to-skin contact. Diagnosis is only confirmed by microscopic observation of skin scrapings. It is highly contagious following intimate or close personal contact with individuals, bedding, clothing, bedsharing, or even handshaking. Clinical signs include crusty lesions in skin folds, axilla, genital areas, buttocks, scrotum in males, or interdigital web areas. Observe for subcutaneous linear burrowing on the skin.

Treatment of scabies is primarily by the use of external insecticides. Patients with eczematous inflammation or signs of infections should be treated with appropriate antibiotics.

Treatment

- Permethrin creams on affected areas.

- Ivermectin is reserved for cases resistant to permethrin.

- Lindane is the last choice with higher side effects (neurotoxicity) and should not be used in infants or children.

- Cephalexin for secondary bacterial infections.

- Topical diphenhydramine or hydrocortisone for pruritis.

- All clothing, bedding, and stuffed animals must be washed in hot water.

Medications

- IVERMECTIN   (*Mectizan*)
    - AAP = Maternal Medication Usually Compatible with Breastfeeding
    - LRC = L3
    - RID = 1.3%
    - Pregnancy = C
    - Comment: Ivermectin is now widely used to treat human onchocerciasis, lymphatic filariasis, and other worms and parasites, such as head lice. In a study of four women given 150 µg/kg orally, the maximum breastmilk concentration averaged 14.13 µg/L. Milk/plasma ratios ranged from 0.39 to 0.57, with a mean of 0.51. Highest breastmilk concentration was at four to six hours. Average daily

ingestion of ivermectin was calculated at 2.1 µg/kg, which is 10 fold less than the adult dose. No adverse effects were reported.

- PERMETHRIN   *(Elimite cream)*
  - ◦ AAP = Not reviewed
  - ◦ LRC = L2
  - ◦ RID =
  - ◦ Pregnancy = B
  - ◦ Comment: Permethrin is a synthetic pyrethroid structure of the natural ester pyrethrum, a natural insecticide, and used to treat lice, mites, and fleas. Permethrin absorption through the skin following application of a 5% cream is reported to be less than 2%. Permethrin is rapidly metabolized by serum and tissue enzymes to inactive metabolites and rapidly excreted in the urine. Overt toxicity is very low. It is not known if permethrin is secreted in human milk, although it has been found in animal milk after injection of significant quantities intravenously. In spite of its rapid metabolism, some residuals are sequestered in fat tissue.

Clinical Tips

Permethrin is a synthetic pyrethroid structure derived from the ester pyrethrum, a natural insecticide in plants. Permethrin is very effective against body lice, head lice, and scabies, although some species are becoming resistant.

Permethrin is ideal for breastfeeding mothers because its transcutaneous absorption is minimal, and it is very unlikely to ever enter milk. Further, it is very nontoxic. In adults and children, following a thorough washing, a 5% permethrin cream is applied to the entire body from the neck down. Wash the cream off after 8-14 hours. In infants two months or older, a 5% cream may be used, but must be applied to the entire skin surface, including head and neck. The manufacturer does not provide recommendations for infants < 2 months of age, but most clinicians would use it anyway. Reapplication may be required after seven days if mites reappear. For resistant scabies, ivermectin (200 µg/ kg PO, one dose for adults) is the most recent recommendation. Due to significant transcutaneous absorption and the possibility of seizures, lindane solutions are no longer recommended for breastfeeding mothers. Never use lindane in pregnant women, infants, or children. Permethrin can be safely used in pregnant women and in infants two months or older.

The most common reasons for treatment failure are: 1) other patient contacts have not been treated, 2) bedding and living areas have not been treated and cleaned, 3) areas under the toenail and fingernails have not been treated effectively, 4) eggs are not removed from the hair. Remind the patient that pruritus will probably remain for up to four weeks, even with the dead parasite. This is due to remaining parasite debris in the burrows.

Suggested Reading

Betti, S., Bassi, A., Prignano, F., & Lotti, T. (2009). Scabies: should we always perform dermatoscopy? *G Ital Dermatol Venereol, 144*(3), 313-315.

Chosidow, O. (2006). Clinical practices. Scabies. *N Engl J Med, 354*(16), 1718-1727.

Goyal, N. N., & Wong, G. A. (2008). Psoriasis or crusted scabies. *Clin Exp Dermatol, 33*(2), 211-212.

Hicks, M. I., & Elston, D. M. (2009). Scabies. *Dermatol Ther, 22*(4), 279-292.

Mills, M. (2008). Practice makes perfect. Scabies. *Emerg Nurse, 16*(2), 18-19.

Mounsey, K. E., Holt, D. C., McCarthy, J., Currie, B. J., & Walton, S. F. (2008). Scabies: molecular perspectives and therapeutic implications in the face of emerging drug resistance. *Future Microbiol, 3*(1), 57-66.

Mumcuoglu, K. Y., & Gilead, L. (2008). Treatment of scabies infestations. *Parasite, 15*(3), 248-251.

Rabinowitz, P. M., Gordon, Z., & Odofin, L. (2007). Pet-related infections. *Am Fam Physician, 76*(9), 1314-1322.

Strong, M., & Johnstone, P. W. (2007). Interventions for treating scabies. *Cochrane Database Syst Rev*(3), CD000320.

Schizophrenic Disorders, Psychoses

Principles of Therapy

The schizophrenic disorders are a group of syndromes manifested by formal thought disorders, delusions, hallucinations, disorganized speech and thinking, and loss of contact with reality. Symptoms and signs vary enormously, even within the individual at different times, and can vary from complete catatonic stupor to frenzied excitement. Formerly treated with the older phenothiazines, thioxanthenes, and butyrophenones, the newest treatment is now with the safer "atypical" antipsychotics. Fortunately, we have significant data on the use of antipsychotics, particularly the atypical antipsychotics, in breastfeeding mothers.

Treatment

- Schizophrenics have very high rates of suicide, and some patients experience extremely persistent voices telling them to harm others, including their children. Close monitoring by trained personnel is essential.

- Typical antipsychotics: haloperidol, chlorpromazine, fluphenazine. These agents are effective and inexpensive, but carry a higher side effect profile (extrapyramidal symptoms and tardive dyskinesia) than the atypical antipsychotics.

- Atypical antipsychotics: quetiapine, olanzapine, ziprasidone, aripiprazole, risperidone are generally compatible with breastfeeding. Most, but not all, of these agents cause weight gain, but cause fewer central nervous system side effects.

Medications

- ARIPIPRAZOLE   (*Abilify, Abilitat*)
  - AAP = Not reviewed
  - LRC = L3
  - RID = 1%
  - Pregnancy = C
  - Comment: Aripiprazole is a second-generation antipsychotic, now first-line treatment for schizophrenia. In a small study of a single patient receiving 10 mg/day initially and then 15 mg subsequently, levels of aripiprazole in milk were reported to be 13 and 14 µg/L on two consecutive days (15 and 16 after initiation of therapy). Maternal plasma levels at the same time were 71 and 71 µg/L. Levels were drawn in the morning before aripiprazole administration. Thus it appears from this brief report that they were drawn approximately 24 hours postdose.

    Several reports (personal communication) of somnolence have been reported to this author. The infant should be monitored for somnolence.

- CHLORPROMAZINE   (*Thorazine, Ormazine*)
    - ○ AAP = Drugs whose effect on nursing infants is unknown but may be of concern
    - ○ LRC = L3
    - ○ RID = 0.25%
    - ○ Pregnancy = C
    - ○ Comment: Chlorpromazine is a powerful CNS tranquilizer. Small amounts are known to be secreted into milk. Following a 1200 mg oral dose, samples were taken at 60, 120, and 180 minutes. Breastmilk concentrations were highest at 120 minutes and were 0.29 mg/L at that time. The milk/plasma ratio was less than 0.5. Ayd suggests that in one group of 16 women who took chlorpromazine during, after pregnancy, and while breastfeeding, the side effects were minimal and infant development was normal. In a group of four breastfeeding mothers receiving unspecified amounts of chlorpromazine, milk levels varied from 7 to 98 µg/L. Maternal serum levels ranged from 16 to 52 µg/L. Only the infant who ingested milk with a chlorpromazine level of 92 µg/L showed drowsiness and lethargy.

        Chlorpromazine has a long half-life and is particularly sedating. Long-term use of this product in a lactating mother may be risky to the breastfed infant. There are consistent reports of phenothiazine products increasing the risk of apnea and SIDS. Observe for sedation and lethargy and avoid if possible.

- CHLORPROTHIXENE   (*Taractan*)
    - ○ AAP = Drugs whose effect on nursing infants is unknown but may be of concern
    - ○ LRC = L3
    - ○ RID = 0.3%
    - ○ Pregnancy = C
    - ○ Comment: Sedative commonly used in psychotic or disturbed patients. Chlorprothixene is poorly absorbed orally (<40%) and has been found to increase serum prolactin levels in mothers. Although the milk/plasma ratios are relatively high, only modest levels of chlorprothixene are actually secreted into human milk. In one patient taking 200 mg/day, maximum milk concentrations of the parent and metabolite were 19 µg/L and 28.5 µg/L, respectively. This is approximately 0.1% of the maternal dose.

- CLOZAPINE   (*Clozaril*)
    - ○ AAP = Drugs whose effect on nursing infants is unknown but may be of concern
    - ○ LRC = L3
    - ○ RID = 1.4%
    - ○ Pregnancy = B
    - ○ Comment: Clozapine is an atypical antipsychotic, sedative drug somewhat similar to the phenothiazine family. In a study of one patient receiving 50 mg/d clozapine at delivery, the maternal and fetal plasma were reported to be 14.1 ng/mL and 27 ng/mL, respectively. After 24 hours postpartum, the maternal plasma level was 14.7 ng/mL and maternal milk levels were 63.5 ng/mL. On day seven postpartum and receiving a dose of 100 mg/d clozapine, the maternal plasma and milk levels were 41.1 ng/mL and 115.6 µg/L, respectively. From these data, it is apparent that clozapine concentrates in milk, with a milk/plasma ratio of 4.3 at a dose of 50 mg/d and 2.8 at a dose of 100 mg/d. The change from day one to seven suggests that clozapine entry into mature milk is less. From these data,

the weight-adjusted relative infant dose would be 1.2% of the maternal dose. However, cloazpine carries a risk of seizures and agranulocytosis. Caution is recommended.

- HALOPERIDOL   (*Haldol*)
  - AAP = Drugs whose effect on nursing infants is unknown but may be of concern
  - LRC = L2
  - RID = 2.1-12%
  - Pregnancy = C
  - Comment: Haloperidol is a potent antipsychotic agent that is reported to increase prolactin levels in some patients. In one study of a woman treated for puerperal hypomania and receiving 5 mg twice daily, the concentration of haloperidol in milk was 0.0, 23.5, 18.0, and 3.25 µg/L on day 1, 6, 7, and 21, respectively. The corresponding maternal plasma levels were 0, 40, 26, and 4 µg/L at day 1, 6, 7, and 21, respectively. The milk/plasma ratios were 0.58, 0.69, and 0.81 on days 6, 7, and 21, respectively. After four weeks of therapy, the infant showed no symptoms of sedation and was feeding well.

    In another study after a mean daily dose of 29.2 mg, the concentration of haloperidol in breastmilk was 5 µg/L at 11 hours postdose. In a study of three women on chronic haloperidol therapy receiving 3, 4, and 6 mg daily, milk levels were reported to be 32, 17, and 4.7 ng/mL. The latter levels (4.7) were taken from a patient believed to be noncompliant.

    Bennett calculates the relative infant dose to be 0.2-2.1% to 9.6% of the weight-adjusted maternal daily dose.

- OLANZAPINE   (*Zyprexa, Symbyax*)
  - AAP = Not reviewed
  - LRC = L2
  - RID = 1.2%
  - Pregnancy = C
  - Comment: Olanzapine is a typical antipsychotic agent structurally similar to clozapine and may be used for treating schizophrenia. It is rather unusual in that it blocks serotonin receptors rather than dopamine receptors.

    In a recent and excellent study of seven mother-infant nursing pairs receiving a median dose of olanzapine of 7.5 mg/day (range = 5-20 mg/day), the median infant dose ingested via milk was approximately 1.02% of the maternal dose. The median milk/plasma AUC ratio was 0.38. Olanzapine was undetected in the plasma of six infants tested. All infants were healthy and experienced no observable side effects. The maximum relative infant dose was approximately 1.2%.

    In a case report of a mother taking 20 mg/day, the milk/plasma ratio was 0.35, giving a relative infant dose of about 4% at steady state. This milk was not fed to the infant, so infant plasma levels were not performed.

    A study of five mothers receiving olanzapine at a dose of 2.5-20 mg/day reported milk/plasma ratios of 0.2 to 0.84, with an average relative infant dose of 1.6%. The authors reported no untoward effects on the infants attributable to olanzapine.

    The new product Symbyax contains both fluoxetine and olanzapine for treatment of Bipolar Depression.

- **QUETIAPINE FUMARATE**   (*Seroquel*)

  ◦ AAP = Not reviewed
  ◦ LRC = L2
  ◦ RID   = 0.07-0.1%
  ◦ Pregnancy = C
  ◦ Comment: Quetiapine (Seroquel) is indicated for the treatment of psychotic disorders. It has some affinity for histamine receptors, which may account for its sedative properties. It has been shown to increase the incidence of seizures, prolactin levels, and to lower thyroid levels in adults.

    In a patient (92 kg) receiving 200 mg/day of quetiapine throughout pregnancy, samples were expressed just before dosing, and at one, two, four, and six hours postdose. The average milk concentration (AUC) of quetiapine over the six hours was 13 µg/L, with a maximum concentration of 62 µg/L at one hour. Levels of quetiapine rapidly fell to almost predose levels by two hours. The authors report that an exclusively breastfed infant would ingest only 0.09% of the weight-adjusted maternal dose. At maximum, the infant would ingest 0.43% of the weight-adjusted maternal dose. Although only one patient was studied, the data suggests levels in milk are minimal at this maternal dose.

    One study of six mothers taking a combination of quetiapine, paroxetine, clonazepam, trazodone, and/or venlafaxine showed that no medication was detectable in three of the mothers' milk. In two of the other cases, quetiapine levels were below 0.01 mg/kg/day infant dose, while the final mother expressed an infant dose of less than 0.10 mg/kg/day. The mothers' doses of quetiapine ranged from 25-400 mg. The authors reported that no correlation was noted between drug exposure and developmental outcomes.

    In another study of one mother receiving 400 mg quetiapine per day three months postpartum, expressed milk contained an average drug concentration of 41 µg/L and a milk-to-plasma ratio of 0.29. The relative infant dose reported was 0.09% of the mother's dose. The infant's plasma concentration was 1.4 µg/L, or 6% of the mother's plasma concentration. No adverse effects were reported in the infant, but the authors suggest monitoring the infant's progress and quetiapine serum concentration.

- **RISPERIDONE**   (*Risperdal, Invega*)

  ◦ AAP = Not reviewed
  ◦ LRC = L3
  ◦ RID   = 2.8-9.1%
  ◦ Pregnancy = C
  ◦ Comment: Risperidone is a potent antipsychotic agent, belonging to a new chemical class, and is a dopamine and serotonin antagonist. Risperidone is metabolized to an active metabolite, 9-hydroxyrisperidone. In a study of one patient receiving 6 mg/day of risperidone at steady state, the peak plasma level of approximately 130 µg/L occurred four hours after an oral dose. Peak milk levels of risperidone and 9-hydroxyrisperidone were approximately 12 µg/L and 40 µg/L, respectively. The estimated daily dose of risperidone and metabolite (risperidone equivalents) was 4.3% of the weight-adjusted maternal dose. The milk/plasma ratios calculated from areas under the curve over 24 hours were 0.42 and 0.24, respectively, for risperidone and 6-hydroxyrisperidone.

    In another study, the transfer of risperidone and 9-hydroxyrisperidone into milk was studied in two breastfeeding women and one woman with risperidone-induced galactorrhea. In case two (risperidone dose = 42.1 µg/kg/d), the average concentration of risperidone and 9-hydroxyrisperidone in milk (Cav) was 2.1 and 6 µg/L, respectively. The relative infant dose was 2.8% of the maternal dose. In case three (risperidone dose = 23.1µg/kg/d), the average concentration of risperidone and 9-hydroxyrisperidone in milk (Cav) was 0.39 and 7.06 µg/L, respectively. The milk/plasma ratio determined in two women was <0.5 for both risperidone compounds. The relative infant doses were 2.3%, 2.8%, and 4.7% (as risperidone equivalents) of the maternal weight-adjusted doses in these three cases. Risperidone and 9-hydroxyrisperidone were not detected in the plasma of the two breastfed infants studied, and no adverse effects were noted.

Paliperidone (Invega), the active metabolite of risperidone, is available in extended release tablets. This formulation has a volume of distribution of 6.95 L/kg, 74% protein binding, and a bioavailability of 28%.

- ZIPRASIDONE   (*Geodon*)
    ◦ AAP = Not reviewed
    ◦ LRC = L4
    ◦ RID = 0.1-1.2%
    ◦ Pregnancy = C
    ◦ Comment: Ziprasidone is an atypical antipsychotic agent chemically unrelated to phenothiazines or butyrophenones. No data are available on its transfer into human milk. Until data are available, risperidone or olanzapine should be suggested.

Clinical Tips

The amount of data on the use of phenothiazines in breastfeeding women is very limited, although most papers suggest that the clinical dose transferred is low. Information on chlorpromazine suggests that infants can breastfeed without major complications, due to limited transfer into milk. The only reported side effect has been minimal sedation. Although one report has made the suggestion that phenothiazines may be implicated in an increased risk of sleep apnea and SIDS, in these studies, the medication (promethazine) was administered directly to infants (PO) rather than via breastmilk. Therefore, unless the dose via milk is high enough to induce sedation, an elevated risk of SIDS may be unlikely.

Neurobehavioral development appears normal in a number of these infants exposed to long term phenothiazines via breastmilk. As for haloperidol, levels in milk appear quite low, and this drug would be an optimal choice as a rapid neuroleptic agent.

At present, we have modest literature concerning the use of atypical antipsychotics in breastfeeding women. New data on risperidone and olanzapine indicate milk levels are quite low for both these agents. Aripiprazole, risperidone, quetiapine, and olanzapine are becoming more popular, as they are less likely to induce tardive dyskinesia, extrapyramidal, and other symptoms. Hence, they are replacing the older phenothiazines in treatment of psychosis. New data suggest their milk levels are quite low, and they have not adversely affected the infants in these preliminary studies. The major complication with the new atypical antipsychotics is extraordinary weight gain. With exception of aripiprazole, most of the other atypical antipsychotics induce significant weight gain.

The older clozapine, despite its rather high incidence of agranulocytosis (1-2%), is still commonly used in treatment-refractory patients. Its use in breastfeeding mothers should be viewed very cautiously, and monitoring of the infant for agranulcytosis is probably mandatory.

Suggested Reading

ACOG Practice Bulletin: Clinical management guidelines for obstetrician-gynecologists number 92, April 2008 (replaces practice bulletin number 87, November 2007). Use of psychiatric medications during pregnancy and lactation. (2008). *Obstet Gynecol, 111*(4), 1001-1020.

Bota, R. G., Sagduyu, K., Filin, E. E., Bota, D. A., & Munro, S. (2008). Toward a better identification and treatment of schizophrenia prodrome. *Bull Menninger Clin, 72*(3), 210-227.

Ernst, C. L., & Goldberg, J. F. (2002). The reproductive safety profile of mood stabilizers, atypical antipsychotics, and broad-spectrum psychotropics. *J Clin Psychiatry, 63 Suppl 4*, 42-55.

Fan, X., Goff, D. C., & Henderson, D. C. (2007). Inflammation and schizophrenia. *Expert Rev Neurother, 7*(7), 789-796.

Fruntes, V., & Limosin, F. (2008). Schizophrenia and viral infection during neurodevelopment: a pathogenesis model? *Med Sci Monit, 14*(6), RA71-77.

Gentile, S. (2004). Clinical utilization of atypical antipsychotics in pregnancy and lactation. *Ann Pharmacother, 38*(7-8), 1265-1271.

Hudson, T. J., Owen, R. R., Thrush, C. R., Armitage, T. L., & Thapa, P. (2008). Guideline implementation and patient-tailoring strategies to improve medication adherence for schizophrenia. *J Clin Psychiatry, 69*(1), 74-80.

Kertzman, S., Reznik, I., Grinspan, H., Weizman, A., & Kotler, M. (2008). Antipsychotic treatment in schizophrenia: the role of computerized neuropsychological assessment. *Isr J Psychiatry Relat Sci, 45*(2), 114-120.

Owen, R. R., Hudson, T., Thrush, C., Thapa, P., Armitage, T., & Landes, R. D. (2008). The effectiveness of guideline implementation strategies on improving antipsychotic medication management for schizophrenia. *Med Care, 46*(7), 686-691.

Seeman, M. V. (2004). Gender differences in the prescribing of antipsychotic drugs. *Am J Psychiatry, 161*(8), 1324-1333.

Sit, D., Rothschild, A. J., & Wisner, K. L. (2006). A review of postpartum psychosis. *J Womens Health (Larchmt), 15*(4), 352-368.

Susser, E., St Clair, D., & He, L. (2008). Latent effects of prenatal malnutrition on adult health: the example of schizophrenia. *Ann N Y Acad Sci, 1136*, 185-192.

Toprac, M. G., Dennehy, E. B., Carmody, T. J., Crismon, M. L., Miller, A. L., Trivedi, M. H., et al. (2006). Implementation of the Texas Medication Algorithm Project patient and family education program. *J Clin Psychiatry, 67*(9), 1362-1372.

Xu, M. Q., Sun, W. S., Liu, B. X., Feng, G. Y., Yu, L., Yang, L., et al. (2009). Prenatal malnutrition and adult schizophrenia: further evidence from the 1959-1961 Chinese famine. *Schizophr Bull, 35*(3), 568-576.

Seizure Disorders

Principles of Therapy

The term epilepsy denotes any disorder characterized by recurrent or chronic seizures. A seizure is a transient involuntary disturbance of CNS function due to synchronous abnormal neuronal discharge across the brain. Approximately 1% of the population has epilepsy, with the incidence of epilepsy higher in children and the elderly. Eighty percent of patients with proper doses of anticonvulsants will remain refractory to convulsive seizures. Seizures have innumerable causes, many of which are not yet understood. Specific types of seizures require specific medications, so the selection of medication largely depends on the type of seizure. The medications listed below are used for many seizures, ranging from partial, simple partial, complex partial, absence (petit mal), myoclonic, tonic-clonic, etc. Therefore, it is important to understand that the medications listed are for all of the various seizures and may not be interchangeable. Most of these medications have been thoroughly studied and used in breastfeeding women for years, with exception of gabapentin and lamotrigine. More recently, we have significant data on their use in breastfeeding mothers.

Treatment

- Patients with recurrent seizures should optimally be cared for by a neurologist.

- Termination of an acute seizure: Glucose; lorazepam or diazepam as first-line agent; phenytoin or phosphenytoin as second-line agent; phenobarbital as third-line agent.

- Epilepsy is treated with many different medications, including valproic acid, carbamazepine, topiramate, lamotrigine, oxcarbazepine, levetiracetam, gabapentin, pregabalin, ethosuximide, felbamate, and clonazepam.

Medications

- CARBAMAZEPINE   (*Tegretol, Epitol, Carbatrol*)
    - AAP = Maternal Medication Usually Compatible with Breastfeeding
    - LRC = L2
    - RID = 3.8-5.9%
    - Pregnancy = D
    - Comment: Carbamazepine (CBZ) is a unique anticonvulsant commonly used for grand mal, clonic-tonic, simple, and complex seizures. It is also used in manic depression and a number of other neurologic syndromes. It is one of the most commonly used anticonvulsants in pediatric patients.

      In a brief study by Kaneko, with maternal plasma levels averaging 4.3 μg/mL, milk levels were 1.9 mg/L. In a study of three patients who received from 5.8 to 7.3 mg/kg/day carbamazepine, milk levels were reported to vary from 1.3 to 1.8 mg/L, while the epoxide metabolite varied from 0.5 to 1.1 mg/L. No adverse effects were noted in any of the infants. In another study by Niebyl, breastmilk levels were 1.4 mg/L in the lipid fraction and 2.3 mg/L in the skim fraction in a mother receiving 1000 mg daily of carbamazepine. This author estimated that the daily intake of 2 mg carbamazepine daily (0.5 mg/kg) in an infant ingesting 1 L of milk per day.

In a study of CBZ and its epoxide metabolite (ECBZ) in milk, 16 patients received an average dose of 13.8 mg/kg/d. The average maternal serum levels of CBZ and ECBZ were 7.1 and 2.6 µg/mL, respectively. The average milk levels of CBZ and ECBZ were 2.5 and 1.5 mg/L, respectively. The relative percent of CBZ and ECBZ in milk were 36.4% and 53% of the maternal serum levels. A total of 50 milk samples in 19 patients were analyzed. Of these, the lowest CBZ concentration in milk was 1.0 mg/L; the highest was 4.8 mg/L. The CBZ level was determined in seven infants four to seven days postpartum. All infants have CBZ levels below 1.5 µg/mL.

In a study of seven women receiving 250-800 mg/d carbamazepine, the CBZ level ranged from 2.8-4.5 mg/L in milk to 3.2-15.0 mg/L in plasma. The levels of ECBZ ranged from 0.5-1.7 mg/L in milk to 0.8-4.8 mg/L in plasma.

The amount of CBZ transferred to the infant is apparently quite low. Although the half-life of CBZ in infants appears shorter than in adults, infants should still be monitored for sedative effects.

- ETHOSUXIMIDE (*Zarontin*)

  ○ AAP = Maternal Medication Usually Compatible with Breastfeeding

  ○ LRC = L4

  ○ RID = 31.5%

  ○ Pregnancy = C

  ○ Comment: Ethosuximide is an anticonvulsant used in epilepsy. Rane's data suggest that although significant levels of ethosuximide are transferred into human milk, the plasma level in the infant is quite low. A peak milk concentration of approximately 55 mg/L was reported at one month postpartum. Milk/plasma ratios were reported to be 1.03 on day three postpartum and 0.8 during the first three months of therapy. The infant's plasma reached a peak (2.9 mg/dl) at approximately 1.5 months postpartum, and then declined significantly over the next three months, suggesting increased clearance by the infant. Although these levels are considered subtherapeutic, it is suggested that the infant's plasma levels be occasionally tested.

  In another study of a woman receiving 500 mg twice daily, her milk levels, as estimated from a graph, averaged 60-70 mg/L. A total daily exposure to ethosuximide of 3.6-11 mg/kg as a result of nursing was predicted.

  In a study by Kuhnz of ten epileptic breastfeeding mothers (and 13 infants) receiving 3.5 to 23.6 mg/kg/day, the breastmilk concentrations were similar to those of the maternal plasma (milk/serum: 0.86) and the breastfed infants maintained serum levels between 15 and 40 µg/mL. Maximum milk concentration reported was 77 mg/L, although the average was 49.54 mg/L. Neonatal behavior complications, such as poor suckling, sedation, and hyperexcitability, occurred in 7 of the 12 infants. Interestingly, one infant who was not breastfed, exhibited severe withdrawal symptoms, such as tremors, restlessness, insomnia, crying, and vomiting which lasted for eight weeks, causing a slow weight gain. Thus the question remains, is it safer to breastfeed and avoid these severe withdrawal reactions?

  These studies clearly indicate that the amount of ethosuximide transferred to the infant is significant. With milk/plasma ratios of approximately 0.86-1.0 and relatively high maternal plasma levels, the maternal plasma levels are a good indication of the dose transferred to the infant. Milk levels are generally high. Caution is recommended.

- GABAPENTIN   (*Neurontin*)
  - AAP = Not reviewed
  - LRC = L2
  - RID = 6.6%
  - Pregnancy = C
  - Comment: Gabapentin is an older anticonvulsant used primarily for partial (focal) seizures, with or without secondary generalization. It is also used for postherpetic neuralgia or neuropathic pain. Unlike many anticonvulsants, gabapentin is almost completely excreted renally without metabolism; it does not induce hepatic enzymes and is remarkably well tolerated. In a study of one breastfeeding mother who was receiving 1800 mg/d, milk levels were 11.1, 11.3, and 11.0 mg/L at two, four, and eight hours, respectively, following a dose of 600 mg. The milk-plasma ratio was calculated to be 0.86 and the relative infant dose was 2.34%. No adverse effects to gabapentin were noted in the infant. In another patient receiving 2400 mg/d, milk levels were 9.8, 9.0, and 7.2 mg/L at two, four, and eight hours, respectively, after a dose of 800 mg. Using these data, an infant would consume approximately 3.7% to 6.5% of the weight-adjusted maternal dose per day. No adverse events were noted in these two infants.

    In another study of five mother-infant pairs receiving 900-3200 mg gabapentin per day, the mean milk/plasma ratio ranged from 0.7 to 1.3 from two weeks to three months postpartum. At two to three weeks, two of the five infants had detectable concentrations of gabapentin (1.3 and 1.5 uM) and one was undetectable. These levels were far below the normal plasma levels in the mothers (11-45 uM). Assuming a daily milk intake of 150 mL/kg/day, the infant dose of gabapentin was estimated to be 0.2-1.3 mg/kg/day, which is equivalent to 1.3-3.8% of the weight-normalized dose received by the mother. The plasma levels of gabapentin collected after three months of breastfeeding in another infant was 1.9 μM. The authors concluded that the plasma levels measured were low, if at all detectable in the infants, and no adverse effects were reported in these infants.

- LAMOTRIGINE   (*Lamictal*)
  - AAP = Drugs whose effect on nursing infants is unknown but may be of concern
  - LRC = L3
  - RID = 9.2 – 18.3%
  - Pregnancy = C
  - Comment: Lamotrigine is a newer anticonvulsant primarily indicated for treatment of simple and complex partial seizures.

    In a study of a 24-year-old female receiving 300 mg/day lamotrigine during pregnancy, maternal serum levels and cord levels of lamotrigine at birth were 3.88 μg/mL in the mother and 3.26 μg/mL in the cord blood. By day 22, the maternal serum levels were 9.61 μg/mL, the milk concentration was 6.51 mg/L, and the infant's serum level was 2.25 μg/mL. Following a reduction in dose, the prior levels decreased significantly over the next weeks. The milk/plasma ratio at the highest maternal serum level was 0.562. The estimated dose to infant would be approximately 2-5 mg per day assuming a maternal dose of 200-300 mg per day. The infant developed normally in every way.

    In another study of a single mother receiving 200 mg/day lamotrigine, milk levels of lamotrigine immediately prior to the next dose (trough) at steady state were 3.48 mg/L (13.6 uM). The authors estimated the daily dose to infant to be 0.5 mg/kg/day. The above authors suggest that infants, while developing normally, should probably be monitored periodically for plasma levels of lamotrigine.

The manufacturer reports that in a group of five women (no dose listed), breastmilk concentrations of lamotrigine ranged from 0.07-5.03 mg/L. Breastmilk levels averaged 40-45% of maternal plasma levels. No untoward effects were noted in the infants.

In a study by Ohman of nine breastfeeding women at three weeks postpartum, the median milk/plasma ratio was 0.61, and the breastfed infants maintained lamotrigine concentrations of approximately 30% of the mothers' plasma levels. The authors estimated the dose to the infant at 0.2-1 mg/kg/d. No adverse effects were noted in the infants.

One further study of six breastfeeding women consuming from 175-800 (mean = 400) mg/day resulted in average infant doses of 0.45 mg/kg/day, and an average infant plasma concentration of 0.6 mg/L. No adverse effects in the infants were noted.

In a study of four mothers with partial epilepsy on lamotrigine monotherapy, serum levels of lamotrigine in nursing newborns ranged from <1.0 to 2.0 µg/mL on day 10 of life. Three babies had lamotrigine levels >1.0 µg/mL. Lamotrigine levels in newborns were on average 30% (range 20-43%) of the maternal drug level. Unfortunately, no decline was noted in two children with repeat levels at two months. The authors suggested significant genetic variability in the infants' ability to metabolize this drug. Close monitoring of the infant plasma levels was recommended.

In a recent and well-done study of 30 women under treatment with lamotrigine for seizure disorders, the average milk/plasma ratio was 0.413. Infant plasma levels were 18.3% of maternal plasma levels. The theoretical daily infant dose was 0.51 mg/kg/day and the relative infant dose was 9.2% (range=3.1-21.1%). Most important, this study indicates that there is wide variability in milk levels that seem to be more related to the pharmacogenetic makeup of the individual than the dose.

It is important to remember, that the theoretic infant dose in these studies, that ranges from 0.51 mg/kg/day to perhaps as high as 1 mg/kg/day, is still significantly less than the therapeutic dose (4.4 mg/k/day) administered to 17-day-old infants with neonatal seizures. However, one case of severe apnea has been recently reported in a 16-day-old breastfed infant. In this case, the mother was receiving 850 mg/day and had a plasma level of 14.93 µg/mL. The plasma level of the infant was 4.87 µg/mL. Interestingly, the milk/plasma ratio was higher, 0.79 to 0.96, suggesting higher transfer into milk than in the above studies.

The use of lamotrigine in breastfeeding mothers produces significant plasma levels in some breastfed infants, although they are apparently not high enough to produce side effects in most cases. Exposure in utero is considerably higher, and levels will probably drop in newborn breastfed infants. Nevertheless, it is advisable to monitor the infant's plasma levels closely to insure safety.

- LEVETIRACETAM   (*Keppra*)
  - ○ AAP = Not reviewed
  - ○ LRC = L3
  - ○ RID = 3.4% - 7.8%
  - ○ Pregnancy = C
  - ○ Comment: Levetiracetam is a popular broad-spectrum antiepileptic agent. In a study of a single patient who received levetiracetam at seven days postpartum (dose unreported), the breastmilk concentrations of levetiracetam were 99 µM three hours after administration. The corresponding plasma levels were 32 µM (milk/plasma ratio= 3.09). The mother was also ingesting phenytoin

(3 x 100 mg/day) as well as valproic acid (4 x 500 mg/d). The infant was preterm (36 weeks) and unstable at birth. After the addition of levetiracetam at day seven, the infant became increasingly hypotonic and drank poorly. The infant was removed from the breast, and 96 hours later the infant's plasma levetiracetam levels were 6 μM. The authors strongly advise avoidance of levetiracetam, and close monitoring of the infant in breastfeeding mothers. In this case, the infant was exposed to three anticonvulsants, and it is difficult to suggest that levetiracetam was solely responsible for the hypnotic condition. This is further supported by the study below.

In a new study of eight women receiving from 1500 to 3500 mg/day who were studied at birth (seven patients) and one at ten months, the mean umbilical cord serum/maternal serum ratio was 1.14 (n= 4) at birth, suggesting extensive transport of levetiracetam to the fetus. The mean milk/maternal serum concentration ratio was 1.00 (range, 0.7-1.33) at three to five days after delivery (n= 7). Maternal milk levels ranged from 28 to 153 μM (4.8-26 μg/mL), but averaged 74 μM (12.6 mg/L). At three to five days after delivery, the infants had very low levetiracetam serum concentrations (<10-15 μM) (1.7-2.5 μg/mL), a finding that persisted during continued breastfeeding. One infant had a levetiracetam level of 77 uM (13 μg/mL) at day one, but <10 μM at day four, suggesting infants clear this product rapidly, and that breastfeeding contributes only a minimal dose. No malformations were detected at birth. No adverse effects were noted in any of the breastfeeding infants. The authors conclude that levetiracetam passes to the infant, but breastfed infants have very low serum concentrations, suggesting a rapid elimination of levetiracetam.

Another study of 14 women receiving 1,000 to 3,000 mg per day had a milk-to-plasma ratio of 1.05, with an infant dose of 2.4 mg/kg/day, or 7.9% of the maternal dose. Plasma concentrations in the infants were 13% of those in the mother's plasma, ranging from 4 to 20 μmol/L. There was no evidence of accumulation of levetiracetam in this study. The authors suggest that this study should be reassuring for breastfeeding mothers taking levetiracetam.

- OXCARBAZEPINE   (*Trileptal*)
  ○ AAP = Not reviewed
  ○ LRC = L3
  ○ RID =
  ○ Pregnancy = C
  ○ Comment: Oxcarbazepine is a derivative of carbamazepine and is used in the treatment of partial seizures in adults, and as adjunctive therapy in the treatment of partial seizures in children. It is rapidly metabolized to a longer half-life active metabolite, 10-hydroxy-carbazepine (MHD). In a brief and somewhat incomplete study of a pregnant patient who received 300 mg three times daily while pregnant, plasma levels were studied in her infant for the first five days postpartum, while the infant was breastfeeding. While no breastmilk levels were reported, plasma levels of MHD were essentially the same as the mother's immediately after delivery, suggesting complete transfer transplacentally of the drug. However, while breastfeeding for the next five days, plasma levels of MHD in the infant declined significantly from approximately 7 μg/mL to 0.2 μg/mL on the fifth day. The decay of MHD concentrations in neonatal plasma during the first four days postpartum indicated first order elimination. The plasma MHD levels on day five amounted to 7% of those on day one postpartum (93% drop in five days). The authors estimated the milk/plasma ratio to be 0.5. No neonatal side effects were reported by the authors.

- **PHENOBARBITAL** (*Luminal*)
  - AAP = Drugs associated with significant side effects and should be given with caution
  - LRC = L3
  - RID = 24%
  - Pregnancy = D
  - Comment: Phenobarbital is a long half-life barbiturate frequently used as an anticonvulsant in adults and during the neonatal period. Its long half-life in infants may lead to significant accumulation and blood levels higher than in the mother, although this is infrequent. During the first three to four weeks of life, phenobarbital is poorly absorbed by the neonatal GI tract. However, protein binding by neonatal albumin is poor, 36-43%, as compared to the adult, 51%. Thus the volume of distribution is higher in neonates, and the tissue concentrations of phenobarbital may be significantly higher. The half-life in premature infants can be extremely long (100-500 hours) and plasma levels must be closely monitored. Although varied, milk/plasma ratios vary from 0.46 to 0.6.

    In one study, following a dose of 30 mg four times daily, the milk concentration of phenobarbital averaged 2.74 mg/L 16 hours after the last dose. The dose an infant would receive was estimated at 2-4 mg/day.

    Phenobarbital should be administered with caution and close observation of the infant is required, including plasma drug levels. One should generally expect the infant's plasma level to be approximately 30-40% of the maternal level. In some reported cases, the infant plasma levels have reached twice what the maternal plasma levels were 2.5 hours after the maternal dose.

- **PHENYTOIN** (*Dilantin*)
  - AAP = Maternal Medication Usually Compatible with Breastfeeding
  - LRC = L2
  - RID = 0.6-7.7%
  - Pregnancy = D
  - Comment: Phenytoin is an old and efficient anticonvulsant. It is secreted in small amounts into breastmilk. The effect on the infant is generally considered minimal if the levels in the maternal circulation are kept in low-normal range (10 µg/mL). Phenytoin levels peak in milk at 3.5 hours.

    In one study of six women receiving 200-400 mg/day, plasma concentrations varied from 12.8 to 78.5 µmol/L, while their milk levels ranged from 1.61 to 2.95 mg/L. The milk/plasma ratios were low, ranging from 0.06 to 0.18. In only two of these infants were plasma concentrations of phenytoin detectible (0.46 and 0.72 µmol/L). No untoward effects were noted in any of these infants.

    Others have reported milk levels of 6 µg/mL, or 0.8 µg/mL. Although the actual concentration in milk varies significantly between studies, the milk/plasma ratio appears relatively similar at 0.13 to 0.45. Breastmilk concentrations varied from 0.26 to 1.5 mg/L, depending on the maternal dose.

    In a mother receiving 250 mg twice daily, milk levels were 0.26 and the milk/plasma ratio was 0.45. The maternal plasma level of phenytoin was 0.58. In another study of two patients receiving 300-600 mg/d, the average milk level was 1.9 mg/L. The maximum observed milk level was 2.6 mg/L.

    The neonatal half-life of phenytoin is highly variable for the first week of life. Monitoring of the infants' plasma may be useful, although it is not definitely required. All of the current studies indicate rather low levels of phenytoin in breastmilk and minimal plasma levels in breastfeeding infants.

- PRIMIDONE   (*Mysoline*)
  - AAP = Drugs associated with significant side effects and should be given with caution
  - LRC = L3
  - RID = 8.4-8.6%
  - Pregnancy = D
  - Comment: Primidone is metabolized in adults to several derivatives, including phenobarbital. After chronic therapy, levels of phenobarbital rise to a therapeutic range. Hence, problems for the infant would not only include primidone, but, subsequently, phenobarbital. In one study of two women receiving primidone, the steady-state concentrations of primidone in neonatal serum via ingestion of breastmilk were 0.7 and 2.5 μg/mL. The steady-state "phenobarbital" levels in neonatal serum were between 2.0 to 13.0 μg/mL. The calculated dose of phenobarbital per day received by each infant ranged from 1.8 to 8.9 mg/day. Some sedation has been reported, particularly during the neonatal period. See phenobarbital.

- TOPIRAMATE   (*Topamax*)
  - AAP = Not reviewed
  - LRC = L3
  - RID = 24.5%
  - Pregnancy = C
  - Comment: Topiramate is an anticonvulsant used in controlling refractory partial seizures. In a group of two women receiving topiramate (150-200 mg/day) at three weeks postpartum, the mean milk/plasma ratio was 0.86 (range=0.67-1.1). The concentration of topiramate in milk averaged 7.9 uM (range = 1.6 to 13.7). The weight normalized relative infant dose (RID), assuming a milk intake of 150 mL/kg/d, was 3-23% of the maternal dose/day. The absolute infant dose was 0.1 to 0.7 mg/kg/day. The plasma concentrations of topiramate in two infants were 1.4 and 1.6 uM, respectively. The plasma level in another infant was undetectable. The plasma concentrations in the two infants were 10-20% of the maternal plasma level. At four weeks, the milk/plasma ratio had dropped to 0.69, and plasma levels in the infant were <0.9 uM and 2.1 uM, respectively.

    Topiramate has become increasingly popular due to its fewer adverse side effects. Since plasma levels found in breastfeeding infants were significantly less than in maternal plasma, the risk of using this product in breastfeeding mothers is probably acceptable. Close observation for sedation is advised.

- VALPROIC ACID   (*Depakene, Depakote*)
  - AAP = Maternal Medication Usually Compatible with Breastfeeding
  - LRC = L2
  - RID = 1.4-1.7%
  - Pregnancy = D
  - Comment: Valproic acid is a popular anticonvulsant used in grand mal, petit mal, myoclonic, and temporal lobe seizures. In a study of 16 patients receiving 300-2400 mg/d, valproic acid concentrations ranged from 0.4 to 3.9 mg/L (mean=1.9 mg/L). The milk/plasma ratio averaged 0.05.

In a study of one patient receiving 250 mg twice daily, milk levels ranged from 0.18 to 0.47 mg/L. The milk/plasma ratio ranged from 0.01 to 0.02. Alexander reports milk levels of 5.1 mg/L following a larger dose of up to 1600 mg/d.

In a study of six women receiving 9.5 to 31 mg/kg/d valproic acid, milk levels averaged 1.4 mg/L, while serum levels averaged 45.1 mg/L. The average milk/serum ratio was 0.027.

Most authors agree that the amount of valproic acid transferring to the infant via milk is low. Breastfeeding would appear safe. However, the infant may need monitoring for liver and platelet changes.

Clinical Tips

Phenytoin is an old and efficient anticonvulsant. Present studies show that the amount transferred into milk is rather low and may be too low to be detected in most infants. Published milk levels suggest levels in the range of 0.26 to 1.9 mg per liter of milk. If maternal plasma levels are kept in the 10 µg/mL range, the amount transferred to the infant should be very low. Carbamazepine is an excellent anticonvulsant, particularly in pediatric patients, due to its limited sedative properties. When used in breastfeeding mothers in doses of 200-800 mg/day, breastmilk levels varied from 1.3 to 3.6 mg per liter of milk. Plasma levels in these infants were subclinical, less than 1 µg/ml. Accumulation in the infant has not been reported. While carbamazepine may induce blood dyscrasia in adults, it has not been reported in children.

Phenobarbital has been studied extensively in breastfeeding women. The amount ingested by breastfeeding infants varies from 2 to 4 mg per day. While in an older infant, this may not prove problematic; in a newborn, it could produce accumulation the first month postpartum. Further, the half-life of phenobarbital in newborns is quite long (100-500 hours), and some accumulation and sedation has been reported. Therefore, when using phenobarbital in breastfeeding mothers early postpartum, the infants' plasma levels should be monitored closely for toxic levels. Primidone is metabolized to phenobarbital and should be used with similar precautions to phenobarbital. Valproic acid transfers poorly into human milk. Reported milk levels are generally less than 0.17 to 0.47 mg per liter of milk. No untoward effects have been reported. Reported levels of ethosuximide in milk are 55 mg per liter, with reported peak infant plasma levels of 29 µg/mL after one month, which is subclinical. These data suggested that nursing was safe with normal maternal doses of ethosuximide.

Gabapentin levels in milk range as a function of dose. Reported levels in milk range from 11.1 mg/L (dose =1800 mg/d) to 9.8 mg/L (dose = 2400 mg/d). Relative infant doses range from 2.34% to as high as 6.5%. No adverse side effects were noted in these studies.

We have a number of studies suggesting that lamotrigine is a suitable anticonvulsant for breastfeeding mothers, but due to higher milk levels, caution is still recommended. Topiramate levels in milk are high, but levels in infants appear low. Some caution is recommended with this product as well, particularly in an infant with poor clearance.

Levels of levetiracetam in breastmilk appears somewhat lower than with topiramate or lamotrigine. In some studies, it does not appear to concentrate in infants.

Suggested Reading

Aylward, R. L. (2008). Epilepsy: a review of reports, guidelines, recommendations and models for the provision of care for patients with epilepsy. *Clin Med, 8*(4), 433-438.

French, J. A., & Pedley, T. A. (2008). Clinical practice. Initial management of epilepsy. *N Engl J Med, 359*(2), 166-176.

Noe, K. H. (2007). Gender-specific challenges in the management of epilepsy in women. *Semin Neurol, 27*(4), 331-339.

Roste, L. S., & Tauboll, E. (2007). Women and epilepsy: review and practical recommendations. *Expert Rev Neurother, 7*(3), 289-300.

Somerville, E. R., Cook, M. J., & O'Brien, T. J. (2009). Pregnancy treatment guidelines: throwing the baby out with the bath water. *Epilepsia, 50*(9), 2172.

Stein, M. A., & Kanner, A. M. (2009). Management of newly diagnosed epilepsy: a practical guide to monotherapy. *Drugs, 69*(2), 199-222.

Tettenborn, B. (2006). Management of epilepsy in women of childbearing age: practical recommendations. *CNS Drugs, 20*(5), 373-387.

Vajda, F. J. (2008). Treatment options for pregnant women with epilepsy. *Expert Opin Pharmacother, 9*(11), 1859-1868.

Septic Pelvic Thrombophlebitis / Ovarian Vein Thrombophlebitis

Principles of Therapy

These rare conditions may occur separately or simultaneously. The diagnosis may be considered in postpartum women (usually within one to two weeks from delivery) with persistent fevers. The differential diagnosis includes endometritis. Septic pelvic thrombophlebitis is usually diagnosed when fevers persist after antibiotic treatment for suspected endometritis. A clot visualized by CT may make the diagnosis earlier, but is not commonly seen. Women with ovarian vein thrombophlebitis may have abdominal pain, but those with septic pelvic thrombophlebitis often lack symptoms outside of persistent fevers. Septic pelvic thrombophlebitis is usually a diagnosis of exclusion in situations of persistent spiking fevers when the patient appears otherwise well. Clinical evidence of septic embolization from these syndromes is rare. Risk factors include: surgery, pregnancy, infection, fibroids, and malignancy. In the postpartum population, it occurs most commonly in the setting of cesarean delivery complicated by infection. CT is useful, even when the clot is not visualized, to exclude other etiologies for infection such as pelvic abscess. CT and MRI are of similar effectiveness in diagnosis, whereas pelvic ultrasound is less optimal.

Treatment includes broad spectrum antibiotics to cover common causes of endometritis. Typically ampicillin, gentamycin, and clindamycin. The optimal duration of treatment is not known, but typically antibiotics are continued for at least 48 hours after the patient has defervesced. Often the use of anticoagulation is also employed. Unfractionated heparin is most commonly used, but optimal duration of therapy is unclear. Anticoagulation is usually continued until the patient has defervesced and antibiotics are discontinued. Some authors favor continued anticoagulation after hospital discharge for a period of four to six weeks if a clot is visualized, while other authors do not support the use of anticoagulation for the condition at all.

Treatment

- Broad spectrum antibiotics (ampicillin, gentamycin, clindamycin, ertapenem, imipenem)

- Possible anticoagulation (typically with enoxaparin)

- CT frequently does not visualize the thrombus (noted in approximately 20% of cases), but is useful to exclude other etiology for fever.

Medications

- AMPICILLIN   (*Polycillin, Omnipen*)
    - ◦ AAP = Not reviewed
    - ◦ LRC = L1

- ◦ RID = 0.2-0.5%
- ◦ Pregnancy = B
- ◦ Comment: Low milk/plasma ratios of 0.2 have been reported. In a study by Matsuda of three breastfeeding patients who received 500 mg of ampicillin orally, levels in milk peaked at six hours and averaged only 0.14 mg/L of milk. The milk/plasma ratio was reported to be 0.03 at two hours. In a group of nine breastfeeding women sampled at various times and who received doses of 350 mg TID orally, milk concentrations ranged from 0.06 to 0.17 mg/L, with peak milk levels at three to four hours after the dose. Milk/plasma ratios varied between 0.01 and 0.58. The highest reported milk level (1.02 mg/L) was in a patient receiving 700 mg TID. Ampicillin was not detected in the plasma of any infant.

- AMPICILLIN + SULBACTAM   (*Unasyn*)
  - ◦ AAP = Not reviewed
  - ◦ LRC = L1
  - ◦ RID = 0.5-1.5%
  - ◦ Pregnancy = B
  - ◦ Comment: Small amounts of ampicillin may transfer (1 mg/L). Possible rash, sensitization, diarrhea, or candidiasis could occur, but is unlikely. This drug may alter GI flora. After a dose of 0.5 to 1 gram, sulbactam is secreted into milk at an average concentration of 0.52 μg/mL. This would lead to a maximal dose of 0.7 mg/kg/day in a breastfeeding infant, which equates to less than 1% of the maternal dose. Therefore, untoward effects are unlikely in a breastfeeding infant.

- CEFOTETAN   (*Cefotan*)
  - ◦ AAP = Not reviewed
  - ◦ LRC = L2
  - ◦ RID = 0.2-0.3%
  - ◦ Pregnancy = B
  - ◦ Comment: Cefotetan is a third generation cephalosporin that is poorly absorbed orally and is only available via IM and IV injection. The drug is distributed into human milk in low concentrations. Following a maternal dose of 1000 mg IM every 12 hours in five patients, breastmilk concentrations ranged from 0.29 to 0.59 mg/L. Plasma concentrations were almost 100 times higher. In a group of two to three women who received 1000 mg IV, the maximum average milk level reported was 0.2 mg/L at four hours, with a milk/plasma ratio of 0.02.

- CEFOXITIN   (*Mefoxin*)
  - ◦ AAP = Maternal Medication Usually Compatible with Breastfeeding
  - ◦ LRC = L1
  - ◦ RID = 0.1-0.3%
  - ◦ Pregnancy = B
  - ◦ Comment: Cefoxitin is a cephalosporin antibiotic with a spectrum similar to the second generation family. It is transferred into human milk in very low levels. In a study of 18 women receiving 2000-4000 mg doses, only one breastmilk sample contained cefoxitin (0.9 mg/L), all the rest were too low to be detected. In another study of two to three women who received 1000 mg IV, only trace amounts were reported in milk over six hours. In a group of five women who received an IM

injection of 2000 mg, the highest milk levels were reported at four hours after dose. The maternal plasma levels varied from 22.5 at two hours to 77.6 µg/mL at four hours. Maternal milk levels ranged from <0.25 to 0.65 mg/L. Observe for changes in gut flora.

- CLINDAMYCIN   (*Cleocin, Cleocin T*)
  - ◦ AAP = Maternal Medication Usually Compatible with Breastfeeding
  - ◦ LRC = L2
  - ◦ RID   = 1.7%
  - ◦ Pregnancy = B
  - ◦ Comment: Clindamycin is a broad-spectrum antibiotic frequently used for anaerobic infections. In one study of two nursing mothers and following doses of 600 mg IV every six hours, the concentration of clindamycin in breastmilk was 3.1 to 3.8 mg/L at 0.2 to 0.5 hours after dosing. Following oral doses of 300 mg every six hours, the breastmilk levels averaged 1.0 to 1.7 mg/L at 1.5 to seven hours after dosing. In another study of two to three women who received a single oral dose of 150 mg, milk levels averaged 0.9 mg/L at four hours, with a milk/plasma ratio of 0.47.

    An alteration of GI flora is possible, even though the dose is low. One case of bloody stools (pseudomembranous colitis) has been associated with clindamycin and gentamicin therapy on day five postpartum, but this is considered rare. In this case, the mother of a newborn infant was given 600 mg IV every six hours. In rare cases, pseudomembranous colitis can appear several weeks later.

    In a study by Steen, in five breastfeeding patients who received 150 mg three times daily for seven days, milk concentrations ranged from <0.5 to 3.1 mg/L, with the majority of levels <0.5 mg/L. There are a number of pediatric clinical uses of clindamycin (anaerobic infections, bacterial endocarditis, pelvic inflammatory disease, and bacterial vaginosis). The current pediatric dosage recommendation is 10-40 mg/kg/day divided every six to eight hours. In a study of 15 women who received 600 mg clindamycin intravenously, levels of clindamycin in milk averaged 1.03 mg/L at two hours following the dose. The amount of clindamycin in milk is unlikely to harm a breastfeeding infant.

- DALTEPARIN SODIUM   (*Fragmin, Low Molecular Weight Heparin*)
  - ◦ AAP = Not reviewed
  - ◦ LRC = L2
  - ◦ RID   = 15%
  - ◦ Pregnancy = B
  - ◦ Comment: Dalteparin is a low molecular weight polysaccharide fragment of heparin used clinically as an anticoagulant. In a study of two patients who received 5000-10,000 IU of dalteparin, none was found in human milk. In another study of 15 post-cesarean patients early postpartum (mean = 5.7 days), blood and milk levels of dalteparin were determined three to four hours post-treatment. Following subcutaneous doses of 2500 IU, maternal plasma levels averaged 0.074 to 0.308 IU/mL. Breastmilk levels of dalteparin ranged from <0.005 to 0.037 IU/mL of milk. Using these data, an infant ingesting 150 mL/kg/day would ingest approximately 5.5 IU/kg/day. Unfortunately, this study was done during the colostral phase, when virtually anything can enter milk. Thus the high RID is probably only for the first few days postpartum and would drop significantly after one week. More importantly, however, due to the polysaccharide nature of this production, oral absorption is unlikely, even in an infant.

- ENOXAPARIN   (*Lovenox, Low Molecular Weight Heparin*)
  - ○ AAP = Not reviewed
  - ○ LRC = L3
  - ○ RID =
  - ○ Pregnancy = B
  - ○ Comment: Enoxaparin is a low molecular weight fraction of heparin used clinically as an anticoagulant. In a study of 12 women receiving 20-40 mg of enoxaparin daily for up to five days postpartum for venous pathology (n = 4) or cesarean section (n = 8), no change in anti-Xa activity was noted in the breastfed infants. Because it is a peptide fragment of heparin, its molecular weight is large (2000-8000 daltons). The size alone would largely preclude its entry into human milk at levels clinically relevant. Due to minimal oral bioavailability, any present in milk would not be orally absorbed by the infant. A similar compound, dalteparin, has been studied and milk levels are extremely low as well. See dalteparin.

- ERTAPENEM   (*Invanz*)
  - ○ AAP = Not reviewed
  - ○ LRC = L2
  - ○ RID = 0.1-0.4%
  - ○ Pregnancy = B
  - ○ Comment: The manufacturer reports the concentration of ertapenem in breastmilk from five lactating women with pelvic infections (5 to 14 days postpartum) was measured at random time points daily for five consecutive days following the last 1 gm dose of intravenous therapy (three to ten days of therapy). The concentration of ertapenem in breastmilk within 24 hours of the last dose of therapy in all five women ranged from <0.13 (lower limit of quantitation) to 0.38 mg/L; peak concentrations were not assessed. By day five after discontinuation of therapy, the level of ertapenem was undetectable in the breastmilk of four women and below the lower limit of quantitation (<0.13 μg/mL) in one woman.

    The above data does not report Cmax concentrations in milk nor the time samples were collected, so it is virtually worthless for determining infant exposure to the medication during the day and following the administration.

    Using the above data and an assumed average weight of 70 kg, the mothers received about 14.28 mg/kg/day. After 24 hours, the infant would ingest about 57 μg/kg/day. The relative infant dose would be 0.4% of the maternal dose at this time. Without good data it is not possible to estimate clinical dose to the infant, but it is likely small and its oral bioavailability is poor. Most all the penicillins and the carbapenems are safe to use in breastfeeding mothers.

- GENTAMICIN   (*Garamycin*)
  - ○ AAP = Maternal Medication Usually Compatible with Breastfeeding
  - ○ LRC = L2
  - ○ RID = 2.1%
  - ○ Pregnancy = C
  - ○ Comment: Gentamicin is a narrow spectrum antibiotic generally used for gram negative infections. The oral absorption of gentamicin (<1%) is generally nil with the exception of premature neonates,

where small amounts may be absorbed. In one study of ten women given 80 mg three times daily IM for five days postpartum, milk levels were measured on day four. Gentamicin levels in milk were 0.42, 0.48, 0.49, and 0.41 mg/L at one, three, five, and seven hours, respectively. The milk/plasma ratios were 0.11 at one hour and 0.44 at seven hours. Plasma gentamicin levels in neonates were small, were found in only five of the ten neonates, and averaged 0.41 µg/mL. The authors estimate that daily ingestion via breastmilk would be 307 µg for a 3.6 kg neonate (normal neonatal dose = 2.5 mg/kg every 12 hours). These amounts would be clinically irrelevant in most infants.

- HEPARIN (*Heparin*)
  - ◦ AAP = Not reviewed
  - ◦ LRC = L1
  - ◦ RID =
  - ◦ Pregnancy = C
  - ◦ Comment: Although rarely used in angina, it may be initially used in some cases. Heparin is a large molecular weight protein used as an anticoagulant. It is used SC, IM, and IV because it is not absorbed orally. Due to its high molecular weight (range = 12,000-15,000 daltons), it is unlikely any would transfer into breastmilk. Any that did enter the milk would be rapidly destroyed in the gastric contents of the infant.

- IMIPENEM-CILASTATIN (*Primaxin*)
  - ◦ AAP = Not reviewed
  - ◦ LRC = L2
  - ◦ RID =
  - ◦ Pregnancy = C
  - ◦ Comment: Imipenem is structurally similar to penicillins and acts similarly. Cilastatin is added to extend the half-life of imipenem. Both imipenem and cilastatin are poorly absorbed orally and must be administered IM or IV. Imipenem is destroyed by gastric acidity. Transfer into breastmilk is probably minimal, but no data are available. Changes in GI flora could occur, but is probably remote.

- VANCOMYCIN (*Vancocin*)
  - ◦ AAP = Not reviewed
  - ◦ LRC = L1
  - ◦ RID = 6.7%
  - ◦ Pregnancy = C
  - ◦ Comment: Vancomycin is an antimicrobial agent. Only low levels are secreted into human milk. Milk levels were 12.7 mg/L four hours after infusion in one woman receiving 1 gm every 12 hours for seven days. Its poor absorption from the infant's GI tract would limit its systemic absorption. Low levels in the infant could provide alterations of GI flora.

Clinical Tips

A suspicion of septic pelvic thrombophlebitis (SPT) should arise when spiking fevers early postpartum, or in rarer cases following abortions, fail to respond to standard antibiotic therapy. Patients often complain of flank and lower pain which is constant. Now it is recognized that pelvic thromboplebitis is the probable diagnosis and can be confirmed by CT and MRI. While antibiotic management varies, more recent data suggests that ertapenem, or gentamicin, ampicillin or clindamycin for seven days is suitable. Earlier studies recommended clindamycin, gentamycin, and ampicillin, the so called "triple antibiotic regimen." While most institutions still recommend this therapy, if fever persists past five days of triple therapy, therapy with imipenim or ertapenem is now recommended.

Anticoagulation with enoxaparin (1 mg/Kg), or warfarin (INR 2.5) for longer durations, is also mandatory. Because therapy with heparin is controversial, the newer low molecular weight heparins (enoxaparin, dalteparin) are preferred. Length of treatment with antibiotics is variable, but seven to ten days is normal. The length of anticoagulation totally depends on CT or MRI findings. With confirmed right ovarian vein thrombosis, three to six months of anticoagulation is required. With pelvic branch vein thrombosis, two weeks for longer is required. With negative findings for pelvic thrombi, one week of anticoagulation is recommended.

Suggested Reading

Brown C.E., Stettler R.W., Twickler D., Cunningham F.G. (1999). Puerperal septic pelvic thrombophlebitis: incidence and response to heparin therapy. *Am J Obstet and Gynecol.* *181*(1):143-8.

Garcia J. Aboujaoude R., Apuzzio J. Alvarez J.R. (2006). Septic pelvic thrombophlebitis: diagnosis and management. *Infect Dis Obstet gynecol. 2006*: 15614.

Twickler D.M., Setiawan A.T., Evans R.S., Erdman W.A., Stettler R.W., Brown C.E., Cunningham F.G. (1997). Imaging of puerperal septic thrombophlebitis: prospective comparison of MR imaging, CT, and sonography. *AJR Am J roentgenol. 169*(4):1039-43.

Smoking Cessation

Principles of Therapy

Tobacco (smoking and other forms) is considered a substance abuse disorder. Its use is the largest cause of preventable early death in the USA. Nicotine is one of the most addictive substances in existence, and 20-25% of adult Americans smoke cigarettes regularly. Nicotine replacement therapy is designed to replace the plasma levels of nicotine in a form other than tobacco in order to reduce withdrawal symptoms and aid in withdrawal from the use of tobacco. Presently in the USA, nicotine replacements are in the form of chewable gum and nicotine patches for transcutaneous absorption. Nicotine patches are designed to continuously release nicotine into the cutaneous and subcutaneous layers of the skin, which then facilitates systemic absorption. Plasma levels attained are determined by the dose in the patch or gum, but, in general, produce levels significantly less than that obtained by smoking. The dose administered is then gradually reduced. Recently, the introduction of an older antidepressant, bupropion (Wellbutrin, Zyban) in a new dosage form is sometimes used for smoking cessation therapy. A new oral product varenicline (Chantix) appears more effective than placebo, bupropion, and the transdermal nicotine patches, although it has a number of neurologic complications.

Treatment

- Counseling, behavioral therapy, hypnosis, and acupuncture are non-pharmacologic therapies which may be attempted.

- Provider initiated 5A intervention: Ask, Advise, Assess, Assist and Arrange.

- Nicotine replacement therapy is supplied to the patient through nicotine patches, gum, lozenges, intra-nasally, or an inhaler. Many of these formulations are available without a prescription. Generally, the approach is to wean the nicotine dose over a few months.

- Varenicline is a nicotine receptor partial agonist and blocker. It reduces craving and blocks the nicotine effect from exogenous sources (cigarettes, etc.).

- Bupropion treatment has been shown to increase smoking cessation marginally.

Medications

- BUPROPION   (*Wellbutrin, Zyban*)
    - AAP = Drugs whose effect on nursing infants is unknown but may be of concern
    - LRC = L3
    - RID = 0.2-2%
    - Pregnancy = C

- Comment: Bupropion is an older antidepressant, with a structure unrelated to tricyclics. One report in the literature indicates that bupropion probably accumulates in human milk, although the absolute dose transferred appears minimal, as in three infants studied, no bupropion was detected in the plasma compartment.

  Following one 100 mg dose in a mother, the milk/plasma ratio ranged from 2.51 to 8.58, clearly suggesting a concentrating mechanism for this drug in human milk. However, plasma levels of bupropion (or its metabolites) in the infant were undetectable, indicating that the dose transferred to the infant was low, and accumulation in infant plasma apparently did not occur under these conditions (infant was fed 7.5 to 9.5 hours after dosing). The peak milk bupropion level (0.189 mg/L) occurred two hours after a 100 mg dose. This milk level would provide 0.66% of the maternal dose, a dose that is likely to be clinically insignificant to a breastfed infant.

  In a recent study of two breastfeeding patients consuming 75 mg twice daily and 150 mg (sustained release) daily, respectively, no bupropion or metabolite were detected in either breastfed infant. In the first patient at 17 weeks postpartum, plasma levels were drawn at two hours postdose and bupropion or hydroxybupropion levels were undetectable. In the second patient at 29 weeks postpartum, bupropion and hydroxybupropion were undetectable as well. The limit of detection for bupropion was 5-10 ng/mL and for hydroxybupropion was 100-200 ng/mL.

  In a study of 10 breastfeeding patients who received 150 mg bupropion SR daily for two days and then 300 mg bupropion SR daily thereafter for five more days, milk concentrations of bupropion averaged 45 μg/L. The average infant dose via milk was 6.75 μg/kg/day. The reported relative infant dose was 0.14% of the weight-normalized maternal dose. When the active metabolites present in milk were added, the RID would be 2% of the maternal dose. No side effects were noted in any of the infants.

  Seizures in a six-month-old breastfed infant were recently reported four days following administration of 150 mg/day bupropion in the mother. The mother discontinued bupropion and continued breastfeeding. No further seizures were reported.

  Due to persistent case reports to the author, bupropion may, in some women, suppress milk production. Some caution is recommended concerning changes to milk supply.

- NICOTINE PATCHES, GUM, INHALER   (*Habitrol, NicoDerm, Nicotrol, ProStep*)

  - AAP = Not reviewed
  - LRC = L2
  - RID =
  - Pregnancy = X if used in overdose
  - Comment: Nicotine and its metabolite cotinine are both present in milk. Fifteen lactating women (mean age, 32 years; mean weight, 72 kg) who were smokers (mean of 17 cigarettes per day) participated in a trial of the nicotine patch to assist in smoking cessation. Serial milk samples were collected from the women over sequential 24-hour periods when they were smoking and when they were stabilized on the 21-mg/d, 14-mg/d, and 7-mg/d nicotine patches. Nicotine and cotinine concentrations in milk were not significantly different between smoking (mean of 17 cigarettes per day) and the 21-mg/d patch, but concentrations were significantly lower when patients were using the 14-mg/d and 7-mg/d patches than when smoking. There was also a downward trend in absolute infant dose (nicotine equivalents) from smoking or the 21-mg patch through to the 14-mg and 7-mg patches. Milk intake by the breastfed infants was similar while their mothers were smoking (585 mL/d) and subsequently when their mothers were using the 21-mg (717 mL/d), 14-mg (731 mL/d),

and 7-mg (619 mL/d) patches. The authors conclude that the absolute infant dose of nicotine and its metabolite cotinine decreases by about 70% from when subjects were smoking or using the 21-mg patch to when they were using the 7-mg patch. In addition, use of the nicotine patch had no significant influence on the milk intake by the breastfed infant. Undertaking maternal smoking cessation with the nicotine patch is, therefore, a safer option than continued smoking.

With nicotine gum, maternal serum nicotine levels average 30-60% of those found in cigarette smokers. While patches (transdermal systems) produce a sustained and lower nicotine plasma level, nicotine gum may produce large variations in peak levels when the gum is chewed rapidly, fluctuations similar to smoking itself. Mothers who choose to use nicotine gum and breastfeed should be counseled to refrain from breastfeeding for two to three hours after using the gum product.

The nicotine inhaler (Nicotrol) only dispenses about 4 mg of nicotine following 80 inhalations, of which, only 2 mg is actually absorbed. Plasma levels slowly reach levels of about 6 ng/mL, in contrast to those of a cigarette, which reach a Cmax of approximately 49 ng/mL in only five minutes. These levels (6 ng/mL) are probably too low to affect a breastfeeding infant.

Nicotine has been suggested to decrease basal prolactin production. One study clearly suggests that cigarette smoking significantly reduces breastmilk production at two weeks postpartum from 514 mL/day in non-smokers to 406 mL/day in smoking mothers. However, Ilett's well-done study above did not detect any change in milk production at all, although the methods of these two studies were not identical.

Therefore, the risk of using nicotine patches while breastfeeding is much less than the risk of formula feeding. Mothers should be advised to limit smoking as much as possible and to smoke only after they have fed their infant, or to switch to the use of nicotine patches.

- VARENICLINE   (*Chantix*)
  - ○ AAP = Not reviewed
  - ○ LRC = L4
  - ○ RID =
  - ○ Pregnancy = C
  - ○ Comment: Varenicline is used to assist smoking cessation. It is a partial alpha-4-beta-2-nicotinic receptor partial agonist that binds to nicotine receptors in the brain, thus preventing nicotine stimulation. It stimulates dopamine activity, but to a lesser extent than does nicotine, thus reducing craving and withdrawal symptoms. There have been no studies performed on the transfer of varenicline into human milk, but transfer is possible, as it easily passes into the CNS and has an intermediate molecular weight. Caution should be used in breastfeeding mothers.

Clinical Tips

Nicotine transfers into milk readily. Nicotine patches produce maternal plasma levels as a function of dose. The higher doses mimic a one-pack-a-day smoker. Each subsequent reduction in dose produces lower plasma levels in the user. The choice of patch depends on how much a smoker smokes. In individuals who are heavy smokers (one to two packs per day), then the higher dose patch (21-mg/d) should be initiated. In those who smoke less, a lesser dose should be initiated in breastfeeding mothers. Patches generally produce plasma (and milk) levels significantly less than that of smoking one pack of cigarettes daily, so they are, in essence, preferred over smoking and would offer less risk to a breastfed infant than smoking. It is imperative that the patient be warned to not smoke while using these preparations, as maternal plasma nicotine levels could rise dangerously.

The use of nicotine patches at night is known to induce nightmares. Removal at bedtime is suggested. Another therapy in the form of an older antidepressant, bupropion is also available. Current studies suggest an increased rate of smoking cessation with bupropion use (about 15%). Bupropion is a unique case in which the milk/plasma ratio is quite high (2.5 to 8.58), but the absolute amount transferred to milk is quite low, as none was detected in the infant. It should not be used in mothers with seizure disorders, as bupropion is known to reduce the seizure threshold. Patients should be monitored for increased risk of suicidality, seizures, increased risk of bipolar disorder, agitation, etc.

Varenicline has yet to be studied in breastfeeding mothers. It is a partial nicotine receptor blocker and agonist. Studies suggest a higher rate of smoking cessation, but patients complain of numerous side effects, including nausea (30-40%), vomiting, flatulence, and severely abnormal dreams. Caution is recommended with this product until we have more data in breastfeeding women.

Suggested Reading

Smoking and infertility. (2008). *Fertil Steril, 90*(5 Suppl), S254-259.

Smoking cessation interventions and strategies. (2008). *Aust Nurs J, 16*(6), 29-32.

Albareda, M., Sanchez, L., Gonzalez, J., Viguera, J., Mestron, A., Vernet, A., et al. (2009). Results of the application of the American Diabetes Association guidelines regarding tobacco dependency in subjects with diabetes mellitus. *Metabolism, 58*(9), 1234-1238.

Ashford, K. B., Hahn, E., Hall, L., Rayens, M. K., & Noland, M. (2009). Postpartum smoking relapse and secondhand smoke. *Public Health Rep, 124*(4), 515-526.

Einarson, A., & Riordan, S. (2009). Smoking in pregnancy and lactation: a review of risks and cessation strategies. *Eur J Clin Pharmacol, 65*(4), 325-330.

Flenady, V., Macphail, J., New, K., Devenish-Meares, P., & Smith, J. (2008). Implementation of a clinical practice guideline for smoking cessation in a public antenatal care setting. *Aust N Z J Obstet Gynaecol, 48*(6), 552-558.

Forest, S. (2009). Preventing postpartum smoking relapse: an opportunity for neonatal nurses. *Adv Neonatal Care, 9*(4), 148-155.

Gaffney, K. F. (2006). Postpartum smoking relapse and becoming a mother. *J Nurs Scholarsh, 38*(1), 26-30.

Hannover, W., Thyrian, J. R., Roske, K., Grempler, J., Rumpf, H. J., John, U., et al. (2009). Smoking cessation and relapse prevention for postpartum women: results from a randomized controlled trial at 6, 12, 18 and 24 months. *Addict Behav, 34*(1), 1-8.

Hays, J. T., Ebbert, J. O., & Sood, A. (2009). Treating tobacco dependence in light of the 2008 US Department of Health and Human Services clinical practice guideline. *Mayo Clin Proc, 84*(8), 730-735; quiz 735-736.

Lumley, J., Chamberlain, C., Dowswell, T., Oliver, S., Oakley, L., & Watson, L. (2009). Interventions for promoting smoking cessation during pregnancy. *Cochrane Database Syst Rev*(3), CD001055.

McIvor, A., Kayser, J., Assaad, J. M., Brosky, G., Demarest, P., Desmarais, P., et al. (2009). Best practices for smoking cessation interventions in primary care. *Can Respir J, 16*(4), 129-134.

Solomon, L. J., Higgins, S. T., Heil, S. H., Badger, G. J., Thomas, C. S., & Bernstein, I. M. (2007). Predictors of postpartum relapse to smoking. *Drug Alcohol Depend, 90*(2-3), 224-227.

Syphilis

Principles of Therapy

Syphilis is a sexually transmitted disease caused by the spirochete *Treponema pallidum*. The presentation of this disease varies over time. Primary syphilis manifests as a painless ulcer (chancre) usually one month after exposure that then spontaneously heals in one to two months. This often goes undiagnosed in women. Presentation of secondary syphilis may involve a rash, typically noted on the palm and soles, condylomata lata (velvet like vulvar lesions), lymphadenopathy, fever, and malaise. This occurs from one to six months after the initial chancre. Spontaneous regression occurs after one month, but tertiary syphilis may then present many years later if left untreated. Effects related to tertiary syphilis include skin lesions, aortic aneurysm, tabes dorsales (CNS lesions), and bone lesions (gummas). Diagnosis of primary syphilis can be done using dark field microscopy or direct fluorescent antibody tests of exudates from the lesion. Blood testing is ineffective for primary syphilis. Serologic testing can be done with either a VDRL or RPR test. A confirmatory MHA-TP test is indicated to confirm diagnosis, as the other tests are indirect and can be falsely positive. VDRL or RPR titers are used in monitoring therapy over time. Treatment involves the use of Benzathine penicillin G.

Treatment

- Penicillin G IM as Bicillin L-A (2.4 million units IM once).

- Doxycycline (100 mg orally twice daily for 14 days).

- Ceftriaxone (1 g daily IM or IV for eight to ten days).

- Azithromycin (2 gm single oral dose). But some case failures have been reported.

Medications

- AZITHROMYCIN   (*Zithromax*)
    ◦ AAP = Not reviewed
    ◦ LRC = L2
    ◦ RID = 5.9%
    ◦ Pregnancy = B
    ◦ Comment: Azithromycin belongs to the erythromycin family. It has an extremely long half-life, particularly in tissues. Azithromycin is concentrated for long periods in phagocytes, which are known to be present in human milk. In one study of a patient who received 1 gm initially followed by 500 mg doses each at 24 hour intervals, the concentration of azithromycin in breastmilk varied from 0.64 mg/L (initially) to 2.8 mg/L on day three. The predicted dose of azithromycin received by the infant would be approximately 0.4 mg/kg/day. This would suggest that the level of azithromycin ingested

by a breastfeeding infant is not clinically relevant. New pediatric formulations of azithromycin have been recently introduced.

- BENZATHINE PENICILLIN G (*Bicillin*)
  - AAP = Maternal Medication Usually Compatible with Breastfeeding
  - LRC = L1
  - RID =
  - Pregnancy = B
  - Comment: Penicillins generally penetrate into breastmilk in small concentrations, which is largely determined by class. Following IM doses of 100,000 units, the milk/plasma ratios varied between 0.03 - 0.13. Milk levels varied from 7 units to 60 units/L. Possible side effects in infants would include alterations in GI flora or allergic responses in a hypersensitive infant. It is compatible with breastfeeding in non-hypersensitive infants.

- CEFTRIAXONE (*Rocephin*)
  - AAP = Maternal Medication Usually Compatible with Breastfeeding
  - LRC = L2
  - RID = 4.1-4.2%
  - Pregnancy = B
  - Comment: Ceftriaxone is a very popular third-generation broad-spectrum cephalosporin antibiotic. Small amounts are transferred into milk (3-4% of maternal serum level). Following a 1 gm IM dose, breastmilk levels were approximately 0.5-0.7 mg/L at between four to eight hours. The estimated mean milk levels at steady state were 3-4 mg/L. Another source indicates that following a 2 g/d dose and at steady state, approximately 4.4% of dose penetrates into milk. In this study, the maximum breastmilk concentration was 7.89 mg/L after prolonged therapy (seven days). Poor oral absorption of ceftriaxone would further limit systemic absorption by the infant. The half-life of ceftriaxone in human milk varies from 12.8 to 17.3 hours (longer than maternal serum). Even at this high dose, no adverse effects were noted in the infant. Ceftriaxone levels in breastmilk are probably too low to be clinically relevant, except for changes in GI flora. Ceftriaxone is commonly used in neonates.

- DOXYCYCLINE (*Doxychel, Vibramycin, Periostat*)
  - AAP = Not reviewed
  - LRC = L3
  - RID = 4.2-13.3%
  - Pregnancy = D
  - Comment: Doxycycline is a long half-life tetracycline antibiotic. In a study of 15 subjects, the average doxycycline level in milk was 0.77 mg/L following a 200 mg oral dose. One oral dose of 100 mg was administered 24 hours later, and the breastmilk levels were 0.380 mg/L. Following a dose of 100 mg daily in 10 mothers, doxycycline levels in milk on day two averaged 0.82 mg/L (range 0.37- 1.24 mg/L) at three hours after the dose, and 0.46 mg/L (range 0.3-0.91 mg/L) 24 hours after the dose. The relative infant dose in an infant would be < 6% of the maternal weight-adjusted dosage. Following a single dose of 100 mg in three women or 200 mg in three women, peak milk levels occurred between two and four hours following the dose. The average "peak" milk levels were 0.96 mg/L (100 mg dose) or 1.8 mg/L (200 mg dose). After repeated dosing for five days, milk levels

averaged 3.6 mg/L at doses of 100 mg twice daily. In a study of 13 women receiving 100-200 mg doses of doxycycline, peak levels in milk were 0.6 mg/L (n=3 @100 mg dose) and 1.1 mg/L (n=11 @ 200 mg dose).

Tetracyclines administered orally to infants are known to bind in teeth, producing discoloration and inhibiting bone growth, although doxycycline and oxytetracycline stain teeth the least severe. Although most tetracyclines secreted into milk are generally bound to calcium, thus inhibiting their absorption, doxycycline is the least bound (20%), and may be better absorbed in a breastfeeding infant than the older tetracyclines. While the absolute absorption of older tetracyclines may be dramatically reduced by calcium salts, the newer doxycycline and minocycline analogs bind less and their overall absorption while slowed, may be significantly higher than earlier versions. Prolonged use (months) could potentially alter GI flora and induce dental staining, although doxycycline produces the least dental staining. Short term use (three-four weeks) is not contraindicated. No harmful effects have yet been reported in breastfeeding infants, but prolonged use (> 4 weeks) is not advised. For prolonged administration, such as for exposure to anthrax, check the CDC web site as they have published specific dosing guidelines.

Clinical Tips

The only proven effective treatment for syphilis is penicillin G. During pregnancy, no alternative is acceptable, and penicillin allergic patients should be desensitized to allow for penicillin therapy. Non-pregnant penicillin allergic patients can be treated with doxycycline 100 mg twice daily or tetracycline 500 mg four times daily for two weeks. Treatment with penicillin G is preferred, and this would be of little concern for lactation. Primary and secondary syphilis can be treated with a single injection of 2.4 million units of penicillin G intramuscularly. This single injection is also used for treatment of early latent disease. Early latent disease is diagnosed when there is no demonstrable evidence of disease, but the serologic testing is now positive and was known to be negative within the preceding year. Late latent disease or disease present for an unknown duration is treated with three weekly injections of 2.4 million units of penicillin G for a total of 7.2 million units. Most breastfeeding women and newborn infants would have had serologic testing done at the time of delivery in the United States. It is likely that the breastfed infant will require treatment for syphilis as well, and the infant should be referred for evaluation.

Suggested Reading

Angus, J., Langan, S. M., Stanway, A., Leach, I. H., Littlewood, S. M., & English, J. S. (2006). The many faces of secondary syphilis: a re-emergence of an old disease. *Clin Exp Dermatol, 31*(5), 741-745.

Dayan, L., & Ooi, C. (2005). Syphilis treatment: old and new. *Expert Opin Pharmacother, 6*(13), 2271-2280.

Doroshenko, A., Sherrard, J., & Pollard, A. J. (2006). Syphilis in pregnancy and the neonatal period. *Int J STD AIDS, 17*(4), 221-227; quiz 228.

Eccleston, K., Collins, L., & Higgins, S. P. (2008). Primary syphilis. *Int J STD AIDS, 19*(3), 145-151.

Hercogova, J., & Vanousova, D. (2008). Syphilis and borreliosis during pregnancy. *Dermatol Ther, 21*(3), 205-209.

Kropp, R. Y., Latham-Carmanico, C., Steben, M., Wong, T., & Duarte-Franco, E. (2007). What's new in management of sexually transmitted infections? Canadian Guidelines on Sexually Transmitted Infections, 2006 Edition. *Can Fam Physician, 53*(10), 1739-1741.

Lee, V., & Kinghorn, G. (2008). Syphilis: an update. *Clin Med, 8*(3), 330-333.

Trichomoniasis

Principles of Therapy

Trichomoniasis is a vaginal infection caused by the flagellated protozoan, *Trichomonas vaginalis*. While most common in women, it can infect the bladder and urethra of men, as well, and can be sexually transmitted. Trichomoniasis is frequently asymptomatic in both women and men, although 50-75% of infected women complain of a frothy off-white, purulent green or yellow vaginal discharge. There may be a fishy amine odor, as well as itching, irritation, dyspareunia, and dysuria. The diagnosis is established by visualizing the mobile protozoan in a saline preparation of vaginal secretions under the microscope. Effective therapy is limited to oral metronidazole. Metronidazole gel is useful for treatment of bacterial vaginosis, but is less effective than oral metronidazole for trichomonas and is not recommended. Although somewhat less effective, intravaginal clotrimazole suppositories or povidone vaginal douches may be effective, but are not preferred in pregnant or breastfeeding women. Male sexual partners should be treated as well. Resistance to metronidazole is rising and may require special treatment regimens.

Treatment

- Metronidazole (1.5-2 gm orally once) is treatment of choice.

- Alternate dosing is 500 orally twice daily for seven days.

- Tinidazole (2 gm orally single dose). Suggested only for metronidazole-resistant species.

Medications

- METRONIDAZOLE   (*Flagyl, Metizol, Trikacide, Protostat, Noritate*)
  - AAP = Drugs whose effect on nursing infants is unknown but may be of concern
  - LRC = L2
  - RID = 12.6-13.5%
  - Pregnancy = B
  - Comment: Metronidazole is indicated in the treatment of vaginitis due to *Trichomonas vaginalis* and various anaerobic bacterial infections, including Giardiasis, H. pylori, B. fragilis, and Gardnerella vaginalis. Metronidazole has become the treatment of choice for pediatric giardiasis (AAP). Metronidazole absorption is time and dose dependent and also depends on the route of administration (oral vs. vaginal). Following a 2 gm oral dose, milk levels were reported to peak at 50-57 mg/L at two hours. Milk levels after 12 hours were approximately 19 mg/L and at 24 hours were approximately 10 mg/L. The average drug concentration reported in milk at 2, 8, 12, and 12-24 hours was 45.8, 27.9, 19.1, and 12.6 mg/L, respectively. If breastfeeding were to continue

uninterrupted, an infant would consume 21.8 mg via breastmilk. With a 12 hour discontinuation, an infant would consume only 9.8 mg. In a group of 12 nursing mothers receiving 400 mg three times daily, the mean milk/plasma ratio was 0.91. The mean milk metronidazole concentration was 15.5 mg/L. Infant plasma metronidazole levels ranged from 1.27 to 2.41 µg/mL. No adverse effects were attributable to metronidazole therapy in these infants. In another study in patients receiving 600 and 1200 mg daily, the average milk metronidazole concentration was 5.7 and 14.4 mg/L, respectively. The plasma levels of metronidazole (two hours) at the 600 mg/d dose were 5 µg/mL (mother) and 0.8 µg/mL (infant). At the 1200 mg/d dose (two hours), plasma levels were 12.5 µg/mL (mother) and 2.4 µg/mL (infant). The authors estimated the daily metronidazole dose received by the infant at 3.0 mg/kg, with 500 mL milk intake per day, which is well below the advocated 10-20 mg/kg recommended therapeutic dose for infants.

It is true that the relative infant dose via milk is moderately high, depending on the dose and timing. Infants whose mothers ingest 1.2 gm/d will receive approximately 13.5% or less of the maternal dose or approximately 2.3 mg/kg/day. Bennett has calculated the relative infant dose from 11.7% to as high as 24% of the maternal dose. Heisterberg found metronidazole levels in infant plasma to be 16% and 19% of the maternal plasma levels following doses of 600 mg/d and 1200 mg/d. While these levels seem significant, it is still pertinent to remember that metronidazole is a commonly used drug in premature neonates, infants, and children, and 2.3 mg/kg/d is still much less than the therapeutic dose used in infants/children (7.5-30 mg/kg/d). Thus far, virtually no adverse effects have been reported.

- METRONIDAZOLE VAGINAL GEL   (*MetroGel Vaginal*)
  - ○ AAP = Drugs whose effect on nursing infants is unknown but may be of concern
  - ○ LRC = L2
  - ○ RID =
  - ○ Pregnancy = B
  - ○ Comment: Both topical and vaginal preparations of metronidazole contain only 0.75% metronidazole. Plasma levels following administration are exceedingly low. This metronidazole vaginal product produces only 2% of the mean peak serum level concentration of a 500 mg oral metronidazole tablet. The maternal plasma level following use of each dose of vaginal gel averaged 237 µg/L compared to 12,785 µg/L following an oral 500 mg tablet. Milk levels following intravaginal use would probably be exceeding low.

    Milk/plasma ratios, although published for oral metronidazole, may be different for this route of administration, primarily due to the low plasma levels attained with this product. Topical and intravaginal metronidazole gels are indicated for bacterial vaginosis.

- TINIDAZOLE   (*Tindamax*)
  - ○ AAP = Drugs whose effect on nursing infants is unknown but may be of concern
  - ○ LRC = L2
  - ○ RID = 12.2%
  - ○ Pregnancy = C
  - ○ Comment: Tinidazole is an antimicrobial agent that is sometimes used for the treatment of anaerobic infections and protozoal infections, such as intestinal amebiasis, Giardia, and trichomoniasis. It is similar to metronidazole. Tinidazole is highly lipophilic and passes membranes easily, attaining high concentrations in virtually all body tissues. Concentrations in saliva and bile are equivalent

to that of the plasma compartment. In a study of 24 women, who received a single IV infusion immediately postpartum of 500 mg, aliquots of milk and serum were collected at 12, 24, 48, 72, and 96 hours after the injection. At 48 and 72 hours, fore and hind milk samples were also taken, whereas at 12 and 24 hours only mixed milk samples were collected. Milk levels at 12 and 24 hours were 5.8 and 3.5 mg/L, respectively. Serum levels at 12 and 24 hours averaged 6.1 and 3.7 mg/L, respectively. The milk/serum ratios at 12 and 24 hours were 0.94 and 0.95, respectively, further suggesting the high lipid solubility of this product. At 48 and 72 hours, the foremilk levels were 1.28 and 0.32 mg/L, respectively. Hindmilk levels at these same times were 1.2 and 0.3, respectively. At 96 hours only trace amounts were present in milk and none in serum. In another study of five women taking a dose of 1600 mg IV, milk-to-plasma ratios of between 0.62 and 1.39 were reported. After 72 hours, the majority of the milk samples were below 0.5 µg/mL. The authors, therefore, concluded that breastfeeding should be withheld for 72 hours after a 1600 mg IV dose of tinidazole. Please recognize that the studies above were done using IV tinidazole, not the oral formulation recommended for Giardia infections. Orally, levels would be much lower than intravenous studies.

Clinical Tips

The standard of care is presently limited to oral metronidazole. Vaginal metronidazole should never be used for this syndrome. Three possible regimens are generally used, a one-time 1.5 - 2 gram STAT dose of metronidazole, or 375-500 mg twice daily for seven days, or 250 mg orally three times daily for seven days. The 2-gram dose is about 84% effective in women. Because the effectiveness of the single dose regimen in males is unclear, male partners should be treated with the 500 mg dose twice daily for seven days, unless non-compliance is a concern. Retreatment using metronidazole 500 mgs twice daily is recommended for initial failures. Subsequent treatment for metronidazole-resistant species includes Tinidazole at 2 gm oral single dose.

Metronidazole transfer into human milk is moderate to low. Several treatment regimens can be recommended. The 2-gram STAT dose, followed by pumping and discarding of milk for 12-24 hours is preferred. At 12 hours, the maternal plasma levels of metronidazole are approaching the trough. At 24 hours, the reported peak dose of metronidazole via milk (following a 2000 mg maternal dose) would be less than 10 mg per liter of milk. Thus far, no reports of untoward effects have been found following the use of this protocol in breastfeeding mothers.

Alternate protocols, such as 400 mg three times daily, have also been studied. The dose to the infant via milk was less than 15 mg per liter of milk. While most infants ingest far less than a liter of milk daily (estimated intake = 150 ml/kg), the dose received by the infant would be correspondingly lower. Other recommended doses include 375 mg twice daily or 500 mg twice daily. Metronidazole may induce disulfiram-like reactions with alcohol, unusual metallic taste, and darkened urine. While metronidazole is not FDA approved for pediatric use, the published pediatric dose in term infants is 15 mg/kg/day. In those patients unable to take metronidazole, clotrimazole vaginal suppositories may be effective. While povidone iodine douches have been used in the past, they may lead to significant absorption of iodine by the mother and breastfeeding infant. Povidone iodine should be avoided in breastfeeding mothers. A single dose regimen of tinidazole (2 gm) has been approved for treatment of trichomoniasis.

Suggested Reading

Cleveland, A. (2000). Vaginitis: finding the cause prevents treatment failure. *Cleve Clin J Med, 67*(9), 634, 637-642, 645-636.

Dailey, R. H. (1996). Vaginal discharge in the adult: a practice guideline. *J Emerg Med, 14*(2), 227-232.

Davies, J. E. (1998). All that itches is not yeast. *Adv Nurse Pract, 6*(11), 35-38, 47, 93.

Eckert, L. O. (2006). Clinical practice. Acute vulvovaginitis. *N Engl J Med, 355*(12), 1244-1252.

Fieg, E. L. (1999). Prophylaxis for STDs after sexual assault. *Am Fam Physician, 59*(11), 2983-2984.

Johnston, V. J., & Mabey, D. C. (2008). Global epidemiology and control of Trichomonas vaginalis. *Curr Opin Infect Dis, 21*(1), 56-64.

Van Vranken, M. (2007). Prevention and treatment of sexually transmitted diseases: an update. *Am Fam Physician, 76*(12), 1827-1832.

Wendel, K. A., & Workowski, K. A. (2007). Trichomoniasis: challenges to appropriate management. *Clin Infect Dis, 44*(Suppl 3), S123-129.

Zuger, A. (2006). Updated guidelines for treatment of STDs. *AIDS Clin Care, 18*(10), 91.

Tuberculosis

Principles of Therapy

The incidence of tuberculosis is rising due to the emergence of HIV/AIDS, immigration of people from areas with a high prevalence of tuberculosis, increased poverty and homelessness among this population, and a deterioration of healthcare systems which previously monitored tuberculosis care. Current estimates are that one third of the world's population is infected with *TB bacillus*. Diagnosis is more or less straightforward with the Mantoux tuberculin skin test, chest radiographs, and sputum cultures. Symptoms include fatigue, weight loss, fever, night sweats, productive cough, and pulmonary infiltrates on chest radiograph. The Mantoux skin test (PPD) is highly predictive of infection with *Mycobacterium tuberculosis* (MTB), as judged by the size of the induration surrounding the injection site. The treatment of MTB has become increasingly difficult with the emergence of multidrug resistant strains. Multidrug therapy is the standard, using isoniazid, rifampin, pyrazinamide initially, followed in two months by isoniazid and rifampin (one of many regimens). Ethambutol or streptomycin is reserved for resistant species. Most of the anti-tubercular drugs pass into milk, but the levels transmitted are generally less than 20% of the therapeutic (pediatric) dose used in children, and thus far has not been reported to be a major problem in breastfed infants. Mothers can continue to breastfeed, according to the American Academy of Pediatrics, while undergoing isoniazid or rifampin therapy.

Tuberculosis (TB) is caused by *Mycobacterium tuberculosis*, and typically starts as a pulmonary disease. In later stages, TB can infect virtually any part of the human body. TB is spread through airborne droplets, and infected persons typically have chronic cough. TB is common in many parts of the world. In the USA, TB is not very common, although cases are becoming more resistant to treatment and multidrug-resistant TB is quickly becoming a serious health concern.

Treatment

- Multiple drug treatments for prolonged periods are recommended.

- Initial treatment is with a 4-drug regimen for at least two months, including isoniazid, rifampicin, pyrazinamide and ethambutol.

- Alternate dosing also exists.

Medications

- CYCLOSERINE (*Seromycin*)
  - AAP = Maternal Medication Usually Compatible with Breastfeeding
  - LRC = L3
  - RID = 14.1%

- ○ Pregnancy = C
- ○ Comment: Cycloserine is an antibiotic primarily used for treating tuberculosis. It is also effective against various staphylococcal infections. It is a small molecule with a structure similar to the amino acid, D-alanine. Following 250 mg oral dose given four times daily to mothers, milk levels ranged from 6 to 19 mg/L, an average of 72% of maternal serum levels.

- **ETHAMBUTOL**   (*Ethambutol, Myambutol*)
  - ○ AAP = Maternal Medication Usually Compatible with Breastfeeding
  - ○ LRC = L2
  - ○ RID   = 1.5%
  - ○ Pregnancy = B
  - ○ Comment: Ethambutol is an antimicrobial used for tuberculosis. Small amounts are secreted in milk, although no studies are available which clearly document levels. In one unpublished study, the mother had an ethambutol plasma level of 1.5 mg/L three hours after a dose of 15 mg/kg daily. Following a similar dose, the concentration in milk was 1.4 mg/L. In another patient, the plasma level was 4.62 mg/L and the corresponding milk concentration was 4.6 mg/L (no dose available).

- **ISONIAZID**   (*INH, Laniazid*)
  - ○ AAP = Maternal Medication Usually Compatible with Breastfeeding
  - ○ LRC = L3
  - ○ RID   = 1.2-18%
  - ○ Pregnancy = C
  - ○ Comment: Isoniazid (INH) is an antimicrobial agent primarily used to treat tuberculosis. It is secreted into milk in quantities ranging from 0.75 to 2.3% of the maternal dose. Following doses of 5 and 10 mg/kg, one report measured peak milk levels at 6 mg/L and 9 mg/L, respectively. Isoniazid was not measurable in the infant's serum, but was detected in the urine of several infants. In another study, following a maternal dose of 300 mg of isoniazid, the concentration of isoniazid in milk peaked at three hours at 16.6 mg/L, while the acetyl derivative (AcINH) was 3.76 mg/L. The 24-hour excretion of INH in milk was estimated at 7 mg. The authors felt this dose was potentially hazardous to a breastfed infant.

    In a recent and well-done study in seven exclusively lactating women (at 33 days or steady state) who were receiving 300 mg isoniazid daily in a single dose (and rifampin and ethambutol), the mean (AUC) of isoniazid in plasma and milk was 18.4 µg/mL/24 hours and 14.4 µg/mL/24 hours, respectively. The mean Milk/Plasma ratio (AUC) was 0.89, and the calculated relative infant dose was 1.2%. In this nicely done study, peak levels are clearly evident at one hour and fall rapidly at four hours.

    Caution and close monitoring of infant for liver toxicity and neuritis are suggested. Peripheral neuropathies, common in INH therapy, can be treated with 10-50 mg/day pyridoxine in adults. Suggest the mom breastfeed and then take isoniazid in an attempt to avoid the Cmax (peak) at one to two hours.

- **RIFAMPIN**   (*Rifadin, Rimactane*)
  - ○ AAP = Maternal Medication Usually Compatible with Breastfeeding
  - ○ LRC = L2

- RID = 11.4%
- Pregnancy = C
- Comment: Rifampin is a broad-spectrum antibiotic with particular activity against tuberculosis. It is secreted into breastmilk in very small levels. One report indicates that following a single 450 mg oral dose, maternal plasma levels averaged 21.3 mg/L and milk levels averaged 3.4 - 4.9 mg/L. Vorherr reported that after a 600 mg dose of rifampin, peak plasma levels were 50 mg/L, while milk levels were 10-30 mg/L.

- PYRAZINAMIDE   (*Pyrazinamide, D-50, MK-56*)
  - AAP = Not reviewed
  - LRC = L3
  - RID = 1.5%
  - Pregnancy = C
  - Comment: Pyrazinamide is a typical antituberculosis antibiotic used as first-line therapy in tuberculosis infections. In one patient three hours following an oral dose of 1000 mg, peak milk levels were 1.5 mg/L of milk. Peak maternal plasma levels at two hours were 42 µg/mL.

- STREPTOMYCIN
  - AAP = Maternal Medication Usually Compatible with Breastfeeding
  - LRC = L3
  - RID = 0.3-0.6%
  - Pregnancy = D
  - Comment: Streptomycin is an aminoglycoside antibiotic from the same family as gentamicin. It is primarily administered IM or IV, although it is seldom used today with exception of the treatment of tuberculosis. One report suggests that following a 1 g dose (IM), levels in breastmilk were 0.3 to 0.6 mg/L (2-3% of plasma level). Another report suggests that only 0.5% of a 1 gm IM dose is excreted in breastmilk within 24 hours. Because the oral absorption of streptomycin is very poor, absorption by infant is probably minimal (unless premature or early neonate).

Clinical Tips

The CDC has extensive guidelines on the therapy of tuberculosis, and readers are urged to follow these guidelines. Initial therapy for individuals with "positive PPD screens" is chemoprophylaxis with Isoniazid (INH) 5 mg/kg or 300mg/day for six to nine months for adults. Chemoprophylaxis is primarily for individuals whose PPD skin test has converted from negative to positive within the last two years. Isoniazid passes into human milk in low levels, but over an extended time, may produce moderate plasma levels in some infants. Infants should periodically be monitored for elevated INH plasma levels and liver transaminases. Breastfeeding should be scheduled to avoid the peak maternal plasma levels at one to three hours postdose. This will significantly reduce exposure of the infant to higher breastmilk levels. Maternal pyridoxine therapy (B-6 10 mg daily) is recommended.

Treatment of active infection includes the following: INH, RIF, PZA, and EMB for 56 doses or eight weeks. Rifampin levels in breastmilk have been reported and are quite low. Following a 450 mg dose, milk levels were less than 4.9 mg per liter. Following a 600 mg dose, peak milk levels were 10-30 mg per liter. Pyrazinamide and ethambutol are also considered first-line therapy. Milk levels of pyrazinamide are low (1.5 mg/L of milk), but we have limited data. Reported milk levels of ethambutol range from a low of 1.5 to 4.6 mg/L.

Cycloserine works similarly to ethambutol. Its milk levels range to a peak as high as 19 mg per liter following a 250 mg maternal dose. Please refer to the CDC guidelines for complete recommendations, including treatment of multi-drug resistant forms.

Suggested Reading

Abubakar, I., Chalkley, D., McEvoy, M., Stanley, N., & Alshafi, K. (2006). Evaluating compliance with national guidelines for the clinical, laboratory and public health management of tuberculosis in a low-prevalence English district. *Public Health, 120*(2), 155-160.

Aquilina, S., & Winkelman, T. (2008). Tuberculosis: a breast-feeding challenge. *J Perinat Neonatal Nurs, 22*(3), 205-213.

Burrill, J., Williams, C. J., Bain, G., Conder, G., Hine, A. L., & Misra, R. R. (2007). Tuberculosis: a radiologic review. *Radiographics, 27*(5), 1255-1273.

Chan, E. D., & Iseman, M. D. (2008). Multidrug-resistant and extensively drug-resistant tuberculosis: a review. *Curr Opin Infect Dis, 21*(6), 587-595.

Potter, B., Rindfleisch, K., & Kraus, C. K. (2005). Management of active tuberculosis. *Am Fam Physician, 72*(11), 2225-2232.

Walker, N. F., Kliner, M., Turner, D., Bhagani, S., Cropley, I., Hopkins, S., et al. (2009). Hepatotoxicity and antituberculosis therapy: time to revise UK guidance? *Thorax, 64*(10), 918.

Wei, X., Walley, J. D., Liang, X., Liu, F., Zhang, X., & Li, R. (2008). Adapting a generic tuberculosis control operational guideline and scaling it up in China: a qualitative case study. *BMC Public Health, 8*, 260.

Urinary Tract Infection / Pyelonephritis

Principles of Therapy

Urinary tract infections (UTI) are one of the most common of infections. The term 'Urinary tract infection' encompasses an enormous array of diagnoses, including cystitis, pyelonephritis, bacteruria, infections of catheters, and recurrent infections. Treatment of UTI depends on the delineation of upper or lower tract infection. Lower tract infections are those of the urethra (urethritis) or bladder (cystitis) and are characterized by pyuria, dysuria, frequency, or urgency. Upper tract infections, pyelonephritis, may involve both the kidney and bladder. Symptoms include fever, flank pain, and signs of lower tract infection. Most urinary infections are monomicrobial. The most common bacteria (85%) is *Escherichia coli*, followed by *Proteus, Enterobacter, Klebsiella* and *Pseudomonas* species. Infections are generally labeled as an uncomplicated UTI if it occurs in a patient who has no functional or structural anomalies of the kidneys, ureters, bladder, or urethra. Complicated UTIs occur in those patients with structural abnormalities. The incidence of UTI is increased during pregnancy and the postpartum period, owing to both the local obstructive effect of the enlarged uterus and to the progesterone effect on ureteral mobility. Urinary stasis is more common and vesicoureteral reflux is more likely to occur. Mild ureteral dilatation and hydronephrosis, especially on the right, may be a normal finding during this time and will usually resort to normal between two to eight weeks postpartum. Additionally, the use of catheterization and birth trauma increase the risk of UTI after delivery. Cystitis during pregnancy is considered to be a complicated infection and this may also be applicable to the early postpartum period mentioned above. The therapy of an uncomplicated UTI generally requires only three days of treatment, while a complicated UTI often requires longer (10 to 14 days) treatment and may be recurrent.

Treatment

- Acute uncomplicated UTI: trimethoprim, trimethoprim/sulfamethoxazole or ciprofloxacin for three days; nitrofurantoin as second-line agent for five to seven days. Acute complicated UTI: ciprofloxacin or levofloxacin for 7-14 days.

- Recurrent UTI: Lifestyle changes such as postcoital voiding, cranberry juice, continuous or postcoital prophylaxis with TMP/SMX or nitrofurantoin.

- Pyelonephritis: Ciprofloxacin, levofloxacin or ceftriaxone (decision guided by local susceptibility studies) with continuation of oral therapy for a total of 7-14 days based on sensitivity testing of cultured organisms and treatment used.

Medications

- AMOXICILLIN + CLAVULANATE   (*Augmentin*)
  - AAP = Not reviewed

- ◦ LRC = L1
- ◦ RID = 1%
- ◦ Pregnancy = B
- ◦ Comment: Addition of clavulanate extends spectrum of amoxicillin by inhibiting beta lactamase enzymes. Small amounts of amoxicillin (0.9 mg/L milk) are secreted in breastmilk. No harmful effects were reported in one report.

    In another study of 67 breastfeeding mothers, 27 mothers were treated with amoxicillin/ clavulanic acid and 40 mothers were treated with only amoxicillin. In the amoxicillin/ clavulanic acid group, 22.3% of the infants had mild adverse effects. Only 7.5% of the control group (amoxicillin-only) infants had adverse effects. However, the authors suggest that this difference in untoward effects is not clinically significant. The reported side effects included constipation, rash, diarrhea, and irritability.

- • CEFTRIAXONE (*Rocephin*)
  - ◦ AAP = Maternal Medication Usually Compatible with Breastfeeding
  - ◦ LRC = L2
  - ◦ RID = 4.1-4.2%
  - ◦ Pregnancy = B
  - ◦ Comment: Ceftriaxone is a very popular third-generation broad-spectrum cephalosporin antibiotic. Small amounts are transferred into milk (3-4% of maternal serum level). Following a 1 gm IM dose, breastmilk levels were approximately 0.5-0.7 mg/L at between four to eight hours. The estimated mean milk levels at steady state were 3-4 mg/L. Another source indicates that following a 2 g/d dose and at steady state, approximately 4.4% of dose penetrates into milk. In this study, the maximum breastmilk concentration was 7.89 mg/L after prolonged therapy (seven days). Poor oral absorption of ceftriaxone would further limit systemic absorption by the infant. The half-life of ceftriaxone in human milk varies from 12.8 to 17.3 hours (longer than maternal serum). Even at this high dose, no adverse effects were noted in the infant. Ceftriaxone levels in breastmilk are probably too low to be clinically relevant, except for changes in GI flora. Ceftriaxone is commonly used in neonates.

- • CIPROFLOXACIN (*Cipro, Ciloxan*)
  - ◦ AAP = Maternal Medication Usually Compatible with Breastfeeding
  - ◦ LRC = L3
  - ◦ RID = 2.1-6.3%
  - ◦ Pregnancy = C
  - ◦ Comment: Ciprofloxacin is a fluoroquinolone antibiotic primarily used for gram negative coverage and is presently the drug of choice for anthrax treatment and prophylaxis. Because it has been implicated in arthropathy in newborn animals, it is not normally used in pediatric patients. Levels secreted into breastmilk (2.26 to 3.79 mg/L) are somewhat conflicting. They vary from the low to moderate range to levels that are higher than maternal serum up to 12 hours after a dose. In one study of ten women who received 750 mg every 12 hours, milk levels of ciprofloxacin ranged from 3.79 mg/L at two hours postdose to 0.02 mg/L at 24 hours. In another study of a single patient receiving one 500 mg tablet daily at bedtime, the concentrations in maternal serum and breastmilk were 0.21 μg/mL and 0.98 μg/mL, respectively. Plasma levels were undetectable (<0.03 μg/mL) in

the infant. The dose to the four-month-old infant was estimated to be 0.92 mg/day or 0.15 mg/kg/day. No adverse effects were noted in this infant. There has been one reported case of severe pseudomembranous colitis in an infant of a mother who self-medicated with ciprofloxacin for six days. In a patient 17 days postpartum, who received 500 mg orally, ciprofloxacin levels in milk were 3.02, 3.02, 3.02, and 1.98 mg/L at 4, 8, 12, and 16 hours postdose, respectively.

If used in lactating mothers, observe the infant closely for GI symptoms, such as diarrhea. Current studies seem to suggest that the amount of ciprofloxacin present in milk is quite low. Ciprofloxacin was recently approved by the American Academy of Pediatrics for use in breastfeeding women, and it is becoming increasingly popular for use in pediatric patients.

- GENTAMICIN   (*Garamycin*)
    - AAP =   Maternal Medication Usually Compatible with Breastfeeding
    - LRC = L2
    - RID   = 2.1%
    - Pregnancy = C
    - Comment: Gentamicin is a narrow spectrum antibiotic generally used for gram negative infections. The oral absorption of gentamicin (<1%) is generally nil, with the exception of premature neonates, where small amounts may be absorbed. In one study of 10 women given 80 mg three times daily IM for five days postpartum, milk levels were measured on day four. Gentamicin levels in milk were 0.42, 0.48, 0.49, and 0.41 mg/L at one, three, five, and seven hours, respectively. The milk/plasma ratios were 0.11 at one hour and 0.44 at seven hours. Plasma gentamicin levels in neonates were small, found in only five of the ten neonates, and averaged 0.41 μg/mL. The authors estimate that daily ingestion via breastmilk would be 307 μg for a 3.6 kgneonate (normal neonatal dose = 2.5 mg/kg every 12 hours). These amounts would be clinically irrelevant in most infants.

- LEVOFLOXACIN   (*Levaquin, Quixin*)
    - AAP =   Not reviewed
    - LRC = L3
    - RID   = 10.5-17.2%
    - Pregnancy = C
    - Comment: Levofloxacin is a pure (S) enantiomer of the racemic fluoroquinolone Ofloxacin. Its kinetics, including milk levels, should be identical to Ofloxacin. In one case report of a mother receiving 500 mg/day, the 24 hour average milk level was reported to be approximately 5 μg/mL. A peak level of 8.2 μg/mL was reported, and occurred at five hours after the dose. The half-life of levofloxacin in milk was estimated to be seven hours, which would result in undetectable amounts in milk after 48 hours. The authors report the absolute infant dose would be 1.23 mg/kg/day, although this was calculated from the highest milk level of eight samples. While the peak levels were reported to be 8.2 μg/mL, the average milk level reported was 5 μg/mL. Using these data, the relative infant dose would range from 10.5% to 17%. However, the time-to-peak interval reported in this case was five hours, rather than 1-1.8 hours reported following both oral and IV doses in the prescribing information. Of the 10 reported levels in this study, only one was above 5 μg/mL. Thus the reported average level of 5 μg/mL is probably consistent with other data. This suggests a Milk/Plasma ratio of approximately 0.95, which is probably correct. Thus levofloxacin concentrations in milk peak around 1-1.8 hours and at levels close to plasma levels. Observe the infant for changes in gut flora, candida overgrowth, or diarrhea.

- NITROFURANTOIN   (*Furadantin, Macrodantin, Furan, Macrobid*)
  - ◦ AAP = Maternal Medication Usually Compatible with Breastfeeding
  - ◦ LRC = L2
  - ◦ RID = 6.8%
  - ◦ Pregnancy = B
  - ◦ Comment: Nitrofurantoin is an old urinary tract antimicrobial. It is secreted in breastmilk, but in very small amounts. In one study of 20 women receiving 100 mg four times daily, none was detected in milk. In another group of nine nursing women who received 100-200 mg every six hours, nitrofurantoin was undetectable in the milk of those treated with 100 mg, and only trace amounts were found in those treated with 200 mg (0.3-0.5 mg/L milk). In these two patients, the milk/plasma ratio ranged from 0.27 to 0.31.

    In a well-done study of four breastfeeding mothers who ingested 100 mg nitrofurantoin with a meal, the milk/serum ratio averaged 6.21, suggesting an active transfer into milk. Regardless of an active transfer, the average milk concentration throughout the day (AUC) was only 1.3 mg/L. According to the authors, the estimated dose an infant would ingest was 0.2 mg/kg/day or 6.8% of the weight-adjusted maternal dose if they consumed 200 mg/d nitrofurantoin. The therapeutic dose administered to infants is 5-7 mg/kg/day.

    Use with caution in infants with G6PD or in infants less than one month of age with hyperbilirubinemia, due to displacement of bilirubin from albumin binding sites.

- SULFAMETHOXAZOLE   (*Gantanol*)
  - ◦ AAP = Not reviewed
  - ◦ LRC = L3
  - ◦ RID =
  - ◦ Pregnancy = C
  - ◦ Comment: Sulfamethoxazole is a common and popular sulfonamide antimicrobial. It is secreted in breastmilk in small amounts. It has a longer half-life than other sulfonamides. Use with caution in weakened infants and premature infants or neonates with hyperbilirubinemia. Gantrisin (Sulfisoxazole) is considered the best choice of sulfonamides due to reduced transfer to infant. Compatible but exercise caution. PHL= 14.7-36.5 hours (neonate), eight to nine hours (older infants).

- TRIMETHOPRIM   (*Proloprim, Trimpex*)
  - ◦ AAP = Maternal Medication Usually Compatible with Breastfeeding
  - ◦ LRC = L2
  - ◦ RID = 9.0%
  - ◦ Pregnancy = C
  - ◦ Comment: Trimethoprim is an inhibitor of folic acid production in bacteria. In one study of 50 patients, average milk levels were 2.0 mg/L. Milk/plasma ratio was 1.25. In another group of mothers receiving 160 mg two to four times daily, concentrations of 1.2 to 5.5 mg/L were reported in milk. Because it may interfere with folate metabolism, its long-term use should be avoided in breastfeeding mothers, or the infant should be supplemented with folic acid. However, trimethoprim apparently poses few problems in full term or older infants where it is commonly used clinically.

Clinical Tips

Initial therapy of uncomplicated acute UTI in breastfeeding mothers is generally trimethoprim/sulfamethoxazole double strength (160/800mg) twice daily for three days, or ciprofloxacin (250 mg every 12 hours) for three days. Due to the possibility of jaundice and kernicterus in newborns, sulfonamides should not be used in premature infants, infants with hyperbilirubinemia or G-6-PD deficiency, or infants that have elevated bilirubin levels. They should not be used at term or during the first 30 days postpartum. Nitrofurantoin is another oral therapy useful for uncomplicated lower tract infections, although it should not be used during the neonatal period. Ofloxacin (300 mg BID) for three days is equally effective as the sulfonamides. It is unlikely this brief exposure to this fluoroquinolone would be detrimental to breastfed infants. Due to the emergence of resistance (30-40% of E.coli), amoxicillin is not generally recommended for UTI. Culture with sensitivity testing is indicated for directing therapy for complicated or recurrent UTI. Treatment of complicated UTI generally requires TMP-SMX or a fluoroquinolone for up to 14 days or longer. This may be slightly more risky for breastfed infants as the emergence of *C. difficile* overgrowth in the infant has been reported, but only in one case. Caution is urged with longer therapies with the fluoroquinolones. Watch for bloody diarrhea or indications of overgrowth of *C. difficile*.

Upper tract infections (pyelonephritis) are predominately caused by *E. coli*. Outpatient treatment can be given to the non-pregnant patient who does not have evidence of sepsis. TMP-SMX (160/800mg) orally twice daily can be used for a 14 day course. Sepsis requires hospitalization until afebrile for 24 to 48 hours of antibiotics. Antibiotics can be adjusted if needed based on sensitivity testing from culture results. Pregnancy may also be an indication for hospitalization. TMP-SMZ, ceftriaxone, gentamycin with ampicillin, or a fluoroquinolone (not during pregnancy) may be used during breastfeeding, though the latter would be less desirable for reasons previously discussed. TMP-SMZ is a less desirable choice near term pregnancy and in the immediate postpartum period due to the competition of sulfonamides with bilirubin and potential for toxicity and kernicterus.

In some patients, changes in lifestyle are recommended. These include voiding after sexual intercourse, not using douches, taking a shower rather than a bath, not using hot tubs, increasing fluid intake, including cranberry juice. Chronic reinfections may require prolonged use of sulfonamides, such as TMP/SMX for up to several years.

Suggested Reading

Guay, D. R. (2008). Contemporary management of uncomplicated urinary tract infections. *Drugs, 68*(9), 1169-1205.

Head, K. A. (2008). Natural approaches to prevention and treatment of infections of the lower urinary tract. *Altern Med Rev, 13*(3), 227-244.

Jackson, M. A. (2007). Evidence-based practice for evaluation and management of female urinary tract infection. *Urol Nurs, 27*(2), 133-136.

Kaiser, J., McPherson, V., Kaufman, L., & Huber, T. (2007). Clinical inquiries. Which UTI therapies are safe and effective during breastfeeding? *J Fam Pract, 56*(3), 225-228.

Nicolle, L., Anderson, P. A., Conly, J., Mainprize, T. C., Meuser, J., Nickel, J. C., et al. (2006). Uncomplicated urinary tract infection in women. Current practice and the effect of antibiotic resistance on empiric treatment. *Can Fam Physician, 52*, 612-618.

Rahn, D. D. (2008). Urinary tract infections: contemporary management. *Urol Nurs, 28*(5), 333-341; quiz 342.

Varicella

Principles of Therapy

Varicella (chickenpox or shingles) is caused by the varicella-zoster DNA herpes virus, which typically affects children, although the use of the vaccine has reduced the incidence in children. There are still a significant number of adults who either have not had this infection or have not retained their immunity to this disease. Antibody testing on women who do not recall having chickenpox will have evidence of immunity in 70-90% of cases. Routine vaccination of children between 12 and 18 months of life is now given.

Varicalla is very contagious and is spread by contact with vesicular fluid or respiratory droplets. During adulthood and especially pregnancy, the risk of more serious complications from this infection increases. Immunosuppression also increases the risk associated with this infection. Incubation varies from 10 to 21 days after exposure until lesions appear. The virus may be spread 24-48 hours prior to the appearance of lesions. If a known exposure has occurred, it is possible to give postexposure vaccination to a breastfeeding woman. Women of childbearing potential who have no history of chickenpox should be offered testing and vaccination prior to pregnancy. As the vaccination is a live attenuated virus, it should not be given within one month preceding or during pregnancy. A critical time period for this infection to occur is within five days prior to or 48 hours after delivery of the infant. This allows potential transmission of the virus, but not maternal antibodies to the infant. Infants born to mothers with active varicella should be isolated from the mother and given varicella zoster immune globulin.

Treatment

- Prevention through the varicella vaccine. Varicella vaccination is safe for breastfeeding mothers.

- Cool compresses, warm Aveeno baths, calamine lotion

- Acetaminophen. Do NOT use aspirin or any salicylate.

- Acyclovir (20 mg/kg by mouth four times daily for five days) (not more than 800mg).

- Valacyclovir or famciclovir for cases in those who are immunocompromised or have CNS involvement. Treatment within 24 hours of lesion development reduces symptoms and severity. Little or no benefit after 24 hours.

- Valacyclovir or possibly IVIG for pregnant women or neonates

Medications

- ACYCLOVIR   (*Zovirax*)

- ◦ AAP = Maternal Medication Usually Compatible with Breastfeeding
- ◦ LRC = L2
- ◦ RID = 1.1-1.5%
- ◦ Pregnancy = B
- ◦ Comment: Acyclovir is converted by herpes simplex and varicella zoster virus to acyclovir triphosphate, which interferes with viral HSV DNA polymerase. It is currently cleared for use in HSV infections, Varicella-Zoster, and under certain instances, such as cytomegalovirus and Epstein-Barr infections. There is virtually no percutaneous absorption following topical application, and plasma levels are undetectable. The pharmacokinetics in children are similar to adults. In neonates, the half-life is 3.8-4.1 hours, and in children one year and older, it is 1.9-3.6 hours. Acyclovir levels in breastmilk are reported to be 0.6 to 4.1 times the maternal plasma levels. Maximum ingested dose was calculated to be 1500 μg/day, assuming 750 mL milk intake. This level produced no overt side effects in one infant. In a study by Meyer, a patient receiving 200 mg five times daily produced breastmilk concentrations averaging 1.06 mg/L. Using these data, an infant would ingest less than 1 mg acyclovir daily. In another study, doses of 800 mg five times daily produced milk levels that ranged from 4.16 to 5.81 mg/L (total estimated infant ingestion per day = 0.73 mg/kg/day).

- VALACYCLOVIR (*Valtrex*)
  - ◦ AAP = Not reviewed
  - ◦ LRC = L1
  - ◦ RID = 4.7%
  - ◦ Pregnancy = B
  - ◦ Comment: Valacyclovir is a prodrug that is rapidly metabolized in the plasma to acyclovir. In a study of five women who received 500 mg twice daily for seven days after delivery, the median peak acyclovir concentration in breastmilk was 4.2 mg/L at four hours, while the average concentration (AUC) was 2.24 mg/L if 12 hour dosing intervals were used. Thus the relative infant dose would be 4.7% of the weight-normalized maternal dose. The ratio of milk/serum ratio was highest four hours after the initial dose at 3.4 and reached steady state ratio at 1.85. Valacyclovir is rapidly converted to acyclovir, which transfers into breastmilk. However, the amount of acyclovir in breastmilk after valacyclovir administration is considerably less than that used in therapeutic dosing of neonates.

- VARICELLA VIRUS VACCINE (*Varivax*)
  - ◦ AAP = Not reviewed
  - ◦ LRC = L2
  - ◦ RID =
  - ◦ Pregnancy = C
  - ◦ Comment: A live attenuated varicella vaccine (Varivax - Merck) was recently approved for marketing by the US Food and Drug Administration. Although effective, it does not apparently provide the immunity attained from infection with the parent virus and may not provide life-long immunity. The Oka/Merck strain used in the vaccine is attenuated by passage in human and embryonic guinea pig cell cultures. It is not known if the vaccine-acquired VZV is secreted in human milk, nor its infectiousness to infants. Interestingly, in two women with varicella-zoster infections, the virus was not culturable from milk. Mothers of immunodeficient infants should not breastfeed following

use of this vaccine. Recommendations for Use: Varicella vaccine is only recommended for children >1 year of age up to 12 years of age with no history of varicella infection. Both the AAP and the Centers for Disease Control approve the use of varicella-zoster vaccines in breastfeeding mothers, if the risk of infection is high.

- VARICELLA-ZOSTER VIRUS (*Chickenpox*)
  - ° AAP = Not reviewed
  - ° LRC = L4
  - ° RID =
  - ° Pregnancy =
  - ° Comment: Chickenpox virus has been reported to be transferred via breastmilk in one 27-year-old mother who developed chickenpox postpartum. Her two-month-old son also developed the disease 16 days after the mother. Chickenpox virus was detected in the mother's milk and may suggest that transmission can occur via breastmilk. However, in a study of two breastfeeding patients who developed varicella-herpes zoster infections, in neither case was the virus isolated and cultured from their milk. According to the American Academy of Pediatrics, neonates born to mothers with active varicella should be placed in isolation at birth and, if still hospitalized, until 21 or 28 days of age, depending on whether they received VZIG (Varicella Zoster Immune Globulin). Candidates for VZIG include immunocompromised children, pregnant women, and a newborn infant whose mother has onset of VZV within five days before or 48 hours after delivery.

Clinical Tips

Infants born to mothers with active chickenpox at delivery should be isolated from other infants and given varicella zoster immune globulin (VZIG). It is unclear if transmission via breastmilk can occur, but transmission by close contact is well documented. Ideally, in breastfeeding mothers exposed to infection, postexposure vaccination can be given to the mother, potentially avoiding both maternal chickenpox and any disruption in lactation. For breastfed infants greater than one year of age, vaccination of the child is recommended. Shingles is not a contraindication for breastfeeding, provided that the lesions can be adequately covered to avoid contact with the infant. If lesions are on the nipple, mothers should not breastfeed. VZIG may also be given to the infant in cases of maternal shingles as a precaution.

Level of acyclovir in milk is not high, and that present would not likely be absorbed orally by an infant. Because valacyclovir is rapidly converted by the mother to acyclovir, this product would not be contraindicated in a breastfeeding mother.

Suggested Reading

Campos-Outcalt, D. (2008). Varicella vaccination: 2 doses now the standard. *J Fam Pract, 57*(1), 38-40.

Daley, A. J., Thorpe, S., & Garland, S. M. (2008). Varicella and the pregnant woman: prevention and management. *Aust N Z J Obstet Gynaecol, 48*(1), 26-33.

Marin, M., Meissner, H. C., & Seward, J. F. (2008). Varicella prevention in the United States: a review of successes and challenges. *Pediatrics, 122*(3), e744-751.

Mueller, N. H., Gilden, D. H., Cohrs, R. J., Mahalingam, R., & Nagel, M. A. (2008). Varicella zoster virus infection: clinical features, molecular pathogenesis of disease, and latency. *Neurol Clin, 26*(3), 675-697, viii.

Sauerbrei, A., & Wutzler, P. (2007). Herpes simplex and varicella-zoster virus infections during pregnancy: current concepts of prevention, diagnosis and therapy. Part 2: Varicella-zoster virus infections. *Med Microbiol Immunol, 196*(2), 95-102.

Wound Infection

Principles of Therapy

Wound infections frequently occur with an incidence of approximately 4 to 12% of patients undergoing cesarean delivery. Longer operating time and maternal obesity (BMI > 30) have both been associated with an increased risk of surgical site infection after cesarean. Typically wound infections present four to five days after surgery, often occuring after hospital discharge. The wound is found to be erythematous and tender. Fever may also be present. Treatment involves opening, draining, debriding, and cleaning of the wound. Various techniques are used to assist with wound healing. Some advocate the use of secondary closure of the wound after the infection has been cleared, while others recommend healing by secondary intent and the use of vacuum devices. Antibiotics typically used to treat wound infections should have coverage for staphylococcus and streptococcus species. Again, many different antibiotics may be used for this common infection. Oral or intravenous antibiotics may be chosen, depending on the clinical situation. Some of the commonly used antibiotics for wound infections are listed below.

Treatment

- Opening and draining the incision is often curative in many wounds.

- Most, but certainly not all, skin infections are probably due to staphylococcal infections.

- Antibiotics that cover gram positive and staphylococcal species are recommended.

- Some advocate the use of secondary closure of the wound after the infection has been cleared.

- Others recommend healing by secondary intent and the use of vacuum devices.

Medications

- AMOXICILLIN + CLAVULANATE   (*Augmentin*)
  - AAP = Not reviewed
  - LRC = L1
  - RID = 1%
  - Pregnancy = B
  - Comment: Small amounts of amoxicillin (0.9 mg/L milk) are secreted in breastmilk. No harmful effects were reported in one report. In another study of 67 breastfeeding mothers, 27 mothers were treated with amoxicillin/ clavulanic acid and 40 mothers were treated with only amoxicillin. In the amoxicillin/ clavulanic acid group, 22.3% of the infants had mild adverse effects. Only 7.5% of the control group (amoxicillin-only) infants had adverse effects. However, the authors suggest that

this difference in untoward effects is not clinically significant. The reported side effects included constipation, rash, diarrhea, and irritability.

- **CEFAZOLIN** (*Ancef, Kefzol*)
  - AAP = Maternal Medication Usually Compatible with Breastfeeding
  - LRC = L1
  - RID = 0.8%
  - Pregnancy = B
  - Comment: Cefazolin is a typical first-generation, cephalosporin antibiotic that has adult and pediatric indications. It is only used IM or IV, never orally. In 20 patients who received a 2 gm STAT dose over ten minutes, the average concentration of cefazolin in milk two, three, and four hours after the dose was 1.25, 1.51, and 1.16 mg/L, respectively. A very small milk/plasma ratio (0.023) indicates insignificant transfer into milk. Cefazolin is poorly absorbed orally; therefore, the infant would absorb a minimal amount. Plasma levels in infants are reported to be too small to be detected.

- **CEFOTETAN** (*Cefotan*)
  - AAP = Not reviewed
  - LRC = L2
  - RID = 0.2-0.3%
  - Pregnancy = B
  - Comment: Cefotetan is a third generation cephalosporin that is poorly absorbed orally and is only available via IM and IV injection. The drug is distributed into human milk in low concentrations. Following a maternal dose of 1000mg IM every 12 hours in five patients, breastmilk concentrations ranged from 0.29 to 0.59 mg/L. Plasma concentrations were almost 100 times higher. In a group of two to three women who received 1000 mg IV, the maximum average milk level reported was 0.2 mg/L at four hours, with a milk/plasma ratio of 0.02.

- **CEFOXITIN** (*Mefoxin*)
  - AAP = Maternal Medication Usually Compatible with Breastfeeding
  - LRC = L1
  - RID = 0.1-0.3%
  - Pregnancy = B
  - Comment: Cefoxitin is a cephalosporin antibiotic with a spectrum similar to the second generation family. It is transferred into human milk in very low levels. In a study of 18 women receiving 2000-4000 mg doses, only one breastmilk sample contained cefoxitin (0.9 mg/L), all the rest were too low to be detected. In another study of two to three women who received 1000 mg IV, only trace amounts were reported in milk over six hours. In a group of five women who received an IM injection of 2000 mg, the highest milk levels were reported at four hours after dose. The maternal plasma levels varied from 22.5 at two hours to 77.6 μg/mL at four hours. Maternal milk levels ranged from <0.25 to 0.65 mg/L. Observe for changes in gut flora.

- **CEPHALEXIN** (*Keflex*)
  - AAP = Not reviewed
  - LRC = L1

- ◦ RID = 0.5-1.5%
- ◦ Pregnancy = B
- ◦ Comment: Cephalexin is a typical first-generation, cephalosporin antibiotic. Only minimal concentrations are secreted into human milk. Following a 1000 mg maternal oral dose, milk levels at one, two, three, four, and five hours ranged from 0.20, 0.28, 0.39, 0.50, and 0.47 mg/L, respectively. Milk/serum ratios varied from 0.008 at one hour to 0.140 at three hours. These levels are probably too low to be clinically relevant. In a group of two to three patients who received 500 mg orally, milk levels averaged 0.7 mg/L at four hours, although the average milk level was 0.36 mg/L over six hours. The milk/plasma ratio was 0.25. In another case report of a mother taking probenecid along with cephalexin to prolong the half-life of the cephalexin, the baby developed severe diarrhea. The average milk concentration of probenecid and cephalexin was 964 µg/L and 0.745 µg/L, respectively. This corresponds to a relative infant dose of 0.7% for probenecid and 0.5% for cephalexin. The authors concluded that when using this combination of drugs in breastfeeding women, clinicians should expect the possibility of adverse GI effects in the infant.

- CLINDAMYCIN   (*Cleocin*)
  - ◦ AAP =   Maternal Medication Usually Compatible with Breastfeeding
  - ◦ LRC = L2
  - ◦ RID   = 1.7%
  - ◦ Pregnancy = B
  - ◦ Comment: Clindamycin is a broad-spectrum antibiotic frequently used for anaerobic infections. In one study of two nursing mothers and following doses of 600 mg IV every six hours, the concentration of clindamycin in breastmilk was 3.1 to 3.8 mg/L at 0.2 to 0.5 hours after dosing. Following oral doses of 300 mg every six hours, the breastmilk levels averaged 1.0 to 1.7 mg/L at 1.5 to 7 hours after dosing. In another study of two to three women who received a single oral dose of 150 mg, milk levels averaged 0.9 mg/L at four hours, with a milk/plasma ratio of 0.47. An alteration of GI flora is possible, even though the dose is low. One case of bloody stools (pseudomembranous colitis) has been associated with clindamycin and gentamicin therapy on day five postpartum, but this is considered rare. In this case, the mother of a newborn infant was given 600 mg IV every six hours. In rare cases, pseudomembranous colitis can appear several weeks later.

    In a study by Steen, in five breastfeeding patients who received 150 mg three times daily for seven days, milk concentrations ranged from <0.5 to 3.1 mg/L, with the majority of levels <0.5 mg/L. There are a number of pediatric clinical uses of clindamycin (anaerobic infections, bacterial endocarditis, pelvic inflammatory disease, and bacterial vaginosis). The current pediatric dosage recommendation is 10-40 mg/kg/day divided every six to eight hours. In a study of 15 women who received 600 mg clindamycin intravenously, levels of clindamycin in milk averaged 1.03 mg/L at two hours following the dose.

    With the rise of resistant Staphlococcal infections, clindamycin use in infants has risen enormously. The amount in milk is unlikely to harm a breastfeeding infant.

- DAPTOMYCIN   (*Cubicin*)
  - ◦ AAP =   Not reviewed
  - ◦ LRC = L3
  - ◦ RID   =   0.1%

- ◦ Pregnancy = B
- ◦ Comment: Daptomycin is used intravenously for the treatment of complicated skin and skin structure infections caused by susceptible strains of *Staphylococcus aureus* (including methicillin-resistant or MRSA strains), *Streptococcus pyogenes, S. agalactiae, S. dysgalactiae, Equisimilis,* and *Enterococcus faecalis.* In a mother five months postpartum who received 500 mg IV daily (6.7 mg/kg/d), the highest concentration measured in milk was 44.7 ng/mL at eight hours following administration. Reported levels in milk were 33.5, 44.7, 40.8, 39.3, and 29.2 ng/mL at 4, 8, 12, 16, and 20 hours, respectively. The mother and infant received therapy for four weeks, and no adverse events were noted in mother or infant. In addition, the daptomycin present in milk is poorly absorbed orally.

- **DICLOXACILLIN**   (*Pathocil, Dycill, Dynapen*)
  - ◦ AAP = Not reviewed
  - ◦ LRC = L1
  - ◦ RID = 0.6-1.4%
  - ◦ Pregnancy = B
  - ◦ Comment: Dicloxacillin is an oral penicillinase-resistant penicillin frequently used for peripheral (non CNS) infections caused by *Staph. aureus* and *Staph. epidermidis* infections, particularly mastitis. Following oral administration of a 250 mg dose, milk concentrations of the drug were 0.1, and 0.3 mg/L at two and four hours after the dose, respectively. Levels were undetectable after one to six hours. Compatible with breastfeeding. Observe for diarrhea or candida diaper rash.

- **LINEZOLID**   (*Zyvox, Zyvoxam, Zyvoxid*)
  - ◦ AAP = Not reviewed
  - ◦ LRC = L3
  - ◦ RID =
  - ◦ Pregnancy = C
  - ◦ Comment: Linezolid is a new oxazolidinone family of antibiotics primarily used for gram positive infections, but it has some spectrum for gram negative and anaerobic bacteria. It is active against many strains, including resistant *staph aureus* (MRSA), *streptococcus pneumonia, streptococcus pyogenes*, and others. It is indicated for use in patients with vancomycin resistant enterococcus faecium infections, *staph aureus pneumonia*s, resistant *streptococcus pneumonia* infections, etc.

    Linezolid was found in the milk of lactating rats at concentrations similar to plasma levels, although the dose was not indicated (rat milk levels are always higher than humans). Using these data, with an average maternal plasma concentration of 11.5 µg/mL and a theoretical milk/plasma ratio of 1.0, an infant would ingest approximately 1.7 mg/kg/day following a maternal dose of 1200 mg/day. This amount is likely a high estimate, as doses given animals are extraordinarily high, and rodent milk levels are generally many times higher than human milk. A number of recent studies in children have found linezolid safe. The half-life is shorter in children, which requires dosing more often. Side effects in children are the same as adults and are significant. Observe for changes in gut flora and diarrhea.

- **MOXIFLOXACIN**   (*Avelox, Vigamox*)
  - ◦ AAP = Not reviewed
  - ◦ LRC = L2 Ophthalmically
  - ◦ RID =

- ○ Pregnancy = C
- ○ Comment: Moxifloxacin is a quinolone antibiotic for use orally, intravenously, and in the eye. It is a new-generation fluoroquinolone which exhibits improved activity against *S. pneumonia* and other species. No data are available on its transfer into human milk so until we have data, one should opt for using ofloxacin or levofloxacin for which published data are available.

- **NAFCILLIN** (*Unipen, Nafcil*)
  - ○ AAP = Not reviewed
  - ○ LRC = L1
  - ○ RID =
  - ○ Pregnancy = B
  - ○ Comment: Nafcillin is a penicillin antibiotic that is poorly and erratically absorbed orally. The only formulations are IV and IM. No data are available on concentration in milk, but it is likely small. Oral absorption in the infant would be minimal. See other penicillins.

- **VANCOMYCIN** (*Vancocin*)
  - ○ AAP = Not reviewed
  - ○ LRC = L1
  - ○ RID = 6.7%
  - ○ Pregnancy = C
  - ○ Comment: Vancomycin is an antimicrobial agent. Only low levels are secreted into human milk. Milk levels were 12.7 mg/L four hours after infusion in one woman receiving 1 gm every 12 hours for seven days. Its poor absorption from the infant's GI tract would limit its systemic absorption. Low levels in infant could provide alterations of GI flora.

Clinical Tips

Antibiotics are not required in all cases of wound infections. Virtually all of the above antibiotics have extensive use in breastfeeding mothers and are probably compatible with breastfeeding. The clinical situation dictates when wound care is sufficient, but in some situations, oral or intravenous antibiotics may be needed to treat cellulitus. Many antibiotics provide adequate coverage for the suspected organisms and are compatible with breastfeeding. Clindamycin has risen in popularity for skin-based staphylococcal infections, particularly MRSA. Linezolid has numerous and signficiant side effects, including anemia, thrombocytopenia, leukopenia, pure red cell aplasia, and pancytopenia. It should be used cautiously for resistant species, particularly MRSA.

Suggested Reading

Atiyeh, B. S., Dibo, S. A., & Hayek, S. N. (2009). Wound cleansing, topical antiseptics and wound healing. *Int Wound J, 6*(6), 420-430.

Hellums, E. K., Lin, M. G., & Ramsey, P. S. (2007). Prophylactic subcutaneous drainage for prevention of wound complications after cesarean delivery--a metaanalysis. *Am J Obstet Gynecol, 197*(3), 229-235.

Maida, V., Ennis, M., & Kuziemsky, C. (2009). The toronto symptom assessment system for wounds: a new clinical and research tool. *Adv Skin Wound Care, 22*(10), 468-474.

Menke, M. N., Menke, N. B., Boardman, C. H., & Diegelmann, R. F. (2008). Biologic therapeutics and molecular profiling to optimize wound healing. *Gynecol Oncol, 111*(2 Suppl), S87-91.

Opoien H.K., Valbo A., Grinde-Andersen A., Walberg M. (2007). Post-cesarean surgical site infections according to CDC standards: rates and risk factors. A prospective cohort study. *Acta Obstet Gynecol Scand. 2007.* 86(9): 1097-102.

Pan, A., Ambrosini, L., Patroni, A., Soavi, L., Signorini, L., Carosi, G., et al. (2009). Adherence to surgical site infection guidelines in Italian cardiac surgery units. *Infection, 37*(2), 148-152.

Stojadinovic, A., Carlson, J. W., Schultz, G. S., Davis, T. A., & Elster, E. A. (2008). Topical advances in wound care. *Gynecol Oncol, 111*(2 Suppl), S70-80.

APPENDICES

Systematic Equivalencies of Typical Corticosteroids

Glucocorticoid	Approx. Equivalent Dose (mg)	Relative Anti-Inflammatory Potency	Relative Mineralo-corticoid Potency	Half-life	
				Plasma (min)	Biologic (hrs)
Short-Acting					
Cortisone	25	0.8	2	30	8-12
Hydrocortisone	20	1	2	80-118	
Intermediate Acting					
Prednisone	5	4	1	60	18-36
Prednisolone	5	4	1	115-212	
Triamcinolone	4	5	0	200+	
Methyl-prednisolone	4	5	0	78-188	
Long-Acting					
Dexamethasone	0.75	25-30	0	110-210	36-54
Betamethasone	0.6-0.75	25	0	300+	

Potency of Topical Corticosteroids

Steroid	Vehicle

Lowest Potency (may be ineffective for some indications)

0.1%	Betamethasone	cream
0.2%	Betamethasone (Celestone®)	cream
0.04%	Dexamethasone (Hexadrol®)	cream
0.05%	Desonide	cream
0.1%	Dexamethasone (Decadron®, Phosphate, Decaderm®)	cream, gel
1%	Hydrocortisone	cream, ointment, lotion
2.5%	Hydrocortisone	cream, ointment
0.25%	Methylprednisolone acetate (Medrol®)	ointment
1%	Methylprednisolone acetate (Medrol®)	ointment

Low Potency

0.01%	Betamethasone valerate (Valisone®, Reduced Strength)	cream
0.1%	Clocortolone (Cloderm®)	cream
0.01%	Fluocinolone acetonide (Synalar®)	cream, solution
0.025%	Fluorometholone (Oxylone)	cream
0.025%	Flurandrenolide (Cordran®, Cordran®, SP)*	cream, ointment
0.2%	Hydrocortisone valerate (Westcort®)	cream
0.025%	Triamcinolone acetonide (Kenalog®)*	cream

Intermediate Potency

0.025%	Betamethasone benzoate	cream, gel, lotion
0.1%	Betamethasone valerate (Valisone®)*	cream ointment, lotion
0.05%	Desoximetasone (Topicort® LP)	cream
0.025%	Fluocinolone acetonide*	cream, ointment
0.05%	Flurandrenolide (Cordran®, Cordran® SP)*	cream, lotion, ointment
0.05%	Fluticasone propionate (Cutivate®)	cream
0.025%	Halcinonide (Halog®)	cream, ointment
0.1%	Triamcinolone acetonide (Kenalog®)*	cream, ointment

High Potency

0.1%	Amcinonide (Cyclocort®)	cream ointment
0.05%	Betamethasone dipropionate (Diprosone®)	cream ointment, lotion
0.05%	Clobetasol dipropionate	cream ointment
0.25%	Desoximetasone (Topicort®)	cream
0.25%	Diflorasone diacetate (Florone®, Maxiflor®)	cream ointment
0.2%	Fluocinolone (Synalar-HP®)	cream
0.05%	Fluocinonide (Lidex®)*	cream ointment
0.1%	Halcinonide (Halog®)	cream ointment solution
0.05%	Halobetasol propionate (Ultravate®)	cream ointment
0.5%	Triamcinolone acetonide*	cream ointment

From *Medical Letter,* 1982 (Nov 26):104

Therapeutic Drug Levels

Reference (Normal) Values

Drug	Therapeutic Range	
Acetaminophen	10-20	µg/ml
Theophylline	0-20	µg/ml
Carbamazepine	4-10	µg/ml
Ethosuximide	40-100	µg/ml
Phenobarbital	15-40	µg/ml
Phenytoin		
Neonates	6-14	µg/ml
Children, adults	10-20	µg/ml
Primidone	5-15	µg/ml
Valproic Acid	50-100	µg/ml
Gentamicin		
Peak	5-12	µg/ml
Trough	< 2.0	µg/ml
Vancomycin		
Peak	20-40	µg/ml
Trough	5-10	µg/ml
Digoxin	0.9-2.2	µg/ml
Lithium	0.3-1.3	mmol/L
Salicylates	20-25	mg/dL

From Therapeutic Drug Monitoring Guide, WE Evan, Editor, Abbott Laboratories, 1988.

Managing Hyperbilirubinemia in Healthy Term Newborns:
The AAP Practice Standard

Age (hours)	Total Serum Bilirubin (mg/dl)	Recommended Treatment
24 or under		Term infants who are clinically jaundiced at 24 hours of age or under are not considered healthy and need further evaluation
25-48	≥ 12	Consider phototherapy (based on individual clinical judgement)
	≥ 15	Phototherapy
	≥ 20	Exchange transfusion if intensive phototherapy fails*
	≥ 25	Exchange transfusion and intensive phototherapy
49-72	≥ 15	Consider phototherapy
	≥ 18	Phototherapy
	≥ 25	Exchange transfusion if intensive phototherapy fails
	≥ 30	Exchange transfusion and intensive phototherapy
Over 72	≥ 17	Consider phototherapy
	≥ 20	Phototherapy
	≥ 25	Exchange transfusion if intensive phototherapy fails
	≥ 30	Exchange transfusion and intensive phototherapy

*Intensive phototherapy should reduce total serum bilirubin by 1-2 mg/dl within 4-6 h. Serum bilirubin should continue to decrease and remain below the threshold level for exchange transfusion. If this does not happen, phototherapy is considered to have failed.
Adapted from American Academy of Pediatrics.

Drug Interactions with Oral Contraceptives

Contraceptives	Anticoagulants Heparin, Warfarin	Oral contraceptives sometimes increase and in some cases decrease clotting factors. Anticoagulant therapy may be altered by addition of contraceptives.
Contraceptives	Barbiturates Griseofulvin Felbamate Carbamazepine Phenytoin Primidone Rifampin	These agents may increase the hepatic cytochrome P450 metabolic enzymes and subsequently reduce levels of estrogens/progestins, thereby reducing efficacy of the oral contraceptives. Pregnancy or symptoms of breakthrough bleeding may occur.
Contraceptives	Antibiotics Griseofulvin Penicillins Tetracycline	Many antibiotics alter gut metabolism of OCs thus reducing their absorption and production of clinical levels. Pregnancy or symptoms of breakthrough bleeding may occur.
Contraceptives	Benzodiazepines Lorazepam Oxazepam Temazepam Alrazolam Diazepam Triazolam	OCs may enhance the metabolism and excretion of lorazepam, temazepam or oxazepam. OCs may also inhibit metabolism of certain benzodiazepines such as: alprazolam, diazepam, triazolam. This may lead to increased half-lives and reduced clearance.
Contraceptives	Beta-Blockers Tricyclics Antidepressants Caffeine Steroids Theophylline	OCs may reduce metabolism and clearance of these agents thus leading to increased plasma levels and side effects.
Contraceptives	Smoking	Smoking significantly increases the risk of major cardiovascular side effects. This is a function of number of cigarettes/day and age.

Guidelines for Glucose Monitoring and Treatment of Hypoglycemia in Term Breastfed Neonates*

Clinical Manifestations of Hypoglycemia

It cannot be emphasized enough that all the clinical signs of hypoglycemia are non-specific, and the physician must assess the general status of the infant by observation and physical examination to rule out disease entities and processes that may need additional laboratory evaluation and treatment.

Some common signs include:
1. Tremors, irritability, jitteriness, exaggerated reflexes
2. High pitched cry
3. Seizures
4. Lethargy, listlessness, limpness, hypotonia
5. Cyanosis, apnea, irregular rapid breathing
6. Hypothermia, temperature instability, vasomotor instability
7. Poor suck and refusal to feed

Management of Documented Hypoglycemia

Asymptomatic Infant
1. Continue breastfeeding (approximately every one to two hours) or feed expressed breast milk or breast milk substitute (approximately 10-15 ml/kg).
2. Recheck blood glucose concentration before subsequent feedings until value is stable in normal range.
3. If neonate is unable to suck, avoid intragastric feeding and begin intravenous therapy. Such an infant is not normal and requires very careful examination and evaluation in addition to more intensive therapy.
4. If enteral feeding is not tolerated, begin intravenous glucose infusion. Such an infant is not normal and requires careful examination and evaluation as well as more intensive treatment.
5. Intravenous therapy: 2cc/kg of 10% glucose by bolus followed by a continuous infusion of 6-8 mg/kg/min of glucose (approximately 100 cc/kg/day). Repeat serum glucose within 30 minutes, and serially thereafter until stable in normal range.

6. If glucose is low despite oral feedings, begin intravenous 10% glucose infusion of 6-8 mg/kg/min (approximately 100 cc/kg/day)
7. Adjust intravenous rate according to blood glucose concentration.
8. Once blood sugar is stabilized in the normal range, resume breastfeeding and slowly reduce intravenous infusion. Check glucose concentrations before feedings until values are stabilized off intravenous fluid.
9. Carefully document signs, physical examination, screening values, laboratory confirmation, treatment and changes in clinical condition.

Symptomatic Infant

1. Initiate intravenous glucose using 2 cc/kg 10% glucose bolus followed by a continuous infusion of 6-8 mg/kg/min glucose (approximately 100 cc/kg/day). Do not rely on oral or intragastric feeding to correct hypoglycemia. Such an infant is not normal and requires careful examination and evaluation.
2. Encourage frequent breastfeeding after relief of symptoms.
3. Adjust intravenous rate by blood glucose concentration.
4. Once blood glucose is stabilized, resume breastfeeding and slowly reduce intravenous infusion. Check glucose concentrations before feedings until values are stabilized off intravenous fluid.
5. Carefully document signs, physical examination, screening values, laboratory confirmation, treatment and changes in clinical condition.

*Adapted from Academy of Breastfeeding Medicine guidelines. Clinical Protocol # 1, with permission.

Using Radiopharmaceutical Products in Breastfeeding Mothers

The use of radioactive products in breastfeeding mothers must be approached with great care. Invariably, the administration of a radiopharmaceutical to a lactating mother will result in some transfer of radioactivity into her milk. The relative dose received by the infant is dependent on a number of factors, but most importantly by the radioactive dose administered, the absorption and distribution of the radioisotope, the biological and radioactive half-life of the product, and the amount that enters milk. The following table presents data from some of the best sources in the world and provides their recommendations on interrupting breastfeeding to allow for the decay and/or clearance of the radiopharmaceutical. Most of their decisions were based on the probable radioactive 'dose' transferred to the infant, and whether or not it was considered hazardous. Please note that some of their recommendations conflict. Ultimately, the mother and her radiologist will have to assess the relevancy of these data in their own situation.

- When evaluating radiopharmaceuticals, it is important to understand that all of these products have "two" half-lives. One is the radioactive half-life of the isotope. This half-life is set and invariable. While we prefer shorter half-life products like ^{99m}Technetium (6.02 h), many other isotopes have important uses in medicine. The second half-life is the 'biological' or 'effective' half-life of the specific product. Many of these products are rapidly eliminated from the body via the kidney, some within minutes to hours. Thus the 'biological or effective' half-life is critical and sometimes is so fast that the radiopharmaceutical is gone from the body long before its isotope is decayed (see ^{111}In-Octreotide). However, some isotopes, such as the radioactive iodides (^{131}I, ^{125}I), may be retained in the body for long periods and present extraordinary hazards to the breastfeeding infant. Lastly, two units of radioactivity are commonly used by differing sources. Just remember that one mCi (millicurie) is equal to 37 MBq (megabecquerel). Regardless of the unit you are given, you can now convert them easily.

1 millicurie = 37 megabecquerel

Some important points to remember about evaluating these products in breastfeeding mothers are:

- Use the shortest half-life product permitted, such as ^{99m}Technetium. It's half-life is so short, and its radioactive emissions are so weak, that it poses little risk (but this depends on dose). While the table below often does not even require interrupting breastfeeding, I still suggest that waiting even 12-24 hours before breastfeeding would virtually eliminate all possible risks associated with this isotope.

- Regardless of the isotope used, if the dose is extremely high, then withholding breastfeeding for a minimum of five to as many as ten radioactive half-lives is probably advisable.

- Measuring the radioactivity present in milk is the most accurate way to determine risk. This often requires sophisticated equipment not available in most hospitals, but it is the "final" determinant of risk to the infant. If the isotope present in milk approaches 'background' levels, there is no risk.

- Use great caution before returning to breastfeeding if the Iodides are used. Iodine is selectively concentrated in the thyroid gland, the lactating breast (17% of dose), and breastmilk, and high doses could potentially lead to thyroid cancer in the infant. ^{131}I and ^{125}I are potentially of high risk due to their long radioactive half-lives and their affinity for thyroid tissues. ^{123}I has a much shorter half-life, and brief interruptions may eliminate most risks.

- Because radioactivity decays at a set rate, milk can be stored in the freezer for at least eight to ten half-lives and then fed to the infant without problem. All of the radioactivity will be gone.

Typical Radioactive Half-Lives

Radioactive Element	Half-Life
Mo-99	2.75 days
TI-201	3.05 days
TI-201	73.1 hours
Ga-67	3.26 days
Ga-67	78.3 hours
I-131	8.02 days
Xe-133	5.24 days
In-111	2.80 days
Cr-51	27.7 days
I-125	60.1 days
Sr-89	50.5 days
Tc-^{99m}	6.02 hours
I-123	13.2 hours
Sm-153	47.0 hours

Activities of Radiopharmaceuticals That Require Instructions and Records When Administered to Patients Who Are Breastfeeding an Infant or Child.*

Radiopharmaceutical	COLUMN 1 Activity Above Which Instructions Are Required		COLUMN 3 Examples of Recommended Duration of Interruption of Breastfeeding*
	MBq	mCi	
I-131 NaI	0.01	0.0004	Complete cessation (for this infant or child)
I-123 NaI	20	0.5	
I-123 OIH	100	4	
I-123 mIBG	70	2	24 hour for 370 MBq (10mCi) 12 hour for 150 MBq (4 mCi)
I-125 OIH	3	0.08	
I-131 OIH	10	0.30	
Tc-99m DTPA	1,000	30	
Tc-99m MAA	50	1.3	12.6 hour for 150 Mbq (4mCi)
Tc-99m Pertechnetate	100	3	24 hour for 1,100 Mbq (30mCi) 12 hour for 440 Mbq (12 mCi)
Tc-99m DISIDA	1,000	30	
Tc-99m Glucoheptonate	1,000	30	
Tc-99m HAM	400	10	
Tc-99m MIBI	1,000	30	
Tc-99m MDP	1,000	30	
Tc-99m PYP	900	25	
Tc-99m Red Blood Cell In Vivo Labeling	400	10	6 hour for 740 Mbq (20 mCi)

Radiopharmaceutical	COLUMN 1 Activity Above Which Instructions Are Required		COLUMN 3 Examples of Recommended Duration of Interruption of Breastfeeding*
Tc-99m Red Blood Cell In Vitro Labeling	1,000	30	
Tc-99m Sulphur Colloid	300	7	6 hour for 440 Mbq (12 mCi)
Tc-99m DTPA Aerosol	1,000	30	
Tc-99m MAG3	1,000	30	
Tc-99m White Blood Cells	100	4	24 hour for 1,100 Mbq (5 mCi) 12 hour for 440 Mbq (2 mCi)
Ga-67 Citrate	1	0.04	1 month for 150 Mbq (4 mCi) 2 weeks for 50 Mbq (1.3 mCi) 1 week for 7 Mbq (0.2 mCi)
Cr-51 EDTA	60	1.6	
In-111 White Blood Cells	10	0.2	1 week for 20 Mbq (0.5 mCi)
T1-201 Chloride	40	1	2 weeks for 110 Mbq (3 mCi)

* The duration of interruption of breastfeeding is selected to reduce the maximum dose to a newborn infant to less than 1 millisievert (0.1 rem), although the regulatory limit is 5 millisieverts (0.5 rem). The actual doses that would be received by most infants would be far below 1 millisievert (0.1 rem). Of course, the physician may use discretion in the recommendation, increasing or decreasing the duration of the interruption.

If there is no recommendation in Column 3 of this table, the maximum activity normally administered is below the activities that require instructions on interruption or discontinuation of breastfeeding.

*Source: Nuclear Regulatory Commission. For a more complete table see : http://www.infantrisk. org

Radioactive Diagnostic Procedures

Diagnostic Procedure	Radiopharmaceutical	Dosing Range (mCi)	Comments*
Brain Serotonin levels	^{11}C-WAY 100635	14.2	100 minute interruption
	^{11}C-RACLOPRIDE	10.3	100 minute interruption (see monograph). No interruption[8]
WBC scan	^{99m}Tc-WBC	10-15	12-24 hour interruption for 2-5 mCi or more
	^{99m}Tc-Ceretec	10-24	
	^{111}In-WBC	0.5	1 week interruption for 0.5 mCi[1]
Cystogram (voiding)	^{99m}Tc-SC, ^{99m}Tc-O$_4$-	0.5-1	6 hour interruption for 12 mCi[1]
Liver/spleen scan	^{99m}Tc-SC (sulfur colloid)	2-4	6 hour interruption for 12 mCi[1]
Bone marrow scan	^{99m}Tc-SC	<20	6 hour interruption for 12 mCi[1]
Lymphoscintigraphy	^{99m}Tc-SC	100-800 µCi	No interruption[1]
Liver SPECT (hemangioma)	^{99m}Tc-pyp-RBCs	20-30	12 hour interruption for 25-30 mCi[3]
Myocardial (MI) scan	^{99m}Tc-pyp	20-30	12 hour interruption for 25-30 mCi[3]
Meckel's diverticulum	^{99m}Tc-O$_4$	10-15	24 hours for 30 mCi[1] 12 hours for 12 mCi[1]
Testicular scan	^{99m}TcO$_4$	0-25	24 hours for 30 mCi[1] 12 hours for 12 mCi[1]
Thyroid scan	^{99m}TcO$_4$	1-2	24 hours for 30 mCi[1] 12 hours for 12 mCi[1]
Bone scan	^{99m}Tc-MDP, -HDP	<30	No interruption for 30 mCi or less[1]
MUGA scan	^{99m}Tc-labeled-RBCs	20-30	6 hour interruption of breastfeeding for 20 mCi[1]
Lung ventilation imaging	^{99m}Tc-DTPA (labeled aerosol)	30	No interruption for 30 mCi or less[1]
Renal scan	^{99m}Tc-DTPA	10-15	No interruption for 30 mCi or less[1]
Renal scan	^{99m}Tc-DMSA	3-10	No interruption for 2-5 mCi or less[1]

Radioactive Diagnostic Procedures

Diagnostic Procedure	Radiopharmaceutical	Dosing Range (mCi)	Comments*
Brain scan	^{99m}Tc-D$_4$-, -DTPA, -GH	<20-30	No interruption for 30 mCi or less[1]
HIDA (cholescintigraphy)	^{99m}Tc-Choletec, Hepatolite,	3-5	No interruption for 4 mCi or less[2]
Brain scan-SPEC	^{99m}Tc-Ceretec or Neurolite	20-30	24 hours for 30 mCi[1]
Parathyroid scan Subtraction:	^{99m}Tc-Cardiolite ^{201}Tl ^{99m}Tc-D$_4$-	16-30 2-3 5-12	No interruption for < 30 mCi[3] 2 week interruption for 3 mCi[1]
Scintimammography	^{99m}Tc-Cardiolite	20	No interruption for < 30 mCi[3]
CEA-Scan^R	^{99m}Tc-arcitumomab	20-30	24 hours for 30 mCi[3]
Cardiac Studies	^{99m}Tc, Cardiolite or Myoview	7- 30	No interruption for < 30 mCi[3]
Infections – labeled with HMPAO	^{99m}Tc WBC	3-10	24 hour interruption for 5 mCi[1] 12 hour interruption for 2 mCi[1]
Gastroesophageal emptying time-liquids	^{99m}Tc Sulfur Colloid	1	6 hours for 12 mCi[1]
Gastroesophageal emptying time-solids		0.5	6 hours for 12 mCi[1]
SPECT Analysis – Liver		5	6 hours for 12 mCi[1]
		2	No interruption period[2]
Perfusion study –cardiac Adenoma- parathyroid	^{99m}Tc Sestamibi Teboroxime	25 20	No interruption for < 30 mCi[3]
MUGA Scan for cardiac gated ventriculography	^{99m}Tc RBC	20	6 hour interruption of breastfeeding[1]
Bleeding Scan of GI tract Liver Scan for Hemangioma			
Bleeding Scan of GI tract Liver Scan for Hemangioma	^{99m}Tc RBC	20 20	6-12 hour interruption of breastfeeding[1,4]

Radioactive Diagnostic Procedures

Diagnostic Procedure	Radiopharmaceutical	Dosing Range (mCi)	Comments*
Myocardial Infarct	99mTc Pyrophosphate	15	No interruption required[1]
		20	No interruption required[4]
	99mTc Plasmin	0.5	No interruption[2]
Diagnostic Imaging of thyroid	99mTc Pertechnetate	5	12 hour interruption of breastfeeding[1]
Meckel's Scan of GI tract		21	47 hour interruption[2]
		2	25 hour interruption[2]
	99mTc Microspheres	2.7	17 hour interruption[2]
	99mTc MIBI	27	No interruption[2]
Bone – osteomyelitis	99mTc MDP	20	No interruption for 30 mCi or less[1]
	99mTc Leukoscan	20.3	10 hour interruption[9]
Renal Blood Flow, Clearance	99mTc MAG3	10	No interruption for 30 mCi or less[1]
		11	Interruption for 5 hours[2]
		2.7	No interruption[2]
Perfusion studies of Lung	99mTc-MAA (microaggregated albumin)		12.6 hours for 4 mCi[1]
Biliary Atresia - Cholecystitis -HIDA	99mTc IDA derivative	5	No interruption required[1]
SPECT Analysis of Brain Perfusion	99mTc HMPAO	20	No interruption required[1]
		13.5	No interruption required[2]
	99mTc Glucoheptonate	22	No interruption[2]
	99mTc HAM	8	No interruption[4]
	99mTc Sulfur colloid	12	No interruption[4]
	99mTc Ferrous hydroxide MA		Interruption with measurment[2]

Radioactive Diagnostic Procedures

Diagnostic Procedure	Radiopharmaceutical	Dosing Range (mCi)	Comments*
	^{99m}Tc Erythrocytes	22	17 hour interruption[2]
	^{99m}Tc EDTA	10	No interruption[2]
CNS Perfusion Renal perfusion/filtration	^{99m}Tc DTPA	30 10 or 20 22	No interruption for 30 mCi or less[1] No interruption[2] No interruption[2]
	^{99m}Tc DMSA	2.2	No interruption[2]
Kidney parenchyma imaging kidney DTPA + DMSA	^{99m}Tc DMSA Glucoheptonate	5 10 2.2	No interruption required No interruption required No interruption[1,2]
Unspecific uses	^{99m}Tc DISIDA	4-8	No interruption[2]
	^{99m}Tc Diphosphonate	16.2	No interruption[2]
	^{75}Se Methionine	0.3	450 hour interruption or complete cessation[2]
Infections Tumors imaging	^{67}Ga Citrate	5 5 4	1 month interruption for 4 mCi[1] 2 weeks interruption for 1.3 mCi[1] 1 weeks interruption for 0.2 mCi[1] 20 day interruption[2]
Gallium scan (tumor)	^{67}Ga	5-10	1 month interruption for 4 mCi[1]
Gallium scan for infections	^{67}Ga	5-10	1 month interruption for 4 mCi[1]
Schilling	^{57}Co- B$_{12}$	0.3-0.5	Feed infant following B12 loading. Avoid feeding at 24 hour peak if possible.[5]
Unspecified	^{51}Cr EDTA	0.1	No interruption[2]

Radioactive Diagnostic Procedures

Diagnostic Procedure	Radiopharmaceutical	Dosing Range (mCi)	Comments*
	^{32}P Na phosphate	Any	Complete cessation of breastfeeding[2]
Cardiac perfusion and stress tests	^{201}Tl Chloride	3+1	2 week interruption for 3 mCi[1]
		2.2	No interruption[2]
Cardiac stress test	^{201}Tl	2.5-3.5	2 week interruption for 3 mCi[1]
		3	96 hours[4]
Brain Scan		3	48 hour interruption[7]
Glucose Metabolism Tumor Imaging	^{18}F-FDG	1.35-4.32	Risk from proximity to breast, not milk itself[10]
Lung ventilation	^{133}Xe Gas	10-30	1 hour interruption for washout[1]
Lung ventilation imaging	^{133}Xe	10-15	1 hour interruption[1]
Renogram	^{131}I-OIH	0.15-0.3	No interruption needed[1]
MIBG (adrenal medulla)	^{131}I-MIBG	0.5	25 days interruption[3]
Adrenocortical Scan	^{131}I-Iodomethyinorcholesterol	2	Complete cessation of breastfeeding or until counts are baseline[3]
Thyroid hyperthyroid therapy	^{131}I Sodium diffuse nodular	1-10	Complete cessation of breastfeeding or until counts are baseline[1]
		<30	
Thyroid ablation		30-300	Complete cessation of breastfeeding or until counts are baseline[1]
		108	52 days[6]
Thyroid Diagnostic imaging – (post thyroidectomy)	^{131}I Sodium	5	Complete cessation of breastfeeding or until counts are baseline.[1]
Tumor Imaging	^{131}I MIBG	1.5	Complete cessation of breastfeeding or until counts are baseline.[3]

Radioactive Diagnostic Procedures

Diagnostic Procedure	Radiopharmaceutical	Dosing Range (mCi)	Comments*
	131I HSA	0.25	Complete cessation of breastfeeding or until counts are baseline.[2]
Renal Blood flow and clearance	131I Hippuran	0.05	34 hours interruption[2]
Thyroid scan (substernal)	131I	<0.1	Complete cessation of breastfeeding or until counts are baseline.[1]
Whole-body 131I carcinoma work-up	131I	1-5	Complete cessation of breastfeeding or until counts are baseline.[1]
	125I HSA	0.2	277 hour interruption or complete cessation[2]
	125I Hippuran	0.05	23 hour cessation[2]
	125I Fibrinogen	0.1	620 hour interruption or complete cessation.[2]
Pheochromocytoma scan	123I	3-10	Complete cessation of breastfeeding or until counts are baseline.[3]
Thyroid Imaging Scans	123I Sodium	0.4	Complete cessation of breastfeeding or until counts are baseline.[1]
	123I Hippuran	0.5	27 hour interruption[2]
	123I MIBG	0.5	11 hour interruption[2]
		11	21 hour interruption[2]
Thyroid uptake and scan	123I	<0.35	No interruption of breastfeeding[1]
OncoScint	111In-satumomab pendetide	4-6	14 day interruption[3]
OctreoScan	111In-pentetriotide	6	72 hour interruption[3]
Cisternogram	111Indium-DTPA	0.5-1.5	14 day interruption[3]

Radioactive Diagnostic Procedures

Diagnostic Procedure	Radiopharmaceutical	Dosing Range (mCi)	Comments*
ProstaScint	^{111}In-CYT-356	5-17	14 day interruption[3]
Infections	[111]In WBC	0.5	1 week interruption for 0.5 mCi[1]
CSF – imaging neuroendocrine tumors	[111]In Octreotide	5.3	<10 day interruption (see monograph)
CSF – cisternogram, shunt patency	[111]In DTPA	0.5	1 week interruption for 0.5 mCi[1]
	[111]In Leucocytes	0.5	No interruption[2]

The recommendations in the table above were derived by calculating the dose and time required to limit the ingested effective dose to the infant below 1 mSv. Please be advised, these recommendations still permit a minimal amount of radiation transfer to the infant that is considered safe by the authorities. The only way to totally avoid any radiation is to wait for all of it to decay (5-10 half-lives).

*Recommendations by the following sources:

1. Activities of Radiopharmaceuticals from the Nuclear Regulatory Commission.

2. Montford PI. Textbook of Radiopharmacy. Third Edition. Gordon and Breach Publishers 1999.

3. T.W. Hale Ph.D.

4. Stabin MG, Breitz HB. Breast milk excretion of radiopharmaceuticals: mechanisms, findings, and radiation dosimetry. J Nucl Med 2000 41(5):863-73.

5. Pomeroy KM, Sawyer LJ, Evans MJ. Estimated radiation dose to breast feeding infant following maternal administration of 57Co labelled to vitamin B12. Nucl Med Commun 2005 Sep;26(9):839-41.

6. Robinson PS, Barker P, Campbell A, Henson P, Surveyor I, Young PR. Iodine-131 in breast milk following therapy for thyroid carcinoma. J Nucl Med 1994 Nov;35(11):1797-801.

7. Johnson RE, Mukherji SK, Perry RJ, Stabin MG. Radiation dose from breastfeeding following administration of thallium-201. J. Nucl Med 1996 Dec;37(12):2079-82.

8. Moses-Kolko EL, Meltzer CC, Helsel JC, Sheetz M, Mathis C, Ruszkiewicz J et al. No interruption of lactation is needed after (11)C-WAY 100635 or (11)C-raclopride PET. J Nucl Med 2005 Oct;46(10):1765.

9. Prince JR, Rose MR. Measurement of radioactivity in breast milk following 99mTc-Leukoscan injection. Nucl Med Commun 2004 Sep;25(9):963-6.

10. Hicks RJ, Binns D, Stabin MG. Pattern of uptake and excretion of (18)F-FDG in the lactating breast. J Nucl Med 2001 Aug;42(8):1238-42.

Administration of Contrast Media to Breastfeeding Mothers

Administration of either an iodinated or a gadolinium-based contrast media occasionally is indicated for an imaging study on a woman who is breast-feeding. Both the patient and the patient's physician may have concerns regarding potential toxicity to the infant from contrast media that is excreted into the breastmilk.

The literature on the excretion into breastmilk of iodinated and gadolinium-based contrast media and the gastrointestinal absorption of these agents from breastmilk is very limited however, several studies have shown that 1) less than 1% of the administered maternal dose of contrast medium is excreted into breastmilk; and 2) less than 1% of the contrast medium in breastmilk ingested by an infant is absorbed from the gastrointestinal tract. Therefore, the expected dose of contrast medium absorbed by an infant from ingested breastmilk is extremely low.

Iodinated X-ray Contrast Media (Ionic and Nonionic)

Background

The plasma half-life of intravenously administered iodinated contrast medium is approximately two hours, with nearly 100% of the media cleared from the bloodstream within 24 hours. Because of its low lipid solubility, less than 1% of the administered maternal dose of iodinated contrast medium is excreted into the breastmilk in the first 24 hours. Because less than 1% of the contrast medium ingested by the infant is absorbed from its gastrointestinal tract, the expected dose absorbed by the infant from the breastmilk is less than 0.01% of the intravascular dose given to the mother. This amount represents less than 1% of the recommended dose for an infant undergoing an imaging study, which is 2 mL/kg. The potential risks to the infant include direct toxicity and allergic sensitization or reaction, which are theoretical concerns but have not been reported.

Recommendation

Mothers who are breast-feeding should be given the opportunity to make an informed decision as to whether to continue or temporarily abstain from breast-feeding after receiving intravascularly administered iodinated contrast media. Because of the very small percentage of iodinated contrast medium that is excreted into the breastmilk and absorbed by the infant's gut, we believe that the available data suggest that it is safe for the mother and infant to continue breast-feeding after receiving such an agent. If the mother remains concerned about any potential ill effects to the infant, she may abstain from breast-feeding for 24 hours with active expression and discarding of breastmilk from both breasts during that period. In anticipation of this, she may wish to use a breast pump to obtain milk before the contrast study to feed the infant during the 24-hour period following the examination.

Gadolinium-Based Contrast Agents

Background

Gadolinium compounds are safe and useful as magnetic resonance imaging contrast media. Although free gadolinium is neurotoxic, when complexed to one of a variety of chelates it is safe for use in most adults and children. These hydrophilic gadolinium chelate agents have pharmacokinetic properties very similar to those of iodinated X-ray contrast media. Like iodinated contrast media, gadolinium contrast media have a plasma half-life of approximately 2 hours and are nearly completely cleared from the bloodstream within 24 hours.

Less than 0.04% of the intravascular dose given to the mother is excreted into the breastmilk in the first 24 hours. Because less than 1% of the contrast medium ingested by the infant is absorbed from its gastrointestinal tract, the expected dose absorbed by the infant from the breastmilk is less than 0.0004% of the intravascular dose given to the mother. Even in the extreme circumstance of a mother weighing 150 kg and receiving a dose of 0.2 mmol/kg, the absolute amount of gadolinium excreted in the breastmilk in the first 24-hours after administration would be no more than 0.012 mmol. Thus the dose of gadolinium absorbed from the gastrointestinal tract of a breast-feeding infant weighing 1,500 grams or more would be no more than 0.00008 mmol/kg, or 0.04% (four ten-thousandths) of the permitted adult or pediatric (2 years of age or older) intravenous dose of 0.2 mmol/kg. The potential risks to the infant include direct toxicity (including toxicity from free gadolinium, because it is unknown how much, if any, of the gadolinium in breastmilk is in the unchelated form) and allergic sensitization or reaction, which are theoretical concerns but have not been reported.

Recommendation

Review of the literature shows no evidence to suggest that oral ingestion by an infant of the tiny amount of gadolinium contrast medium excreted into breastmilk would cause toxic effects. We believe, therefore, that the available data suggest that it is safe for the mother and infant to continue breast-feeding after receiving such an agent.

If the mother remains concerned about any potential ill effects, she should be given the opportunity to make an informed decision as to whether to continue or temporarily abstain from breast-feeding after receiving a gadolinium contrast medium. If the mother so desires, she may abstain from breast-feeding for 24 hours with active expression and discarding of breastmilk from both breasts during that period. In anticipation of this, she may wish to use a breast pump to obtain milk before the contrast study to feed the infant during the 24-hour period following the examination.

References

1. Ilett KF, Hackett LP, Paterson JW, McCormick CC. Excretion of metrizamide in milk. Br J Radiol 1981; 54:537-538.

2. Johansen JG. Assessment of a non-ionic contrast medium (Amipaque) in the gastrointestinal tract. Invest Radiol 1978; 13:523-527.

3. Kubik-Huch RA, Gottstein-Aalame NM, Frenzel T, et al. Gadopentetate dimeglumine excretion into human breastmilk during lactation. Radiology 2000; 216:555-558.

4. Nielsen ST, Matheson I, Rasmussen JN, Skinnemoen K, Andrew E, Hafsahl G. Excretion of iohexol and metrizoate in human breastmilk. Acta Radiol 1987; 28:523-526.

5. Rofsky NM, Weinreb JC, Litt AW. Quantitative analysis of gadopentetate dimeglumine excreted in breastmilk. J Magn Reson Imaging 1993; 3:131-132.

6. Schmiedl U, Maravilla KR, Gerlach R, Dowling CA. Excretion of gadopentetate dimeglumine in human breastmilk. AJR Am J Roentgenol 1990; 154:1305-1306.

7. Weinmann HJ, Brasch RC, Press WR, Wesbey GE. Characteristics of gadolinium-DTPA complex: a potential NMR contrast agent. AJR Am J Roentgenol 1984; 142:619-624.

8. Hylton NM. Suspension of breast-feeding following gadopentetate dimeglumine administration. Radiology 2000; 216:325-326.

Radiocontrast Agents

Iodinated Radiocontrast Agents:

As a group, Iodinated Radiocontrast Agents are used as contrast agents in Computed Axial Tomography or CAT scans. In this procedure, X-rays are passed through the body, while the contrast agent is circulating. The iodine in the contrast agent absorbs the X-ray and thus appears white or dense, consequently highlighting hemorrhages or other lesions with high vascularity. With virtually all the iodinated contrast agents, the iodine is covalently bound to the molecule; hence, it is not free to move into other compartments like free iodine. As a result, these contrast agents generally are restricted to plasma and body water and are virtually excluded from the milk compartment. However, very small amounts of iodine may be metabolized and released as "free" iodine. This is usually very small and would not affect thyroid function in a newborn, other than transiently.

Gadolinium-Containing Radiocontrast Agents:

Gadolinium-containing contrast agents are used for Magnetic Resonance Imaging (MRI). As with the iodinated products, the gadolinium metal is tightly bound to the molecule and is unable to become free in the plasma. Just as with the above contrast agents, this product is largely restricted to plasma and body water, although it is able to penetrate tissues to a greater degree than the iodinated products. Unlike CAT scans, MRI uses a powerful magnetic field to align the magnetization of hydrogen atoms in the body which is detected by the scanner. To date, we have a few studies suggesting that gadolinium-containing contrast agents penetrate milk poorly and would be virtually unabsorbed orally. Therefore, they are of little risk to a breastfeeding infant.

The American College of Radiology has reviewed these agents and generally suggests that they are of little or no risk to a breastfeeding infant.[1]

Reference:

1. http://www.acr.org/MainMenuCategories/about_us/committees/gpr-srp/AdministrationofContrastM ediumtoNursingMothersDoc1.aspx

Barium Sulfate

Trade: Baro-cat, Prepcat, Bear-E-Yum CT, Cheetah, Medescan, Enecat CT, Tomocat, EntroEase, Entrobar, Liquid Barosperse, Bear-E-Yum GI, HD 85, Imager ac, Flo-Coat, Medebar Plus, Epi-C, Liqui-Coat HD, EntroEase Dry, Barosperse, Tonopaque, Barobag, Baricon, Enhancer, HD 200 Plus, Intropaste, Anatrast

Barium sulfate is available in a wide variety of concentrations, from 1.5% to 210%, under many trade names. It is not absorbed orally; therefore, none will enter the maternal milk compartment or cause harm to a breastfeeding infant. No interruption in breastfeeding is necessary.

Kinetics: Oral Bioavailability = None

Lactation Risk Category: L1

References:

1. Pharmaceutical Manufacturers prescribing information, 2008.

Diatrizoate

Trade: Angiovist, Cardiografin, Cystografin, Ethibloc, Gastrovist, Hypaque, Reno-30, Reno-60, Reno-Dip, Renografin, Reno-M, Retrografin, Sinografin, Urovist

Diatrizoate is an iodinated containing radiopaque medium used in a wide variety of x-rays. These radiocontrast agents range from 8.5 to 59.87% iodine.[1] However, the iodine is covalently bound to the molecule and is poorly released after injection, most being eliminated in the urine rapidly. Reported levels in breastmilk are very low. In a study of a single patient who received 18.5 grams of iodine in the form of sodium and meglumine salts of diatrizoate, diatrizoate levels were undetectable (LOD < 2 mg/L).[2] In another woman who received 93 grams of Iodine as diatrizoate, total iodine transferred into breastmilk in the first 24 hours was 0.03% or 31 mg.[3]

Based on kinetic data, the American College of Radiology suggests that it is safe for mothers to continue breastfeeding after receiving iodinated x-ray contrast media.[4]

Kinetics: T½ = 120 minutes

Oral Bioavailability = 0.04-1.2%

Protein Binding = 0-10%

MW=614

Lactation Risk Category: L2

References:

1. Pharmaceutical Manufacturers prescribing information, 2002.

2. Fitz John, T. P., Williams, D. G., Laker, M. F., and Owen, J. P. Intravenous urography during lactation. Br. J Radiol. 55(656): 603-605, 1982.

3. Texier, F., Roque, d. O., and Etling, N. [Stable iodine level in human milk after pulmonary angiography]. Presse Med.%19;12(12): 769, 1983.

4. ACR Committee on Drugs and Contrast Media. Administration of contrast medium to breastfeeding mothers. 2004;42-43.

Gadobenate

Trade: MultiHance

Gadobenate is a gadolinium-containing radiocontrast agent used in MRIs. Although free gadolinium is neurotoxic, it is safe when bound to the parent molecule in the contrast medium. There have been no studies on its transfer into human milk, but it is unlikely that it would accumulate in therapeutic levels.[1] The American College of Radiology concludes that it is safe for a mother-infant dyad to continue breastfeeding after the administration of a gadolinium-containing contrast medium.[2]

Kinetics: $T\frac{1}{2}$ = 1.17-2.02 hours

Oral Bioavailability = Poor

Protein Binding = Low

Lactation Risk Category: L3

References:

1. Pharmaceutical Manufacturers prescribing information, 2007.

2. ACR Committee on Drugs and Contrast Media. Administration of contrast medium to breastfeeding mothers. 2004;42-43.

Gadodiamide

Trade: Omniscan

Gadodiamide is a gadolinium-containing nonionic, non-iodinated water soluble contrast medium commonly used in Magnetic Resonance Imaging scans.[1] It is quite similar to Magnevist, another gadolinium-containing agent. These agents penetrate peripheral compartments poorly, especially the brain. As such, they are extremely unlikely to enter milk as well. Data for gadopentetate (Magnevist) support this, as its transfer into milk is negligible (<0.04%). Neither of these compounds is well absorbed orally, and neither is metabolized to any degree. It is likely that gadodiamide will penetrate milk only minimally.

Kinetics: $T\frac{1}{2}$ = 77 minutes

Oral Bioavailability = Nil

Protein Binding = 0%

Lactation Risk Category: L3

References:

1. Pharmaceutical Manufacturers prescribing information, 2007.

Gadopentetate

Trade: Magnevist, Magnevistan, Magnograf, Viewgam

Gadopentetate is a radiopaque agent used in magnetic resonance imaging of the kidney. It is non-ionic, non-iodinated, has low osmolarity and contains a gadolinium ion as the radiopaque entity. Following a dose of 7 mmol (6.5 gm), the amount of gadopentetate secreted in breastmilk was 3.09, 2.8, 1.08, and 0.5 μmol/L at 2, 11, 17, and 24 hours respectively.[1] The cumulative amount excreted from both breasts in 24 hours was only 0.023% of the administered dose. Oral absorption is minimal, only 0.8% of gadopentetate is absorbed. These authors suggest that only 0.013 micromole of a gadolinium-containing compound would be absorbed by the infant in 24 hours, which is incredibly low. They further suggest that 24 hours of pumping would eliminate risks, although this seems rather extreme in view of the short (1.6 hr) half-life, poor oral bioavailability, and limited milk levels.

In another study of 19 lactating women who received 0.1 mmol/kg and one additional woman who received 0.2 mmol/kg, the cumulative amount of gadolinium excreted in breastmilk during 24 hours was 0.57 μmol.[2] This resulted in an excreted dose of <0.04% of the IV administered maternal dose. A similar amount was noted in the patient receiving a double dose (0.2 mmol/kg). As a result, for any neonate weighing more than 1000 gm, the maximal orally ingested dose would be less than 1% of the permitted intravenous dose of 0.2 mmol/kg. According to the authors, "…that the very small amount of gadopentetate dimeglumine transferred to a nursing infant does not warrant a potentially traumatic 24-hour suspension of breastfeeding for lactating women."

Kinetics: T½ = 1.5-1.7 hours

Oral Bioavailability = 0.8%

Lactation Risk Category: L2

References:

1. Rofsky NM, Weinreb JC, Litt AW. Quantitative analysis of gadopentetate dimeglumine excreted in breastmilk. J Magn Reson Imaging 1993; 3(1):131-132.

2. Kubik-Huch RA, Gottstein-Aalame NM, Frenzel T, Seifert B, Puchert E, Wittek S, Debatin JF. Gadopentetate dimeglumine excretion into human breastmilk during lactation. Radiology 2000; 216(2):555-558.

Gadoteridol

Trade: Prohance

Gadoteridol is a non-ionic, non-iodinated gadolinium chelate complex used as a radiocontrast agent in MRI scans. The metabolism of gadoteridol is unknown, but a similar gadolinium salt (gadopentetate) is not metabolized at all. The half-life is brief (1.6 hours), and the volume of distribution is very small. This suggests that gadoteridol does not penetrate tissues well and is unlikely to penetrate milk in significant quantities. A similar compound, gadopentetate, is barely detectable in breastmilk. Although not reported, the oral bioavailability is probably similar to gadopentetate, which is minimal to none. No data are available on the transfer of gadoteridol into human milk, although it is probably minimal.

Kinetics: $T\frac{1}{2}$ = 1.57 hours

Oral Bioavailability = Poor

Lactation Risk Category: L3

References:

1. Pharmaceutical Manufacturers prescribing information, 2007.

Gadoversetamide

Trade: Optimark

Gadoversetamide is a paramagnetic agent used as a contrast agent in magnetic resonance imaging (MRI). It does not enter most compartments and is confined to extracellular water with a low volume of distribution.[1] As with gadopentetate, this agent is very unlikely to penetrate milk or be orally bioavailable. However, no human data are available. Rat studies show some penetration of gadoversetamide into rat milk, but rodent lactation studies do not correlate with humans.

Kinetics: $T\frac{1}{2}$ = 1.7 hours

Oral Bioavailability = Nil

Protein Binding = None

Lactation Risk Category: L3

References:

1. Pharmaceutical Manufacturers prescribing information, 2003.

Iodamide

Trade: Isteropac, Renovue-Dip, Renovue-65

Not available in the US. Iodamide is an ionic contrast medium. No data are available on the transfer into human milk; however, levels would likely be quite low. Due to a poor oral bioavailability, it is unlikely that it would transfer to the infant during breastfeeding.

Kinetics: $T\frac{1}{2}$ = 1.3 hours[1]

Oral Bioavailability = poor

Protein Binding = 5%

Lactation Risk Category: L3

References:

1. Difazio LT, Singhvi SM, Heald AF, et.al. Pharmacokinetics of iodamide in normal subjects and in patients with renal impairment. J Clin Pharmacol. 1978 Jan; 18(1):35-41.

Iodipamide

Trade: Cholografin, Sinografin

Iodipamide is an ionic radiopaque contrast agent used to view the gallbladder and biliary tract. It is used in both adults and pediatric patients.[1] No data are available on the transfer of iodipamide into human milk; however, it is unlikely when compared to other similar agents. It has a very short half life, and it is highly protein bound. Based on kinetic data, the American College of Radiology suggests that it is safe for a mother to continue breastfeeding after receiving iodinated x-ray contrast media.[2]

Kinetics: $T\frac{1}{2}$ = 30 minutes

Oral Bioavailability = 10%

Protein Binding = Very high

Lactation Risk Category: L3

References:

1. Pharmaceutical Manufacturers prescribing information, 2003.

2. ACR Committee on Drugs and Contrast Media. Administration of contrast medium to breastfeeding mothers. 2004;42-43.

Iodixanol

Trade: Visipaque

Iodixanol is an intravenous, nonionic, water soluble radiocontrast medium with iodine concentrations of 270 and 320 mg/mL.[1] It has been studied and approved in children one year of age and older, as well as adults. There are no studies on the transfer of iodixanol into human milk; however, it is unlikely that iodixanol would transfer into milk in any therapeutic level. Its poor oral bioavailability would further reduce any risk to an infant. Based on kinetic data, the American College of Radiology suggests that it is safe for a mother to continue breastfeeding after receiving iodinated x-ray contrast media.[2]

Kinetics: $T\frac{1}{2}$ = 123 minutes

Oral Bioavailability = Poor

Protein Binding = None

Lactation Risk Category: L3

References:

1. Pharmaceutical Manufacturers prescribing information, 2006

2. ACR Committee on Drugs and Contrast Media. Administration of contrast medium to breastfeeding mothers. 2004;42-43.

Iohexol

Trade: Accupaque, Myelo-Kit, Omnigraf, Omnipaque, Omnitrast

Iohexol is a nonionic radiocontrast agent. Radiopaque agents (except barium) are iodinated compounds used to visualize various organs during X-ray, CAT scans, and other radiological procedures. These compounds are highly-iodinated, benzoic acid derivatives. Although under usual circumstances iodine products are contraindicated in nursing mothers (due to ion trapping in milk), these products are unique, in that they are extremely inert and are largely cleared without metabolism. The iodine is organically bound to the structure and is not biologically active.

In a study of four women who received 0.755 g/kg (350 mg iodine/mL) of iohexol IV, the mean peak level of iohexol in milk was 35 mg/L at three hours post-injection.[1] The average concentration in milk was only 11.4 mg/L over 24 hours. Assuming a daily milk intake of 150 mL/kg body weight, the amount of iohexol transferred to an infant during the first 24 hours would be 1.7 mg/kg which corresponds to 0.23% of the maternal dose.

As a group, these radiocontrast agents are virtually unabsorbed after oral administration (<0.1%).[2] Iohexol has a brief half-life of just two hours, and the estimated dose ingested by the infant is only 0.2% of the radiocontrast dose used clinically for various scanning procedures in infants. Although most company package inserts suggest that an infant be removed from the breast for 24 hours, no untoward effects have been reported with these products in breastfed infants. Because the amount of iohexol transferred into milk is so small, the authors conclude that breastfeeding is acceptable after intravenously administered iohexol.

Kinetics: $T\frac{1}{2}$ = 2-3.4 hours

Oral Bioavailability = Poor

Protein Binding = None

Lactation Risk Category: L2

References:

1. Nielsen ST, Matheson I, Rasmussen JN, Skinnemoen K, Andrew E, Hafsahl G. Excretion of iohexol and metrizoate in human breastmilk. Acta Radiol 1987; 28(5):523-526.

2. Pharmaceutical Manufacturer Prescribing Information. 2006.

Iopamidol

Trade: Gastromiro, Iopamiro, Iopamiron, Iopasen, Isovue, Isovue-M, Jopamiro, Niopam, Pamiray, Radiomiron, Scanlux, Solutrast

Unilux Iopamidol is a nonionic radiocontrast agent used for numerous radiological procedures. Although it contains significant iodine content (20-37%), the iodine is covalently bound to the parent molecule, and the bioavailability of the iodine molecule is miniscule. As with other ionic and nonionic radiocontrast agents, it is primarily extracellular and intravascular, it does not pass the blood-brain barrier, and it would be extremely unlikely that it would penetrate into human milk. However, no data are available on its transfer into human milk. As with most of these products, it is poorly absorbed from the GI tract and rapidly excreted from the maternal circulation, due to an extremely short half-life.

Kinetics: $T\frac{1}{2} = 2$ hours

Oral Bioavailability = None

Protein Binding = Very low

Lactation Risk Category: L3

References:

1. Pharmaceutical Manufacturers prescribing information, 2004.

Iopanoic Acid

Trade: Biliopaco, Cistobil, Colegraf, Colepak, Neocontrast, Telepaque

Iopanoic acid is a radiopaque organic iodine compound similar to dozens of other radiocontrast agents. It contains 66.7% by weight of iodine. As with all of these compounds, the iodine is organically bound to the parent molecule, and only minimal amounts are free in solution or metabolized by the body. In a group of five breastfeeding mothers who received an average of 2.77 gm of iodine (as Iopanoic acid), the amount of iopanoic acid excreted into human milk during the following 19-29 hours was 20.8 mg or about 0.08% of the maternal dose.[1] No untoward effects were noted in the infants.

Kinetics: $T\frac{1}{2} = 33\%$ eliminated in 24 hours

Oral Bioavailability = Well absorbed

Protein Binding = High

Lactation Risk Category: L2

References:

1. Holmdahl KH. Cholecystography during lactation. Acta Radiol 1956; 45(4):305-307.

Iopentol

Trade: Imagopaque, Ivepaque

Not available in the US. There are no studies on the transfer of iopentol into human milk; however, it is unlikely that iopentol would transfer into milk in any therapeutic level. The poor oral bioavailability further reduces risk to an infant.[1]

Kinetics: $T\frac{1}{2}$ = 2 hours

Oral Bioavailability = poor

Protein Binding = 3%

Lactation Risk Category: L3

References:

1. Pharmaceutical Manufacturers prescribing information, 2006.

Iopromide

Trade: Clarograf, Proscope, Ultravist

Iopromide is a nonionic, water soluble x-ray contrast agent. Its iodine content is 48.12%, and it is available in 150, 240, 300, and 370 mg iodine/mL.[1] No data are available on the transfer of ioversol into human milk, but others in this family transfer at extraordinarily low levels, and none are orally bioavailable. Therefore, iopromide use is not likely to pose a threat to an infant and should not be a contraindication for breastfeeding.

Kinetics: $T\frac{1}{2}$ = 2 hours

Oral Bioavailability = Poor

Protein Binding = 1%

Lactation Risk Category: L3

References:

1. Pharmaceutical Manufacturers prescribing information, 2002.

Iothalamate

Trade: Angio-Conray, Conray-30, Conray-43, Conray-60, Conray 325, Conray-400, Cysto-Conray, Cysto-Conray II, Vascoray

Iothalamate is an iodinate contrast medium, available in iodine concentrations ranging from 81 mg iodine/mL to 400 mg iodine/mL.[1] No data are available on the transfer into human milk; however, levels in milk are expected to be low to undetectable, and oral bioavailability is low. Therefore, risk to the infant would be minimal. Based on kinetic data, the American College of Radiology suggests that it is safe for a mother to continue breastfeeding after receiving iodinated x-ray contrast media.[2]

Kinetics: $T\frac{1}{2} = 90\text{-}92$ minutes

Protein Binding = Low

Lactation Risk Category: L3

References:

1. Pharmaceutical Manufacturers prescribing information, 2003.

2. ACR Committee on Drugs and Contrast Media. Administration of contrast medium to breastfeeding mothers. 2004;42-43.

Ioversol

Trade: Optiject, Optiray

Ioversol is a typical iodinated radiocontrast agent used in computed tomographic imaging (CT scans). The concentration of iodine varies from 16% organically bound iodine (160) to 35% iodine (350).[1] Ioversol is not metabolized, but it is excreted largely unchanged. Iodine is only minimally released; therefore, thyroid function tests remain unchanged with exception of iodine uptake studies (PBI, radioactive iodine uptake). The vascular half-life is brief, only 20 minutes. No data are available on its transfer into milk, but many others in this family have been studied and transfer to milk at extraordinarily low levels. Further, none of these agents are orally bioavailable.

Kinetics: $T\frac{1}{2} = 1.5$ hours

Oral Bioavailability = Nil

Protein Binding = Very low

Lactation Risk Category: L3

References:

1. Pharmaceutical Manufacturers prescribing information, 2003.

Ioxaglate

Trade: Hexabrix 160, Hexabrix 200, Hexabrix 320, Hexabrix

Ioxaglate is an ionic dimer that offers a lower osmolarity and consequently less pain upon injection. It contains 32% iodine and is approved for both pediatrics and adults. No data are available on the transfer into human milk; however, levels are expected to be below therapeutic levels, and oral bioavailability is low. Based on kinetic data, the American College of Radiology suggests that it is safe for a mother to continue breastfeeding after receiving iodinated x-ray contrast media.[1]

Kinetics: $T\frac{1}{2}$ = 60-140 minutes

Protein Binding = Low

Lactation Risk Category: L3

References:

1. ACR Committee on Drugs and Contrast Media. Administration of contrast medium to breastfeeding mothers. 2004;42-43.

Ioxitalamic Acid

Trade: Telebrix

Ioxitalamic acid is available in both an oral solution and an injectable solution, in concentrations ranging from 12% to 38% iodine.[1] It is used in both adults and pediatrics. There are no data available on the transfer of ioxitalamic acid into breastmilk, although levels are likely to be low. Also, oral bioavailability is extremely low. As a result, any small ingested amount would pose little threat to a breastfeeding infant. Based on kinetic data, the American College of Radiology suggests that it is safe for a mother to continue breastfeeding after receiving iodinated x-ray contrast media.[2]

Kinetics: Oral Bioavailability = None

Lactation Risk Category: L3

References:

1. Pharmaceutical Manufacturers prescribing information, 1999a.

2. ACR Committee on Drugs and Contrast Media. Administration of contrast medium to breastfeeding mothers. 2004;42-43.

Ipodate

Trade: Bilivist, Biloptin, Oragrafin, Solu-Biloptin, Solubiloptine

Not available in the US. Ipodate is an oral contrast agent used for examining the gallbladder and bile ducts when gallstones are suspected. There have been no studies on the transfer of tyropanoate into human breastmilk. It is likely that minimal drug would transfer into the milk compartment; however, levels are unknown. Caution should be used.

Kinetics: $T\frac{1}{2}$ = 45% gone in 24 hours

Oral Bioavailability = High

Protein Binding = High

Lactation Risk Category: L3

References:

1. Pharmaceutical Manufacturers prescribing information, 2008.

Mangafodipir Trisodium

Trade: Teslascan

Mangafodipir is a manganese-containing radiocontrast agent used in Magnetic Resonance Imaging. It is rapidly redistributed to liver and less so to other tissues.[1] The release of manganese is significant, and whole-body stores are approximately doubled with infusion of this product. Elevated plasma manganese levels drop rapidly, with a redistribution half-life of about 25 minutes, while the terminal elimination half-life of manganese is more on the order of 10.1 hours. Manganese is effectively transported into human milk, and milk levels are apparently a function of oral intake in the mother. Consequently, manganese levels in milk could temporarily be elevated. Infants are somewhat deficient in manganese and have higher oral bioavailability of manganese, due to the relative state of deficiency.[2] For this reason, it is reasonable to assume that the use of this product in a breastfeeding woman could conceivably elevate the levels of her milk significantly, although briefly. A brief interruption of breastfeeding for a few hours (four or more), followed by pumping and discarding, would significantly reduce any risk to the infant.

Kinetics: $T\frac{1}{2}$ = 10 hours

Oral Bioavailability = Low

Protein Binding = Nil

Lactation Risk Category: L3

References:

1. Pharmaceutical Manufacturers prescribing information, 2003.

2. Vuori E, Makinen SM, Kara R, Kuitunen P. The effects of the dietary intakes of copper, iron, manganese, and zinc on the trace element content of human milk. Am J Clin Nutr 1980; 33(2):227-231.

Metrizamide

Trade: Amipaque

Metrizamide is a radiographic contrast medium used mainly in myelography. It is water soluble and nonionic. Metrizamide contains 48% bound iodine. The iodine molecule is organically bound and is not available for uptake into breastmilk due to minimal metabolism. Following subarachnoid administration of 5.06 gm, the peak plasma level of 32.9 µg/mL occurred at six hours. Cumulative excretion in milk increased with time, but was extremely small, with only 1.1 mg or 0.02% of the dose being recovered in milk within 44.3 hours.[1] The drug's high water solubility, nonionic characteristic, and its high molecular weight (789) also support minimal excretion into breastmilk. This agent is sometimes used as an oral radiocontrast agent.[2] Only minimal oral absorption occurs (<0.4%). The authors suggest that the very small amount of metrizamide secreted in human milk is unlikely to be hazardous to the infant.

Kinetics: $T\frac{1}{2}$ = >24 hours

Oral Bioavailability = <0.4%

Lactation Risk Category: L2

References:

1. Ilett KF, Hackett LP, Paterson JW, McCormick CC. Excretion of metrizamide in milk. Br J Radiol 1981; 54(642):537-538.

2. Johansen JG. Assessment of a non-ionic contrast medium (Amipaque) in the gastrointestinal tract. Invest Radiol 1978; 13(6):523-527.

Metrizoate

Trade: Angiocontrast, Isopaque

Metrizoate is an ionic radiocontrast agent. Radiopaque agents (except barium) are iodinated compounds used to visualize various organs during X-ray, CAT scans, and other radiological procedures. These compounds are highly iodinated benzoic acid derivatives. While iodine products are generally contraindicated in nursing mothers, these products are unique, because they are extremely inert and are largely cleared without metabolism.

In a study of four women who received metrizoate 0.58 g/kg (350 mg Iodine/mL) IV, the peak level of metrizoate in milk was 14 mg/L at three and six hours post-injection.[1] The average milk concentration during the first 24 hours was only 11.4 mg/L. During the first 24 hours following injection, it is estimated that a total of 1.7 mg/kg would be transferred to the infant, which is only 0.3% of the maternal dose.

As a group, radiocontrast agents are virtually unabsorbed after oral administration (<0.1%). Metrizoate has a brief half-life of just two hours, and the estimated dose ingested by the infant is only 0.2% of the radiocontrast dose used clinically for various scanning procedures in infants. Although most company package inserts suggest that an infant be removed from the breast for 24 hours, no untoward effects have been reported with these products in breastfed infants. Because the amount of metrizoate transferred into milk is so small, the authors conclude that breastfeeding is acceptable after intravenously administered metrizoate.

Kinetics: $T\frac{1}{2}$ = 60-140 minutes

Oral Bioavailability = Nil

Protein Binding = Very low

Lactation Risk Category: L2

References:

1. Nielsen ST, Matheson I, Rasmussen JN, Skinnemoen K, Andrew E, Hafsahl G. Excretion of iohexol and metrizoate in human breastmilk. Acta Radiol 1987; 28(5):523-526.

Tyropanoate

Trade: Bilopaque

Tyropanoate is an oral contrast agent used for examining the gallbladder, when gallstones are suspected. It contains 57.4% bound iodine and is only used in adults.[1] Safety in pediatrics has not been established. There have been no studies done on the transfer of tyropanoate into human breastmilk. It is possible that minimal drug would transfer into the milk compartment; however, levels are unknown.

Kinetics: $T\frac{1}{2}$ = 45% gone in 24 hours

Oral Bioavailability = Well absorbed

Protein Binding = Moderate

MW= 641

Lactation Risk Category: L3

References:

1. Pharmaceutical Manufacturers prescribing information, 1997.

GLOSSARY

$T\frac{1}{2}$	Adult elimination half-life
T_{max}	Time to peak plasma level (PK)
M/P	Milk/Plasma ratio
RID	Relative Infant Dose
C_{max}	Plasma or milk concentration at peak
Vd	Volume of distribution
PB	Percent of protein binding in maternal circulation
PHL	Pediatric elimination half-life
Oral	Oral bioavailability (adult)
µg/L	Microgram per liter
ng/L	Nanogram per liter
mg/L	Milligram per liter
mL	Milliliter. One cc
NSAIDs	Non-steroidal anti-inflammatory
ACEi	Angiotensin converting enzyme inhibitor
MAOI	Monoamine oxidase inhibitors
MW	Molecular weight
µCi	Microcurie of radioactivity
mmol	Millimole of weight
µmol	Micromole of weight
X	Times
AUC	Area under the curve
BID	Twice daily
TID	Three times daily
QID	Four times daily
PRN	As needed
QD	Daily
d	Day

INDEX

Uppercase = generic drug name

Q

Ordering Information

Hale Publishing, L.P.

1712 N. Forest Street

Amarillo, Texas, USA 79106

8:00 am To 5:00 pm CST

Call » 806.376.9900

Sales » 800.378.1317

Fax » 806.376.9901

Online Orders

www.ibreastfeeding.com